Mental Health Nursing in the Community

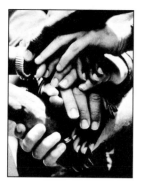

Mental Health Nursing in the Community

Nancy K. Worley, RN, PhD

Associate Professor
Coordinator, Graduate Psychiatric-Mental Health Program
College of Nursing
Medical University of South Carolina
Charleston, South Carolina

Illustrated

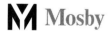 Mosby

St. Louis Baltimore Boston Carlsbad Chicago Naples New York Philadelphia Portland
London Madrid Mexico City Singapore Sydney Tokyo Toronto Wiesbaden

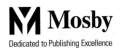

Mosby
Dedicated to Publishing Excellence

A Times Mirror
Company

Vice President and Publisher: Nancy L. Coon
Editor: Jeff Burnham
Developmental Editor: Linda Caldwell
Project Manager: John Rogers
Production Editor: Jennifer Furey
Interior Design: Yael Kats
Manufacturing Manager: Linda Ierardi
Cover Art: © Patrisha Thomson/Tony Stone Images

Printed in the United States of America
Composition by Carlisle Communications, Ltd.
Printing/binding by R.R. Donnelley & Sons Company

Mosby–Year Book, Inc.
11830 Westline Industrial Drive
St. Louis, Missouri 63146

Library of Congress Cataloging in Publication Data

Mental health nursing in the community / [edited by] Nancy K. Worley.
    p.   cm.
    Includes bibliographical references and index.
    ISBN 0-8151-9429-3 (pbk.)
    1. Psychiatric nursing.   2. Community mental health services.
   3. Community health nursing.   I. Worley, Nancy K.
    [DNLM: 1. Psychiatric Nursing—methods. 2. Community Health
Nursing—methods. 3. Mental Disorders—nursing. WY 160 M5486
1996]
RC440.M3544 1996
610.73'68—dc20
DNLM/DLC
for Library of Congress   96-25537
                                          CIP

96 97 98 99 00 / 9 8 7 6 5 4 3 2 1

Contributors

Donna C. Aguilera, PhD, FAAN, MFC, FIAEP
Consultant in Private Practice
Beverly Hills and Sherman Oaks, California

Philip S. Allard, MSW (candidate)
Regional Director–Southeastern Massachusetts
New England Fellowship for Rehabilitation
    Alternatives, Inc.
Fall River, Massachusetts

Share DeCroix Bane, MEd
Director
National Resource Center for Rural Aging
University of Missouri—Kansas City
Kansas City, Missouri

Richard C. Baron, MA
Executive Director
Matrix Research Institute
Philadelphia, Pennsylvania

Jeff Blum
Program Specialist
Office of the Public Defender
Nashville, Tennessee

Kathleen C. Buckwalter, PhD, RN
Professor
College of Nursing
University of Iowa
Iowa City, Iowa

James A. Cates, PhD
Clinical Rehabilitation Psychologist
Fort Wayne, Indiana

Susan E. Caverly, ARNP, MA, CS
Research and Clinical Faculty
Department of Psychosocial and Community Health
    Nursing
University of Washington
Seattle, Washington

Sara J. Corse, PhD
Department of Psychiatry
Center for Mental Health Policy and Services Research
University of Pennsylvania
Philadelphia, Pennsylvania

Phillippe B. Cunningham, PhD
Instructor
Family Services Research Center
Medical University of South Carolina
Charleston, South Carolina

Barbara L. Garrison, MSW, CCSW
Director of Administrative and Clinical Services
Linden Vale Hospital
St. Joseph Mishawaka Healthcare Services
Mishawaka, Indiana

Linda L. Graham, MSN, RN, C
Associate Professor of Nursing
Indiana University—Purdue University at Fort Wayne
Fort Wayne, Indiana

Dan E. Harris, RN, MSN
Birmingham, Alabama

Karen Hellwig, MN, RN, C
Professor, Nursing Department, El Camino College
Torrance, California
Case Manager, Hospital Home Health Care Agency
    of California
Torrance, California
Clinical Nurse Specialist, Centinela Hospital Home Care
Inglewood, California

Scott W. Henggeler, PhD
Director
Family Services Research Center
Professor
Department of Psychiatry and Behavioral Sciences
Medical University of South Carolina
Charleston, South Carolina

Elizabeth A. Huggins, PhD, RN, CS
Assistant Professor
College of Nursing
Medical University of South Carolina
Charleston, South Carolina

Norman L. Keltner, RN, CRNP, EdD
Associate Professor
School of Nursing
University of Alabama at Birmingham
Birmingham, Alabama

Michael G. Kennedy, PhD, ARNP, CS
Assistant Professor
School of Nursing
Seattle University
Adult Psychiatric/Mental Health Nurse Practitioner
Asian Counseling and Referral Service
Seattle, Washington

Diane K. Kjervik, JD, RN, FAAN
Professor and Associate Dean for Community
  Outreach and Practice
University of North Carolina—Chapel Hill
Chapel Hill, North Carolina

Joyce K. Laben, RN, MSN, JD, FAAN
Professor
School of Nursing
Vanderbilt University
Nashville, Tennessee

Neil Meisler, MSW
Assistant Professor of Psychiatry
Administrative Director of Public Psychiatry
Department of Psychiatry and Behavioral Sciences
Medical University of South Carolina
Charleston, South Carolina

Cynthia A. O'Neil, ACSW
Vice-President/Chief Operating Officer
New England Fellowship for Rehabilitation
  Alternatives, Inc.
Lincoln, Rhode Island

V. Jann Owens, MSN, RN, CS
Assistant Professor
College of Nursing
Medical University of South Carolina
Clinical Director, Burke School-Based Clinic
Charleston, South Carolina

Marianne Smith, MS, RN
Geropsychiatric Clinical Nurse Specialist
Abbe, Inc.
Cedar Rapids, Iowa

Sara-Ann Steber, MSS, MLSP
Director
Technical Assistance and Education Center
Lecturer
Center for Mental Health Policy and Services
  Research
University of Pennsylvania Medical Center
Philadelphia, Pennsylvania

Cynthia Cupit Swenson, PhD
Assistant Professor
Medical University of South Carolina
Charleston, South Carolina

Sandra L. Talley, APRN/PP, CS, MN
Associate Instructor
Psychiatric Mental Health Nursing Program
Doctoral Student
College of Nursing
University of Utah
Salt Lake City, Utah

Carol A. Williams, DSN, RN
Associate Professor
College of Nursing
University of South Carolina
Columbia, South Carolina

Lore K. Wright, PhD, RN, CS
Associate Professor and Chair, Department of
    Mental Health and Psychiatric Nursing
School of Nursing
Medical College of Georgia
Augusta, Georgia

Cynthia D. Zubritsky, PhD
Department of Psychiatry
University of Pennsylvania
Philadelphia, Pennsylvania

Reviewers

Lorna Mill Barrell, PhD, RN
Associate Professor
Virginia Commonwealth University
School of Nursing
Richmond, Virginia

Sharon E. Beck, DNSc, RN
Assistant Hospital Director for Nursing Education
   and Quality Improvement
Temple University Hospital
Philadelphia, Pennsylvania

Andrea Bostrom, PhD, RN
Associate Professor
Kirkhof School of Nursing
Grand Valley State University
Allendale, Michigan

Marcia Carr, BN, MSc, RN
Director of Resident Care/Administrator
Cherington Place
Surrey, British Columbia

Judith A. Chaney, PhD, RN
Private Practice
Highland, Illinois

Marjorie Childers, PhD, RN, CS
Associate Professor of Nursing
College of Our Lady of the Elms
Chicopee, Massachusetts

Jeanne Clement, EdD, RN, CS, FAAN
Associate Professor of Nursing and Psychiatry
Ohio State University
Columbus, Ohio

Marga Simon Coler, EdD, RN, CS, CTN, FAAN
Professor and Coordinator
Community Mental Health and Psychiatric Nursing
School of Nursing
University of Connecticut
Storrs, Connecticut

Mickie W. Crimone, MS, RN, CS-P
Psychiatric Clinical Specialist, Private Practice
Rockville, Maryland
Director, Retired
Southern Community Mental Health Center
Potomac, Maryland

Ruth Davidhizar, RN, DNS, CS, FAAN
Assistant Dean and Chairperson of Nursing
Bethel College
Mishawaka, Indiana

Kathleen Shannon Dorcy, RN, BSN, MN
Adjunct Faculty
University of Washington
Tacoma, Washington

Cheryl Graham Eason, RN, MEd, MS, CS, CRRN
Professor of Nursing and Anthropology
Community College of Allegheny County,
   North Campus
Pittsburgh, Pennsylvania

Marlene Farrell, RN, MSN
Professor
California State University, Los Angeles
Los Angeles, California
Academic Coordinator
Center for International Nursing Education
California State University
Dominguez Hills, California

Janice Cooke Feigenbaum, MSN, PhD, RN
Professor of Psychiatric/Mental Health Nursing
Coordinator of Graduate Program in Community
   Addictions
Department of Nursing
D'Youville College
Buffalo, New York

E. A. Furlong, RN, C, PhD
Coordinator
Community Health/Community Mental Health
  Nursing
School of Nursing
Creighton University
Omaha, Nebraska

Elaine Gallien, RN, MSN, CS
Assistant Professor
University of Alabama
Capstone College of Nursing
Tuscaloosa, Alabama

Rauda Gelazis, PhD, RN, CS, CTN
Associate Professor
Ursuline College
Pepper Pike, Ohio

Deanne Gilmur, MEd
Patient Education Director
Western State Hospital
Tacoma, Washington
Faculty
University of Washington/Washington Institute
Tacoma, Washington

Mary E. Halupa, RN, MSN
Psychosocial Nursing Instructor
Pottsville Hospital School of Nursing
Pottsville, Pennsylvania

Lynn Hanson, RN, MS
Assistant Professor
Department of Nursing
Shepherd College
Shepherdstown, West Virginia

Donna F. Hecke, RN, MA, CPNP
School Health Coordinator
College of Nursing and Allied Health
Jewish Hospital
St. Louis, Missouri

Dixie Koldjeski, PhD, RN, FAAN
President and CEO
Health Education Seminars & Consultation, Inc.
Morehead City, North Carolina
Interim Associate Dean, School of Nursing
East Carolina University
Greenville, North Carolina

Jeanne B. Kozlak, RN, MSN, CS
Professor of Mental Health Nursing
Department of Nursing
Humboldt State University
Arcata, California

Courtney H. Lyder, ND, APRN, CS, GNP
Coordinator and Assistant Professor
Gerontology Concentration, Adult Advanced Practice
  Nursing Program
Yale University
New Haven, Connecticut

Betty Margolis, RN, MSN, CS
Assistant Professor, Retired
Chicago City Colleges
Chicago, Illinois

Susan McCabe, MS, RN, CS
Instructor
College of Nursing
East Tennessee State University
Johnson City, Tennessee

Rebecca Michaels, RN, MSN, CS
Clinical Specialist
Neighborhood HealthCare Centers
Clinical Instructor
Georgia College
Macon, Georgia

Wendy Noble, RN, MSN
Instructor, Associate Degree Nursing
Western Wisconsin Technical College
La Crosse, Wisconsin

Cindy A. Peternelj-Taylor, RN, BScN, MSc
Associate Professor
College of Nursing
University of Saskatchewan
Saskatoon, Saskatchewan

Ardyce A. Plumlee, RN, MN, CARN
Assistant Professor, Retired
School of Nursing
University of Kansas
Kansas City, Kansas

Rozann M. Reyerson, RN, BSN, MSEd
Instructor
University of South Dakota
Department of Nursing
Watertown Outreach Site
Watertown, South Dakota

Mary Rode, BNS, MSN
Associate Professor
Department of Nursing
University of Evansville
Evansville, Indiana

Betty W. Ross, PhD, RN, CS
Assistant Professor, Retired
School of Nursing
Fairleigh Dickinson University
Teaneck, New Jersey

Carol Sherwood, MSN, RN, CS
Assistant Professor
Simmons College
Boston, Massachusetts

Linda Sue Smith, RN, MSN
Nurse Educator
Gateway Technical College
Kenosha, Wisconsin

Anita Throwe, MS, BSN, CS
Associate Professor
Medical University of South Carolina
College of Nursing Satellite Program
    at Francis Marion University
Florence, South Carolina

Anna Tichy, BS, MS, PhD, RN
Professor
Department of Administrative Studies
College of Nursing
University of Illinois at Chicago
Chicago, Illinois

Linda G. Trabucco, JD, RN
Partner
Kelly, McLaughlin & Foster
Philadelphia, Pennsylvania

Mary G. Trainor, PhD, RN, CS
Associate Professor
College of Nursing and Health Science
George Mason University
Fairfax, Virginia

Joyce Van Nostrand, RN, PhD
Associate Professor and Department Head
Northeastern State University
Department of Nursing
Tahlequah, Oklahoma

Jean E. Wold, RN, MSN
Professor of Nursing
California State University
Chico, California

Susan Klasson Zareski, MN, RN, C
Assistant Director
Professor of Nursing
Nursing Department
El Camino College
Torrance, California

Preface

As I began the planning of this book, it occurred to me that less than a decade ago, a book on mental health in the community would have focused primarily on community mental health centers. Other than the private practice offices of psychiatrists and other mental health practitioners, the community mental health centers were where the "action" in community mental health took place. It is a sign of the rapidity with which a system of community-based services has evolved that this book contains 27 chapters, only one of which is devoted to community mental health centers.

In the current era of health care reform, much attention is being paid to a system of community-based services designed to help improve the quality of life for people with serious mental illness. Essential services in this rapidly evolving continuum of care include case management, rehabilitation, family and peer support, housing, and crisis stabilization, services that received little attention in the more traditional hospital-focused mental health system.

This book was conceived as a practical, clinically focused guide for psychiatric nurses who are making the transition from inpatient to community-based practice and for students in psychiatric-mental health nursing who will be starting new careers in the many opportunities now available in the community. This is an exciting time for psychiatric-mental health nursing. I hope this book will serve as a guide to those of you who accept the challenges of the new adventure into community-based practice.

ORGANIZATION OF THE BOOK

The book is divided into six units. Unit 1, The Context of Community Psychiatric Care, explores the evolution of mental health care in the community from the reform led by Dorothea Dix to the modern community mental health movement. The present state of health care in the United States, the concept of managed mental health care, and the evolving roles for psychiatric nurses in this era of health care reform are discussed.

Unit 2, Client Advocacy, focuses on the responsibilities of the nurse in the role of client advocate. The legal and ethical issues faced by psychiatric nurses working in a newly evolving health care system are discussed. Chapter 3 traces the evolution of family and consumer movements from their inception as advocates for people with mental illness to their present-day emergence as a strong political force in mental health. Chapter 4 provides guidance for working successfully with clients from various ethnic and cultural backgrounds.

Unit 3, Models, Roles, and Responsibilities, presents the theoretical foundation for the chapters that follow. Chapter 5 provides an in-depth discussion of the principles of prevention at the primary, secondary, and tertiary levels and includes examples of mental health prevention at each of these levels. Chapter 6 discusses the changing role of psychiatric nursing as the profession moves toward community-based practice.

Unit 4, Intervention in the Community, concentrates on commonly used community-based interventions. It begins with a review of basic assessment skills, then presents the theory and practice of crisis stabilization. The next four chapters discuss modalities that have been found to be particularly effective in working with clients who have severe and persistent mental illnesses: supportive psychotherapy, case management, psychoeducation, and psychosocial rehabilitation. This unit concludes with a chapter on the management of medications in the community setting.

Unit 5, Community Settings, consists of the many community settings in which mental health is now practiced. It begins with a chapter on home care, one of the fastest-growing opportunities for psychiatric nurses. Chapter 15 contains explanations of the often confusing issue of managed care. School-based clinics are discussed as a newly emerging opportunity for psychiatric nurses to work as clinicians and consultants. Chapters describe community mental health centers, partial hospital programs, and residential treatment agencies, rapidly expanding settings for the care of people with severe and persistent mental illnesses. A chapter is devoted to the special problems and opportunities that are found in practicing in rural settings. The unit concludes with practical advice for those interested in starting their own practices.

Unit 6, At-Risk Populations, is devoted to populations in the community that are especially vulnerable. The family preservation model of treating children, adolescents, and their families is a central focus of Chapter 22. The rapidly growing problem of comorbidity is discussed in the chapters on persons with mental illness and substance abuse and mental illness and HIV disease. Persons with mental illnesses who are homeless or housed in jails are particularly at risk and have recently gained the attention of practitioners and policy makers. Chapters 24 and 26 explain the scope of the problems and the efforts being made to alleviate them. Chapter 27 is devoted to the special problems faced by elderly people with mental illness.

FEATURES

This book is a practical guide for working with clients in community settings and includes in the appendixes tools for assessment, screening, and diagnosis. The *DSM-IV* classification system of medical diagnoses is included to offer quick access to the diagnostic codes needed for most record keeping. An outline for conducting a psychiatric history and mental status examination is presented. The Global Assessment of Functioning Scale is included because it is used to report overall functioning on Axis V of the *DSM-IV*

multiaxial classification. It also is useful in planning treatment and following progress. The Specific Level of Functioning Scale has been found to be useful in assessing social, occupational, and behavioral functioning and tracking progress in rehabilitation. The Brief Psychiatric Rating Scale is a commonly used tool for assessing psychopathology. Two disorder-specific scales are included to assess conditions that are commonly encountered: depression and alcoholism. The last four assessment tools have been developed specifically for the elderly. The Geriatric Depression Scale and the Global Deterioration Scale measure clinical status, whereas the Risk of Elder Abuse in the Home (REAH) Scale is designed to aid the practitioner in assessing the risk for elder abuse and the Stress Assessment Score of the Caregiver (SASC) measures stress in the caregiver.

In keeping with the public health theory of prevention that guides this book, whenever practical the chapters include sections on the following principles:

- Levels of prevention
- Epidemiology
- Etiology
- Target groups
- Interventions
- Model programs
- Role of the nurse
- Future directions

A final unique feature of the book is the inclusion of chapters written by individuals who are not nurses. This was done for several reasons. We wanted to provide readers with the best available and most current information on all the topics covered in this book and therefore sought the best-known experts in a particular field and invited them to contribute a chapter. In addition, changes in health care delivery will be likely to promote increasing collaboration with other mental health disciplines in a less hierarchical structure than is presently in place. As nurses, we must be willing to share our expertise with others and allow others to share their expertise with us.

ACKNOWLEDGMENTS

The author and contributors would like to acknowledge the assistance of several individuals:

Barbara Etzel, RN, MSN, Supervisor, Ramsey County Public Health Nursing Service, St. Paul, Minnesota, for case examples included in Chapter 2, Legal and Ethical Issues

Mary McBride, Chapter 14, Home Care

Brian M. Block, MA, Chapter 18, Partial Hospital Programs

Debra M. Sparks, RN, C, BSN, Chapter 18, Partial Hospital Programs

TERMINOLOGY

The term *client* instead of *patient* has been used predominately throughout the book to recognize individuals receiving mental health treatment as significant participants in the reciprocal process of treatment.

Nancy K. Worley

Brief Contents

Detailed Contents

The Context of Community Psychiatric Care

Chapter 1

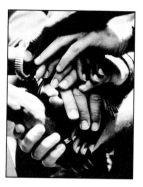

Political and Economic Perspectives

Nancy K. Worley

It will be said by a few, perhaps, that each state shall establish and sustain its own institutions; that it is not obligatory upon the general government to legislate for maintenance of state charities.... but may it not be demonstrated as the soundest policy of the federal government to assist in the accomplishment of great moral obligations, by diminishing and arresting wide spread miseries which mar the face of society, and weaken the strength of communities?

I confide to you the cause and the claims of the destitute and the desolate...who through the providence of God, are wards of the nation, claimants on the sympathy and care of the public, through the miseries and disqualifications brought upon them by the sorest afflictions with which humanity can be visited.

Dorothea Dix
Address to the U.S. Congress
Washington, D.C., 1848

THE EVOLUTION OF COMMUNITY MENTAL HEALTH CARE

From reform to "the shame of the states" in 100 years

In making this eloquent and emotional appeal, Dorothea Dix attempted to convince Congress to assume responsibility for the development of mental hospitals. When this attempt failed because of congressional uneasiness about tampering with states' rights, Dix turned to state-by-state lobbying. She was extraordinarily successful and was given credit for establishing state mental hospitals in more than 30 states. When Dix began her campaign, "moral treatment"—the care of people with mental illness in a humane and sympathetic environment far from the stresses of modern life—was available only to wealthy people. Poor people who were mentally ill were housed in workhouses, almshouses, and jails. Dorothea Dix envisioned the establishment of state hospitals that would house no more than 250 patients as a way of providing the same care to poor people that was available to the wealthy. For a while it seemed her vision would be realized; between 1850 and 1890, 94 state mental hospitals were built.

> The abandonment of depletion, external irritants, drastic purges, and starvation, and the substitution of baths, narcotics, tonics, and generous diet, is not less to be appreciated in the improved condition of the insane than the change from manacles, chains, by locks, and confining chairs, to the present system of kindness, confidence, social intercourse, labor, religious teaching, and freedom from restraint. In this age of improvement, no class of mankind has felt its influence more favorably than the insane.
>
> Samuel B. Woodward, President of the American Psychiatric Association, 1846

However, the "retreats" that Dix and her colleagues envisioned as quiet pastoral refuges for small numbers of patients rapidly became huge and overcrowded custodial institutions, some of which held as many as 15,000 patients. Close personal relationships between staff and patients, which had been a hallmark of moral treatment, gave way to custodial care and social control. Cities and towns that supported jails and almshouses were eager to send people to these new hospitals where the state bore the cost. The flood of immigrants into the United States during the late 19th century worsened the overcrowding. Many immigrants were poor and unable to speak English. The stress of relocation and the need to learn a new language, adjust to new customs, and find employment overwhelmed many and resulted in the admission of large numbers of immigrants to state mental hospitals.

> The overcrowding goes on, cots are brought out at night and laid down on corridor floors, at first one or two in nooks and alcoves that seem designed for this sort of thing, but the business grows, the special adaptation of recesses and alcoves becomes less apparent as the line of beds side by side stretches in lengthening vista down the hall. And still the floors fill up until one, two, three hundred are thus nightly—not accommodated but provided for...Day by day, year after year, I have seen the individualized treatment of special cases swamped by the rising tide of indiscriminate lunacy pouring through the wards,

> filling every crevice, rising higher and higher until gradually most distinctions and landmarks have been blotted out.
>
> W.W. Godding, President of the American Psychiatric Association, 1890

The wretched conditions in state hospitals exposed by journalists and patients caused some public outcry, and sporadic attempts were made to improve the lives of patients in these institutions. However, it would take nearly 100 years for real reform of state mental hospitals to take place. The major impetus for that reform would come from Congress, the body to which Dorothea Dix had appealed in 1848. A chronology of defining events in the history of mental health care in the United States is provided in Box 1-1.

The beginning of federal government involvement

Why did the federal government, which had long resisted involvement in the plight of people with mental illness, reconsider its stance? The roots of this policy change can in part be traced to the economic and social upheaval caused by the Great Depression of 1930-1939. The Depression marked the federal government's first massive intervention into social welfare. The success of Franklin D. Roosevelt's New Deal programs in diminishing the misery of joblessness, homelessness, and hunger resulted in a new acceptance of the federal government's role in helping to solve national problems (Foley & Sharfstein, 1983). World War II also increased national concern about mental illness. The conscription process for the armed services revealed a worrisome level of mental and emotional disorder in the country: 12 out of every 100 men examined were rejected for military service for neuropsychiatric reasons (Grob, 1991).

The plight of people with mental illness in state hospitals became even more desperate as the already inadequate number of mental health professionals in these institutions was further depleted as doctors and nurses left to join the war effort.

Box 1-1. Community mental health chronology of events

1848 Dorothea Dix appeals to the U.S. Congress to build federally funded mental hospitals. The bill authorizing construction is vetoed.

1850-1890 94 state mental hospitals are built.

1941-1945 World War II. 12 of every 100 men examined for service are rejected for psychological problems.

1946 National Institute of Mental Health (NIMH) is established.

1946 *The Snake Pit,* a popular novel about conditions in a mental hospital, is published.

1949 Albert Deutch writes *The Shame of the States,* an exposé of conditions in state mental hospitals.

1955 The Joint Commission on Mental Illness and Health is appointed by Congress.

1961 The report of the Joint Commission, *Action for Mental Health,* is published.

1963 President Kennedy signs PL-88-164, the Mental Retardation Facilities and Community Mental Health Centers Construction Act, establishing community mental health centers.

1973 The Health Maintenance Organization Act is passed by Congress. The law mandates the inclusion of mental health benefits to all HMO subscribers.

1975 Extensive amendments to the original Community Mental Health Centers Act expand service requirements from 5 to 12 "essential services."

1980 President Carter signs the Mental Health Systems Act to expand the community mental health center system.

1981 President Reagan signs the Omnibus Budget Reconciliation Act that provides "block grants" to the states for alcohol, drug abuse, and mental health services, repealing the Mental Health Systems Act and ending federal oversight of community mental health centers. In the private sector the first managed care organization that specializes in mental health is established.

1982 The Tax Equity and Fiscal Responsibility Act (TEFRA) is passed by Congress in an attempt to control Medicare and Medicaid costs. The act established diagnosis-related groups (DRGs) that reimburse a flat fee for all costs accrued during an episode of hospitalization. Most psychiatric hospital care is excluded from DRG regulations, leading to a proliferation of large for-profit "chains" of specialty psychiatric and chemical dependency hospitals. Between 1979 and 1986 the number of psychiatric hospitals grows by 40%.

1985 The growth in direct costs for mental health care exceeds the growth of all other health care costs.

1986-1990 Behavioral managed care organizations proliferate as attempts are made to slow the growth rate of expenditures for mental health and substance abuse.

1992 NIMH is reorganized. It retains its research and training functions but becomes an institute under the National Institutes of Health (NIH). Its service functions, along with those of the alcohol and drug abuse institutes, are combined into a new agency—the Substance Abuse and Mental Health Services Administration (SAMHSA). President-elect Clinton appoints the Health Task Force, which is charged with reforming health care in the United States.

1993 President Clinton presents the Health Task Force's results to Congress in a bill entitled the American Health Security Act.

1994 The 103rd Congress adjourns without voting on health care reform.

1995 Republicans gain a majority in the House of Representatives and the Senate, making substantial health care reform at the federal level unlikely.

Public outcry over deplorable conditions might never have been aroused had it not been for exposés by journalists and other writers during the immediate postwar period. Albert Deutch, a journalist who toured many state mental hospitals during and after the war, wrote that during a 1947 visit "the writer heard state hospital doctors frankly admit that the animals of nearby piggeries were better fed, housed and treated than many of the patients in their wards" (Deutch, 1949). The best-selling novel *The Snake Pit* (Ward, 1946), with its depiction of horrifying conditions and inhumane attendants in a state mental hospital, was published in 1946.

> At present there are being cared for in the Massachusetts state hospital system (mentally ill, mentally defective and epileptic) approximately 23,000 patients, at a per capita expenditure of approximately $1.00 per day. The total cost of this is so great that unless we are resolved to face the prospect of a steadily increasing expenditure we are compelled to ascertain whether the present work is being done efficiently.
>
> George M. Kline, President of the American Psychiatric Association, 1927

The birth of the National Institute of Mental Health

The confluence of these events—federal involvement in social policy, continued deterioration of state mental hospitals, and the public's awakening to deplorable hospital conditions—led to the National Mental Health Act's passage in 1946. In accordance with this legislation, the National Institute of Mental Health (NIMH) was established in 1949. Since then, NIMH has been a national focal point of concern, leadership, and effort for people with mental illness. Unlike other health institutes in the National Institutes of Health (NIH), NIMH's responsibilities extend far beyond research. The legislation that created NIMH mandated that in addition to promoting research, the Institute also spearhead the training of mental health professionals in psychiatry, psychology, social work, and nursing, and aid in the development of new services. This mandate resulted in a powerful organization that was able to chart the direction of mental health in the United States for many decades. Through its research branch, NIMH fostered rapid advancement in the pharmacological treatment of depression, schizophrenia, and drug and alcohol addiction, and in the systematic study of child mental health, mental retardation, and aging. Through its training branch, it supported graduate education in the four core mental health disciplines and increased

the number of mental health professionals at a rate ten times greater than that of all other health professionals combined (Foley & Sharfstein, 1983). Psychiatric nursing benefited enormously from this educational support. In 1947 NIMH provided funding to six universities that initiated graduate programs in psychiatric nursing. Over the next several decades many more universities were added to the original list; a large cadre of psychiatric nurses graduated from these programs and went on to become leaders in the specialty and in nursing in general. NIMH continues to supply some educational funds to nursing, although the amount has been drastically curtailed in recent years (Mereness, 1990). The National Institute of Mental Health's service branch made grants to states to assist in the establishment of clinics and treatment centers, and to fund demonstration studies dealing with the prevention and treatment of psychiatric disorders.

The community mental health movement

NIMH's early leaders were reform-minded professionals who had been given the opportunity to control national research, training, and service initiatives. Most had served in World War II, which had caused a basic intellectual shift in their assumptions about treatment. Their experience in working with men in combat helped crystallize beliefs that environmental stress contributed to mental maladjustment, and that changes in environmental stress decreased symptoms. They also had observed that they were most successful in preventing prolonged debilitating effects when they treated soldiers with psychological symptoms near the battlefield. These psychiatrists became convinced that their success in rapid, intensive treatment of impaired servicemen in proximity to their comrades could be translated to the treatment of civilians after the war. Using their professional, technical, and public relations skills, they influenced the movement toward early intervention and community treatment. NIMH's leaders urged Congress to initiate a national study on the state of mental health care in the United States. In 1955 Congress passed the Mental Health Study

Act, which funded the Joint Commission on Mental Illness and Health. The Commission existed for 5 years. Its final report recommended establishment of community mental health centers (CMHCs) and a decrease in the size of state mental hospitals. The Commission report was well received and led to the passage of the Community Mental Health Centers Act of 1963.

Unfortunately, the legislation also had some unintentional outcomes. As Mosher (1994) and others have pointed out, new federal support for people with mental illness created a care system parallel to that provided by state hospitals. Funding for the new community mental health system was provided directly from the federal government (through NIMH) to local entities that applied for funds and could assure the federal government that they could provide the five essential required services:

1. Inpatient care
2. Outpatient care
3. Emergency services
4. Partial hospitalization programs
5. Consultation and education services

It quickly became apparent that the conflict the original legislation fomented between the goals of preserving the mental health of communities through prevention and treating individual cases of mental illness was becoming more pronounced. Althouth one goal of the NIMH leadership in proposing community care was to empty the state hospitals, care of people with chronic mental illness was not mentioned in the original legislation. As a result of this oversight, the administrations of new community mental health centers did not perceive long-term care as a primary responsibility, and in many cases avoided working with clients with chronic mental illness, who were considered unrewarding and difficult. Realizing that moving clients into the community would transfer the financial burden to the federal government, states rapidly began to reduce inpatient populations and close their mental hospitals. Through this process of deinstitutionalization, tens of thousands of patients, many of whom had been institutionalized

for years, were moved into the community, where they received little care because community mental health centers were reluctant to treat them.

This situation led to the passage of major amendments to the original Community Mental Health Centers Act in 1975. Seven additional mandated services were added to the original five, thus requiring a community mental health center to provide 12 services in order to be funded. Some of the newly mandated services follow:

- Requirements for community mental health centers to assist the courts in screening people being considered for admission to a state hospital
- Aftercare and transitional halfway house services for people being discharged from state hospitals
- Formal coordination agreements between state hospitals and community mental health centers

Centers were given 2 years to comply with the new mandates or risk losing federal support. However, the centers were not given sufficient resources to comply with these mandates and began to cut back on preventive services. Since 1975 community mental health centers have been primarily treatment and rehabilitation centers for people with severe mental illness.

Chapter 17, Community Mental Health Centers, provides more detailed information on community mental health centers. Specific issues concerning the treatment of people with severe mental illness are discussed later in this book.

HEALTH CARE REFORM IN THE 1990s
The cost of health care

Health care expenditures in the United States have grown from less than 6% of national domestic spending in 1965 to more than 12% today; it is estimated that by the year 2000 health care costs will consume at least 15% of the nation's total spending (Gray, 1991).

In spite of the enormous amount of money spent on health care in the United States, life expectancy is shorter than in 15 other countries, and infant mortality is higher than in 22 other countries (Hilts, 1991). Thirty-seven million people in this country have either no health insurance or inadequate insurance and thus little or no access to care (Pardes, 1995).

Sporadic attempts made by the federal government in the 1970s and 1980s to inhibit the growth rate of health care costs met with little success. Concern about the ever-increasing cost of a health care system that is generally perceived as inefficient caused renewed interest in reform. This issue occupied much of the 1992 election campaign and continues to the present. While government struggles with the political and legislative complexity of increasing access and containing costs, basic reform is already underway in the business sector, which has watched health care devour ever larger portions of its profits. In the 1960s business spent between 4 cents and 8 cents of each dollar of profit on health care. By 1990 the cost of health care had grown to 50 cents per dollar; without massive intervention, it is expected to reach 60 cents per dollar by the year 2000 (Hilts, 1991).

The advent of managed care

By 1990, in response to escalating costs, most large firms in the United States had implemented managed care programs to provide health insurance coverage to their employees. In general managed care attempts to control health care costs by reimbursing only necessary and appropriate care delivered in the least restrictive, least intensive treatment setting. Figure 1-1 illustrates the massive change in the type and location of services that proponents of managed health care envision for the future. A glossary of key managed health care terms is provided in Box 1-2.

Health maintenance organizations

Managed care has itself become a growth industry, and its complexity is related to the variety of organizational configurations and reimbursement mechanisms used. One model of managed care is the health maintenance organization (HMO). HMOs

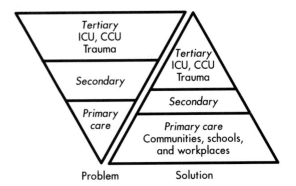

Figure 1–1. The goal of health care reform. Proponents of health care reform hope to emphasize health care services in primary settings, with a focus on prevention, in an effort to decrease the need for services at the tertiary level.

have existed since 1973; however, only 6% of people in the United States were enrolled in HMOs as late as 1982 (Luft, 1982). Loss of physician choice was a complaint cited by the majority of people reluctant to join HMOs at that time. Recently HMOs have grown in popularity as research demonstrates that they can reduce cost without adverse effect on health outcomes, and as consumers have shown greater readiness to sacrifice choice for cost reduction in their health care plans. Currently, the 540 HMOs in the United States enroll 42 million people (Christianson & Osher, 1994).

Although HMO plans vary greatly, most operate under the following assumptions:

1. In return for an annual fee per person or per family, the HMO provides the enrollee with comprehensive medical care.
2. Each enrollee is assigned to a primary care practitioner who acts as a gatekeeper for expensive specialty care. All visits to a specialist and all inpatient care must be approved by the primary care practitioner.
3. Because all health care must be provided from a prearranged annual amount (prospective payment), effort is focused on prevention and early intervention.

4. Because hospitalization is the single most expensive locus of care, substitutions such as outpatient surgery, transitional care, and home care are used whenever possible. Patients are hospitalized for the fewest number of days possible.

In the public sector (government-funded programs such as Medicaid and Medicare, and federal, state, and local appropriations) experimentation with managed care is underway. Although significant differences exist between managed care in the public and private sectors, all managed care arrangements attempt to shift the locus of care away from hospitals to a continuum of treatment options in the community.

The cost of mental health care

Although general health care costs rose rapidly in the 1980s, the fastest growth in costs occurred in the mental health care sector. In 1980 the cost to treat mental illness and chemical dependency was $35 billion. The cost spiraled to $50 billion by 1983 and to $80 billion by 1989 (Kessler, 1989). A recent study that estimated direct costs (expenditures for institutional care, professional services, medication, and rehabilitation services) and indirect costs (estimated value of lost work, lost productivity, and losses from premature death) put the total cost of alcohol, drug, and mental health disorders at $168 billion a year (Rice et al., 1990). Twenty-five percent of all hospital beds in the United States are occupied by people with mental illness, and 58% of the treatment costs of mental illness are for institutional care.

What are some of the reasons for the increasing cost of mental health care? The decreasing number of state hospital residents shifted the cost of care from the states to the federal government through the community mental health centers. The centers were mandated to provide inpatient services for their clients. The most common way to provide this service was (and continues to be) through a contractual arrangement with a community hospital with a psychiatric unit or with a freestanding psychiatric hospital in the community. This shifting of

---

Box 1–2. Definitions of key health care terms

Capitation　The paying to a provider of a fixed sum per person served for a defined range of services for a specific time period, usually 1 year.

Carve-out　The separation of mental health from general medical benefits.

Fee-for-service　A method of reimbursing on the basis of services rendered. This is the most common method of reimbursement for medical services. It is considered a major factor in the escalation of health care costs.

Gatekeeper　A primary care practitioner to whom a defined insured population is assigned and who is required to provide all health care or to authorize care from other specialists, if necessary, for the assigned individuals.

Health maintenance organization (HMO) Any organization that through an organized system of health care provides or insures the provision of an agreed-upon set of health maintenance and treatment services for an enrolled group of people under a prepaid fixed sum or capitation arrangement.

Managed care　The oversight by insurers or their designates to monitor the utilization of care and in so doing to contain or reduce the associated cost.

Prospective payment　Providers receive a predetermined fixed fee for care delivered during a defined episode of illness. Diagnosis-related groups (DRGs) are the most common example of prospective payment in the general health sector. In mental health the most common example is the fixed "target rate" per discharge that private hospitals receive for the inpatient care of Medicare-insured patients, regardless of how long the patient stays or the amount of services the patient uses.

inpatient mental health care from state hospitals to community hospitals resulted in an increase in the number of inpatient episodes paid for by the community mental health centers from 27,000 in 1967 to 254,000 in 1980 (when the federal government discontinued direct federal funding for CMHCs) (Kiesler & Sibulkin, 1987).

Private psychiatric hospitals also increased in size and number with the scaling-down of state hospitals. The most dramatic growth, however, occurred in the general hospital sector, presently the largest provider of acute psychiatric inpatient care. Supported by the expansion of public and private mental health insurance benefits, admissions to psychiatric units in general hospitals increased 84% between 1969 and 1988. This growth in inpatient care cannot be attributed solely to the shift from state to community hospitalization. The reimbursement system for care of people with mental illness in private health insurance and public programs provided strong incentives for inpatient care but little inducement for aftercare and follow-up services. Outpatient providers have little incentive to address the needs of people with chronic mental illness covered by Medicaid because reimbursement is low and noncompetitive. Repeated short-term hospitalization with little or no follow-up became the norm in the care of people with severe and persistent mental illness.

Employers and insurers responded to rapidly escalating costs by slashing coverage, or in some cases eliminating coverage for mental health services. However, even with these radical measures the spiral of spending showed little or no sign of abating. Despite 35 years of deinstitutionalization, programs providing alternatives to hospital care have grown slowly. As recently as 1986 70% of state mental health funds (excluding Medicaid) were allocated to state and county hospitals. In the private sector the reliance on hospitalization for treatment was just as problematic.

Managed mental health care

The major impetus for reform has come from the business sector, which now spends as much as 20 cents of every health care dollar on mental health services (Hilts, 1991). In response to the inability to slow the growth of mental health costs, the public and private sectors have begun to experiment with managed care as a more cost-effective method of delivering mental health services. Managed care in the mental health sector is more complex than in the general health care sector because of the need to establish relations between acute and long-term care, between medical and social services, and between services provided by physicians and those provided by other health care professionals (Mechanic, 1993). Because of the differences between delivering general health care and mental health care, most insurance companies and other managed care organizations have "carved out" the mental health benefit package and capitated it separately from other medical services. As a result, providers of mental health benefits fear heavy use of these services. Therefore almost all insurance policies establish different limits for psychiatric services than for other medical services. Psychiatric services tend to have higher deductibles, higher coinsurance (the percentage of the cost paid by the insured at the time of service), and lower utilization limits. At present, managed care of mental health appears to allow greater access to mental health services than fee-for-service reimbursement but limits the intensity of service (particularly hospitalization), and it tends to substitute other mental health professionals for psychiatrists and group therapy for individual therapy (Mechanic, 1993).

Evidence suggests that managed mental health care in the private sector is slowing the growth of the cost of care (especially the cost of hospitalization), but progress in the public sector is problematic. Public sector clients, by definition, depend on Medicaid or a variety of government-funded disability and social service benefits for their subsistence. Unlike the private sector, which serves primarily a low-risk population of healthy and employed people, the public mental health sector serves a preponderance of people who are seriously and persistently mentally ill. These people need not only medical care, but also a variety of services such as case management, supported housing, and psychosocial rehabilitation. Many states are experimenting with managed care for their Medicaid populations, including people who are severely and persistently mentally ill. Some states are experimenting with HMOs created specifically to serve people with chronic mental illness (Babigian et al., 1992).

> Without any additional expenditure of monies, we could pool the various existing medical, social, vocational, housing, and rehabilitative service funds that flow from federal, state, and local agencies and distribute them on a capitation basis.
>
> John A. Talbott, President of the American Psychiatric Association, 1985

Cities also are moving toward managed care for their Medicaid populations. For the past 5 years, about half of the 509,000 Philadelphia residents on medical assistance have been enrolled in HMOs. In 1995 everyone on medical assistance was moved into managed care plans (Collins & Uhlman, 1995). See Chapter 15, Managed Behavioral Health Services, for more detailed information on managed care.

PSYCHIATRIC NURSING IN THE 1990s

Psychiatric nursing has historically been a hospital-based specialty. The health care system's rapid transformation from one in which the hospital plays a major role to one in which the hospital is no longer central to the delivery of health care has had a tremendous impact on psychiatry and psychiatric nursing. The immediate outcome has been the closing or downsizing of psychiatric hospitals and psychiatric units in general hospitals, and the dislocation of many workers, including psychiatric nurses (Himali, 1995). Although this shrinking of the hospital market is distressing in the short term, it also is forcing an expansion of the boundaries of practice that in the long term will be beneficial to the profession. Opportunities

for practice along the entire continuum of care are rapidly becoming available to psychiatric nurses. As patients are hospitalized for shorter periods of time, the market for home care services increases. Partial hospitalization and other rehabilitative services, case management, and supportive therapies as alternatives to hospitalization are expanding rapidly.

Many opportunities in managed care are becoming available at both the organizational and clinical levels. At the organizational level nurses perform preadmission certification, continuing hospital certification, retrospective medical record audits, and case management (Waugh, 1993). At the clinical level managed care will continue to develop innovative treatment programs that in the past would not have been reimbursed under traditional fee-for-service arrangements. Because providers need not be concerned about whether they will be reimbursed for a specific service, they have the flexibility to develop individualized treatment plans. Interventions that emphasize family support (including education on client disorders and practical information about medications) and offer clients and families information about school, hospital, and vocational systems are likely to flourish under managed care programs. Nurses who typically have had major responsibility for patient and family education in the hospital setting will have the opportunity to transfer these skills to working with families in the community.

Managed care has forced a shift in emphasis from medical diagnosis to interest in the client's ability to participate successfully in interpersonal relationships, function within a family or social group, perform useful work, maintain an independent existence, and attend to basic needs for food, shelter, and self-care. Traditionally, "ways of living" or functional patterns have been an important focus of nursing's health promotion, intervention, and rehabilitation (Gordon, 1994). It is up to nurses to capitalize on their expertise in these areas. See Chapter 15, Managed Behavioral Health Services, for more detailed information on nursing opportunities in managed care.

Short intensive hospital stays will bring new challenges for nurses who continue to practice in hospital settings. The increased use of technology and the increasing attention paid to the biological aspects of a client's illness call for nurses with skills in these areas. The recognition by the general medical community that ignoring the interplay between medical illness and psychological response increases both complications and length of stay will expand the opportunity for psychiatric liaison nursing in general hospitals.

The aging of the population in the United States increases the need for psychiatric nurses who have special skill in working with older people. Interest in geropsychiatric nursing is increasing.

The change in the health care reimbursement system from fee-for-service to capitation rewards preventive efforts. Psychiatric nurses skilled at client education will find their skills in great demand in this new environment. Wellness programs, stress management workshops, and parenting classes are just a few of the preventive programs that businesses and managed care organizations will encourage their clients to attend.

As the concept of a continuum of care moves from theory to reality, psychiatric nurses with a background in the biological and psychosocial sciences have an exciting opportunity to provide primary care in a variety of new service settings. Significant clinical roles for psychiatric nurses are emerging in the schools. Drug and alcohol abuse, adolescent pregnancy, school violence, and a myriad of other social and psychological problems have led to increased interest in providing expanded health services in the schools. Presently, an estimated 300 school-based health centers in the United States are located in secondary schools. School nurses in California and New York are forming their own school health companies and contracting directly with schools. Hospitals, as part of their search for new markets, have begun to contract with schools to administer health programs (Igoe & Speer, 1992). The large number of people with mental illness in jails and the lack of treatment for this population, first exposed by Torrey et al. (1992), has led to a proliferation of programs that either divert people with mental illness from jail to appropriate treatment in community-based services or provide in-jail mental health services. These programs provide opportunities for psychiatric nurses in the screening, assessment, and treatment of this growing population. Homelessness, which began to receive attention from the government and the media in the 1980s, shows no sign of abating in the 1990s. It is estimated that as many as one third of homeless people are mentally ill (Federal Task Force on Homelessness and Severe Mental Illness, 1992). Psychiatric nurses have been providing and will continue to provide services in such nontraditional sites as in shelters, on the streets, in soup kitchens, and in drop-in centers.

As new clinical opportunities emerge, the search for innovative service delivery models continues. The decentralization of services in the community has increased the complexity of providing and integrating a full range of service according to each client's needs. The realization that people with severe psychiatric disorders are often unable to locate and negotiate services on their own has led to increasing interest in case management. Psychiatric nurses who have traditionally coordinated and managed the delivery of services in the hospital environment will have the opportunity to transfer many of these skills to positions in the relatively new and expanding field of case management.

SUMMARY

Exciting changes and opportunities are occurring in the care and treatment of people with mental illness. Fundamental changes in mental health delivery systems mean that the major portion of mental health care and treatment will take place in the community. New treatment sites, new treatment modalities, and new methods of delivering services are developing rapidly. The chapters that follow will expand on these developments and introduce an exciting new world of psychiatric nursing in the community.

REFERENCES

Babigian, H., Mitchell, O., Marshall, P., & Reed, S. (1992). A mental health capitation experiment: Evaluating the Monroe-Livingston experience. In R. G. Frank, & W. G. Manning (Eds.), *Economics and mental health*. Baltimore: Johns Hopkins.

Christianson, J. B., & Osher, F. C. (1994). Health maintenance organizations, health care reform and persons with serious mental illness. *Hospital and Community Psychiatry* 45, 898-905.

Collins, H., & Uhlman, M. (1995, February 5). The new world of mental health. *The Philadelphia Inquirer*, pp. A1, A12.

Deutch, A. (1949). *The mentally ill in America: A history of their care and treatment from colonial times*. New York: Columbia University Press.

Dix, D. (1848). *Address to the United States Congress*. Washington, DC.

Federal Task Force on Homelessness and Severe Mental Illness: Outcasts on Main Street (1992). Washington, DC: Interagency Council on the Homeless.

Foley, H., & Sharfstein, S. (1983). *Madness and government: who cares for the mentally ill?* Washington, DC: American Psychiatric Press.

Godding, W. (1890). Aspects and outlook of insanity in America. *American Journal of Insanity, 47,* 1-16.

Gordon, M. (1994). *Nursing diagnosis, process and application* (3rd ed.). St. Louis: Mosby.

Gray, B. (1991). *The profit motive and patient care*. Cambridge, MA: Harvard University Press.

Grob, G. N. (1991). *From asylum to community*. Princeton, NJ: Princeton University Press.

Hilts, P. (1991, May 19). Demands to fix U.S. health care reach crescendo. *New York Times,* Section 4, pp. 1,5.

Himali, U. (1995, March). ANA sounds alarm about unsafe staffing levels. *The American Nurse, 27*(2), 1,7.

Igoe, J., & Speer, S. (1992). The community health nurse in schools. In M. Stanhope, & J. Lancaster (Eds.), *Community health nursing* (Ch. 40). St. Louis: Mosby.

Kessler, W. K. (1989). Managed psychiatric care will continue to boom. *Clinical Psychiatry News,* 17, 6-7.

Kiesler, C., & Sibulkin, A. (1987). *Mental hospitalization, myths and facts about a national crisis*. Newbury Park, CA: Sage Publications.

Kline, G. (1927). Presidential address. *American Journal of Psychiatry,* 84, 1-22.

Luft, H. (1982). Health maintenance organizations and the rationing of medical care. *Milbank Quarterly,* 60, 2.

Mechanic, D. (1993). Mental health services in the context of health care reform. *Milbank Quarterly,* 71, 349-364.

Mereness, D. (1990). Foreword in C. Taylor (Ed.), *Essentials of psychiatric nursing* (13th ed.). St. Louis: Mosby.

Mosher, L. (1994). *Community mental health, a practical guide*. New York: W.W. Norton.

Pardes, H. (1995, September). *Psychiatry and health care reform*. Paper presented at the 46th Institute on Hospital and Community Psychiatry, San Diego, CA.

Rice, D., Kelman, S., Miller, L., & Dunmeyer, S. (1990). *The economic costs of alcohol and drug abuse and mental illness: 1985.* (DHHS Publication No. ADM 90-1694). Rockville, MD: National Institute of Mental Health.

Talbott, J. (1985). Presidential address: Our patients' future in a changing world: the imperative for psychiatric involvement in public policy. *American Journal of Psychiatry,* 142, 1003-1008.

Torrey, E., Stieber, J., Ezekiel, J., Wolfe, S., & Flynn, L. (1992). *Criminalizing the seriously mentally ill: the abuse of jails as hospitals*. Arlington, VA: National Alliance for the Mentally Ill.

Ward, M. (1946). *The snake pit*. New York: Random House.

Waugh, J. (1993). Role in a managed care setting. In *Advanced nursing practice roles in an era of health care reform*. Proceedings of the Southern Council on Collegiate Education for Nursing.

Woodward, S. B. (1850). Observations on the medical treatment of insanity. (Read at a meeting of the Association of medical Superintendents of American Institutions for the Insane, May 1846) *American Journal of Insanity,* 7, 1-34.

Client Advocacy

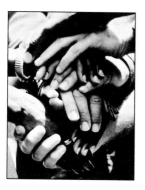

Chapter 2

Legal and Ethical Issues

Diane K. Kjervik

During this time of cost containment and managed care, health care available and accessible to people with mental illness is jeopardized. Emphasis on client outcomes rewards the quick fix and overlooks long-term care and community-based solutions. This new emphasis chooses superficial behavioral and drug-based approaches to mental health care over more traditional psychodynamic and psychoanalytical modes, de-emphasizing the client's understanding of the problem and valuing superficial evidence of improvement. Clients of mental health services, as with clients of other health care services, are discharged sicker and quicker to the community without adequate community resources to handle their needs. Homelessness, drug and alcohol abuse, domestic violence, and high levels of mental illness continue unabated (Torrey, 1993). Without adequate insurance coverage for mental problems, only wealthy people can afford the treatment required for lasting change.

Primary mental health care has not been given the stature of primary physical health care within the discipline of nursing. Thus although mental health nurses are responding to the market by learning physical assessment skills, pathophysiology, and advanced pharmacology, nurse practitioner students are not learning mental health assessment, psychopathology, and psychopharmacology. Mental health nursing therefore continues to be treated as the "other" in relation to the rest of nursing. Marginalization of mental health nursing to a certain degree reflects the marginalizaton of people with mental illness generally and the value (or lack of value) placed on their treatment.

Legal and ethical concerns abound in the health care environment. How can adequate care be given if it is not reimbursed? How can a prudent mental health nurse behave reasonably in an environment in which care of the person with mental illness is devalued? How can the nurse maintain client confidentiality and yet carry out a duty to protect society from potential harm from the client? Compassion is a necessary virtue when considering the roles of the nurse and the community in mental health care. Compassion, as Kerr (1995) points out, was sorely lacking in deinstitutionalization programs that dismantled inpatient facilities and left little more than prisons or homelessness for clients in the community. Certainly a darker side of caring exists (Aroskar, 1991), and even nurses with benevolent intentions need to face the realities of this side. The urge to control, rather than to enable independent action, is one aspect of this dark side. Even reassurance, as Kashka and Keyser (1995) point out, can be coercive. Do mental health care policies truly show compassion, or are they not-so-benign neglect?

This chapter will address legal and ethical concerns mental health nurses face. Frameworks for ethical and legal analysis will be discussed, and a virtue ethics model of analysis will be suggested as an approach to resolving many of the problems mental health nurses confront in the community. Two cases from a public health nurse's caseload provide examples of contemporary mental health problems nurses may face in the community. Recent legal cases that involve mental health nursing will demonstrate the need to attend carefully to standards of practice to prevent legal problems.

LEGAL AND ETHICAL FRAMEWORKS

The United States legal system is a political framework for decision making on a community level. Legislative enactments, judicial decisions, and executive orders reflect community values held by a majority of people. The law also attempts to address minority groups in civil rights legislation that empowers less powerful groups, including racial and ethnic minorities. The U.S. Constitution, federal and state legislation, court opinions, and executive branch decisions provide sources of law. The law examines value-laden issues (such as abortion) and pragmatic societal concerns (such as automobile traffic), and makes and enforces decisions to minimize conflict and respect community standards.

Ethics is philosophical inquiry into the nature of right and wrong. Ethicists give recommendations but no mandates. Beauchamp and Childress (1994) discuss the following eight theoretical orientations to ethics in health care:

1. **Obligation-based theory** (Kantianism) examines objective principles that display rightness, specifically Kant's categorical imperative that one should do that which one would want all people to do.
2. **Consequence-based theory** (teleology) examines an action's end point for rightness (for example, maximum utility). Its primary orientation is that rightness promotes the greatest good for the greatest number.
3. **Virtue-based ethics** assesses the character of the moral agent for compassion, trustworthiness, and respectfulness. The intent of the moral agent is considered, and in that sense, the subjectivity of the decision-maker matters. Pellegrino (1991) identifies temperance, justice, courage, and prudence as cardinal virtues.
4. **Rights-based theories** (liberal individualism) emphasize individual rights over obligations. The right of the individual to have the space to pursue personal projects is basic to this view.
5. **Communitarianism** (community-based theory) assesses an act's rightness based on whether it promotes the common good, supports community standards, and enhances social norms. This view deemphasizes the individual and values actions that promote the group.
6. **Ethics of care** measures an act's rightness according to its impact on intimate relationships among people. Caring is valued above abstract principles.
7. **Casuistry**, or case-based reasoning, focuses on making pragmatic decisions in specific cases. Historical patterns among cases are relevant, but each case is still examined on its own merits. It is analogous to common law, which also is detail-oriented and honors precedent.
8. **Principle-based common morality theories** examine principles but unlike Kantian theories are pluralistic in nature. A balancing among moral norms is carried out to determine rightness.

Beauchamp and Childress (1994) indicate that all of these ethical theories are useful in guiding moral decisions because "in moral reasoning, we often blend appeals to principles, rules, rights, virtues, passions, analogies, paradigms, parables, and interpretations." This chapter emphasizes virtue-based ethics to promote consensus building among mental health nurses about character traits that are especially helpful in resolving ethical and legal problems.

Legal scholars debate the meaning and purpose of the law (metalaw), just as ethicists explore the nature and meaning of morality (metaethics). Both disciplines struggle between absolutism and relativism. Legal realists see laws change with the times and believe it should be this way, but natural law advocates say certain immutable legal tenets are never to be changed. Casuistic ethicists examine the details of each case for unique patterns and requirements, whereas virtue ethicists believe in a set of character traits critical to human function. The tension among these philosophies stimulates creativity in problem solving.

In nursing, philosophical subtleties are lost in the demands of client crises. In mental health nursing, in which the client's judgment is in question, ethical questions prevail as patient autonomy is jeopardized. Likewise, legal concerns arise when the client's will and choice are overruled by the application of restraints and by seclusion, administration of drugs, and electroconvulsive treatment. In these situations questions of consent, manipulation, and coercion can be easily raised but not readily answered. The subtleties are even greater in community settings. Family members and friends are involved in day-to-day client activities, and evaluation of the client's condition is affected by relationships with others. Autonomy and confidentiality are constantly challenged by the presence and influence of others.

Case example

Margaret is a 50-year-old woman with schizoaffective disorder who has had frequent hospitalizations in at least 10 acute care settings in a state in the upper Midwest. Her mental illness manifests in mood lability, hostility, disorganized thinking, obsessive anxiety, and delusions, all of which contribute to poor decision making and lack of insight. Her physical health also is significantly impaired by severe chronic obstructive pulmonary disease (COPD). Although she is on continuous oxygen, she is a chain smoker. She was recently hospitalized with profound respiratory acidosis and respiratory failure. She was placed on a respirator in the ICU but as soon as she recovered sufficiently she demanded to be released—although she had not yet recovered. The hospital discharged her to her apartment, where she lives with her ex-husband.

QUESTIONS RAISED BY PUBLIC HEALTH NURSES

How many times should medical technology be used to rescue clients who significantly impair their health with poor life-style choices?

How often should public dollars pay the bill for clients on medical assistance?

Discussion of case

This case illustrates the tension between the exercise of the client's will (in this case, self-destructive behavior) and the effect on the community (high financial cost) of this behavior. This situation also occurs in general medical settings but in this case the choice of action is complicated by the mental illness. Is Margaret's choice truly voluntary? As far as we know from this case, no one is forcing her to smoke. Does her mental illness impede the voluntariness of her choice? If she can recite the effects of smoking on her condition without distortion of facts, the voluntariness is reason-based. Does she consider the effect on the community? Perhaps not, but how often do we expect clients to examine their behavior in this fashion?

What nursing virtues are served by continuing to care for Margaret? Compassion for the client would require helping her as she struggles for breath, but caring for the community might dictate the opposite. Informing the client about her behavior's effect on her health and the cost to the community would serve the virtue of truth telling.

Withholding care from her or refusing her admission to an ER would not be compassionate, but would support considerations of justice for the community's economic health.

This case illustrates how policy, law, and ethics converge. Legally, issues of abandonment (if care is refused), informed consent, and meeting professional standards of practice intertwine with the ethical concerns already mentioned. Health policy concerns, in terms of resource allocation, accompany ethical and legal concerns. The mental health nurse, who in this case would consult with the public health nurse, must address all three areas.

CONNECTION OF LAW AND ETHICS TO THE CONCEPT OF AGENCY

Law and ethics conceive of agency differently. In law, agency is a major content area, similar to contract, corporate, or tort law. Agency law addresses the relationship and respective authority between the principal (employer) and agent (employee). An agent carries out actions on behalf of the principal within the scope of employment. Agency is similar to advocacy in that the agent carries out tasks and functions to improve the status of the principal.

In ethics, agency concerns the expression of the agent's autonomy toward the agent's own goals (Husted & Husted, 1995). A third view of agency, clinical agency, is described by Benner et al. (in press) as "the sense and possibilities for acting in particular clinical situations," which leaves open the question of the recipient of the agent's acts. The idea that one can act to effect a given change is common to all three views of agency.

Agency is a vital concept in mental health nursing, because nurses must act to reach goals for themselves and for and with clients. The goal of care is to empower clients to act as effective agents on their own behalf. Thus, the restoration of autonomous expression is agency's highest application. Nurses and clients must know their own values and goals and speak clearly about

them with one another. Communication, as Duldt (1995) points out, is a vital component in the synthesis of nursing theory and ethics.

LEGAL AND ETHICAL RESPONSIBILITIES IN THE COMMUNITY

Although many ethical and legal challenges face the mental health nurse working in the community, several particularly notable areas will be discussed here. Because many treatment modalities and variations in approach fall within a reasonable standard of care, lawsuits are not typically generated by the adequacy of the given modality's use. Rather, the client's self-destruction or harm to others, resulting from the inaction of the therapist, creates legal liability. If a therapist oversteps therapeutic boundaries (for example, by engaging in a sexual relationship with a client), legal liability also is created. Mental health nurses are considered expert witnesses in cases involving standards of practice and client competency. Ethical concerns exist within each of the areas of legal involvement, although not always in the foreground.

Duty to warn

Within a therapeutic relationship's security, a client may disclose suicidal or homicidal feelings. Mental health nurses must consider how realistic these threats are and what actions they should take to prevent life-endangering actions. Historically, the law has not held therapists liable for a client's actions that harmed someone outside the therapeutic relationship. However, beginning with *Tarasoff v. Regents of the University of California* (1976), the courts changed the precedent. In *Tarasoff*, a young man who had been a student health center client killed his girlfriend after telling clinic therapists that he would do so as soon as she returned from her vacation. The California court held that the therapists should have acted to prevent the killing by informing the victim so she could act to save her life. Since this decision, many state courts (including Colorado, Kentucky, Louisiana, Minnesota, Montana, New Hampshire,

Utah, Washington, and Michigan) have adopted an approach similar to the California precedent (Geske, 1989). Other states, such as Florida, have not imposed a duty to warn third parties (*Boynton v. Burglass*, 1991).

Concern about preservation of confidentiality creates conflict among states. A 1993 study of duty to warn by Rosenhan et al. found that of 872 California psychotherapists surveyed, 79% thought confidentiality should be breached if a client threatened to kill someone, and 8% thought confidentiality should never be breached. Even in the state that took a leadership position on the topic, some therapists are unwilling to violate confidentiality even if it means violating the law. Interestingly, 63% of the therapists surveyed would not warn for situations involving AIDS, syphilis, or herpes (Rosenhan et al., 1993). The study surveyed only psychiatrists and psychologists, so whether mental health nurses hold the same views is unknown.

Mental health nurses need to know their state law regarding duty to warn and other areas of malpractice, because these matters are clearly within each state's jurisdiction. Knowledge of ethical problems related to confidentiality and prevention of harm to others also warrants the mental health nurse's consideration. Honesty and compassion for the client and for the person being threatened assist the nurse in finding creative solutions. The nurse may wish to commit the client to the hospital rather than warn a third party, thus protecting the third party and providing help for the client to deal with homicidal feelings. If the nurse cannot commit the client because standards for commitment are not met, he or she can inform the client honestly of the professional need to inform the potential victim and possibly the police. In this way clients learn that consequences will result from their actions.

Case example

Melanie is a 32-year-old woman with a diagnosis of major depression, alcohol dependence, polysubstance abuse, and antisocial personality disorder. She was recently discharged from a treatment center where she had been hospitalized following decompensation while off medication for depression and delirium tremens.

Melanie prostitutes to earn money and is a hepatitis C carrier. She states that she uses condoms when sexually active, but the public health nurse doubts that she uses them consistently. Hepatitis C and its consequences for her sexual partners have been explained to Melanie by many health professionals who are concerned that she may be exposing others to harm by her casual attitude about safe sex.

QUESTION RAISED BY PUBLIC HEALTH NURSES

What is the public health nurse's obligation to the community when this type of situation occurs?

Discussion of case

One major distinction exempts this case from the duty to warn obligation—the public health nurse does not actually know whether unsafe sex is occurring. Because the duty to warn is a carefully crafted exception to the rule of confidentiality, the nurse must have a strong reason to violate confidentiality. Assessment of violence typically requires specificity of victim, weapon, time, and place. This specificity is simply lacking for legal duties to arise in Melanie's case.

However, several ethical concerns persist. Melanie is not behaving virtuously (that is, not caring for others or for herself). Whether she is being truthful and fully disclosing her behavior also is open to debate. When suspicious of unlawful or harmful behavior, what actions should the nurse take? Trust between nurse and client is vital to discovering the facts in this situation, and yet to disclose the truth will place the client in legal jeopardy. This situation is similar to child abuse; the abuser must trust the nurse enough to admit to the abuse, which will result in a report to legal authorities. The nurse's honesty from the inception of the relationship will make it easier for the client to disclose these facts and remain open to assistance. Thus the nurse should not promise

blanket confidentiality to clients. Some states require the reporting of sexual activity by HIV
carriers to the department of health, which will
make follow-up contact notification to sexual partners. The law may mandate what the ethical
approach cannot.

Choice to die

Mental health nurses often are confronted by a
client's suicidal wish or plan. Professional standards of practice forbid condoning suicide or
assisting with it. Suicide prevention should be
more the mental health nurse's orientation. The
law also does not condone suicide, but does allow
refusal of treatment by the client or the client's
surrogate. However, the argument can be made
that psychotherapists could be shielded from liability if the suicide results from rational delibera-
tion (Kjervik, 1984; Kjervik, 1991). Indeed, some
courts have shielded therapists from liability because suicide is considered a voluntary act by the
client, an "intervening cause" that breaks the
chain of causation between the therapist's negli-
gent act and the client's injury (*R.D. v. W.H.*, 1994;
Eidson v. Reproductive Health Services, 1994).
Courts in other cases have held that suicide is not
an intervening cause that shields a third party
from liability (*Muse v. Charter Hospital of
Winston-Salem*, 1995; *People v. Velez*, 1993). The
clients did not act voluntarily; they acted as a
result of mental illness.

The gray area of suicide and the therapist's role
in it creates serious ethical tensions. However,
unlike the taking of another life, this situation
involves the taking of one's own life, raising issues
of autonomy and self-determination. In the community setting (as opposed to the hospital environment), the law imposes a less stringent standard for suicide prevention, holding that clients
act more autonomously in the community than in
a hospital, where staff are expected to monitor
suicidal patients closely. If the therapist judges
that a client is highly suicidal, the client should
be committed to the hospital for observation.
The mental health professional must judge the

probability of suicide, although self-violence is
notoriously difficult to predict.

The moral questions regarding suicide involve
the value of life, the value of a person's choices,
and the influence of mental instability on the
client's ability to choose. From the standpoint of
virtue, mental health nurses act with integrity, in
harmony with their values, when they know their
own values about suicide but can separate them
from the client's. As Pellegrino (1989) points out,
effacement of the health professional's self-
interest is an important virtue. If mental problems
impair the client's cognition, nurses will recognize
this and respect it by listening to clients and
helping them explore the threatened suicide's
consequences to family members, friends, and
others. Compassion for the client leads the nurse
to care for all the client's inner voices, including
the wish to die and the corresponding wish to
live.

Diagnosis and treatment: the mental health nurse as witness

Nurses can act as lay or expert witnesses in
trials and hearings (Laben & MacLean, 1989). Lay
witnesses testify to facts, and expert witnesses
provide opinions on adequacy of care. Mental
health nurses are often recognized as expert witnesses in cases brought against psychotherapists.

Mental health nurses assess and treat clients'
health care needs, and have testified on their
diagnoses and assessments in the following situations:

- **Dangerousness:** *State v. Patterson*, 1994
- **Physical and mental health problems**:
  United States v. Watson, 1994
- **Intake assessment for civil commit-
  ment:** *Ziemba v. Riverview Medical Center*,
  1994
- **Hypochondriasis:** *Virakitti v. Oregon De-
  partment of Corrections*, 1994
- **Post-traumatic stress disorder:** *United
  States v. Grimes*, 1994; and *Hill v. Allstate
  Associates*, 1994

- **Childhood sexual abuse:** *State v. Bingham*, 1993; and *Peterson v. Peterson*, 1991
- **Competency in criminal cases:** Taslitz, 1993; *United States v. Herrera-Martinez*, 1993; and Winick, 1985
- **Depressive disorder and schizotypal personality disorder:** *In re Christina D.*, 1991; and *State v. Martin*, 1990
- **Suicidal/homicidal ideation:** *Bramlette v. Charter-Medical-Columbia*, 1990.

Mental health nurses also have testified on treatment they have provided, including treatment for depression in a conservatorship case (*In re Conservatorship of Blikstad*, 1994), individual therapy in a child custody case (*In re Kathleen R.*, 1993), and biofeedback in a worker's compensation case (*Cantu v. J.R. Simplot Company*, 1992).

At times a mental health nurse's credibility as a witness is challenged. In *People in the Interest of E.H. and S.W.* (1992) a psychiatric nurse's testimony on parental fitness for custody was challenged but allowed into evidence. The court said the nurse had the requisite knowledge, skill, and experience to provide the testimony. In *George v. Commonwealth* (1994) the judge questioned the credibility of a psychiatric nurse with a master's degree in social work to testify whether her client, a 12-year-old child, would be traumatized by providing in-court testimony in a child sexual abuse case. The judge said, "In the present case, the sole testimony at the hearing on the motion was that of Dorothy Keller, a psychiatric nurse with a master's degree in social work. Although she was not challenged on her qualifications, she hardly qualified to provide psychiatric evaluation." The judge then decided against the psychiatric nurse's advice and said the 12-year-old should testify in person rather than by closed-circuit television.

The ethicist's concern is that assessment and treatment be carried out carefully (with prudence) and reported honestly to clients and other appropriate recipients. The legal concept of privileged communication, available to nurses in some states, protects the confidentiality of nurse-client communication unless the client waives the privilege. If the client waives the privilege, the nurse may divulge assessment and treatment information in court.

Sometimes nurses become witnesses against their own employers. For instance, in *Baptist Medical Centers v. Trippe* (1994) a mental health nurse testified about a hospital's strip search policy before and after a patient's suicide in the hospital. She was considered an adverse witness because her testimony that the policy changed after the suicide cast a negative light on the hospital.

Informed consent

Treatment of people with mental illness in the community or in an institution requires informed consent. Without it a nurse can be charged with assault and battery or false imprisonment (Aiken & Catalano, 1994). Forced administration of medication denies the client's right to refuse treatment, and must be undertaken with the proper procedures followed as specified within the given state. If an emergency exists or the nurse acts in self-defense, informed consent is no longer necessary (Aiken & Catalano, 1994). Adequate documentation of the necessity for forced treatment is helpful in case court action is taken. However, once given, consent can be revoked by the client (Laben & MacLean, 1989). Ethically, nurses show compassion for their clients when they provide information about proposed treatment. They demonstrate respect by seeking the client's approval for the intervention. Psychiatric clients are often vulnerable, and compassion dictates that special efforts be made to inform them about proposed intervention.

Sexual harassment of clients constitutes an abuse of the nurse's power over the client. Although no reported cases of sexual harassment were found that had been brought against mental health nurses, the possibility exists. Such intentional actions are typically not covered by malpractice insurance, and the nurse will be responsible for payment directly, as in a criminal case.

NURSE SELF-CARE

Self-care is ethically grounded in the ethic of care that values care for self and for others. Compassion as a virtue can reasonably be shown to self and to the client. In the legal system self-care within the nursing profession appears regularly. Nurses receive the privilege to practice nursing through their licensure and certification. Some states give special credentials to clinical nurse specialists that allow advanced practice and protect the public from unsafe practice by unlicensed personnel. Nurses who practice a specialty provide a livelihood for themselves and thus exercise self-care. Mental health nurses obtain staff admitting privileges to hospitals in some states, although they are sometimes refused, as in *Wrable v. Community Memorial Hospital* (1985).

When injured, mental health nurses have the right to receive workers' compensation. In *Fitzgerald v. Open Hands* (1993) a psychiatric nurse was judged totally disabled after having been brutally beaten by a psychotic prisoner in the New Mexico State Penitentiary in Santa Fe. Despite the fact that the nurse was working in another job, she was disabled by the limitations that her psychological state placed upon her nursing activities. In *Agnew-Watson v. County of Alameda* (1994), a psychiatric nurse's child sued a hospital successfully for injuries sustained in utero when his mother, a psychiatric nurse at Highland Hospital in Oakland, California, was kicked in the stomach, causing permanent injury to the fetus. The court held that the Workers' Compensation Act did not preclude this suit.

The value of the work of the mental health nurse appears in the law at times. Comparable worth cases occasionally involve mental health nurses. In *Briscoe v. Prince George's County Health Department* (1991) the court reviewed a state salary scheme challenged by social workers who objected to being paid less than psychiatric nurses. The court held that equal protection principles were not violated, because nurses had additional responsibilities:

Because the nurses are qualified to perform patient care services, the State legitimately may value their services more highly. Assuming that the psychiatric nurses and clinical social workers at the Prince George's County Mental Health Centers and the Regional Institute for Children and Adolescents primarily perform psychotherapy, the nurses are still capable of, and occasionally do perform, other patient care services. The clinical social workers are not able to evaluate patients physically or to administer medication as the nurses are.

The cost of psychiatric nursing care was listed as a specific part of a malpractice settlement in *Steinberg v. Jensen* (1994). Twenty-four hour psychiatric nursing care was estimated at $251,846 annually, as part of a $4 million award against a physician for a patient's brain damage following treatment for hyponatremia.

In Delaware (*Del. Op. Atty. Gen.,* 1991) the state attorney general issued an opinion that different starting salaries of nurses in three hospitals—Delaware State Hospital, the Emily P. Bissell Hospital, and the Stockley Center—were justified because of the shortage of nurses in certain areas of the state.

Mental health nurses also may be named as parties in lawsuits. For example, in *Gibbs v. Waller* (1994), a psychiatric nurse was named as one of several defendants and successfully defended a suit for malpractice. In *Williams v. Secretary of the Executive Office of Human Services* (1993) a psychiatric nurse at Boston City Hospital filed a complaint with the mayor of Boston and the Pine Street Inn on behalf of a group of people with mental illness who were former inpatients. The court found no violation of federal statutes and constitutional provisions in the actions of the state department of mental health. The nurse's acting as a "next friend" by filing this complaint demonstrated courage, compassion, and communitarian values.

Similarly, in *Com. of Pa. ex rel. Rafferty v. Philadelphia Psychiatric Center* (1973) a psychiatric nurse exercised her freedom of speech rights in voicing concerns about conditions in a state hospital where she had previously worked. The public interest in hearing about these problems was greater than the interest of the state mental hospital's employees in allaying their own anxiety.

LEGAL AND ETHICAL DECISION MAKING IN MENTAL HEALTH NURSING

A framework for decision making should address both legal requirements and ethical considerations. Mental health nursing may propose its own legal and ethical orientation to decisions to promote safe and competent care for culturally diverse clients and to care for the discipline of nursing. Character traits to be valued in the nurse and enhanced in the client may serve as the framework's foundation.

Clients employ advanced directives to guide professionals during their decisional incapacity (Kjervik, 1994; Patient Self-Determination Act of 1990, 1990), and these directives may perhaps be used for mentally ill and terminally ill clients (Kjervik, in press). The Office of Mental Health in New York (18 Deaths, 1994) has recommended that clients use written declarations to guide interventions in crisis.

Carpenter (1991) studied how mental health nurses make ethical decisions, and found a 10-stage process, beginning with an emotional response to the event, and then cognitive considerations, behavioral options, and action. Carpenter found that nurses considered emotional components throughout the decision-making process. A model of virtue ethics that recognizes compassion (the ethic of care), honesty, prudence, and courage may be useful in mental health nursing decision making.

SUMMARY

This chapter has reviewed major ethical and legal concerns faced by mental health nurses, and has proposed a virtue ethics orientation for analyzing and resolving problems. The legal and ethical systems can work hand in hand to promote compassionate client care and to ensure the safety of the mental health nurse. In order for nurses and clients to be empowered, they must be able to act on their own behalf and on that of others. Legal, ethical, and clinical agencies can all be employed to reach mental health nursing goals and are foundational to nursing advocacy.

Just as compassion is a worthy virtue in mental health nursing practice, compassion's dark side also should be considered. Further research on the subtleties of manipulation and coercion in mental health settings would be informative for nurses and assist them in avoiding inappropriate statements and actions.

Suicide and homicide continue to be areas of legal and ethical concern in mental health nursing. Tension between the duty to protect the client and the duty to protect the community continues to cause consternation. Courts seem more willing to ask therapists to breach confidentiality to protect innocent third parties from harm. As mental health nurses continue to develop their advanced practice roles, their opinions as expert witnesses in court will be sought more frequently. Both emotional and cognitive aspects of ethical and legal decision making should be incorporated into a mental health nursing framework.

REFERENCES

Agnew-Watson v. County of Alameda, 36 Cal. Rptr.2d 196 (1994).

Aiken, T. D., & Catalano, J. T. (1994). *Legal, ethical, and political issues in nursing.* Philadelphia: F.A. Davis Co.

Aroskar, M. A. (1991). Caring—Another side. *Journal of Professional Nursing, 7*(1), 3.

Baptist Medical Centers v. Trippe, 643 So.2d 955 (1994).

Beauchamp, T., & Childress, J. (1994). *Principles of biomedical ethics* (4th ed.)(p. 111). New York: Oxford University Press.

Benner, P., Tanner, C., & Chesla, C. (1996). *Expertise in nursing practice: Caring, clinic judgment, and ethics* (p. xiii). New York: Springer Publishing.

Boynton v. Burglass, 590 So.2d 446 (1991).

Bramlette v. Charter-Medical-Columbia, 302 S.C. 68, 393 S.E.2d 914 (1990).

Briscoe v. Prince George's County Health Department, 323 Md. 439, 593 A.2d 1109 (1991).

Cantu v. J. R. Simplot Company, 121 Idaho 585, 826 P.2d 1297 (1992).

Carpenter, M. A. (1991). The process of ethical decision making in psychiatric nursing practice. *Issues in Mental Health Nursing, 12,* 179-191.

Com. of Pa. ex rel. Rafferty v. Philadelphia Psychiatric Center, 356 F.Supp. 500 (1973).

Del Op. Atty. Gen. 91-I006, WL 474655 (Del. A.G.) (1991).

Duldt, B. W. (1995). Integrating nursing theory and ethics. *Perspectives in Psychiatric Care, 31*(2), 4-10.

Eidson v. Reproductive Health Services, 863 S.W.2d 621 (1994).

18 deaths in NY psychiatric facilities instigate changes: Ethical concerns about restraints apply equally to mental patients. (1994). *Medical Ethics Advisor, 10* (12), 162-163.

Fitzgerald v. Open Hands, 115 N.M. 210, 848 P.2d 1137 (1993).

George v. Commonwealth, 885 S.W.2d 938 (1994).

Geske, M. R. (1989). Statutes limiting mental health professionals' liability for the violent acts of their patients. *Indiana Law Journal, 64,* 391-422.

Gibbs v. Waller, 28 F.3d 1209, WL 369878 (4th Cir. (N.C.)) (1994).

Hill v. Allstate Associates, WL 119758 (Conn. Super.) (1993).

Husted, G. L., & Husted, J. H. (1995). *Ethical decision making in nursing* (2nd ed.). St. Louis: Mosby.

In re Christina D., WL 30997 (Conn. Super.) (1991).

In re Conservatorship of Blikstad, WL 373481 (Minn. App.) (1994).

In re Kathleen R., WL 392872 (Conn. Super.) (1993).

Kashka, M. S., & Keyser, P. K. (1995). Ethical issues in informed consent and ECT. *Perspectives in Psychiatric Care, 31*(2), 15-21.

Kerr, N. J. (1995). The "ethics" of state hospital closings. *Perspectives in Psychiatric Care, 31*(2), 3.

Kjervik, D. (in press). Advance decision making for psychiatric care. In P. Barker, & B. Davidson (Eds.), *Psychiatric nursing: Ethical strife.* London: Edward Arnold.

Kjervik, D. (1994). Advance directives. In J. McCloskey, & H. Grace, (Eds.), *Current issues in nursing* (4th ed.) (pp. 752-757). St. Louis: Mosby.

Kjervik, D. (1991). The choice to die. *Journal of Professional Nursing, 7*(3), 151.

Kjervik, D. (1984). The psychotherapist's duty to act reasonably to prevent suicide: A proposal to allow rational suicide. *Behavioral Sciences & the Law, 2*(2),207-218.

Laben, J. K., & MacLean, C. P. (1989). *Legal issues and guidelines for nurses who care for the mentally ill* (2nd ed.). Owings Mills, MD: National Health Publishing.

Muse v. Charter Hospital of Winston-Salem, 452 S.E.2d 589 (1995).

Patient Self-Determination Act of 1990, 42 U.S.C.A. Sec. 1395cc (f)(1)(A)(i)(1991 Supp. pam.), PL 101-508 Sec. 4206, 104 Stat. 1388-115 (1990).

Pellegrino, E. D. (1989). Character, virtue, and self-interest in the ethics of the professions. *Journal of Contemporary Health Law and Policy, 5,* 53-73.

Pellegrino, E. D. (1991). Trust and distrust in professional ethics. In E. D. Pellegrino, R. M. Veatch, & J. Langan (Eds.), *Ethics, trust, and the professions: Philosophical and cultural aspects.* Washington, DC: Georgetown University Press.

People in the Interest of E.H. and S. W., 837 P.2d 284 (1992).

People v. Velez, 159 Misc. 2d 38, 602 N.Y.S.2d 758 (1993).

Peterson v. Peterson, 818 P.2d 1305 (1991).

R. D. v. W. H., 875 P.2d 26 (1994).

Rosenhan, D. L., Teitelbaum, T. W., Teitelbaum, K. W., & Davidson, M. (1993). Warning third parties: The ripple effects of *Tarasoff. Pacific Law Journal, 24,* 1165-1232.

State v. Bingham, 124 Idaho 698, 864 P.2d 144 (1993).

State v. Martin, WL 193106 (Ohio App.) (1990).

State v. Patterson, 229 Conn. 328, 641 A.2d 123 (1994).

Steinberg v. Jensen, 519 N.W.2d 753 (1994).

Tarasoff v. Regents of the University of California, 17 Cal. 3d 425, 131 Cal. Rptr. 14, 551 P.2d 334 (1976).

Taslitz, A. E. (1993). Myself alone: Individualizing justice through psychological character evidence. *Maryland Law Review, 52,* 1-121.

Torrey, E. F. (1993). Thirty years of shame: The scandalous neglect of the mentally ill homeless. *National Forum, 73*(1), 4-7, 12.

United States v. Grimes, 17 F.3d 397, WL 5741 (9th Cir. (Or.)) (1994).

United States v. Herrera-Martinez, 985 F.2d 298 (1993).

United States v. Watson, 43 F.3d 1480, WL 703155 (9th Cir. (Or.)) (1994).

Virakitti v. Oregon Department of Corrections, 40 F.3d 1247, WL 655893 (9th Cir. (Or.)) (1994).

Williams v. Secretary of the Executive Office of Human Services, 414 Mass. 551, 609 N.E.2d 447 (1993).

Winick, B. J. (1985). Restructuring competency to stand trial. *UCLA Law Review, 32,* 921-985.

Wrable v. Community Memorial Hospital, 205 N.J. Super. 438, 501 A.2d 187 (Law Div.)(1985).

Ziemba v. Riverview Medical Center, 275 N.J. Super. 293, 645 A.2d 1276 (1994).

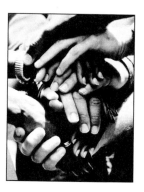

Chapter 3

Family and Consumer Movements

Sara-Ann Steber

Successful outcomes in community treatment of 4people with mental illness often depend on the clinician's ability to communicate effectively with primary consumers (people receiving the service) and secondary consumers (their family members and significant others). The role of both primary and secondary consumers in the design, delivery, and evaluation of mental health services has changed dramatically in the past 15 years. This chapter explores the origins of consumer and family movements, describes the impact these movements have on mental health treatment and service delivery, and offers guidance for the professional in working with consumers and their families.

THE DEVELOPMENT OF THE CONSUMER MOVEMENT

The consumer movement is an outgrowth of complex and interactive factors, including deinstitutionalization, the legislation establishing community mental health centers, new treatment technologies, and landmark legal cases involving the civil rights of people with mental illness. The

interaction of these factors has led to the shifting of mental health services away from a hospital-based medical model to a community-based rehabilitation model; the resulting change in the relationships between professionals and the consumers of mental health services has become known as the consumer movement. A brief synopsis of the historical events and treatment modalities that led to the emergence of the consumer movement follows.

Deinstitutionalization and the implementation of community mental health centers were conceived of as interrelated social movements. Theoretically, the large number of people with mental illness discharged from state hospitals into the community in the 1960s and 1970s were to receive care and treatment in the new community mental health centers. However, the professionals who worked in these centers had no experience in working with chronically mentally ill clients and preferred to serve a clientele that had the kinds of problems with which the clinicians had previous experience and therefore felt the most comfortable. The result was that hundreds of thousands of severely mentally ill people were moved into the community but received little or no treatment and support, while the community mental health centers concentrated on counseling services for life adjustment difficulties such as marital, family, and personal problems. Eventually fiscal incentives enticed the community mental health centers to become the locus of care and treatment for people with severe mental illnesses, but not before thousands of people discharged from state hospitals and their families had endured a great deal of financial and emotional hardship. The failure of community mental health centers to care for the population for which they were created sowed the seeds for the consumer movement in mental health.

At the same time, grassroots movements in other social and consumer services were developing; these too had an impact on the development of the mental health consumer movement. General dissatisfaction and distrust of the "establishment" produced increased efforts to challenge traditional power structures. Ralph Nader's activism related to product liability, the increase in medical malpractice, the Watergate scandal, and disillusionment with the war in Vietnam, to name a few historical factors, led to the empowerment of people, the demand to hold professionals accountable for their actions, and the proliferation of self-help and other consumer organizing groups. Civil libertarians supported these activities through court cases that challenged authority and gained rights for people.

After their successes in the courts with civil rights lawsuits, civil libertarians turned their attention to the rights of criminal suspects, then to prisoners, and finally to mental patients. Involuntary commitment procedures ignored the basic rights of patients and were paternalistic in nature. Commitment criteria were vague, the duration of commitment was indefinite, and commitment procedures provided little or no opportunity for the patient to object. A variety of court cases (*Wyatt v. Stickney*, 1971; *O'Connor v. Donaldson*, 1975; *Lessard v. Schmidt*, 1972 to 1976) were initiated to guarantee due process rights, require that appropriate treatment be provided to confined patients,

and prevent involuntary confinement of nondangerous people with mental illness.

In the 1970s these efforts encouraged some mental health service funding streams to recognize the need for and to support the development of a variety of community-based psychosocial rehabilitation programs. These programs responded to the basic needs of people with serious mental illness and included residential, vocational, and outreach services, access to health and dental care, income supports and entitlements, peer support, and other services traditionally provided in state institutions (Stroul, 1989).

As the deinstitutionalization process accelerated in the 1970s, former patients organized to speed the change. They organized to gain control over their treatment and their lives and to develop self-help groups that focused on personal problems, advocacy, reduction of stigma, and changes in the mental health system (Chamberlin, Rogers, & Sneed, 1989).

The National Institute of Mental Health (NIMH) formally supported these efforts by establishing the Community Support Program (CSP) in 1977. The CSP was the first national program that encouraged the involvement of consumers, families, and advocates in the development of a system of care for providing an array of services for people with mental illness who were capable of living in the community with appropriate rehabilitation and support services (Craig & Wright, 1988). In addition to providing start-up money for model programs that developed new and alternative mental health services, the CSP encouraged the reorientation of existing service models toward a community service system concept that fosters consumer empowerment.

The Community Support Program also has been a major supporter of consumer-operated services, which it defines as consumer-controlled operations in which responsibility, control, and decision making are shared among the consumer membership and participation is voluntary. Projects funded by the CSP encompass the scope of consumer-operated services designed to meet the needs of specific communities and assist in the development of a better understanding of these services and the roles they play in the mental health service system. These activities and other federal initiatives helped establish a formal role for consumers in the design and delivery of mental health services.

However, establishing a formal role for consumers requires more than token representation. Many consumers serve on boards and committees but are often ignored, intimidated, or otherwise rendered ineffective (Leete, 1988). Consumer opinions are frequently sought and just as frequently disregarded by people in power (Blanch, Penny, & Knight, 1995). In the area of service provision the practitioner is often asked to support the establishment of roles for consumers in the existing service system and to determine the appropriate level of their involvement. This is a new task for practitioners and one that must be taken seriously.

Federal legislation and expanded CSP funding for consumer-operated services have further empowered consumers and established a more formal role for them in policy and administration. The Mental Health Planning Act (1986) and the Protection and Advocacy for Mentally Ill Individuals Act (1986) specifically required the inclusion of consumers, families, and advocates in the implementation of activities prescribed in each Act. The Mental Health Planning Act broadened the planning process at the state level and established a formal role for consumers by mandating that each state mental health planning council be composed of residents of the state and include in its membership representatives of the principal state agencies involved in mental health, higher education training facilities, and public and private entities concerned with the planning, operation, funding, and use of mental health and related services and activities. At least one half of the counsel members were to be people who were not state employees or providers of mental health services. The administrative document that described the planning process (NIMH, 1987) stated that "among these

members, States should include a balanced representation of primary consumers and family members."

The Protection and Advocacy for Mentally Ill Individuals Act established the first federally funded advocacy program for each state. Although advocacy service funding had been available for other special need populations (including people with developmental disabilities or physical handicaps, and elderly people), the need for such services for people with mental illness was unmet. The advisory boards formed to implement this legislation were required to include 50% representation of consumers and their families.

Following the federal lead, many states have formally and informally expanded opportunities for consumers to actively participate in design, planning, delivery, and policy development related to mental health services at the state and local levels (Stephens & Belisle, 1993). In many states community mental health and mental retardation boards have been reconceptualized to incorporate the consumer/advocate perspective. State and local mental health committees and work groups consistently balance membership to ensure adequate representation of consumer/advocates.

A final federal initiative was the enactment of the Americans with Disabilities Act (ADA) of 1990 (Pub. L. No. 101-336). Regulations pertaining to this Act were not promulgated until 1991; the public accommodations and employment provisions took effect in 1992. The ADA provides protection from discrimination in employment for people with mental disabilities. This protection prevents employers from asking if a person currently has or has ever had a mental disability, and requires employers to make reasonable workplace accommodations for qualified people with mental disabilities. Examples of reasonable accommodations for people with mental disabilities include flexible scheduling, a trained supervisor who can provide support, clear direction and appropriate feedback, education for co-workers about mental illness, changes in workplace policy, and other types of human assistance such as from a job coach or mentor. These accommodations allow people with disabilities to compete for and maintain employment. The inclusion of people with mental disabilities in the provisions of the ADA resulted from vigorous lobbying on the part of consumers, families, and other advocates, and is another example of the empowerment of mental health consumers.

THE IMPACT OF THE CONSUMER MOVEMENT
Management of services

The development of the consumer movement and the evolution of the mental health service delivery system from a medical to a psychosocial rehabilitation model have created opportunities for consumers to interact with policy makers, professionals, administrators, family members, and others from a position of strength (Chamberlin et al., 1989). These interactions fostered a change in the professional perception of consumers as passive, incompetent people who were not included in discussions about their treatment or their needs because the medical model of care gave control to hospitals, professionals, guardians, and the court system (Leete, 1988).

Another area of change relates to the emergence of the self-help movement among consumers of mental health services. As the consumer movement became more active and more empowered, the growth in the number of self-help agencies has constituted a major development in mental health services (Segal, Silverman, & Temkin, 1995). A survey conducted by the Center for Self-Help Research and the National Association of State Mental Health Program Directors (NASMHPD) showed that 46 states funded 567 self-help groups and agencies for people with mental illness and their families (NASMHPD, 1993). Although self-help agencies run by mental health consumers vary widely in philosophy, mission, and range of services, all are concerned with improving the lives of their members and helping them gain the skills and resources necessary to achieve stability. Many consumer-operated programs were developed because of consumer dissatisfaction or frustration with traditional mental health services.

Drop-in centers have proliferated across the country. Most of these centers were established and are operated by consumers as places to socialize, build networks, and receive material help such as housing, food, food stamps, and clothing. Unlike in community mental health centers, there is no need to register, fill out numerous forms, or agree to participate in counseling or other clinical services in order to participate in drop-in center activities.

Many organizations that began as drop-in centers have evolved into a more formal "clubhouse" model. In 1948 Fountain House in New York City opened as the original clubhouse. Presently there are more than 200 clubhouses modeled after Fountain House throughout the United States. Clubhouses retain the socialization and networking features of the drop-in centers but also offer additional services. Most clubhouses are allied in some way with housing for the clubhouse "members." Typically, the clubhouse sponsors a series of apartments in which several members live together. Employment opportunities are incorporated into almost all clubhouses. Efforts are made to help members locate jobs in the private sector. Staff who serve as job coaches accompany new workers and assist them in learning the job until the clubhouse member and the staff are satisfied that the member can perform satisfactorily. Often two clubhouse members will share a full-time job to decrease the stress of full-time employment. Some members work in the clubhouse, where they operate the cafeteria, put out a weekly newsletter, administer the housing units, or do other chores associated with the upkeep of the clubhouse.

Not all consumers want to enter the mental health workforce, but many are interested and support is growing to provide additional opportunities for this group. Although literature on consumer participation in professionally run mental health agencies is scant, a national survey of supported housing programs operated primarily by professionals revealed that 38% of these organizations had mental health consumers on their staffs. These organizations reported that consumer staff empathized with clients and understood their emotional, psychological, and day-to-day struggles because of their own experience with psychiatric disability; that consumer staff were more tolerant of unusual behavior and less likely than nonconsumer staff to feel the need to maintain a professional distance (Besio & Mahler, 1993).

Sherman and Porter (1991) report on the training of mental health consumers as case management aides in a psychiatric rehabilitation project. Surveys of the aides and their supervisors indicated that both groups were highly satisfied with the program. Interestingly, this project and the Besio and Mahler survey reported a pronounced positive effect on staff attitudes toward the potential abilities of clients who have chronic mental illness.

Consumer and practitioner relationships

The growth of the self-help movement in mental health care and the development of alternative models of service have produced an increase in nontraditional interactions between consumers and professionals. In the past, clients (especially those who relied on publicly funded services) had little recourse if they objected to the treatment they received. The perception was that the professional was always right and consumers, if they complained, were considered "treatment resistant."

Borkman (1976) describes the distinction between consumers and professionals as the difference between experiential and professional knowledge. Members of a self-help group or movement either in general health care or in mental health develop knowledge and wisdom through the experience of sharing a common problem. The focus of control in self-help is more diverse or decentralized; all members of the group are equally valued, and the leadership responsibility is shared. The primary goals of such groups are to empower members to understand their condition, make informed decisions about their treatment, and lobby for change.

Professionals, on the other hand, learn through a structured educational or training program and base their knowledge on theory and practical academic examples of what works. Most training reinforces the role of the professional as a leader who provides services to or for a client. The leader is expected to control the situation and direct the treatment process. These disparate experiences and philosophical points of view have caused a great deal of tension between many consumers of mental health services and professionals. A genuine effort on the part of consumers and practitioners to communicate more effectively has begun. In 1989 the first national symposium of self-help groups and providers was held in Chicago. Emerick (1995) hailed this meeting as a step forward in tempering the strong antiprofessional sentiments in consumer groups and the anti–self-help attitudes of professionals.

In an effort to better understand the unmet needs of consumers, Uttaro and Mechanic (1994) surveyed 552 primary consumers of mental health services. Information was obtained from the consumers on their perceived needs in finance, employment, personal relationships, and other aspects of daily living. Table 3-1 shows the percentages of the consumers who had a perceived need for help, were receiving help, and wanted more help. Although this study was conducted exclusively with the mentally ill relatives of members of the National Alliance for the Mentally Ill (NAMI) and therefore has limited generalizability, it nevertheless shows that it is useful for practitioners and program designers to have input from the consumers of their services.

Table 3-1.   Consumers' need for help and receipt of help in 15 areas, in percentages (*n* = 552)

AREA OF NEED	PERCEIVED NEED	RECEIVING HELP	WANT MORE HELP
Keeping busy so you don't get bored or lonely	51	25	37
Recognizing and controlling symptoms	46	37	35
Finding or getting along with boyfriend or girlfriend, husband or wife	53	16	33
Making or getting along with friends	51	19	30
Controlling anger or temper	48	30	27
Getting or keeping a job	61	29	19
Managing your money	50	27	19
Housing problems	28	18	19
Maintaining the place where you live	36	18	18
Obtaining Social Security Disability Insurance, Supplemental Security Income, or other benefits	29	20	18
Getting around your town	26	14	16
Shopping for groceries, preparing meals	27	14	12
Keeping aftercare appointments	26	15	10
Personal care, getting haircuts, looking good	20	7	8
Taking medications	87	88	5

Modified from "The NAMI Consumer Survey: Analysis of Unmet Need," by T. Uttaro and D. Mechanic, 1994, *Hospital and Community Psychiatry, 45,* p. 372.

SECONDARY CONSUMERS: THE FAMILIES OF PEOPLE WITH MENTAL ILLNESS

As with the development and growth of the mental health consumer movement, the organization of family members, significant others, and advocates evolved at the grassroots level. Dissatisfaction with their interactions with professionals and concern about the lack of community services for their family members with mental illness resulted in the organization of many family groups throughout the United States. In an effort to speak in a more powerful voice at the national level, approximately 100 self-help groups for the families of people with serious mental illness came together in 1979 to form the National Alliance for the Mentally Ill (NAMI). This movement has grown and expanded dramatically over time to include more than 1000 local and state affiliates with over 140,000 members (Mosher & Burti, 1994). NAMI provides advocacy and support for

many federal, state, and local initiatives designed to improve the quality of life of people with mental illness, and supports family members who are coping with their roles as caregivers to mentally ill family members.

Mental illness is often as devastating for the family as it is for the person afflicted. Family schedules, social life, and finances are frequently put in total disarray. Compounding the problems for many families is their perception that they are viewed by mental health professionals as the cause of the mental illness of their family member. Traditional psychoanalytical and family systems theories that are still taught in many professional schools view the family of a person with mental illness in a negative light. In these theories families (and especially mothers) are seen as noxious elements that set into motion the eventual mental illness of the ill member. A logical outcome of these theories was a great deal of tension and distrust between family members and professionals; this situation is slowly being rectified as new evidence of a strong biological factor in mental illness emerges, making some of the old causative theories obsolete. The organized protest of family members regarding their treatment by mental health professionals also has contributed to the beginning of a new sense of partnership between professionals and families.

One source of tension between family members and professionals that continues to go largely unresolved is the issue of confidentiality. The reluctance of mental health professionals to share information with the family about a family member's illness because of fear of violating confidentiality laws is a valid issue. However, families who are the primary caregivers for their mentally ill members argue that confidentiality laws have been invoked by mental health professionals to an absurd degree. The following highlight from an article in the *Philadelphia Inquirer* illustrates this problem (Acker & Fine, 1989).

Case example

A 38-year-old woman diagnosed with schizophrenia was released from an inpatient mental health unit with tokens for public transportation to an intake center for homeless adults 30 blocks away. The woman never arrived. For 3 ½ months, she moved in and out of boarding homes and lived on the street while her mother tried to discover her whereabouts and make certain she was safe and in treatment.

During this time, the mental health system refused to let the mother know where they had placed her daughter or what her condition was, citing the client's expressed right to confidentiality. While the daughter was in the inpatient unit for 16 days, the same lack of information sharing occurred at the daughter's request.

After living with her daughter's illness for 19 years, the mother and primary caretaker is shut out of meaningful discussions regarding her care and treatment. If the mental health system fails

and the daughter slips through the cracks, the mother wonders if anyone will notice or care.

The issues of the family's right to know and to participate in treatment planning and the primary consumer's right to self-determination pose a challenge for practitioners and require a thoughtful balancing of perspectives.

Family burden

The majority of people with chronic psychiatric illnesses reside with their families (Halford, Schweitzer, & Varghese, 1991). Researchers have studied the burden of caregiving with a view to developing interventions to help these families (Bulger, Wandersman, & Goldman, 1993). Their studies suggest that families of psychiatric clients tend to exhibit significant levels of chronic stress, a concept referred to as objective and subjective burden. Objective burden refers to concrete problems such as financial hardships, limitations in social life, and disruptions in other areas of family life. Subjective burden refers to psychological strain and includes emotional reactions to caregiving such as worry, tension, grief, guilt, sadness, and resentment (Peternelj-Taylor & Hartley, 1993; Bulger et al., 1993). Self-help groups such as NAMI and the National Depressive and Manic Depressive Association (NDMDA) can be useful for families in decreasing the objective and subjective burdens of caregiving.

Stigma

Most dictionaries define stigma as "a mark of disgrace." Consumer and family movements have made combating the stigma of mental illness a major priority. The effects of stigma have made it difficult for people with mental illness to obtain employment, find adequate housing, and become truly integrated in the communities in which they reside. Consumer and family movements have been particularly alert to the portrayal of people with mental illness in the media. Consumer and family groups argue that the consistent linkage of violence and mental illness in the media has perpetuated the myth that most people with mental illness are dangerous and should be avoided. Consumer and family groups have formed media watches that are active and effective in calling for correction when the media misrepresent people with mental illness and in applauding them for accurate coverage.

IMPLICATIONS FOR WORKING WITH CONSUMERS AND FAMILIES

The family and consumer movements have empowered their members to change their traditional relationships with mental health professionals. They are no longer satisfied to be passive recipients of professional help but are insisting on being active members of the treatment team and of the mental health system. They are asking that professionals provide them with information about mental illness, including treatment options.

Working with primary consumers

Psychiatric nurses who work with consumers who have severe and persistent mental illness need to be aware of the treatment and social service options and consumer self-help groups available in the community in order to refer clients to appropriate services (Box 3-1). Mosher and Burti (1994) urge that staff work with clients on their goals. The nurse's goal should be to work in partnership with the client to facilitate the process of normalization and integration into the community. Practitioners should supply information on the client's diagnosis and medications, aid the client in recognizing early symptoms of recurring illness, and help the client form a plan of action when these symptoms occur.

Working with families

Family caregivers have reported a variety of problems in their interactions with the mental health system, including communication difficulties, a lack of involvement in treatment decisions, a lack of knowledge of community resources by professionals, and conflicts about caregivers' roles as client advocates. A recent study (Biegel, Song, &

Box 3-1. Resources for consumers and families

Organizations

National Alliance for the Mentally Ill (NAMI)
1901 North Fort Myer Drive
Arlington, VA 22209
(703) 524-7600
National Mental Health Consumers Association (NMHCA)
311 South Juniper Street
Room 902
Philadelphia, PA 19107
(215) 735-6082

Publications

Surviving Mental Illness by Agnes B. Hatfield and Harriet Lefley. New York: Guilford Press, 1993.
Surviving Schizophrenia: A Family Manual by E. Fuller Torrey. New York: Harper & Row, 1995.

Milligan, 1995) obtained information from family caregivers of relatives with mental illness about the caregivers' contacts with mental health professionals and their opinions about those contacts. Analysis of the data showed that a significant minority (30%) of the caregivers was dissatisfied with their degree of involvement with mental health professionals. Many were not consulted about their family member's treatment, and were not given adequate information about the family member's illness and treatment, specific assistance in managing disruptive behaviors, or general assistance in coping with their caregiving role. The results of the study led the authors to recommend the following:

- Educational programs for caregivers that include written information and videotapes
- Workshops focusing on behavior management, stress management, community resources, and psychoeducational interventions
- Support group affiliation with the National Alliance for the Mentally Ill or independent family support groups

An issue that continues to cause difficulty between professionals and families is the right to self-determination and the right of confidentiality for the primary consumer. When the primary consumer and the family are in disagreement, the practitioner must balance the perspectives of both on issues related to medication, hospitalization, rehabilitation services, and living arrangements. The practitioner can play an important role in supporting the empowerment of consumers by working with consumers and family members to resolve conflicts and protect the consumer's right to self-determination. Parker (1993) suggests that mental health professionals have a responsibility to explain to the family member with mental illness that if the family is to be involved in caregiving or as support, the client should consent to the family's inclusion as team members.

The role of the nurse

Families of people with mental illness are usually unprepared to be caregivers. Nurses can be useful to the family by helping it learn about the illness of the family member. Non-compliance with medications is a common problem for people who have a mental illness. Nurses should aid the family in understanding medications, including dosages, side effects, and strategies to increase compliance. Family members can be extremely helpful in monitoring the effects of medications and the signs and symptoms of relapse. In the Biegel et al. (1995) study, families ranked the need for communication with health care professionals above housing, job training, day treatment, and other resources for their mentally ill family members.

SUMMARY

Primary consumers and their families have become increasingly vocal about the failure of mental health professionals to include them in treatment decisions and in service planning. In response, mental health services are beginning to implement policies that reflect the inclusion of consumers and their families. Consumers and families are asking professionals to share their expertise about diagnosis, medication, and treatment options and to work with them as equal partners in improving quality of life for consumers with mental illness. Equality of partnership requires that practitioners also listen to and learn from the experiences that consumers and their families have encountered while learning to cope with serious illness. Psychiatric nurses, who have always considered client and family education an important aspect of their nursing role, can be pivotal in modeling the partnership approach to working with consumers, families, and practitioners in other disciplines.

REFERENCES

Acker, C., & Fine, M.J. (1989, September 10). Families under siege: A mental health crisis. *Philadelphia Inquirer,* p. A1.

Americans with Disabilities Act of 1990, Pub. L. No. 101-336, Washington, DC: U.S. Government Printing Office.

Besio, S., & Mahler, J. (1993). Benefits and challenges of using consumer staff in supported housing services. *Hospital and Community Psychiatry, 44,* 490-491.

Biegel, D., Song, L., & Milligan, S. (1995). A comparative analysis of family caregivers' perceived relationships with mental health professionals. *Psychiatric Services, 46,* 477-482.

Blanch, A., Penny, D., & Knight, E. (1995). Identity politics: Close to home. *American Psychologist, 50,* 49-50.

Borkman, T. (1976). Experiential knowledge: New concept for the analysis of self-help groups. *Social Service Review, 50,* 446-456.

Bulger, M., Wandersman, A., & Goldman, C. (1993). Burdens and gratifications of caregiving: Appraisal of parental care of adults with schizophrenia. *American Journal of Orthopsychiatry, 63,* 255-265.

Chamberlin, J., Rogers, J., & Sneed, C. S. (1989). Consumers, families, and consumer support systems. *Psychosocial Rehabilitation Journal, 12*(3), 95-106.

Craig, R. T., & Wright, B. (1988). *Mental health financing and programming* (pp. 6-12). Denver, CO, and Washington, DC: National Conference of State Legislatures.

Emerick, R. E. (1995). Clients as claims makers in the self-help movement: Individual and social change ideologies in former mental patient self-help newsletters. *Psychosocial Rehabilitation Journal, 18* (3), 17-35.

Halford, W., Schweitzer, R., & Varghese, F. (1991). Effects of family environment on negative symptoms and quality of life of psychotic patients. *Hospital and Community Psychiatry, 42,* 1241-1247.

Leete, E. (1988). The role of the consumer movement and persons with mental illness. Presented at Rehabilitation Support Services for Persons with Long-Term Mental Illness: Preparing for the Next Decade. Mary Switzer Memorial Seminar, Washington, DC.

Lessard v. Schmidt, 340 F. Supp. 1078 (E.D. Wisc. 1972); vacated and remanded on procedural grounds, 414 U.S. 473 (1973); judgment reinstated, 179 F. Supp. 1376 (1974); vacated and remanded on procedural grounds, 421 U.S. 957 (1975); judgment reinstated, 413 F. Supp. 1318 (1976).

The Mental Health Planning Act of 1986, Pub. L. No. 99-660. Washington, DC: U.S. Government Printing Office.

Mosher, L., & Burti, L. (1994). *Community Mental Health* (p. 27). New York: W.W. Norton and Company.

National Association of State Mental Health Program Directors. (1993). *Putting their money where their mouths are: SMHA support of consumer and family-run programs.* Alexandria, VA: Author.

National Institute of Mental Health. (1987, October). *Toward a model plan.* Administrative document in response to Public Law 99-660, Title V—The State Comprehensive Mental Health Plan Act of 1986.

O'Connor v. Donaldson, 422 U.S. 563, 95 S. Ct. 2486 (1975).

Parker, B. (1993). Mental illness: The family as caregiver. *Journal of Psychosocial Nursing, 31,* 19-21.

Peternelj-Taylor, C., & Hartley, V. (1993). Living with mental illness: Professional/family collaboration. *Journal of Psychosocial Nursing, 31,* 23-28.

Protection and Advocacy for Mentally Ill Individuals Act of 1986, Pub. L. No. 99-319. Washington, DC: U.S. Government Printing Office.

Segal, S., Silverman, C., & Temkin, T. (1995). Characteristics and service use of self-help agencies for mental health clients. *Psychiatric Services, 46,* 269-274.

Sherman, P., & Porter, R. (1991). Mental health consumers as case management aides. *Hospital and Community Psychiatry, 42,* 494-498.

Stephens, C. L., & Belisle, K. C. (1993). The consumer-as-provider initiative. *The Journal of Mental Health Administration, 20,* 178-182.

Stroul, B. (1989). Community support systems for persons with long-term mental illness: A conceptual framework. *Psychosocial Rehabilitation Journal, 12* (3), 9-27.

Uttaro, T., & Mechanic, D. (1994). The NAMI consumer survey: Analysis of unmet need. *Hospital and Community Psychiatry, 45,* 372-374.

Wyatt v. Stickney, 325 F. Supp. 781 (MD Ala 1971); 344 F.Supp. 373 (MD Ala 1972).

Chapter 4

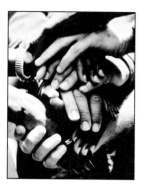

Cultural Competency

Michael G. Kennedy

By the year 2080 ethnic minorities will comprise roughly 51% of the U.S. population (U.S. Bureau of the Census, 1990). As the United States becomes increasingly diverse, this trend will have significant consequences for nursing practice. Culturally diverse clients bring beliefs and practices to the health care system that can be confusing and disconcerting to health care providers. Misunderstandings about cultural differences may result in clients being labeled difficult or uncooperative. Language and cultural barriers can cause frustration and dissatisfaction for care providers and their clients. Most nurses will eventually encounter clients whose health beliefs and practices differ markedly from their own. Thus it is important that nurses, the health care providers who have the most contact with clients, become culturally sensitive.

Culture-sensitive care has been defined as "a practice style that includes a positive professional focus on culture in health care" (Chrisman, 1991a). Three principles of culture-sensitive care follow (Chrisman, 1991b):

1. Knowledge about a client's cultural context
2. Mutual respect between client and nurse

3. Negotiation around important cultural factors

Before these three principles can be put into action, however, it is necessary to have a basic understanding of essential cultural concepts.

CULTURAL CONCEPTS

Culture is a complex and frequently misunderstood phenomenon. Sociocultural context informs every aspect of life, including family and household composition, work, education, gender relations, social networks, religious practices, health beliefs, and use of health care services. Although culture has a profound influence on human behavior, like oxygen, its subtle presence is rarely acknowledged.

Definitions of culture abound, but a useful one may be "the shared values, norms, traditions, customs, arts, history, folklore, and institutions of a group of people" (Orlandi, 1992). This definition is neither too broad nor too narrow but includes the major components of most widely accepted definitions of culture.

Culture has four basic characteristics (Herberg, 1995):

1. It is learned from birth, both formally and informally, through enculturation.
2. It is shared by all members of the cultural group.
3. It is adapted and integrated to the specific conditions of the cultural group.
4. It is dynamic and changing.

Culture is universal, but the cultural aspects that define a specific group are unique and distinctive to that group. Culture shapes a society's values, beliefs, practices, role relationships, laws, customs, artifacts, and knowledge (Hartog & Hartog, 1983). Values are a common feature of all cultures, but not all members of a society share the same values. Every culture has dominant values that a majority of its members embrace and variant values that distinguish individuals or groups. Three common variant value orientations in the United States are ethnic, class, and role differences (Kluckhohn, 1990). Cultural values shape a society's beliefs and practices, including those related to health and illness.

Culture should not be confused with ethnicity, which generally refers to identification with a common group linked by race, nationality, and language. Culture also is distinct from race, which is determined by genetically transmitted physical characteristics. Finally, culture is not the same as nationality, which is linked to an identified country or homeland. In summary (Tripp-Reimer, 1984):

- Culture is not defined by racial or biological characteristics.
- Cultures are not static but dynamic and continuously evolving.
- Cultural characteristics are acquired early and are not easily changed.
- Cultures are not deterministic, and intracultural variance exists in all groups.
- Culture influences all of us.

Box 4-1 lists key terms in understanding culture.

Box 4-1.   Definitions of key cultural terms

- **Culture**   Knowledge, beliefs, and rules that generate and interpret social behavior and shape the material products of a group of people
- **Ethnicity**   Group identity based on common culture, language, religion, geography, or familial relations
- **Ethnocentrism**   Interpreting the beliefs and behavior of others in terms of one's own cultural values and traditions, and assuming the superiority of one's own culture
- **Cultural relativism**   Interpreting the beliefs and behavior of others in terms of their own traditions and experiences
- **Acculturation**   Change in one or more cultures that results from prolonged contact

Modified from "Race, Culture, and Ethnicity, Unit I," by A. Monroe, R. Goldman, & C. Dube, 1994, in *Race, Culture, and Ethnicity: Curriculum for Health Care Professionals,* by C. E. Dube, & D. C. Lewis (Eds.), 1994, Providence: Project ADEPT.

CULTURE AND HEALTH CARE

Definitions of health and disease vary widely, not only between various cultural groups, but also within a specified culture (Kleinman, Eisenberg, & Good, 1978). Intracultural factors that influence definitions of health and disease include age, gender, educational level, and socioeconomic status (Herberg, 1995). A society's dominant values also help define illness or disease; symptoms are significant within the social context in which they occur. If a particular condition is widespread in a specific population, it may not be considered a health problem (Herberg, 1995). For example, malnutrition, intestinal parasites, and poor dentition are so widespread in some societies that they are not identified as health problems needing attention. Nurses who encounter these conditions and beliefs among disadvantaged people often mistakenly assume they are caused by ignorance and neglect. Such assumptions may engender prejudice and hinder the nurse-client relationship.

Health care systems are culturally constructed and generally include the popular, professional, and folk sectors (Kleinman, 1980). The popular sector is usually the first source of health care; it includes individual, family, and community non-professional health networks. It is estimated that the popular sector manages 70% to 90% of all illnesses (Kleinman, 1980). The professional sector comprises the organized healing professions and may include both indigenous medical systems and modern scientific health care. The folk sector is a mixture of various components, including sacred and secular beliefs about illness and health care. It is not unusual for individuals to use all three sectors simultaneously. Nurses, as part of the professional sector, tend to devalue the popular and folk sectors. They frequently assume that everyone shares their professional belief in the preeminence of the biomedical model. When clients violate this assumption, nurses may feel anger and frustration toward them. The following case example illustrates how this can happen.

Case example

A young Somali woman with high fever, delirium, and muscular rigidity was brought to the emergency room by her family. The nurse quickly recognized the symptoms as suggestive of meningitis. When questioned, family members stated that the symptoms had been present for 10 days. The nurse realized that significant neurological damage might already have occurred and was angry with the family for not bringing the patient to the hospital immediately after they noticed the symptoms. The nurse explained the gravity of the situation, and implicitly blamed the family for the daughter's poor prognosis.

A nurse who had better understood the family's culture and had done a culturally sensitive assessment would have realized that the family had sought treatment for the daughter in a culturally prescribed manner. When the symptoms first ap-

peared, the family tried various foods, charms, and other popular remedies. As the symptoms persisted and the daughter's condition deteriorated, the family consulted an indigenous healer who prescribed traditional herbal remedies. Only after all other remedies had failed and the daughter's condition had worsened did the family bring her to the emergency room. Like many of their neighbors they knew that sick people who went to the Western hospital sometimes died. This family considered the hospital the treatment of last resort. They had no knowledge of bacteria or antibiotics, nor would they have considered such information particularly relevant. They were willing to undertake Western medical treatment, but only within the context of their own cultural understanding.

As this example illustrates, cultural beliefs may profoundly affect health-seeking behaviors. Box 4-2 lists basic cultural values that influence health care.

> **Box 4-2.** Cultural value orientations affecting health care
>
> - Relationship to nature: subjugating, submitting, or harmony
> - View of individuals as basically good or honest
> - Interpersonal relationships: vertical (authoritarian cultures); horizontal (communal cultures); egalitarian (sharing cultures); or individualistic
> - Time orientation toward the past, present, or future
> - Basic orientation of being, doing, or being-in-becoming
> - Child-oriented versus elder-oriented
> - Dependence orientation versus independence orientation
> - Orientation toward community

Modified from "Cultural Aspects of Health and Illness Behavior in Hospitals," by J. Hartog and E. Hartog, 1983, *The Western Journal of Medicine, 139* (6), pp. 106-112.

CULTURE AND MENTAL HEALTH NURSING
Problems with normal and abnormal behavior

Tripp-Reimer (1984) has identified three reasons why cultural variables are important for mental health nursing. First, culture determines how mental health and mental illness are defined, what are appropriate health-seeking behaviors, and how members of the cultural group perceive and treat people with mental illness. Second, the culture itself may cause stress for some individuals. Third, cultural misunderstanding between the nurse and client may impede the therapeutic relationship.

Mental disorders are more difficult to delineate than physical disorders because they generally lack observable organic phenomena (Kavanagh, 1995). Major psychiatric disorders such as schizophrenia, bipolar disorder, major depressions, and anxiety disorders are found in all cultural groups. However, the culture largely determines how these disorders are expressed and interpreted. Societal beliefs about mental health and mental illness are intricately linked to prevailing social norms and the labeling of deviant behavior. Definitions of normal and abnormal behavior are not absolute; rather, they are socially and culturally determined. Hearing voices may not be considered pathological in a culture that values contact with spirits or ghosts. To contemporary Western culture, however, which values reason, hearing disembodied voices indicates mental illness. The content of delusions and hallucinations and the expression of other psychiatric symptoms are particularly susceptible to cultural nuances. Chronic mental illness may itself be a cultural artifact that is intimately related to sick role expectations (Lefley, 1990). The following case example illustrates the difficulties of assessing abnormal behavior in a cross-cultural context.

Case example

A 34-year-old Laotian man was referred to a community mental health center for psychiatric evaluation. Throughout the initial interview with the nurse the client exhibited inordinate interest in the moon. He answered most questions with some reference to the moon. The client discussed at great length the phases of the moon and how they related to various aspects of his own life and recent behavior. The client acknowledged seeing and hearing "ghosts," some of which frightened him and interfered with his sleep. Nevertheless, he denied that he had any problems or needed treatment.

This presentation could easily lead nurses to make two erroneous assumptions. The first is an ethnocentric assumption that the client is obviously psychotic because what he says sounds deviant by Western standards. The opposite assumption, equally dangerous, is based on excessive cultural relativism, which could lead nurses to disregard their own knowledge and experience and assume that a client's unusual behavior is due entirely to cultural factors rather than underlying pathology. Neither assumption facilitates culturally competent care.

Problems with mind-body dualism

Mind-body dichotomy and the separation of illnesses into physical and mental categories dominate Western thinking. The language and structure of our health care system reflect this dualism. Many cultures, however, do not share this dichotomy and frequently lack a psychological language to describe emotional states. Western health care practitioners unaware of this phenomenon may have difficulty assessing clients from non-Western cultures. A review of clinical studies of depression in non-Western cultures (Marsella et al., 1985) found a marked absence of psychological symptoms of depression but a dominance of somatic complaints. The lack of physical cause for these complaints and poor treatment response may frustrate clients and health care providers. Western perceptions of self, cognition, and human subjectivity have profoundly influenced our understanding of schizophrenia (Fabrega, 1989). Culture-bound syndromes (disorders that exist within specific cultural groups) further contribute to misunderstanding between Western health care providers and non-Western clients. Many culture-bound syndromes are culturally approved expressions of psychosocial distress. Table 4-1 lists selected culture-bound syndromes.

Culturally competent assessment

Madeleine Leininger was an early advocate of culturally competent nursing care. Her Sunrise Model of transcultural nursing offers a theoretical framework for the provision of culturally sensitive nursing care. This transcultural nursing model has profoundly influenced the development of culturally competent nursing care. Leininger (1978) defined transcultural nursing as:

The area of nursing which focuses upon the comparative study and analysis of different cultures and subcultures with respect to nursing and health-illness caring practices, beliefs, and values with the goal of generating scientific and humanistic knowledge, and of using this knowledge to provide culture-specific and culture-universal nursing care practices.

The culturological nursing assessment is crucial to Leininger's model. Leininger (1978) defines a culturological nursing assessment as:

A systematic appraisal or examination of individuals, groups, and communities as to their cultural beliefs, values, and practices to determine explicit nursing needs and intervention practices within the cultural context of the people being evaluated.

Table 4-1.   Selected culture-bound syndromes

GROUP	DISORDER	EXPLANATION
Caucasian	Anorexia nervosa	Preoccupation with body weight and image
	Bulimia	Binge eating followed by self-imposed vomiting
African-American	Low blood	Not enough blood or weakness of blood
	High blood	Blood that is too rich
	Thin blood	Susceptibility to illness
Chinese/Southeast Asian	*Koro*	Fear that penis is retracting into body
	Amok	Acute reaction to loss, grief, or hostility
Hispanic	*Empacho*	Food clings to stomach and intestines, causing pain and cramping
	Mal ojo ("evil eye")	Illness in children caused by a stranger's attention
	Susto	Anxiety, phobias
	Pasmo	Pseudo-paralysis of face or limbs
Native American	Ghost	Hallucinations, terror
Japanese	*Wagamama*	Childish behavior
Korean	*Hwa-byung*	Multiple somatic and psychological symptoms
Cambodian	*Koucharang* ("Thinking too much")	Headaches, chest pain, palpitations, shortness of breath, insomnia

Modified from "Transcultural Nursing Care," by M. M. Andrews, 1995, in *Transcultural Concepts in Nursing Care,* 2nd ed., pp. 49-96, by M. M. Andrews and J. S. Boyle (Eds.), 1995, Philadelphia: Lippincott; "The Theoretical Implications of Converging Research on Depression and the Culture-Bound Syndromes," by J. E. Carr and P. P. Vitaliano, 1985, in *Culture and Depression,* pp. 244-266, by A. Kleinman and B. Good (Eds.), 1985, Berkeley: University of California Press; and "Cultural Themes in Family Stress and Violence among Cambodian Refugee Women in the Inner City," by B. A. Frye and C. D. D'Avanzo, 1994, *Advances in Nursing Science, 16,* pp. 64-77.

Box 4-3. Culturological assessment domains

1. Life pattern or life-style of an individual or a cultural group
2. Specific cultural values, norms, and individual or group experiences regarding health and caring
3. Cultural taboos and myths
4. World view and ethnocentric tendencies of an individual or group
5. Cultural diversities, similarities, and variations
6. Health and life care rituals and rites of passage to maintain health and avoid illness
7. Folk and professional illness systems
8. Caring behaviors, values, and beliefs
9. Cultural changes and acculturation processes

Modified from "Culturological Assessment Domains for Nursing Practices," by M. Leininger, ed., 1978, in *Transcultural Nursing: Theories, Concepts, Practices,* New York: Wiley.

Leininger (1978) identifies seven principles to guide the nurse in making a culturological assessment:

1. Maintain a broad, objective, and open attitude.
2. Avoid seeing all people as alike.
3. Be aware of cultural variations among individuals, groups, and communities.
4. Focus on one individual or one culture.
5. Select a culture that contrasts with one's own in order to recognize and understand cultural differences.
6. Reflect on reasons for behavior and verify observations and interpretations with a reliable cultural observer.
7. Listen attentively and act in a caring manner.

A culturological assessment includes the nine domains listed in Box 4-3.

Another method for conducting a culturally sensitive assessment is the Explanatory Model Interview (Chrisman, 1991b; Kleinman, 1980; Kleinman, Eisenberg, & Good, 1978). This technique, presented in Box 4-4, encourages nurses to attend to related aspects of an individual's illness. In an Explanatory Model Interview the nurse listens to the client's fundamental beliefs about health and illness. Principles from both the Ex-

Box 4-4. Explanatory Model Interview

- What do you call your illness?
- When did it start? What else was going on?
- What do you think caused it?
- How does your illness work?
- How severe is it? How long will it last?
- What have you been doing to treat the illness?
- What treatment should you receive now?
- What do you fear most about your illness?

Modified from "Cultural Systems," by N. J. Chrisman, 1991, in *Cancer Nursing: A Comprehensive Textbook,* pp. 45-54, by S. Baird, R. McCorkle, & M. Grant (Eds.), 1991, Philadelphia: W. B. Saunders.

Box 4-5. Stages of cultural awareness

- Fear of other ethnic groups
- Denial of cultural differences
- Feeling of superiority of one's own values
- Tendency to minimize the impact of cultural differences
- Increasing respect for cultural differences but little skill for dealing with disparities
- Empathetic understanding of the other's world view and value system
- Balancing an understanding of differing world views and value systems

Modified from "Race, Culture and Ethnicity, Unit I," by A. Monroe, R. Goldman, & C. Dube, 1994, in *Race, Culture and Ethnicity: Curriculum for Health Care Professionals,* by C. E. Dube and D. C. Lewis (Eds.), 1994, Providence: Project ADEPT.

planatory Model Interview and Leininger's culturological assessment can be adapted to elicit data for a psychiatric nursing assessment.

Culturally competent care

Cultural awareness is a continuing process of self-knowledge, sensitivity, and appreciation for individuals or groups from diverse backgrounds. As cultural awareness grows, fear gives way to empathy and respect for the other's world view and value system (Box 4-5). Cultural knowledge is important in moving through cultural awareness toward cultural competence.

Campinha-Bacote (1994) has proposed a Culturally Competent Model of Care that includes cultural awareness, cultural knowledge, cultural skill, and cultural encounter as essential components of cultural competence. Cultural awareness entails a process of sensitivity in interactions with other cultures and a willingness to examine prejudices. Examining prejudices can be humbling and usually requires a willingness to accept constructive feedback from others. Cultural knowledge is an educational process in which the nurse seeks to understand the various world views of other cultures and the relationship between culture and health beliefs and practices. Cultural skill entails learning to conduct the culturological assessment discussed above. Finally, cultural encounter is the process by which the nurse directly interacts with clients from diverse cultures, thus gaining clinical skills in cross-cultural interactions. The Culturally Competent Model of Care is one framework for delivering culturally sensitive psychiatric-mental health nursing care.

Culture-sensitive care involves knowledge, mutual respect, and negotiation (Chrisman, 1991a). Knowledge, as noted above, includes self-knowledge, cultural knowledge, theoretical knowledge, and culture-sensitive skills. Mutual respect implies reciprocal knowledge and is a prerequisite for negotiation. Negotiation is particularly useful when conflict exists between client and provider health care beliefs. The negotiation process includes the following steps (Chrisman, 1991a; Chrisman, 1991b):

- **Listen** to the client's perspective and beliefs about illness and treatment.
- **Teach** from one's own knowledge and experience in language appropriate for client and family.
- **Compare** similarities and differences in views. Disagree with, but do not devalue, the client's perspective.
- **Compromise** When client treatment is not harmful, promote its use. When a treatment is harmful, explain the harm and suggest alternatives.

In summary, culturally sensitive care requires accepting people from diverse backgrounds, avoiding stereotypes, facilitating communication, understanding others' health care beliefs and practices, and negotiating goals and expectations (Kavanagh, 1995).

Working with interpreters

Communication is crucial to psychiatric-mental health nursing. Providing mental health services to clients with limited English language skills often requires language interpreters. However, communication through interpreters can pose special problems in mental health settings, where concepts and terminology do not easily translate across cultures. Psychotic thought processes, cognitive deficits, and paranoia can further complicate the issue. A basic understanding of the principles involved in working with interpreters is essential to providing culturally competent nursing care.

Interpreting is a complex task that requires specialized knowledge and training. A skilled interpreter can assume various roles depending on the needs of the specific situation (Svy, 1995):

- **Advocate** A role in which the interpreter moves from interpreting the communication of the speaker to acting on behalf of the speaker
- **Clarifier** A role that emphasizes the interpreter's ability to assess and identify linguistic differences between unmatched language speakers and to supply linguistic and cultural equivalencies
- **Conduit** A role in which the interpreter provides word-for-word oral interpretation using the closest linguistic equivalent. This is required in legal and court settings
- **Culture broker** A role in which the interpreter provides both cultural information and linguistic interpretation. This role is particularly useful in psychiatric or mental health settings

In addition, there are four different interpretation models (Svy, 1995):

1. **Consecutive** Converting an oral message from one language into an oral message in a different language after each speaker speaks.

Box 4-6.   Activity guidelines for interpreter-dependent interviews

Pre-session activities

- Match language needs with language ability. Make sure you know what language the client speaks—don't make assumptions based on ethnicity.
- Assess the interpreter's level of cultural familiarity with the client—be aware that interpreters also have cultural limitations.
- Meet with the interpreter before meeting together with the client.

In-session activities

- Allow enough time for the meeting—working through an interpreter may take twice as long as a meeting in which a common language is spoken.
- Make sure the seating positions reflect the atmosphere of the meeting.
- Conduct introductions.
- Speak directly to the client—use first and second person pronouns ("I" and "you").
- Speak in short sentences. Stop often to allow the interpreter to interpret.

- Be aware that one English word may require many words in another language to convey the same concept.
- Encourage the interpreter to ask for clarification—pause to make sure the interpreter understands what you are saying.
- Be aware of nonverbal messages. Nonverbal messages vary according to culture and may require interpretation just as spoken language.

Post-session activities

- Plan post-session meetings with the interpreter.
- Discuss in-session difficulties and how best to resolve them.
- Allow discussion of stressful discussions. Interpreters may be personally affected by reliving the emotional or traumatic experiences they interpret.
- Compare notes and clarify any miscommunication that arose during the session.
- Perform any additional service tasks.

Modified from *Bridging Differences: Interpretation and Expressions of Help-Seeking in Southeast Asian Clients,* by D. P. Svy, 1995, November, Paper presented at the Pacific Northwest Conference for Primary Care Practitioners, Seattle, WA.

2. **Simultaneous**   Converting an oral message from one language into an oral message in a different language as the speaker is speaking.
3. **Sight Translation**   Converting written material from one language to a written or oral form in another language.
4. **Summarization**   Summarizing the information the speaker provides when relaying it to the listener.

Interviewing a client through an interpreter in a psychiatric-mental health setting can be difficult and frustrating for everyone involved. Box 4-6 provides guidelines for pre-session, in-session, and post-session activities that will assist the nurse in working with an interpreter. The following guidelines also are helpful in interpreter-dependent interviews (Putsch, 1985):

- Avoid using family members as interpreters. In doing so you confuse role relationships, run the risk of skewed information, and may expose the client to feelings of shame.
- Develop alternatives to direct questions.
- Be alert to seemingly unconnected issues the client raises.
- Use short questions and comments; avoid technical jargon.
- Avoid ambiguous language, abstractions, and idiomatic expressions.
- Be aware that personal information may be difficult to obtain, particularly if the client comes from a small ethnic community.
- Speak slowly and clearly; use repetition as needed.
- Above all—**Be Patient!**

SUMMARY

As our society becomes increasingly diverse, the need to provide culturally sensitive nursing care also increases. The psychiatric-mental health setting poses special challenges in this regard. Psychiatric terms and concepts do not translate easily across cultures. Moreover, culture plays a significant role in determining whether behavior is defined as normal or abnormal, and in shaping societal attitudes toward people with mental illness. Cultural competence involves increasing the nurse's awareness, knowledge, and skill in working with individuals, families, and communities from diverse cultural backgrounds. For nurses willing to take the challenge, cultural competence enhances both the outcomes and the rewards of community mental health nursing.

REFERENCES

Andrews, M. M. (1995). Transcultural nursing care. In M. M. Andrews, & J. S. Boyle (Eds.), *Transcultural concepts in nursing care* (2nd ed.). (pp. 49-96). Philadelphia: Lippincott.

Campinha-Bacote, J. (1994). Cultural competence in psychiatric mental health nursing. *Nursing Clinics of North America, 29,* 1-7.

Carr, J. E., & Vitaliano, P. P. (1985). The theoretical implications of converging research on depression and the culture-bound syndromes. In A. Kleinman, & B. Good (Eds.), *Culture and depression* (pp. 244-266). Berkeley: University of California Press.

Chrisman, N. J. (1991a). Culture-sensitive nursing care. In M. Patrick, S. Woods, R. Craven, J. Rokosky, & P. Bruno (Eds.), *Medical-surgical nursing: Pathophysiologic concepts* (2nd ed.). (pp. 34-47). Philadelphia: Lippincott.

Chrisman, N. J. (1991b). Cultural systems. In S. Baird, R. McCorkle, & M. Grant (Eds.), *Cancer nursing: A comprehensive textbook* (pp. 45-54). Philadelphia: W. B. Saunders.

Fabrega, H., Jr. (1989). The self and schizophrenia: a cultural perspective. *Schizophrenia Bulletin, 15,* 277-290.

Frye, B. A., & D'Avanzo, C. D. (1994). Cultural themes in family stress and violence among Cambodian refugee women in the inner city. *Advances in Nursing Science, 16,* 64-77.

Hartog, J., & Hartog, E. (1983). Cultural aspects of health and illness behavior in hospitals. *The Western Journal of Medicine, 139*(6), 106-112.

Herberg, P. (1995). Theoretical foundations of transcultural nursing. In M. M. Andrews, & J. S. Boyle (Eds.), *Transcultural concepts in nursing care* (2nd. ed.). (pp. 3-48). Philadelphia: Lippincott.

Kavanagh, K. H. (1995). Transcultural perspectives in mental health. In M. M. Andrews, & J. S. Boyle (Eds.), *Transcultural concepts in nursing care* (2nd ed.). (pp. 253-285). Philadelphia: Lippincott.

Kleinman, A. (1980). *Patients and healers in the context of culture.* Berkeley: University of California Press.

Kleinman, A., Eisenberg, L., & Good, B. (1978). Culture, illness, and care. *Annals of Internal Medicine, 88,* 251-258.

Kluckhohn, F. (1990). Dominant and variant value orientations. In P. Brink (Ed.), *Transcultural nursing* (pp. 63-81). Prospect Heights: Waveland Press.

Lefley, H. P. (1990). Culture and chronic mental illness. *Hospital and Community Psychiatry, 41,* 277-286.

Leininger, M. (1978). Culturological assessment domains for nursing practices. In M. Leininger (Ed.), *Transcultural nursing: Theories, concepts, practices.* New York: Wiley.

Marsella, A. J., Sartorius, N., Jablensky, A., & Fenton, F. R. (1985). Cross-cultural studies of depressive disorders: An overview. In A. Kleinman, & B. Good (Eds.), *Culture and depression* (pp. 299-324). Berkeley: University of California Press.

Monroe, A., Goldman, R., & Dube, C. (1994). Race, culture and ethnicity, Unit I. In C. E. Dube, & D. C. Lewis (Eds.), *Race, culture and ethnicity: Curriculum for health care professionals.* Providence: Project ADEPT.

Orlandi, M. (1992). The challenge of evaluating community-based prevention programs: a cross-cultural perspective. In M. Orlandi, R. Weston, & L. Epstein (Eds.), *Cultural competence for evaluators: OSAP cultural competence series I* (pp. 1-22). Rockville: U.S. Department of Health and Human Services.

Putsch, R. W. (1985). Cross-cultural communication. *Journal of the American Medical Association, 254,* 3344-3348.

Svy, D. P. (1995, November). *Bridging differences: interpretation and expressions of help-seeking in Southeast Asian clients.* Paper presented at the Pacific Northwest Conference for Primary Care Practitioners, Seattle, WA.

Tripp-Reimer, T. (1984). Cultural diversity in therapy. In C. Beck, R. Rawlins, & S. Williams (Eds.), *Mental health-psychiatric nursing* (pp. 381-398). St. Louis: Mosby.

U.S. Bureau of the Census. (1990). *General population characteristics.* Washington, DC: U.S. Government Printing Office.

Unit 3

Models, Roles, and Responsibilities

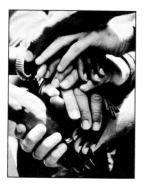

Chapter 5

Levels of Prevention

Nancy K. Worley

THE PUBLIC HEALTH MODEL

The public health model of prevention frames the content of this book. Renewed interest in the public health model has resulted from changes in the organization of health care. Managed care and capitation reimbursement strategies have engendered the rapid expansion in community-based services, mobilized concern about the health status of Americans, and increased interest in promoting health and preventing disease. Diagnosis and treatment of existing disease—the hallmarks of the medical model—are only two components of the public health model. This paradigm shift from a pathology model to a preventive model involves different concepts, target groups, and activities.

Community as client

The public health model addresses the community as client instead of as individual clients treated separately. This concept focuses practice on promoting and preserving the community's health. The transition to treating the community

as client, instead of treating individuals or families separately, entails understanding some key public health concepts. Box 5-1 defines terms commonly used in public health.

Epidemiology

Epidemiology underlies all preventive efforts. Epidemiological studies focus on the relationships among three variables: the host; the agent; and the environment (Figure 5-1). Public health efforts to prevent disease include the following three strategies for intervening in this epidemiological triangle:

1. Remove or neutralize the noxious agent
2. Strengthen the host's resistance
3. Prevent the transmission of the noxious agent to the host

Epidemiological research attempts to identify populations at risk in order to initiate preventive health measures. A major problem in studying the incidence and prevalence of mental disorders in the general population has been the lack of

---

Box 5–1. Definition of terms commonly used in public health

Epidemiology The systematic scientific study of the distribution patterns and determinants of health and disease frequencies in populations. Psychiatric epidemiologists study the distribution and determinants of psychiatric problems in defined populations.

Incidence The rate at which new cases of a disorder develop in a defined population.

Prevalence The number of cases of a disorder in the population at any one time.

Primary prevention Interventions aimed at reducing the incidence of new cases of mental disorder and disability in a population. Efforts are made to modify the environment and strengthen the capacities of people, families, and communities to cope with situations.

Secondary prevention Interventions aimed at reducing the duration of cases of mental disorders. By shortening the duration, the prevalence of mental disorders in the community is reduced.

Tertiary prevention Interventions aimed at reducing the community rate of residual defects that are often sequelae of acute mental illness.

Risk factors Characteristics, variables, or hazards associated with a high probability of onset, greater severity, and longer duration of major mental health problems.

Protective factors Conditions that improve people's resistance to risk factors and disorders.

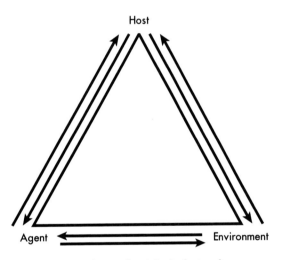

Figure 5–1. The epidemiological triangle.
(Modified from *Comprehensive Family and Community Health Nursing*, (4th ed.), by S. Clemen-Stone, D. Eigsti, & S. McGuire, 1995, St. Louis: Mosby.)

valid diagnostic procedures for large-scale screening of the general public (Dohrenwend, 1995). Semi-structured diagnostic interviews and rating examinations, developed for clinical research with clients and designed to be used by skilled clinicians, have been adapted for epidemiological research. Moreover, attempts have been made to build instruments specific to epidemiological studies. One of these instruments, the NIMH Diagnostic Interview Schedule (DIS), is specifically designed to be administered by trained interviewers who are not clinicians (Robins et al., 1991). This instrument incorporates *DSM-III* diagnostic criteria and is designed for use in the Epidemiologic Catchment Area study.

Epidemiologic Catchment Area (ECA) study

The Epidemiologic Catchment Area (ECA) Study, launched by the National Institute of Mental Health in the 1980s, is the most ambitious psychiatric epidemiological study to date. Between 1979 and 1982, over 18,000 adult residents in five U.S. communities were selected for intensive psychiatric examination. The ECA survey remains the most comprehensive source of information on the prevalence of mental illness in the United States. The ECA survey revealed that diagnosable mental illness is prevalent in the general population.

Approximately one in six adult Americans (15.4%) suffers from a mental disorder during a single month, one in five (19.5%) suffers from a mental disorder during a 6-month period, and one in three (32.7%) meets criteria for a mental disorder at some point during his or her life.

When these prevalence rates are extrapolated to the 1990 U.S. adult population, the results are astonishing. Nearly 30 million adults suffer from a mental disorder during a single month, 35 million during a 6-month period, and 60 million at some point in their lives. Most researchers believe these are conservative estimates. The ECA estimates do not include Alzheimer's disease, childhood and adolescent disorders, generalized anxiety disorder, and many personality disorders (Klerman et al., 1992).

The ultimate goal of epidemiology is to develop effective methods to prevent and control disease in the population. The ECA study, in addition to determining the incidence and prevalence of mental disorders in the general population, also sought to identify persons at increased or decreased risk of developing specific disorders. Variations in risk status may provide clues to possible causes and identify high-risk groups for targeted interventions to prevent or moderate the course of illness (Reiger & Kaelber, 1995). For example, the ECA data indicate that people between 18 and 29 years old and 30 and 44 years old have the highest lifetime rates of psychiatric disorder. African-Americans had higher lifetime and active rates of disorder than whites and Hispanics. However, as Reiger and Kaelber (1995) point out, when socioeconomic status is controlled, rates for African-Americans are no higher than for whites.

The ECA study assessed socioeconomic status based on education, current income, and current occupation. Persons who did not complete high school had an increased risk for psychiatric disorders compared with those who had graduated high school. Nearly half of all people receiving public assistance had a lifetime disorder. The study found the highest rates of lifetime and active disorder among men who were not working full

time; men employed in unskilled jobs had higher rates of disorder than men in more skilled positions. When marital status was examined, it was revealed that 44% of people who had been separated or divorced and 52% of those who had cohabited but never married had experienced a disorder over the lifespan (Robins et al., 1991). Caution must be used in assigning cause and effect relationships to these data because of the cross-sectional nature of the data collection. Observed associations may indeed be risk factors, but they also may be consequences of psychiatric disorders. For example, does the stress of poverty cause one to develop a psychiatric disorder, or does having a psychiatric disorder result in the inability to stay in school and obtain and maintain a well-paying job?

PRIMARY PREVENTION

Currently, the major mental health care thrust in the United States is toward secondary prevention efforts. The relatively recent emphasis on social skills training and other forms of psychosocial rehabilitation for people who suffer from severe or persistent mental illness reflects renewed efforts in tertiary prevention. Primary prevention is just beginning to emerge as a significant force in mental health. The massive reorganization of the health care delivery system is likely to remove many barriers that impeded the widespread development of primary prevention programs. The medical model's preoccupation with treating existing dysfunction, the lack of training of professionals in primary prevention modalities, and the lack of a political constituency have all contributed to disinterest in primary prevention. However, a previously insurmountable barrier has been the fee-for-service reimbursement system that essentially reimburses for illness care. The increasing use of capitated payment systems in which an annual amount is budgeted to take care of health care costs for an individual or a group, will force rethinking prevention as a method of decreasing the amount of money that will have to be spent on ill people. Controversy exists about the definition of primary prevention. Albee et al. (1988) define primary prevention by the following characteristics:

- Primary prevention seeks to build adaptive strengths, coping resources, and health in people.
- Primary prevention is concerned about total populations, especially groups at high risk.
- Primary prevention's main tools are education and social change.
- Primary prevention assumes that equipping people with personal and environmental resources for coping is the best way to avoid maladaptive problems.

Primary prevention contains two key components: health promotion and disease prevention. Health promotion begins with healthy people and seeks to promote community and individual measures to help develop life-styles that will maintain and enhance well-being.

Disease prevention or specific protection responds to a health threat (a disease or environmental hazard) and seeks to protect as many people as possible from the harmful consequences of that threat.

Health promotion

These two components of primary prevention have not developed in a parallel manner in the United States (Cowen, 1994). The prevention of specific disorders and dysfunctions among high-risk groups has received much more attention than health promotion in the general population. Health promotion in mental health encompasses the concept of psychological wellness, which is more than the absence of pathology; it is defined by the presence of positive characteristics such as:

- Effective interpersonal relationships
- Age-appropriate and ability-appropriate tasks
- A sense of belonging and purpose
- A sense of control over one's fate
- Satisfaction with oneself and one's existence

The strengthening of protective factors that mitigate the effects of risk exposure can promote psychological wellness. Cowen (1994) defines these protective factors as:

- Forming wholesome early attachments
- Developing age-appropriate and ability-appropriate competencies
- Developing environments that favor positive adaptation
- Fostering empowerment
- Acquiring skills for coping effectively with stress

The following preventive programs have been implemented to promote positive mental health.

Forming wholesome early attachments

Perhaps the best-known wellness programs are those that deal with pregnancy and parenting. Prenatal and parenting classes are widely available and have proven effective in teaching appropriate caregiving practices and promoting positive parent-child relationships (Cowen, 1994).

Enhancing social competence

Improving Social Awareness—Social Problem Solving Skills (Elias & Clabby, 1992) is a program based on a 2-year social competence training curriculum designed to build and promote self-control, social awareness, group participation, problem solving, and social decision making. An evaluation of the program indicated gains in the participants' sense of efficacy, improvements in social behavior, and reductions in pathology (such as depression) and socially disordered behaviors (such as vandalism and aggression).

Developing environments that favor positive adaptation

Several primary prevention programs have focused on changing school organization and management for children making the transition from elementary to middle school, and from middle school to high school. These programs are based on evidence that school transitions represent a time of increased risk for drug abuse and antisocial behavior (Hamburg, 1992). Several interventions have focused on changing the schools' organizational structure to facilitate shared management and decision making by a team of teachers, parents, school administrators, community agencies, and students (Gottfredson & Gottfredson, 1992; Cowen, 1994). The team reviews policy, school climate, instruction, and organization, and plans and implements change. Evaluations have been generally positive, with students showing significant decreases in delinquent behavior, lower rates of drug use, greater rates of attachment to school, and greater educational expectations than students in comparison schools.

Fostering empowerment

Empowerment refers to people gaining control over and making critical decisions about their lives (Swift, 1992). The field of prevention in mental health has only recently begun to explore empowerment and its relationship to prevention. Empowerment theory includes intrapersonal, interactional, and behavioral components. Wandersman and Florin (1992) describe the positive impact of citizen participation on the community, the organization, and the individual. Specifically, participation is associated with improved physical conditions, decreased deterioration, and increased social services on the community level, and with personal and political efficacy on the individual level.

Acquiring effective coping skills

Selye's (1975) theory of stress and adaptation continues to be the foundation of much of the work in primary prevention. Briefly, Selye's model states that we live in a field of forces. We respond to these forces in ways that ensure our survival, maintain our integrity, and fulfill our basic needs. We adapt or readjust to meet the demands of the stress and maintain equilibrium. Adaptation and readjustment are accomplished through coping. Four major ways of coping follow:

1. Stress avoidance
2. Stress management
3. Stress resistance building
4. Stress reaction management

Stress avoidance is usually the least feasible strategy for coping with stress, but in cases in which it is impossible to modify or eliminate stressors, it may be best to remove vulnerable persons from feeling the impact of such stressors. The use of curfew laws for minors, the imposition of legal drinking ages, and the removal of children from abusive homes are examples of stress avoidance.

Stress management focuses on identifying stressors that can be decreased, modified, or eliminated. A neighborhood crime watch in a high crime area and noise abatement laws are examples of ways in which communities modify stressors. Community-sponsored or corporate-sponsored child care centers modify stress for working parents.

Stress resistance building focuses on strengthening coping abilities through cognitive understanding of the stressor and by providing emotional and social support to help people cope with stressors. Education and anticipatory guidance are often used in this strategy. Premarital counseling, parent training, and preretirement groups are examples of this strategy.

Stress reaction management focuses on preventing the progression of disability in a person who has already felt a stressor's impact; this strategy overlaps with secondary prevention. Grief counseling after the death of a loved one and counseling after a natural disaster are examples of this kind of preventive effort. See Chapter 8, Crisis Stabilization, and Chapter 9, Supportive Psychotherapy, for more information on this topic.

Disease prevention

Risk factors

Risk factors and risk reduction are at the heart of disease prevention strategies. Risk factors are

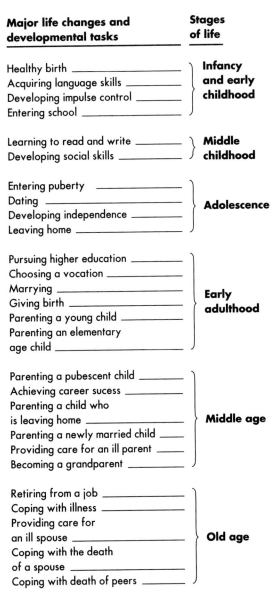

Major life changes and developmental tasks	Stages of life
Healthy birth _____ Acquiring language skills _____ Developing impulse control _____ Entering school _____	Infancy and early childhood
Learning to read and write _____ Developing social skills _____	Middle childhood
Entering puberty _____ Dating _____ Developing independence _____ Leaving home _____	Adolescence
Pursuing higher education _____ Choosing a vocation _____ Marrying _____ Giving birth _____ Parenting a young child _____ Parenting an elementary age child _____	Early adulthood
Parenting a pubescent child _____ Achieving career sucess _____ Parenting a child who is leaving home _____ Parenting a newly married child _____ Providing care for an ill parent _____ Becoming a grandparent _____	Middle age
Retiring from a job _____ Coping with illness _____ Providing care for an ill spouse _____ Coping with the death of a spouse _____ Coping with death of peers _____	Old age

Figure 5-2.   Developmental tasks over the life course.
(Modified from *Mental Health and Going to School,* by S.G. Kellam, J.D. Branch, K.C. Agrawal, & M.E. Ensminger, 1975, Chicago: University of Chicago Press.)

characteristics, variables, or hazards that if present for a given individual make it more likely that that individual (rather than someone selected at random from the general population) will develop a disorder (Werner & Smith, 1992). Risk factors can reside within the individual, the family, or the community, and can be biological or psychosocial (Institute of Medicine, 1994).

Protective factors

Clinicians and researchers have often observed that certain individuals have an unusual or marked capacity to recover from or successfully cope with significant stresses, and appear to escape relatively unscathed from psychosocial environments that cause maladaptive behavior in their peers. These observations of resilience have led to interest in protective factors and ways in which risk factors and protective factors might interact to modify, ameliorate, or alter a person's response to an environmental hazard. Because some risk factors (such as genetic vulnerability) are not readily amenable to change, and other risk factors (such as living in an urban ghetto) are difficult to change without massive social intervention, understanding and promoting protective factors are gaining favor in primary prevention.

Life stages and developmental tasks

A systematic way to organize and plan primary preventive interventions is to consider the major life changes and developmental tasks that need to be accomplished at each stage of life, as shown in Figure 5-2. Because the knowledge of human development throughout the lifespan and of the developmental tasks that need to be accomplished at each stage is well established, preventive interventions can build on this knowledge base. The following sections provide examples of preventive interventions for groups at risk for developing mental disorders.

Birth and infancy.   Evidence suggests that low birth weight babies face difficulty in accomplishing subsequent developmental tasks

(McGauhey et al., 1991). Prenatal and perinatal care aid in preventing prematurity and low birth weight. Strong evidence indicates that adolescent pregnancy, poverty, poorly educated parents, and a stressful environment keep pregnant women from obtaining adequate prenatal care (Center for the Study of Social Policy, 1992). Therefore many interventions have been directed toward pregnant women at great risk for obtaining little or no prenatal or perinatal care. Among the best known of these is the Prenatal/Early Infancy Program (Olds et al., 1988), a selective program targeted to a high-risk geographical area with high rates of poverty and child mistreatment. It consists of home visits by a nurse to prevent a wide range of maternal and child health problems associated with poverty. During the home visits, the nurse carries out three major activities: educating parents about influences on fetal and infant development; encouraging the involvement of family members and friends in the pregnancy, birth, and care of the infant and support for the mother; and linking family members with other health and human services. When compared with a control group, the women in the Prenatal/Early Infancy Program made better use of formal support systems, experienced greater informal support, improved their diets and smoked fewer cigarettes. Birth weight and length of gestation improved for the very young teenagers. The researchers also found a 75% reduction in child abuse and significantly fewer visits to the emergency room for the program children. The mothers were more frequently employed and had fewer subsequent pregnancies compared to controls.

Early childhood.   Language acquisition and the development of impulse control are two of the most important developmental tasks of early childhood. Failure at these tasks has been associated with later behavioral and school maladjustment and with the development of mental health problems (Hawkins, Catalano & Miller, 1992). A variety of preventive programs focus on enhancing economically deprived parents' skills in behavior management and in verbal interactions with their children to strengthen protective factors. One program, Parent-Child Interaction Training, consists of group sessions with instructions and role-playing on parenting skills, including behavioral management. Parents also were trained in play and conducted individual play sessions with their children. Evaluation revealed significant improvement in teacher-rated attention deficit and hyperactivity and in behavior when compared to controls (Strayhorn & Weidman, 1991).

Middle childhood.   Major developmental tasks accomplished during this period include academic success and social competency. Children who cannot perform academic tasks at grade level or who develop social incompetence, impulsivity, and aggressive behavior during this period are at risk for developing mental disorders (especially substance abuse, conduct disorder, and depression) (Institute of Medicine, 1994). Risk factors for developmental difficulties at this stage include poverty, conflict in the family, and lack of bonding between parents and children. As children mature, the interactions among schools, peers, parents, and the social environment become more complex. Preventive programs with components that seek to reduce risk and enhance protective factors seem to be most successful. The Seattle Social Development Project is an example of this kind of intervention (Hawkins et al., 1992). The intervention lasted for 4 years, from the first through the fourth grade. It included teacher training and supervision, and taught classroom management, effective instructional methods, and cooperative learning. The intervention offered parents a skills training program focused on management of their children's behavior and a second program that focused on providing parental support for academic development. Evaluation demonstrated positive results for parent management, family communication, family involvement, family attachment, school attachment, and academic achievement when compared to a control group.

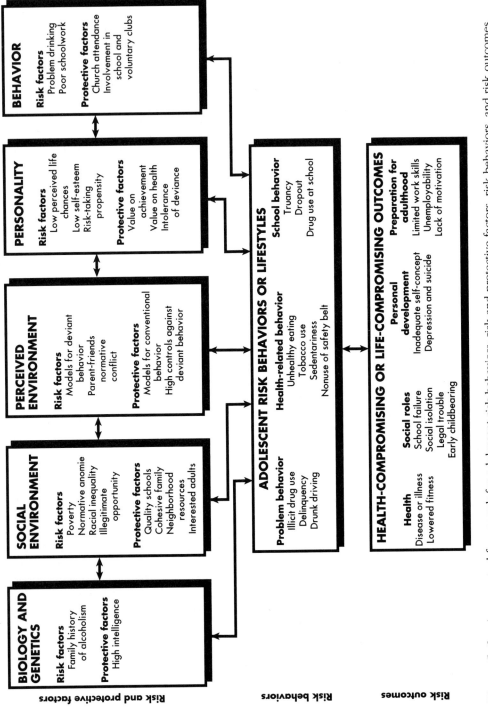

Figure 5–3. A conceptual framework for adolescent risk behaviors: risk and protective factors, risk behaviors, and risk outcomes. (Modified from "Risk Behavior in Adolescence: A Psychosocial Framework for Understanding and Action," by R. Jessor, 1992, in *Adolescents at Risk: Medical and Social Perspectives*, by D.E. Rogers and E. Ginzburg (Eds.), 1992, Boulder, CO: Westview Press.)

Adolescence. The complexity of the developmental tasks that need to be accomplished during adolescence (see Figure 5-2), combined with the interaction of the biological, psychological, and social environments in which these tasks take place, result in a difficult developmental period for most adolescents. Figure 5-3 illustrates the interrelation of risk factors and protective factors that influence these developmental tasks. Although poverty is one risk factor listed in this figure, many other risk factors have their roots in an impoverished environment (racial inequality, models for deviant behavior, and low perceived life chances). Poverty and its associated environmental risks affect large numbers of adolescents. A report by the U.S. Congress Office of Technology Assessment (1991) showed that about 8.5 million of the 31 million adolescents in the United States live at or below 150% of the federal poverty level. The preponderance of preventive interventions for adolescents has been disorder specific, focusing for the most part on substance abuse prevention, or to a lesser extent on conduct disorder prevention (Institute of Medicine, 1994). The formation of the Research Network on Successful Adolescent Development Among Youth in High-Risk Settings has been an exciting development in the study of adolescent behavior (Jessor, 1993). The project seeks to advance knowledge about development among youths growing up in social contexts that put them at risk (including poverty, limited access to opportunity, and racial and ethnic marginality). Rather than focusing primarily on risk factors, research focuses on factors and processes that safeguard and promote success in such environments.

One study in the larger research network is the Family Management Study (Furstenberg, 1993). This study focuses on strategies that families use to protect adolescents from the risks, dangers, and illegitimate opportunities characteristic of disadvantaged neighborhoods. It also studies the strategies families use to manage problematic situations such as negotiations with schools or the police when a child is having difficulties. The study investigates the ways in which parents seek out resources (which despite their scarcity do exist) in the environment and the strategies parents use to provide monitoring and support as insulation against drug use and other deviant behaviors modeled by their children's peers. The study also investigates the methods parents use to locate a safer niche (such as a parochial school) when the neighborhood school and its environment become too dangerous. Understanding these strategies can be useful in developing broad-based preventive programs for youths at risk as a consequence of their social environment.

Young adulthood. In adulthood, psychosocial risk factors that increase the likelihood of mental health problems closely correspond to the developmental tasks depicted in Figure 5-2. Preventive programs that address the developmental tasks of giving birth and parenting are discussed in other sections of this chapter. Other developmental tasks that have been associated with increased risk factors include marital relationships (for example, separation and divorce) and occupational stress (for example, losing a job). Several preventive programs have developed around these issues.

The University of Colorado Separation and Divorce Program aims to help newly separated persons negotiate the transition to single life with new occupational and child-rearing responsibilities. Specialists in child-rearing and single parenting, housing and homemaking, employment and education, and legal and financial issues provide 2-hour workshops with the goal of enhancing coping skills and mobilizing support systems (Bloom et al., 1985). People who participated in the program rated significantly higher in social and psychological adjustment, had fewer separation-related problems, and reported significantly greater separation-related benefits than control group members.

The JOBS Project for the Unemployed was designed to help persons who had recently lost their jobs cope with the stresses of job loss and setbacks in the job search process (Vinokur et al., 1991). The curriculum included skills training and support for dealing with obstacles to reemployment, identifying sources of job leads, practicing and rehearsing interviews, handling emotions related to unemployment, and evaluating a job offer. Evaluation of the impact of the JOBS program through a randomized controlled study demonstrated that people in the program obtained higher paying jobs and higher quality jobs than the controls. Thirty-six months after completing the program, group participants showed greater reduction in depressive symptoms than their counterparts in the control group (Vinokur et al., 1991).

Middle age. One of the middle-age person's most stressful developmental tasks is providing care for ill and elderly parents. As life expectancy continues to increase, more and more middle-age children will face this problem. Peer and Professionally Led Groups to Support Family Caregivers (Toseland, 1990) are preventive interventions that include education, discussion, and problem solving training. The education and discussion groups address caregivers' emotions, the care receiver's reaction to illness, community resources, pharmacology, nursing home placement, and managing care within the home. The interventions were evaluated in a three-group randomized trial that included peer-led sessions, professionally led sessions, and a control group. Both peer-led and professionally led groups produced increases in psychological well-being compared to the control group. At 1-year follow-up both experimental groups had greater success than the control group in helping the caregivers of frail elderly family members reduce the stress of pressing problems, increase formal and informal support systems, and make changes in their caregiving roles (Toseland, 1990). See Chapter 27, Elderly Persons with Mental Illness, for more information on preventive interventions useful to caregivers of persons with Alzheimer's disease.

Late adulthood. Widowhood and bereavement will affect large numbers of elderly people in the coming years (Institute of Medicine, 1994). Bereavement has been studied extensively as a risk factor, and epidemiological studies have found an increased risk for depression, physical deterioration, and death in elderly widows and widowers (Blazer, 1989). Moreover, widows and widowers are more likely than their single or married peers to be socially isolated, to live in poverty, to be emotionally troubled, and to have fewer meaningful social activities (Institute of Medicine, 1984).

Widow-to-Widow: A Mutual Help Program for the Widowed is a preventive program in which widowed helpers reach out to recently widowed persons to help them through the transition. Helpers are recruited by word of mouth or through community action groups. Identification of newly widowed women is done through funeral directors who are involved in the program as sponsors and advisory board members (Silverman, 1988). Widows who participated in the program were more apt to begin new relationships and activities and did so more quickly than members of a control group. They also experienced fewer depressive symptoms (Vachon et al., 1980).

Because women have a longer life expectancy than men, women who have lost a husband far outnumber men who have lost a wife. Well-designed research on the effects of support groups on widowers has yet to be done.

The future of primary prevention

In an investigation of resources spent on primary prevention by the federal government, the Institute of Medicine (1994) concluded that only $20 million per year is spent on rigorous preventive intervention research targeted toward preventing mental disorders. The investigation also concluded that federal agencies researching preventive intervention and providing prevention services were decentralized and uncoordinated and had little awareness of each other's efforts. An investigation of personnel involved in preventive research noted a scarcity of researchers working in mental disorder prevention. Data on researchers working in the field reveal that most are psychologists, with some physicians and sociologists but few social workers or nurses. The report made the following recommendations:

- Build an infrastructure to coordinate research and service programs and to train and support new researchers
- Expand the knowledge base for preventive interventions
- Conduct well-evaluated preventive interventions

SECONDARY PREVENTION

Secondary prevention focuses on reducing the prevalence of a disease or condition. It involves activities aimed at early diagnosis, prompt treatment, and disability limitation. Identification of health needs, health problems, and clients at risk is vital to secondary prevention. Casefinding through screening surveys is an important secondary prevention methodology. Two types of screening programs are used in mental health. The single screening test identifies a specific disorder. Depression screenings are an example of this type of screening. The second type of screening assesses the presence of any psychiatric disorder or the presence of more than one psychiatric disorder in the same person. An example of this type of screening is the Diagnostic Interview Schedule. Caution must be exercised in implementing community-wide casefinding efforts. Facilities for further diagnostic tests and for treatment must be available.

Prompt treatment is a crucial part of secondary prevention. One of the most important contributions of the community mental health movement has been the development and refinement of crisis intervention principles. This brief, direct, and time-limited treatment strategy seeks to return the person who has experienced a crisis to a precrisis level of functioning and thereby avoid or limit disability. See Chapter 8, Crisis Stabilization, for detailed information on crisis intervention.

TERTIARY PREVENTION

Tertiary prevention focuses on rehabilitation and attempts to reduce the severity, discomfort, or disability of a condition. Rehabilitation of persons with severe or persistent mental illness has been an important focus of mental health in community settings for the past 2 decades. Rehabilitation aims to assist the individual in learning or relearning emotional and intellectual skills necessary to function in the environment with the least amount of assistance from the mental health system. Foundations of psychosocial rehabilitation include skills training, drug therapy, and community support (Attkisson et al., 1992). Skills training encompasses social and vocational skills; social skills training has been studied extensively. A National Institute of Mental Health (1992) study noted that the effectiveness of social skills training during the past 15 years has been documented in more than 50 research studies. These studies indicate that social skills training is a feasible treatment strategy, especially for concrete behavioral skills (such as eye contact, voice volume, and appropriate gestures). There are four focal points in social skills training models:

1. Improving basic psychobiological and cognitive functions by training to lengthen attention span and to engage in higher order abstractions
2. Training in the receiving, processing, and sending skills of communication, which involves coaching, reinforcement, modeling, and homework
3. Reprogramming the individual's natural environment so that acquired skills will meet with support and favorable feedback
4. Improving the understanding of social perceptions

During the past decade, the vocational rehabilitation of persons with severe mental illness has emerged as a major rehabilitative focus (Rosenheck, Frisman, & Sindelar, 1995). Various models of vocational rehabilitation exist. Some, such as the Fountain House model, stress arrangements with employers and the presence of nonhandicapped coworkers (Fountain House, 1985). Others, such as Fairweather Lodges and Soteria houses, involve a group of mentally ill persons living and working together in a consumer-owned business.

An important aspect of community support for people with severe mental illness is the availability of residential and independent living services. In the 1950s and early 1960s, deinstitutionalization resulted in the proliferation of community-based residential services. The trend was toward a transitional program structure organized developmentally or functionally. The continuum of services included quarter-way houses, halfway houses, family foster care, crisis residences, and Fairweather Lodges (Carling et al., 1988). Recently this transitional model has been criticized because its time-limited nature forces clients constantly to move to different levels on the continuum of residential services, thereby negating the positive effect of housing stability. In an attempt to overcome this problem and attend to consumer preference for more independent living, the use of normalized housing situations is being investigated.

The client's family and self-help groups are vital components of rehabilitative efforts. Families can speed rehabilitation by providing support and reinforcement of acquired skills. Self-help groups can provide needed peer support during the difficult transition from the hospital to the community. Consumer drop-in centers and consumer-run businesses provide social support and community employment that is interesting and enhances self-esteem. Several chapters in this book discuss rehabilitative interventions (see Chapter 3, Family and Consumer Movements;

Chapter 12, Psychosocial Rehabilitation; Chapter 18, Partial Hospital Programs; and Chapter 19, Residential Treatment).

ASSESSMENT OF THE COMMUNITY

Mental health professionals who work in community settings need to know the resources available in the community and any gaps in the continuum of services. Whether it is undertaken to plan for the service needs of an individual, a family, or a particular population group, community assessment requires the acquisition of specific skills. The depth of the community assessment varies with its purpose and the time and resources available for it. At a minimum, professionals who work in the community should be familiar with the characteristics and components listed in Box 5-2.

Mental health professionals involved in community program planning and development need to be able to perform a more detailed community needs assessment. Table 5-1 lists various approaches used in performing community assessment. Some or all of these approaches should be used in accomplishing the following planning tasks.

Delineate target groups. Epidemiological Catchment Area data revealed that one in five adult Americans met criteria for having an active mental disorder and that the vast majority of these people did not receive treatment for their symptoms (Klerman et al., 1992). In addition, epidemiological studies have demonstrated a strong correlation between emotional disorders and social indicators such as poverty, lack of education, and unemployment. Thus a vast unmet need exists for mental health services for people with diagnosed mental illness and for people at risk for developing such disorders.

Prioritize target groups. Because no community is likely to have sufficient funds to serve all potential target groups adequately, it is necessary to prioritize needs. Community assessment

Box 5-2. Community characteristics

Physical characteristics

Natural resources
Climate
Location
Major roadways
Open space
Waterways

Population characteristics

Overall age, gender, ethnic distribution
Socioeconomic status
Educational status

Basic services

Post office
Banks
Food, drug, clothing stores
Dry cleaners
Restaurants

Health care

Hospitals
Clinics
Ambulance service
Physicians
Dentists
Home health care
Pharmacists
Folk healers

Social services

Social Security offices
Welfare offices
Homeless shelters
Children services
Senior citizen services
Drug and alcohol services
Housing authority

Environmental and safety services

Police department
Fire department
Sanitation services
Animal control

Educational services

Nursery schools
Public and private secondary schools
Colleges
Universities
Vocational schools
Public libraries
Adult education

Social and recreational facilities

Churches
Parks
Sports facilities (ball parks, stadiums, tracks, bicycle
    and walking paths)
YMCA and YWCA
Fitness centers
Theaters (live and cinema)

Public transportation

Buses
Subways
Trains
Taxis

Mental health facilities

Community mental health centers
Psychiatric emergency rooms
Mobile crisis unit
Crisis "hot lines"
Battered women's shelters
Residential treatment facilities
Partial hospital programs
Board and care homes
Sheltered employment

Table 5-1. Community needs assessment approaches

APPROACH	PURPOSE	SPECIFIC TOOLS	OUTCOMES	TIME REQUIRED
I Key Informant	Tap perceptions of persons knowledgeable about characteristics of population under study and needs for mental health services.	Mailed questionnaire, telephone interviews, or personal interview.	Summary perceptions regarding population subgroups, geographic and programmatic areas of need.	4-12 weeks
II Community Forum	Same as I, with citizens at large also included.	Public meetings.	Same as I.	2-6 weeks
III Social Indicators	Utilize social area characteristics that are associated with prevalence of mental disabilities to identify, locate, and describe population with high need for mental health services.	Social area and ecological data; socioeconomic and demographic characteristics.	Description of community (e.g., census tract), inference of level of need, and estimate of number of persons at risk.	1 month (assuming easy access to existing data)
IV Rates Under Treatment	Infer service needs based on use of existing services.	Use of admissions/activity data from existing reports and surveys.	Summary of existing utilization, profile of areas, and use of treated prevalence to estimate true prevalence (gross need).	1-4 months of utilizing already existing data
V Field Survey	Measure need for mental health services via direct assessment of mental status and relevant variables of a sample of population.	Various sampling techniques and survey instruments, typically drawing portions from instruments already used (and proven as to validity and reliability), or same as I.	Mental status and other relevant data (i.e., support system, attitude toward mental health, health history, by geographic areas and target groups.	6-18 months
VI Nominal Group	Same as I.	A technique to elicit opinions from all participants in the group, including usually silent members.	Same as I.	2-6 months

Table 5–1—cont'd

BASIC ASSUMPTIONS	RELATIVE COST	LIMITATIONS	ADVANTAGES
Community leaders are knowledgeable about subject; they also are unbiased.	Inexpensive	Relies on perceptions. Little empirical research reported revalidity. Built in bias from selection of informants, results may not be representative of entire community.	Time and cost. Facilitates communication among service agencies in the community.
Same as I, expanded to include local citizenry.	Inexpensive	Same as I, plus risk of subjecting process to "grievance" sessions.	Same as I, plus input gained directly from the consumer level.
Indicators are good predictors of mental health needs (a casual relationship is not assumed), emphasis on measuring needs of lower-middle and lower socioeconomic groups.	Economical, major cost is in analysis and presentation of data	Indicators represent indirect measures. Unknown validity of indicators. Assumptions of uniform meaning (i.e. of poverty) across areas (i.e. urban vs. rural). Dated census data, and under enumeration and unreliable counts in some areas. May emphasize lower level of social structure.	Employs existing data. Although not able to show causal relationships, correlation between indicators and prevalence of mental illness is backed by literature.
Treated prevalence is a good approximation of true prevalence of mental disorders. Differences between treated and true prevalence are unbiased.	Typically more expensive than Approaches I, II, and VI, but still relatively economical if based on already collected data	Basic assumptions have weaknesses, particularly the assumption that utilization is the same as need.	Employs much "hard" data rather than impressions. Links estimates of future service utilization to present service utilization.
Reliability and validity of instrument determining mental disability, representativeness of the sample, lack of response bias.	Very expensive	Very expensive. Requires extensive publicity and time.	If carefully designed and conducted, provides the most scientifically valid and reliable information about individuals regarding their needs and utilization patterns.
Same as I or II, depending on whether or not local citizenry are involved.	Inexpensive	Same as I or II.	Same as I or II.

for planning purposes involves identifying groups in the community at high risk for the development of mental disorders and then prioritizing these target groups. Criteria for prioritizing target groups include:

- The degree of severity or incapacitation caused by a particular maladaptive behavior
- The degree of neglect a particular target group has suffered relative to other groups in the population
- The degree of impairment as measured by epidemiological studies in a particular category
- The degree of interest on the part of funding sources in a particular target group

A good starting point for the planner is to combine the information presented in Table 5-1 with clinical expertise, research, and theory drawn from the social sciences and empirical observation to understand the social, political, and economic foundations of the community. For example, the physical characteristics of a community dictate to a large extent the character of the economy. The natural resources of some communities appeal to tourists, and the economy of the community is thus organized around the tourist trade. These communities have large numbers of relatively low-skill, low-wage seasonal jobs. How does this affect the mental health of the community? Some communities are centers for high-technology companies, some are banking and finance centers, and others are heavily dependent on military facilities in the community. The presence or absence of major road systems will determine whether the community is isolated or accessible to the outside world. Because communities are dynamic systems, the interactions among physical characteristics and social, political, and economic forces are complex. Understanding these forces and the dynamic interplay among them is fundamental to the coherent planning of mental health services for the community.

SUMMARY

The reorganization of the financing and delivery of mental health services has led to renewed interest in prevention. Although the focus has been on primary prevention, the early diagnosis, treatment, and rehabilitation of persons with severe mental illnesses also have benefited from increased attention to the public health model of prevention.

The concept of community as client is basic to the public health model and encompasses the provision of services to groups of clients based on age-related developmental tasks and at-risk characteristics (Clemen-Stone, Eigsti, & McGuire, 1995). As the focus of care and treatment of persons with mental illness continues to move from the hospital to the community, practitioners with the skills to assess and intervene at the community level will find themselves in demand. The public health concepts of health promotion, health maintenance, health education, and coordination of care are fundamental to nursing. Therefore nursing is well positioned to meet the challenges of a new and evolving health care delivery system.

REFERENCES

Albee, G., Joffe, J., & Dusenbury, L. (1988). *Prevention, powerlessness, and politics, readings on social change.* Newbury Park, CA: Sage Publications.

Attkisson, C., Cook, J., Karno, M., Lehman, A., et al. (1992). Clinical services research. *Schizophrenia Bulletin, 18,* 561-626.

Blazer, D. (1989). The epidemiology of psychiatric disorders in late life. In E. Busseand, & D. Blaser (Eds.), *Geriatric psychiatry.* Washington, DC: American Psychiatric Press.

Bloom, B., Hodges, W., Kern, M., & McFaddin, S. (1985). A preventive intervention program for the newly separated. *American Journal of Orthopsychiatry, 55,* 9-26.

Carling, P., Randolph, F., Blanch, A., & Ridgeway, P. (1988). Review of the research on housing and community integration for people with psychiatric disabilities. *National Rehabilitation Information Center Quarterly, 1,* 6-18.

Center for the Study of Social Policy, Annie E. Casey Foundation. (1992). *Kids count data book*. Washington, DC: Center for the Study of Social Policy.

Clemen-Stone, S., Eigsti, D., & McGuire, S. (1995). *Comprehensive family and community health nursing* (4th ed.). St. Louis: Mosby.

Cowen, E. (1994). The enhancement of psychological wellness: Challenges and opportunities. *American Journal of Community Psychology*, 22, 149-179.

Dohrenwend, B. (1995). The problem of validity in field studies of psychological disorders revisited. In M. Tsuang, M. Tohen, & G. Zahner (Eds.), *Textbook in psychiatric epidemiology* (pp. 3-20). New York: Wiley-Liss.

Elias, M., & Clabby, J. (1992). *Building social problem-solving skills: Guidelines from a school-based program*. San Francisco: Jossey-Bass.

Fountain House. (1985). *Evaluation of clubhouse model community-based psychiatric rehabilitation: Final report to the National Institute of Handicapped Research*. Washington, DC: National Institute of Handicapped Research.

Furstenberg, F. (1993). How families manage risk and opportunity in dangerous neighborhoods. In W. J. Wilson (Ed.), *Sociology and the public agenda*. Newbury Park, CA: Sage Publications.

Gottfredson, D., & Gottfredson, G. (1992). Theory-guided investigation: Three field experiments. In J. McCord, & R. Tremblay (Eds.), *Preventing anti-social behavior: Interventions from birth through adolescence* (pp. 311-329). New York: Guilford Press.

Hamburg, D. (1992). *Today's children: Creating a future for a generation in crisis*. New York: Times Books.

Hawkins, J., Catalano, R., & Miller, J. (1992). Risk and protective factors for alcohol and other drug problems in adolescence and early adulthood: Implications for substance abuse prevention. *Psychological Bulletin, 112*, 64-105.

Institute of Medicine. (1984). *Bereavement: Reactions, consequences and care*. Washington, DC: National Academy Press.

Institute of Medicine. (1994). *Reducing risks for mental disorders, frontiers for preventive intervention research*. Washington, DC: National Academy Press.

Jessor, R. (1993). Successful adolescent development among youth in high risk settings. *American Psychologist, 48*, 117-126.

Jessor, R. (1992). Risk behavior in adolescence: A psychosocial framework for understanding and action. In D.E. Rogers, & E. Ginzburg (Eds.), *Adolescents at risk: Medical and social perspectives*. Boulder, CO: Westview Press.

Kellam, S.G., Branch, J.D., Agrawal, K.C., & Ensminger, M.E. (Eds.)(1975). *Mental health and going to school*. Chicago: University of Chicago Press.

Klerman, G., Olfson, M., Leon, A., & Weissman, M. (1992, Fall). Measuring the need for mental health care. *Health Affairs*, 23-33.

McGauhey, P., Starfield, B., Alexander, C., & Ensminger, M. (1991). Social environment and vulnerability of low birth weight children: A social-epidemiological perspective. *Pediatrics, 88*, 943-953.

National Institute of Mental Health. (1992). Caring for people with severe mental disorders: A national plan to improve services. *Schizophrenia Bulletin, 18*, 559-696.

Olds, D., Henderson, C., Tatlebaum, R., & Chamberlin, R. (1988). Improving the life course development of socially disadvantaged mothers: A randomized trial of nurse home visitations. *American Journal of Public Health, 78*, 1436-1444.

Reiger, D., & Kaelber, C. (1995). The Epidemiologic Catchment Area (ECA) program: Studying the prevalence and incidence of psychopathology. In M. Tsuang, M. Tohen, & G. Zahner (Eds.), *Textbook in psychiatric epidemiology* (pp. 135-155). New York: Wiley-Liss.

Robins, L., Locke, B., & Reiger, D. (1991). An overview of psychiatric disorders in America. In L. Robins, & D. Reiger (Eds.), *Psychiatric disorders in America* (pp. 328-366). New York: Free Press.

Rosenheck, R., Frisman, L., & Sindelar, J. (1995). Disability compensation and work among veterans with psychiatric and nonpsychiatric impairments. *Psychiatric Services, 46*, 359-365.

Selye, H. (1975). *The stress of life*. New York: McGraw-Hill.

Silverman, P. (1988). Widow-to-widow: A mutual self help program for the widowed. In R. Price, E. Cowen, R. Lorin, & J. Ramos-McKay (Eds.), *Fourteen ounces of prevention: A casebook for practitioners* (pp. 175-187). Washington, DC: American Psychological Association.

Strayhorn, J., & Weidman, C. (1991). Follow-up one year after parent-child interaction training: Effects on behavior of preschool children. *Journal of the American Academy of Child and Adolescent Psychiatry, 30*, 138-143.

Swift, C. (1992). Empowerment: An emerging mental health technology. *Journal of Primary Prevention, 8*, 71-94.

Toseland, R. (1990). Long-term effectiveness of peer-led and professionally-led support groups for caregivers. *Social Service Review, 64*, 308-327.

U.S. Congress Office of Technology Assessment. (1991). *Adolescent health: Vol 1. Summary and policy options*. Washington, DC: U.S. Government Printing Office.

Vachon, M., Sheldon, A., Lancee, W., Lyall, W., et al. (1980). A controlled study of self-help intervention for widows. *American Journal of Psychiatry, 137,* 1380-1384.

Vinokur, A., van Ryn, M., Gramlich, E., & Price, R. (1991). Long-term follow-up and cost-benefit analysis of the JOBS project. *Journal of Applied Psychology, 76,* 213-219.

Wandersman, A., & Florin, P. (1992). Citizen participation. In J. Rappaport, & E. Seidman (Eds.), *Handbook of community psychology.* New York: Plenum Press.

Werner, E., & Smith R. (1992). *Overcoming the odds: High risk children from birth to adulthood.* New York: Cornell University Press.

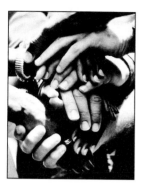

Chapter 6

Roles and Functions of Psychiatric Nurses in the Community

Susan E. Caverly and Sandra L. Talley

The term *psychiatric nurse* is generally used to describe all nurse providers who have experience and expertise in the mental health field. Practice environments for psychiatric nurses include but are not limited to hospital settings, public and private outpatient clinics, home care agencies, drug and alcohol treatment programs, and primary care settings. Because of the wide variation in the opportunities for and the utilization of psychiatric nurses, it is the intent of this chapter to clarify educational backgrounds, expertise of psychiatric nurses, licensure, credentialing processes, and roles. This clarification may assist nurses, consumers, employers, and policy makers in making the best and most appropriate use of this nursing specialty.

By understanding role opportunities and limitations, nurses are better informed to determine if positions and responsibilities are within the scope of their practice or expertise, and conversely if restrictions are being imposed unnecessarily by organizations or other disciplines. Emerging issues in health care and psychiatric-mental health nursing will be addressed, as will

predictions from leaders in nursing and other fields about the future of the profession (Aiken & Salmon, 1994; Safriet, 1994; Safriet, 1992; Lowery, 1992; Pothier et al., 1990; McBride, 1990).

References for professional standards of practice in psychiatric-mental health nursing include the American Nurses Association Statement on Psychiatric-Mental Health Nursing and Standards of Psychiatric Mental Health Nursing Clinical Practice, the ANA Consultation-Liaison Standards, Child Psychiatric Nursing Standards, and Standards of Chemical Dependency. Organizations currently devoted to differing aspects of psychiatric nursing include APNA, SERPN, PCLPMHN, and CHILD. State Nurse Practice Acts further stipulate the scope of practice or licensure requirements for selected nursing groups. These documents should be read to understand definitions of nursing practice, options for advanced practice roles, and educational or supervisory requirements for nursing practice at various educational levels. State Nurse Practice Acts (NPAs) regulate nursing in the respective states; nurses are responsible for knowing the contents of their state's NPA.

HISTORICAL OVERVIEW OF EVENTS SHAPING MENTAL HEALTH POLICIES AND PSYCHIATRIC NURSING

In the years following World War II there was a surge of interest in and funding for the care of people with mental illness. The National Mental Health Act of 1946 established the National Institute of Mental Health (NIMH) with a mandate to foster and aid research into psychiatric disorders, provide for the training of personnel, and aid states in developing clinics and treatment centers for pilot and demonstration projects (Armour, 1981; Foley, 1975). In the 1950s and 1960s federal funding resulted in increased monies for trainees in the four core mental health disciplines: psychiatry, psychology, social work, and psychiatric nursing. This led to a dramatic increase in the numbers of nurses entering the psychiatric-mental health specialty (NIMH, 1987). In 1969, the peak year of funding, 1721 stipends were awarded to students in baccalaureate, master's, and doctoral programs. Graduates of master's programs in psychiatric-mental health nursing accounted for 40% of all master's program nursing graduates. By 1986 only 97 stipends were awarded. The percentage of psychiatric-mental health nurses dropped from 23% of nurses in graduate nursing programs in 1973 to 12.4% in 1983 and 1984 (NIMH, 1987; Chamberlain, 1987). Programs also faced increased competition for monies when funding mandates shifted toward priorities in mental health care. No longer were training grants available for any master's level program, but only for those that were developing a new focus on care of people with chronic mental illness, recruitment of minorities into mental health nursing, and care of children and adolescents (Martin, 1985). A reduction in training monies, lack of a psychiatric rotation in undergraduate nursing education, and increased choices in other specialty programs at the master's level all influenced the numbers of advanced practice psychiatric nurses (NIMH, 1985).

Early training of psychiatric nurses occurred in specialty hospitals or asylums. The first school of nursing for psychiatric nurses opened in 1882 at the McLean Psychiatric Asylum in Waverly, Massachusetts (Martin, 1985; Peplau, 1989). The earliest descriptions of the roles of psychiatric nurses were written by physicians for the purpose of training nurses to provide psychiatric nursing care. In a 1936 volume by Carmichael and Chapman, the primary concern of psychiatric nursing is sympathy, self-sacrifice, and the doctrine of the Golden Rule. By 1941 Sands expanded the focus to include observation, consultation with family members, home visits, and preventive interventions.

During that same time, the National League for Nursing (NLN) required course work in "nervous and mental diseases" in nursing curricula. This ended the separation of psychiatric nursing schools from hospital-based and university-based schools of nursing; by 1949 psychiatric nursing would begin to be integrated into undergraduate nursing programs (NIMH, 1987). Although public health nursing was a strong influence on the construction of the psychiatric nursing role, the affiliation with psychiatry and other mental health professionals drew criticism that psychiatric nursing was no longer affiliated with nursing. This early view of the psychiatric nurse as an extension of the psychiatrist and as the provider of physical treatment and support created barriers to the recognition of nurses as mental health professionals rather than providers of custodial care. In an attempt to overcome this early perception, the psychiatric clinical specialist clarification was developed in 1951. The psychiatric clinical specialist was required to have a master's degree and be prepared to offer psychotherapy, consultation-liaison services, education, and participation in research. Later the authority to prescribe medications was added to the psychiatric clinical specialist role (ANA Council of Psychiatric and Mental Health Nursing et al., 1994).

The wave of deinstitutionalization that began in the 1960s signaled a paradigm shift in the treatment of psychiatric clients. Treatment was viewed as more valuable if provided in the consumer's community, close to family, friends, and treatment providers.

The economic and political pressures of the 1980s and 1990s further increased the demand for management of psychiatric disorders in the community setting. For example, the number of state hospital beds was reduced from a high of 559,000 in 1955 to 109,939 in 1986 (Mechanic & Rochefort, 1990). During this same period the number of private psychiatric hospital beds proliferated. Efforts at cost containment for mental health services soon prevailed within the private sector, and outpatient services became the preferred modality whenever feasible. Issues of cost effectiveness and outcome measures have continued to gain prominence with health insurers, policy makers, and service providers.

The emphasis on biological processes in mental health care began in the 1990s, "the decade of the brain." Increasing evidence has supported biological etiologies for many mental disorders, allowing for more specific intervention strategies. New mental health research funding priorities, changes in service priorities, and pharmacological advances have provided a remarkable opportunity for psychiatric-mental health nurses (Lowery, 1992; McBride, 1990). Some of the evolving roles take a distinct nursing approach, and others are more multidisciplinary in focus (Aiken & Salmon, 1994). For example, nursing is quite comfortable delivering mental health services and case management in community and home care settings; many states have granted prescriptive authority to Clinical Specialists in Psychiatric Nursing. As cost becomes increasingly important, practitioners possessing a broad range of skills will become more attractive to third-party payers, consumers, families, and agencies or businesses that contract for health care services (Valentine, 1995; Lowery, 1992). In fact nurses are already increasingly being sought as providers of mental health services in board and care settings, nursing homes, primary care offices, and community mental health centers.

RESPONSE OF ROLE TO ENVIRONMENT

The nature of nursing education and specialty conceptualization can best be understood as a series of concurrent continua. The continua directly related to this discussion include educational preparation, credentialing, and practice scope and setting. Each continuum is embedded in the environment, a web of subspecialization characterized by the population served, the setting, and the intervention modality. This model recognizes the significant role flexibility available to and required of psychiatric-mental health nurses. This flexibility contributes to the necessity and the potential for expansion of practice boundaries at all levels of psychiatric nursing preparation (Figure 6-1). The use of continua to understand nursing roles demonstrates that at times the continua flow in a synchronous manner; at other times this is not the case. In general, practitioners at all levels of psychiatric-mental health nursing may be found anywhere along the continua of circumstances and variations common to the specialty.

The ecology within which the various continua interact is multilayered and dynamic. The population served, the subspecialization, and even the social, cultural, and political structures may coalesce to form distinct, discrete environments that by design attract and necessitate the development of a specific psychiatric-mental health nursing role. For example, nonspecialty settings also have added psychiatric nursing experts to their staffs for consultation and liaison activities (Lehman, 1995; Titlebaum, Hart, & Romano, 1992).

This model also contains an element of role overlap that is in part a response to unmet community and professional needs for information regarding the scope of practice of psychiatric-mental health nurses. Role overlap also may be secondary to resource scarcity—nursing shortages or agency funding limitations.

The geographic distribution of health care providers of all disciplines has been a focus of concern for policy makers for some time. Efforts to distribute health care personnel resources equitably to rural and underserved populations have resulted in only modest improvements. Increased interest in the preventive and episodic care needs of these populations may perhaps eventually lead

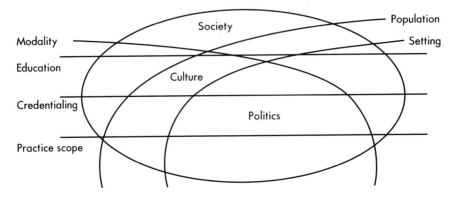

Figure 6-1. Multiple continua influencing psychiatric nursing roles.

to integrated goals for health plans (Aiken & Salmon, 1994). Efforts to expand mental health services in rural areas have used a multidisciplinary approach to identify the skill and resource capabilities of psychology, social work, and psychiatric nursing. An interdisciplinary project funded by the American Psychological Association, the American Nurses Association, and the National Social Work Organization developed a curriculum for rural mental health training (APA, 1995). Follow-up training efforts will provide three regional "train the trainer" workshops to enhance community mental health treatment in an interdisciplinary fashion.

Any reconfiguration of the structure and delivery of health care services will likely have cost management as a key element. The prioritization of "cost" in discussions of "cost effective care" has the potential to increase role and continuum overlap that may limit consumer access to certain resources and providers of specialty care. It is likely that as understanding grows about the mechanisms of managed care, the value of psychiatric-mental health nurses and other mental health professionals will become increasingly apparent. As this chapter is being written, third-party payers are beginning to solicit advanced practice psychiatric-mental health nurses to become preferred providers; in states such as Washington that

authorize prescriptive privileges for advanced practice psychiatric nurses, community mental health centers are increasingly employing these professionals.

With health care reform likely to organize around a primary care model, psychiatric nursing must position itself strategically between the specialty care and primary care needs of its clients. The capacity of the psychiatric-mental health nurse to assess and manage the mental health care needs and many of the physical health care needs of the consumer in a culturally acceptable context positions the profession well for the health care industry transitions ahead (Talley & Caverly, 1994; Worley, Drago, & Hadley, 1990; Aiken, 1987; Talley, 1988). Valentine (1995) predicts greater role autonomy for nurses who have higher levels of skill, which suggests an educational shift and a role shift for psychiatric nursing. These efforts are already underway: several university programs have begun to prepare psychiatric nurse practitioners (for example, the University of Washington, University of Virginia, and University of Pittsburgh).

Changes in modality in the 1990s have highlighted the necessity for nursing to retain the authority to define its practice. The 1990s also have been a time when "turf protection" activities such as efforts to restrict the practice of other mental health specialties have sporadically occurred in a reactive mode. It is interesting to observe nursing striving for ownership of its professional role at the same time as it is becoming an active participant in the discourse framing the role limitations of other groups. Although it is not the purpose of this chapter to enter the debate surrounding the scope of other disciplines, several points relate directly to understanding the new roles that have become available to psychiatric mental health nurses (for example, prescriptive authority and the role of the attending nurse in inpatient settings). The survival of psychiatric-mental health nursing, the rationality and viability of the current credentialing and licensing process, and the expansion of role capacities for all psychiatric-mental health nurses need to fit the needs of consumers and the community. These issues are relevant for nursing education, practice arenas, and the health policy domain (Aiken & Salmon, 1994; Safriet, 1994).

The survival of the psychiatric-mental health specialty has been a topic of discussion in the literature for a number of years (Martin, 1985). The fact that this concern has existed over time reflects its resilience. However, the current issue of survival is different in nature from past crises. In the past difficulties were related to dwindling enrollment in psychiatric nursing graduate programs and the small numbers of nurses choosing to work with mentally ill clients. The current question of survival is related to the professional niche of the psychiatric-mental health nurse. Preparation, credentialing, and licensing will all be required for survival.

Nursing and the public boards regulating nursing have long relied on licensing and certification to maintain standards of competence. Nursing has been relatively successful in gaining the power to define the profession's standards, if not to define the legal scope of practice. Title protection statutes have prevented those who are not nurses from practicing what the statutes designate as nursing. In recent years this title protection has eroded as other professional and paraprofessional groups

have gained the capacity to define alternative practices and legislate the scope of those practices. Some of these groups have practice scopes quite similar to nursing. In some cases alternative provider categories have been developed to cope with a perceived shortage of nurses, to reduce the cost of services, or to avoid empowering the independent practitioner by delegating powers to an ancillary medical provider with a dependent and directed scope of practice.

One example of a role that overlaps with psychiatric-mental health nursing is that of the chemical dependency counselor. This counseling specialty has become prevalent in the community mental health setting. The historical separation of chemical dependency programs from traditional mental health treatment has come under increased scrutiny. In particular, evidence suggests that failing to deal with both the substance abuse and the mental health diagnoses of clients with a dual diagnosis diminishes treatment response. The integration of mental health care and substance abuse care must be a primary focus of treatment planning for this difficult-to-treat population. It also is evident that requiring some standardized program of study for individuals who seek to become chemical dependency counselors is important in providing safe client care. However, when these providers seek licensure in their respective states, debate arises regarding what effect such licenses (complete with title protection) might have on the practice of nurses who assume substance abuse treatment roles. Analyses of consumer safety and scope of practice for other, newer professions must be conducted in a context that acknowledges the intent of nursing to maintain or expand its scope of practice.

The most recent challenge to the roles of psychiatric-mental health nursing lies in the regulatory movement to license by competency rather than by profession. The significant feature of this model of licensing is the lack of specified professional preparation. Nursing would no longer have title protection; it is impossible to predict whether the philosophy that directs nursing education and practice would retain pertinence. The historical efforts of nursing to gain legitimacy by credentialing and the regulatory process would become anachronistic, and the definition of practice constructed in the past could become irrelevant. The model of licensing by competency represents only one possible regulatory alternative that has the potential to simultaneously remove barriers to practice and professional entry and challenge professions to reconsider (and perhaps to justify) the costly and previously mandated preparation for a specified health care practice. An obvious advantage for nursing is the potential for the opening of advanced practice doors that have long been closed or only half opened. One such opportunity would be the granting of prescriptive authority in states in which it had not previously been extended to advanced practice psychiatric nurses (Talley & Brooke, 1992). It also would extend the inconsistent achievement of third-party reimbursement for advanced practice psychiatric nursing services to additional states (Pearson, 1995).

An increased state-to-state consistency of regulation would perhaps rectify "the state by state diversity [that] has resulted in a patchwork of licensing laws and a national fragmentation of nursing titles and practice boundaries" (Carson, 1993). Alternative models such as licensing by competence may or may not improve on existing licensing systems.

EDUCATION AND LEVEL OF PRACTICE

Psychiatric nursing has evolved from an educational system influenced by nursing, psychology, social science, behavioral science, social work, and biological perspectives of mental illness and mental health care. The philosophical differences among these disciplines shape and enrich the practice of psychiatric nursing and the nurse's values and beliefs about mental illness. Interventions are logical extensions of philosophy.

Shifting values and practice opportunities have significantly influenced psychiatric nursing in the last decade. Independent practice has become a more limited option because of managed care contracts, requirements for affiliations with and referrals from primary care, and the need to maintain a wide range of interventions within a practice setting. Prescriptive authority has become available to advanced practice psychiatric nurses in certain states. This practice opportunity brings with it a need for physical health care expertise and integration of psychotherapy with pharmacotherapy or somatic therapy. It is the general assumption of the authors that scope of practice is legitimately based in academic preparation and professional credentialing.

Revisiting the philosophical tenets of psychiatric nursing and the psychiatric mental health specialty may help determine how these underpinnings can be retained during the discipline's process of transformation. The destabilization caused by the shifting health care environment will either result in immobilization or act as a catalyst for growth and attainment of goals. The specialty of psychiatric-mental health nursing has been an innovative force in the nursing profession in the past and is perhaps the best situated of the specialties to lead the way to the future. The multidisciplinary nature of the health care reform discourse is a good fit with the way in which psychiatric-mental health nursing in the community has evolved and defined itself and its many subspecialties. The educational process must provide a strong nursing foundation and promote the development of not only clinical skills that meet the challenges of today, but also the critical thinking abilities practitioners need for the unanticipated role responsibilities of the future, and an understanding of the political and social environments in which health care is delivered.

LEVELS OF ACADEMIC PREPARATION AND TITLES
Psychiatric nursing technician

Any discussion of educational preparation for psychiatric-mental health nurses must include a discussion of the preparation of paraprofessionals who practice under the supervision of nurses. In most instances the training of psychiatric nurse's aides, assistants, or technicians occurs in a certificate community college program or on site at the facility of employment. Education is focused on terminology and procedure rather than on philosophy, foundation knowledge, or professional decision making. The paraprofessional role is modeled after the nursing assistant role in the inpatient medical surgical unit or the hospital. Psychiatric nursing technicians were first employed by psychiatric institutions and community hospitals with psychiatric wards (Gleeson et al., 1992).

Increasingly psychiatric nursing technicians are finding employment in the community mental health system and in the home health care system. Community resources often dictate the extent to which psychiatric nursing technicians are present in these settings. Other factors that influence the use of nonlicensed personnel over licensed professionals is the degree to which the job has a therapeutic impact on the care of the client. If the goal or potential for change is minimal, the level of care borders more closely on a custodial care model. Unfortunately, these decisions are often made without fully appreciating how the expertise of a professional may alter a seemingly custodial role and produce better than expected outcomes.

Case manager

Perhaps the most debated position in community mental health has been that of the case manager. This position has evolved from the deinstitutionalization movement and the need to better manage the care of clients with chronic mental illness in the community. Universal agreement has never been achieved regarding the scope of practice of case managers and the level of education they need. On one end of the spectrum, a case manager is viewed as a therapist, an outreach provider of care, and a maintainer of the most fragile clients in the community. However, in other situations the role is considered administrative; managers help clients adjust to community living, gain benefits, and get to appointments (Maurin, 1990). The latter view of case management is quite common and psychiatric technicians are often hired to fulfill this role. There is no title protection for the case manger role; the role reflects community economics and administrative dictates.

Licensed practical nurse

The next formal level of nursing educational preparation is that of the licensed practical nurse. These nurses have been educated in academic or vocational programs that have an average duration of 18 months. The licensed practical nurse provides nursing care grounded in the theory of health science, physiology, and anatomy, and in practical experience providing bedside care under the direction of a registered nurse.

The degree to which licensed practical nurses function independently rather than under the direct supervision of a registered nurse varies according to the situation. In some geographic or institutional settings little distinction may be made between the role expectations an employer places on a licensed practical nurse as opposed to a registered nurse. State licensing statutes also differ according to the scope of practice granted to a licensed practical nurse. Some states place limitations on the authority to administer medications or intravenous therapies or require a procedure for the licensed practical nurse to meet a standard of competency in pharmacology that permits the administration of medication. There is no certification in psychiatric mental health available at this level of education.

Registered nurse

The title *registered nurse* applies to nurses who are eligible for and successfully complete the national licensing examination that is the prerequisite to state licensure as a registered nurse. The educational preparation of the registered nurse may be a diploma in nursing from a hospital-based school of nursing, an associate degree in nursing from a 2-year school, a 4-year baccalaureate degree in nursing, or a 5-year baccalaureate degree in nursing. This variety of educational levels for entry into the profession as a registered nurse has had both positive and negative effects.

Health care reform will produce an increased need for nursing expertise within hospital settings, home care, and community networks (Aiken & Salmon, 1994). Nurses working in these settings will require higher educational degrees and training, expanded practice scope, and a focus on the community to provide preventive and episodic care. In psychiatric nursing these demands will be even more pronounced as high levels of psychopathology coupled with coexisting social, economic, and physical health problems among people with severe and persistent mental illness are increasingly encountered. Psychiatric nurses trained at the baccalaureate level are educationally and philosophically positioned to care for the mentally ill consumers with the greatest needs.

Master's degree prepared psychiatric-mental health nurse

The master's degree in psychiatric-mental health nursing is the academic requirement for practice as a clinical specialist in psychiatric-mental health nursing. This specialty is in transition as the profession adds curriculum content and clinical practice in areas that will expand the scope of practice under the title of nurse practitioner. Three primary factors have been instrumental in this transition. The first is prescriptive authority. Although most states regulate prescribing by nurses according to area of expertise, there remains a need to understand drug interactions, physical health problems, and management of untoward effects. Thus greater expectation is placed on the advanced practice psychiatric nurse to understand physiological and medical procedures associated with prescribing (Talley & Brooke, 1992).

Second, there is a long documented history of physical health problems in the psychiatric client population (Worley et al., 1990; Talley, 1988). The motivational and behavioral problems of these clients often interfere with their ability to use health care services or obtain appropriate care from their health care providers. To this end, advanced practice psychiatric nurses should articulate interventions that will address primary, secondary, and tertiary prevention of health problems within their constituencies.

Third, public awareness of the nurse practitioner title and role has increased, but the term *clinical specialist* remains largely unknown and many of the clinical specialist's functions are presumed to be consultative or educational. Shifting to a more identifiable title may help produce public recognition. However, in states in which nurse practitioner practice is more restrictive than the practice of the clinical specialist, legitimate concern persists regarding the potential for loss of autonomy and access to third-party reimbursement.

Doctoral preparation

Psychiatric-mental health nurses who choose to seek doctoral education do so in a number of ways. Anthropology, psychology, sociology, or even an individual PhD program of study have been common discipline choices for psychiatric-mental health nurses. This breadth of knowledge has greatly enriched nursing and has been in keeping with the role it has taken in interpreting specialized information for the consumer. The varied expertise within nursing academe permits collaborative work with other professions and prepares nurses to interact in arenas that might otherwise be closed to an outside discipline.

Increasingly nurses are pursuing education through an academic research pathway leading to the PhD or through a more clinically focused program of study leading to a D.N.Sc. Unlike in the master's level of education, the area of specialization or subspecialization is only rarely designated in the focus of the program. Nurses prepared at the doctoral level practice in academic settings, mental health regulatory agencies, private corporations, and private practices or as consultants.

PROFESSIONAL LICENSURE AND CREDENTIALING

Psychiatric-mental health nurse

The American Nurses Association recognizes only two levels of psychiatric-mental health clinical nursing practice: the basic level of specialization and the advanced level of specialization. The basic level may be attained by nurses with baccalaureate degrees in nursing and is described in the 1994 Statement on Psychiatric Mental Health Nursing (ANA Council of Psychiatric and Mental Health Nursing et al., 1994):

> The Psychiatric Mental Health Nurse is a licensed RN who has a baccalaureate degree in nursing and demonstrated clinical skills, within the specialty, exceeding those of a beginning RN or novice in the specialty. The designation Psychiatric Mental Health Nurse applies only to those nurses who are certified within the specialty and who meet the profession's standards of knowledge and experience. Certification is the formal process that validates the nurse's clinical competence. The national certifying body is the American Nurses Credentialing Center. The examination and the eligibility requirements are established in consultation with the American Nurses Association. The letter "C," placed after the RN (that is, RN, C) is the initial that designates basic-level certification status.

Psychiatric-mental health advanced practice nurse

The distinction between the credentialing of the Psychiatric-Mental Health Advanced Practice Nurse and the Certified Psychiatric-Mental Health Nurse lies in education, post-master's experience, and the certification test that the practitioner successfully completes. The American Nurses Association describes the Psychiatric-Mental Health Advanced Practice Nurse as a licensed RN who is educationally prepared at the master's level (at a minimum) and is nationally certified as a clinical specialist in psychiatric and mental health nursing (ANA Council of Psychiatric and Mental Health Nursing et al., 1994).

In 1994 master's or doctorally prepared psychiatric-mental health nurses were required to have an advanced degree in nursing rather than in a related field, and to have obtained the required clinical supervision from an advanced practice psychiatric nurse. Currently there are Clinical Specialist examinations in adult psychiatric-mental health nursing and in child and adolescent psychiatric-mental health nursing. Many Psychiatric-Mental Health Advanced Practice Nurses become certified for both populations; however, the position of the ANA and American Nurses Credentialing Committee (ANCC) is that the nurse need only become certified for advanced practice in one area. The Clinical Specialist will presumably then develop clinical expertise not dependent on the original certification. The responsibility for acquiring subspecialty knowledge to practice in another population lies with the professional nurse.

National certification for psychiatric-mental health advanced practice nursing is a voluntary process at this time. However, it is required by some states that recognize psychiatric-mental health advanced practice nursing. In these states Psychiatric-Mental Health Advanced Practice Nurses may be allowed an expanded scope of practice under the title of Clinical Specialist or may be required to apply for a second license as an Advanced Registered Nurse Practitioner. In either case the scope of practice is usually consistent with the statement developed in 1994 by the American Nurses Association.

SUMMARY

This chapter has provided an overview of factors that have contributed to the current roles open to psychiatric-mental health nurses at all levels of practice and education throughout the United States. It focused on the formal processes of education, credentialing, and licensure that influence the roles available to and embraced by nurses. Specific population issues are addressed elsewhere in this book, but location of practice has been identified as an important aspect of the roles individual nurses will play or have imposed on them. Issues of professional territories and boundaries have been addressed only superficially in this chapter, but the reader is encouraged to look further. Although a number of other topics are relevant to the roles of psychiatric-mental health nurses in the community, this chapter has considered only the discourse related to the "proper" role of the advanced practice psychiatric nurse. The political nature of the advanced practice role and the internal and external harmony or discord that will no doubt chart the future of the role will be attended to in the summary of this chapter.

In earlier sections the struggle to define the psychiatric nursing role within the profession rather than by the authority of regulatory boards was articulated, as was the necessity for the psychiatric-mental health nurse in advanced practice in the community (or in the acute care setting) to be able to meet not only the psychiatric needs but also many of the physical health care needs of mental health clients. However, this is not so easily accomplished as the words imply. The psychiatric nursing community is engaged in debate regarding the boundaries that should be imposed on the practice of psychiatric-mental health nursing. The option for prescriptive authority in many states has fueled this discussion and at times has led to polarization regarding the appropriateness of nurses providing health care services traditionally provided by physicians. More recently the competition between the terms *clinical specialist* and *nurse practitioner* has been a focal point for identifying the direction in which psychiatric-mental health advanced practice nursing should move.

One perspective contends that for the profession to flourish there must be loyalty and safeguarding of traditional nursing roles rather than a subsuming of historical medical roles into the evolving nursing tradition. Such a standpoint is supported by a desire to retain the traditional values and terrain of the nursing profession. It is similar to the view that asserts that nursing must retain the privileged role granted through the nurse practice acts that provide the discipline with title protection (Lego & Caverly, 1995).

The opposite viewpoint distinguishes the values that have strengthened and sustained the profession and led to the development of the myriad roles that serve a diverse population. However, even while recognizing the roots of the profession that have been so positive and influential, there must be an incorporation of the reality of a changing environment in keeping with the notion of flexibility discussed earlier in this chapter. This will provide a mechanism for retaining the primary characteristics of the profession while meeting community need and recognizing that health care practice for professionals and consumers alike is in a state of reconstruction.

The title *Nurse Practitioner* is a symbol of the internal debate regarding the proper role for Psychiatric-Mental Health Advanced Practice Nurses. The assumption of a clear title that carries with it the message that health care is the service offered to the public has a strong appeal for nurses who see a need to become more closely allied with other advanced practice nurses, and for nurses who desire a user-friendly term through which consumers can identify a potential care provider. However, because this title also carries with it a history of being conferred on a lesser educated group of professional nurses, it can be perceived as unacceptable. Furthermore, it can be mistakenly seen as mandating that all Psychiatric-Mental Health Advanced Practice Nurses provide hands-on physical care. This, were it true, would be cause enough for the title to be rejected, because a great many nurses would require extensive retooling to accommodate such a role. The nature of nursing is to meet all expectations; therefore a resistance to imposing onerous expectations will be felt by many advanced practice nurses.

Any requirement for the provision of physical health care by advanced practice psychiatric nurses must be reframed in this debate. It must be made clear that the expectation that a psychiatric nursing expert provide physical health care is limited by the individual's scope of knowledge, skill, and ability. Such a reframing removes institutional barriers to a practice that best suits the client's needs, but it does not press nurses to perform beyond their individual capacities. Professional standards for Psychiatric-Mental Health Advanced Practice Nurses hold them accountable if they practice beyond their abilities. However, the mandate inherent in assuming the practice of prescribing somatic interventions clearly holds a nurse accountable for the skills required to perform these interventions. The ability to perform a health assessment and manage the physiological aspects of pharmacological or other somatic therapy is certainly a reasonable expectation for nurses who elect to practice this expanded role (Lego & Caverly, 1995).

The debate swirling around the nurse's title rather than around the reframing of the issue as given in the above example represents a potential threat to the future of the profession. However, this does not imply that some titles are not likely to have tremendous positive or negative impact; evidence currently indicates that titles do influence the practice scope recognized by state licensing regulation. Rather, significant damage may result from the fragmentation of the collective, and produce a weaker body less capable of promoting the growth and development of the psychiatric-mental health nursing profession. Such a splintering is similar to those that occurred in the past between the educational levels or the specialties within nursing.

The difficulties of maintaining a coalition of nurses are increased in the community setting, where there is a greater multidisciplinary team approach to care, and frequently less nurse-to-nurse interaction. In such environments nurses can begin to negate the distinct characteristics of the nursing discipline and more easily distance themselves from the collective body. Thus the critical mass of nurses necessary to promote nursing and challenge the boundaries and barriers to nursing practice may eventually become inadequate to move the profession forward.

Socialization to the profession, the educational system, the credentialing or licensing processes, the population of interest, and the geography of practice are all important aspects of the roles nurses assume in the community mental health setting. However, it may well be the capacity for maintaining an actively invested and coalesced body of professionals that will define the future viability and enactment of psychiatric-mental health nursing roles in the community. The fact that this is a property over which nursing holds control is a cause for both celebration and conviction on the part of every psychiatric-mental health nurse.

REFERENCES

Aiken, L. H. (1987). Unmet needs of the chronically mentally ill: Will nursing respond? *Image–The Journal of Nursing Scholarship, 19,* 121-125.

Aiken, L. H., & Salmon, M. E. (1994). Health care workforce priorities: What nursing should do now. *Inquiry, 31,* 318-329.

American Nurses Association. (1994). *Psychiatric mental health nursing psychopharmacology project.* Washington, DC: Author.

American Nurses Association Council of Psychiatric and Mental Health Nursing, American Psychiatric Nursing Association, Association of Child and Adolescent Psychiatric Nurses, & Society for Education and Research in Psychiatric-Mental Health Nursing. (1994). *A statement on psychiatric and mental health clinical nursing practice and standards of psychiatric mental health clinical nursing practice.* Washington, DC: Author.

American Psychological Association (APA) Office of Rural Health. (1995). *Caring for the rural community: Interdisciplinary curriculum.* Washington, DC: Author.

Armour, P. K. (1981). *The cycles of social reform.* Washington, DC: University Press of America.

Carmichael, F. A., & Chapman, J. (1936). *A guide to psychiatric nursing.* Philadelphia, PA: Lea & Febiger.

Carson, W. (1993). *Prescriptive practice in the 1990s: A crazy quilt of overregulation.* Unpublished manuscript, Nurse Practice Council, American Nurses Association, Washington, DC.

Chamberlain, J. G. (1987). Update on psychiatric-mental health nursing education at the federal level. *Archives of Psychiatric Nursing, 12,* 132-138.

Foley, H. A. (1975). *Community mental health legislation: The formative process.* Lexington, MA: Lexington Books.

Gleeson, S., Metz, E., McEachen, I., & Sklar, R. (1992). The psychiatric technician: Trespasser or welcomed ally? *Journal of Psychosocial Nursing and Mental Health Services, 30*(12), 28-31.

Lego, S., & Caverly, S. (1995). Point of view: Coming to terms—Psychiatric nurse practitioner versus clinical nurse specialist. *Journal of the American Psychiatric Nursing Association, 1,* 63-65.

Lehman, F. (1995). Consultation liaison psychiatric nursing care. In G. Stuart, & S. Sundeen (Eds.), *Principles and practice of psychiatric nursing* (5th ed.). St. Louis: Mosby.

Lowery, B. (1992). Psychiatric nursing in the 1990s and beyond. *Journal of Psychosocial Nursing and Mental Health Services, 30*(1) 7-13.

Martin, E. J. (1985, January/February). A specialty in decline? Psychiatric-mental health nursing, past, present, and future. *Journal of Professional Nursing,* 48-53.

Maurin, J. T. (1990). Case management: Caring for psychiatric clients. *Journal of Psychosocial Nursing and Mental Health Services, 28*(7), 6-12.

McBride, A. B. (1990). Psychiatric nursing in the 1990s. *Archives of Psychiatric Nursing, 4,* 21-28.

Mechanic, D., & Rochefort, D. A. (1990). Deinstitutionalization: An appraisal of reform. *Annual Review of Sociology, 16,* 301-327.

National Institute of Mental Health. (1985). *Psychiatric mental health proceedings.* Washington, DC: Author.

National Institute of Mental Health. (1987). *Report of the task force on nursing.* Washington, DC: Author.

Pearson, L. J. (1995). Annual update of how each state stands on legislative issues affecting advanced nursing practice: The nurse practitioner. *The American Journal of Primary Health Care, 20*(1), 13-51.

Peplau, H. E. (1989). Future directions in psychiatric nursing from the perspective of history. *Journal of Psychosocial Nursing, 27*(2), 18-28.

Pothier, P., Stuart, G., Puskar, K., & Babich, K. (1990). Dilemmas and directions for psychiatric nursing in the 1990s. *Archives of Psychiatric Nursing, 4,* 284-291.

Safriet, B. J. (1992). Health care dollars and regulatory sense: The role of advanced practice nursing. *Yale Journal of Regulation, 9*(1), 417-487.

Safriet, B. J. (1994). Impediments to progress in health care workforce policy: License and practice laws. *Inquiry, 31,* 310-317.

Sands, I. J. (1941). *Nervous and mental diseases for nurses* (4th ed.). Philadelphia, PA: W.B. Saunders Company.

Talley, S. (1988). Basic health care needs of the mentally ill: Issues for psychiatric nursing. *Issues in Mental Health Nursing, 9,* 409-423.

Talley, S., & Brooke, P. S. (1992). Prescriptive authority for psychiatric clinical specialists: Framing the issues. *Archives of Psychiatric Nursing, 4*(2), 71-82.

Talley, S., & Caverly, S. (1994). Advanced practice psychiatric nursing and health care reform. *Hospital and Community Psychiatry, 45,* 545-547.

Titlebaum, H., Hart, C., & Romano, E. (1992). Interagency psychiatric consultation nursing peer review and peer board quality assurance and empowerment. *Archives of Psychiatric Nursing, 6,* 125.

Valentine, N. (1995). Policy partners—Nursing and psychiatry in the capital: An interview with Dr. Mary Jane England [Interview]. *Journal of the American Psychiatric Nursing Association, 1*(3), 76-82.

Worley, N., Drago, L., & Hadley, T. (1990). Improving the physical health—mental health interface for the chronically mentally ill: Could nurse case managers make a difference? *Archives of Psychiatric Nursing, 4,* 108-113.

Unit 4

Intervention in the Community

Chapter 7

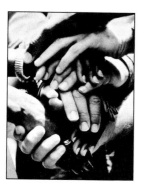

Basic Assessment Skills

Nancy K. Worley and Elizabeth A. Huggins

Thorough and effective assessment of the biological, psychological, social, and cultural components of an individual or family is the foundation of client care. During assessment, the nurse fashions a therapeutic alliance, makes a diagnosis, estimates the severity of the problem, and initiates a treatment plan. Although a mental health assessment may occur in a traditional office setting, it also may occur in the home, in an emergency room, in a homeless shelter, or even on the streets. It may take some creativity on the part of the psychiatric nurse to conduct an assessment interview in the stressful environment of some of these settings. The nurse should try to find a quiet place with as little sensory stimulation as possible under the conditions.

Members of the Coalition of Psychiatric Nursing Organizations, under the leadership of the American Nurses Association's (ANA) Council on Psychiatric and Mental Health Nursing, produced standards of psychiatric-mental health clinical nursing practice (ANA, 1994). Standards relating to assessment include the following:

- Eliciting the client's central complaint, symptom, or focus of concern

- Assessing the physical, developmental, cognitive, mental, and emotional health of the client
- Assessing family, social, cultural, and community systems
- Gathering data on daily activities, functional health status, alcohol and drug use, health habits, and social role functioning
- Exploring interpersonal relationships, communication skills, and coping patterns
- Understanding spiritual and philosophical beliefs, including the client's health beliefs and values
- Discerning economic, political, legal, and environmental factors affecting health
- Evaluating significant support systems
- Assessing strengths and competencies
- Assessing the client's ability to remain safe and not be a danger to self and others
- Collecting pertinent data from many sources using assessment techniques and standardized instruments as appropriate

Diagnostic skills include:

- Devising diagnoses and potential problem statements from assessment data

---

Box 7-1. Guidelines for effective interviewing

1. Do not use a set speech; each person is different.
2. Sit down and establish eye contact if possible and appropriate.
3. Avoid asking questions that can be answered "yes" or "no." Try broad, open-ended statements such as "Tell me what you think about. . . ."
4. Learn how to listen and observe. When silence occurs, allow for it.
5. Respond appropriately, but make sure the client also has time to talk.
6. Monitor your own thoughts; they may mirror the client's.
7. Always ask yourself what the client was like before the client became ill.
8. Use timely, informative, and evocative questions such as:
   - What has bothered you most about this illness?
   - How has it been a problem for you?
   - What have you done (or what are you doing) about the problem?
   - What has been the most difficult thing you've had to face until now? What did you do then?
   - Whom do you rely on most or expect will be most helpful to you?
   - In general, how do things normally turn out for you?
   - What do you think about this whole situation?
9. Include family members or significant others in your assessment.
10. Remember, above all, you have human dignity and so does your client.
11. Be respectful. Regardless of the client's condition, the client deserves to be treated with courtesy.
12. Ask clients how they want to be addressed. Never use a client's first name unless invited to do so.

- Identifying interpersonal, systemic, or environmental circumstances that affect the well-being of the individual, family, or community
- Using accepted classification systems such as NANDA Nursing Diagnosis Classification and the *Diagnostic and Statistical Manual of Mental Disorders* (*DSM-IV*), in the practice setting
- Documenting diagnoses and clinical impressions in a manner that facilitates the identification of client outcomes

This chapter describes interviewing techniques and tools nurses can use to assess clients and families and diagnose actual or potential psychiatric illnesses and mental health problems. Chapter 5, Levels of Prevention, describes techniques and tools for assessing communities.

INDIVIDUAL CLIENT ASSESSMENT

Psychiatric interview

A psychiatric interview consists of a psychiatric history and mental status examination. Skill in interviewing and observation will allow the nurse to obtain much of the information needed for the history and mental status examination during the interview itself, thus keeping formal questions to a minimum. Box 7-1 provides a review of basic interviewing procedure.

Psychiatric history

The psychiatric history allows clients to tell their life stories in their own words from their points of view. Obtaining a careful and comprehensive client history (including if necessary information from other informed sources) is essential to making a correct diagnosis and formulating a specific and effective treatment plan. A comprehensive psychiatric history will reveal the client's personality characteristics, including strengths and weaknesses; it will provide insight into the client's relationships with those close to the client and include all important people in the client's past and present. An important technique in obtaining a psychiatric history is to allow clients to tell their stories in their

---

> **Box 7-2.** Components of the psychiatric history
>
> - Identification
> - Chief complaint
> - History of present illness
> - Past medical and psychiatric history
> - Past personal history
> - Family history

---

own words in the order they feel is most important (Kaplan & Sadock, 1994). The following sections present the traditional order in which the psychiatric history is recorded and can be used as a guide to write up the history after the interview. Box 7-2 lists components of a psychiatric history. Appendix B provides a more detailed guide to the psychiatric history and mental status examination.

Identifying data

This information identifies and describes the client by name, age, marital status, gender, occupation, native language (if first language is other than English), ethnic background, religion, and current living circumstances. The information also can include the place or circumstance in which the interview occurs and whether this is the first episode of its type for the client. Identifying data should provide a thumbnail sketch that people can read and get a picture of the client in their minds. An example of information gathered in an identifying data interview follows.

J. T. is a 60-year-old African-American woman brought to the emergency room by the police, who found her wandering in the middle of a busy city street. She is unkempt, dirty, and foul smelling. Although she knows her name, she is otherwise unresponsive and apparently confused.

The chief complaint

The chief complaint, in the client's own words, states why the client has come or been brought in for help. The client's explanation, no matter how bizarre or seemingly irrelevant, should be recorded verbatim. Examples of chief complaints include the following:

- "I was feeling very depressed and thinking of killing myself"
- "I've been receiving coded messages from television programs revealing a plot to kill the President, and I thought someone else should know about this"
- "I've been having pains in my stomach and my doctor said I should come here to have some tests done"

Each of these examples should alert the interviewer to pay particular attention to certain parts of the interview and mental status examination. In the first example, the interviewer must carefully assess for suicidal intent and decide whether the client should be hospitalized for safety reasons. In the second example, the interviewer immediately becomes alert to the possibility of a thought disorder. The third example is somewhat more complex, but because the client was referred to a mental health professional by a general medical physician, the interviewer should probe for a history of somatization. However, the nurse should not jump to conclusions, but should instead consult the referring physician and obtain information about physical examinations and laboratory tests already conducted.

History of present illness

The history of the present illness should answer the following questions:

- Why now?
- What immediate precipitating events triggered the current episode?
- In what ways has the current illness affected life activities such as work and interpersonal relationships?
- How is the current dysfunction manifested?
- Are there psychophysiological symptoms such as changes in patterns of eating, sleeping, and elimination?

- Have there been major life events during this time, or particular stresses or conflicts?

In a well-organized client, the question "how did this begin?" will elicit a chronological history of the present difficulty. However, in a disorganized client, the chronology will be less clear; it will take skillful interviewing to get a clear picture. This is an excellent point in the interview to explore coping behaviors and strategies. How did the client attempt to manage the situation? What are some ways in which the client has managed distress in the past?

Past medical and psychiatric history

The past medical history should include major medical illnesses, surgeries, and traumas, particularly those requiring hospitalization. Episodes of head trauma, neurological illness, tumors, and seizure disorders are particularly relevant. Interviewers should ask all clients about drug and alcohol use, including quantity and frequency of use. In gauging alcohol use, it is better to ask how many drinks the client has in a typical week than to ask if the client drinks. Asking the question in this way is less judgmental and takes for granted that most people drink socially. A well-recognized screening tool for alchoholism is the Michigan Alcoholism Screening Test (MAST), which is found in Appendix G.

After the medical history, the nurse should ask about any previous psychiatric hospitalizations or encounters with the mental health system. If the client has a past psychiatric history, is the current episode similar to or different from past episodes? What were the frequency and duration of past episodes?

Past personal history

The past personal history is usually divided into the major developmental periods of early and middle childhood, adolescence, and adulthood. The predominant emotions associated with different life periods should be noted. The depth of examination of each developmental stage will depend on the client's age, the time available, and the situation.

Early childhood.   If the client is a young child, more emphasis will be put on information from the prenatal and perinatal periods and very early childhood, most of which will have to be supplied by family members. For adolescents and adults, past history usually begins with middle childhood (from about 3 to 10 years of age). The client's recollection of interactions with parents and siblings is of primary importance. What kinds of punishments were used in the home? Who was the disciplinarian? Early childhood experiences, especially separation from mother or another caregiver, and earliest friendships also are important areas to explore.

Adolescence.   Major milestones in the adolescent client's developmental history usually revolve around school relationships, emerging sexuality, and experimentation with drugs and alcohol. This portion of the past history should include exploration of relationships with teachers and peers, and school interests and extracurricular activities. Feelings about the onset of puberty, preparation for adulthood by parents, attitudes toward the opposite sex, and sexual activity should be explored.

Adulthood.   This part of the history should include information on the client's occupational history, intimate relationships, and social activities. Exploration of the client's occupational history should include choice of occupation, work-related conflicts, long-term ambitions and goals, feelings about the current job, and relationships at work with peers, supervisors, and subordinates.

Relationship history includes a history of marriages or relationships with persons with whom the client has lived for a protracted period of time. The history of the evolution of each relationship and areas of agreement and disagreement (including money management, child rearing, in-laws, and the quality of the sexual relationship) should be explored.

Social activities should include a description of the client's social life and friendships, with an emphasis on the depth, duration, and quality of these friendships.

Family history

Family history should include any psychiatric illnesses, hospitalizations, and treatments of immediate family members. Any family history of alcoholism, drug abuse, or suicide should be elicited. The family history also should include the client's description of the personality of each individual who has lived in the client's home from childhood to present and the role each person has played in the client's childhood and upbringing. Later sections of this chapter will provide a detailed explanation of the methods and rationale for obtaining the family history.

Mental status examination

The mental status examination (MSE) is the psychological counterpart of the physical examination. It sums up the examiner's observations and impressions of the client during the interview and serves as a basis for diagnosis and psychodynamic understanding. The nurse gathers most of the information for the mental status examination through careful observation of the client's responses and behavior during the psychiatric history. Box 7-3 outlines areas to be assessed in the mental status examination.

Appearance, behavior, and attitude

The mental status examination starts with a general description of the client's appearance, behavior, activity, and attitude toward the examiner. The description should be detailed and specific enough to identify and characterize the client.

General appearance describes the client's appearance and the overall physical impression conveyed to the interviewer during the interview. Items the nurse should note in the appearance category include posture, poise, manner of dress, grooming, facial expression, eye contact, and general state of health and nutrition. Common terms

---

Box 7-3. Areas of assessment during a mental status examination

Appearance, behavior, and attitude
Mood and affect
Speech
Thought disturbances
Thought process
Thought content
Perception
Levels of consciousness and cognition
   Orientation
   Memory
   Concentration
   Abstract thinking
   Intellectual functioning
Impulse control
Judgment and insight
Reliability

---

used to describe appearance include healthy, sickly, ill at ease, poised, younger or older than stated age, disheveled, childlike, and bizarre.

Behavior and psychomotor activity refer to the qualitative and quantitative aspects of the client's motor activity. The nurse should include any mannerisms, tics, gestures, hyperactivity, agitation, combativeness, rigidity, gait, and unusual agility in the client's description. Restlessness, wringing of hands, pacing, psychomotor retardation, or general slowing down of movements also should be noted.

Attitude toward examiner can be described as cooperative, friendly, attentive, seductive, defensive, hostile, and evasive, among other terms. The level of rapport established should be recorded.

Mood and affect

Mood is pervasive and sustained emotion that colors a person's perception of the world. Statements about the client's mood should include depth, intensity, duration, and fluctuation. Common adjectives used to describe mood include depressed, angry, and euphoric. Mood may be labile, meaning that it fluctuates or alternates rapidly between extremes.

Affect is the outward manifestation of the client's feelings, tone, or mood. The examiner observes the client's affect in facial expression and body language. Affect may be blunted (emotional expression is reduced), flat (virtually no signs of affective expression—the face is immobile and the voice monotonous), or labile (fluctuating rapidly between extremes).

Speech

Speech can give important clues to the client's emotional state. Speech can be described in terms of quantity, rate of production, and quality. In describing quantity, the client may be talkative, unspontaneous, or normally responsive to cues from the examiner. Assessment of rate of production includes descriptors such as rapid, slow, pressured, or hesitant. Quality may be loud, whispered, slurred, or mumbled.

Thought disturbances

Thought is divided into form or process of thinking (the way in which a person puts together ideas and associations) and content of thoughts, which refers to what a person actually thinks about.

Thought process

The most important question to answer about thought process is whether the client's responses answer the questions asked. Does the client have the capacity for goal-directed thinking? Are responses relevant? Is there a clear cause and effect relationship in the client's explanations? Does the client have loose associations (the ideas expressed seem unrelated or connected in peculiar ways)? Disturbances in thought continuity may produce tangential, circumstantial, rambling, or evasive responses. Blocking (the interruption of thought before an idea is completed) may indicate inability to recall what has been said or what response was intended. Blocking also may be a symptom that hallucinations are interfering with the client's thoughts.

Thought content

Disturbances in thought content include delusions (fixed false beliefs), obsessions (persistent and irresistible thoughts, feelings, or impulses), compulsions (insistent, intrusive, and unwanted urges to perform acts contrary to one's ordinary wishes and standards), and recurrent ideas about suicide or homicide.

Assessing the potential for suicide or for assaultive and violent behavior should always be part of the mental status examination. Assessment of suicidal or homicidal behavior is always important, but is particularly crucial for the client being assessed in the community, where opportunities to carry out suicidal or homicidal plans are more readily available than in a hospital setting and the probability of discovery is less. Nurses should ask all clients about suicidal thoughts. Crucial variables in assessing the potential for suicide include the plan, the method, and the provision for rescue (Keltner, 1995). If the client admits to thoughts of suicide, a thorough exploration of any plans the client may have made to carry out the act must be explored, including the method being contemplated and whether the client has minimized the possibility of rescue. A well thought out suicide plan constitutes a psychiatric emergency and the nurse should take immediate steps to get the client to a safe and secure environment.

Homicidal thoughts are assessed in the same manner as suicidal thoughts. A statement of anger and hostility toward a person or group of people, or the blaming of a person or group of people for the client's situation, should be followed by asking the client if he or she has thoughts of harming another person. If the client answers positively, it is important to thoroughly assess any plan to carry out the act, and the method under contemplation. Legal decisions beginning with the *Tarasoff v. Regents of the University of California* case (1976) indicate that, when a person is foreseeably dangerous to another person, the therapist can (and in some cases must) breach the confidentiality of the therapist-client relationship to protect the third party. For a more detailed discussion of this matter, see Chapter 2, Legal and Ethical Issues.

Perception

Perception is the process by which sensory stimuli are brought to conscious awareness. This part of the mental status examination assesses for perceptual disorders. Hallucinations (sensory perceptions with no external stimuli) and illusions (misperceptions of external stimuli) are the most common perceptual disturbances seen in psychosis, and may be experienced in reference to self or the environment. The sensory systems involved (auditory, visual, tactile, olfactory) and the content of the perceptual experience should be described. Feelings of depersonalization (extreme detachment from oneself) and derealization (extreme detachment from the environment) are other examples of perceptual disturbances.

Level of consciousness and cognition

This part of the MSE assesses comprehension, memory, and reasoning.

Any alteration in the level of consciousness should be noted. The term *clouding of consciousness* describes an overall reduced awareness of the environment. Other terms to describe the client's level of consciousness include clouded, stupor, coma, and lethargy. The client who has an altered state of consciousness often shows some impairment in orientation as well.

Orientation. Orientation disorders are traditionally described in terms of time, person, place, and situation. Questions asked during the assessment interview will usually reveal any problems with orientation. The nurse ascertains orientation to time by asking the time of day, the day of the week, the month, the season, or the year. Questions regarding the client's address or city and state of residence will aid in ascertaining orientation to place. Orientation to person can be determined by asking for the client's name, the names of relatives, or the names or disciplines of health care profes-

sionals who have had frequent contact with the client. Orientation to situation can be determined by asking a question such as "Why are you here?"

Memory. Memory functions have traditionally been divided into four areas, and can be assessed according to the following criteria:

1. Immediate retention and recall   Ask the client to repeat three objects immediately after you have stated them; ask again 5 minutes later.
2. Recent memory   This criterion involves testing what the client remembers in the past few days. Ask clients what they had for breakfast this morning, or how long they have been in the hospital.
3. Recent past memory   This criterion involves memory of the past few months. Ask the client to recall recent news events. Who is President of the United States?
4. Remote memory   This criterion can be tested by asking for childhood data or important historical events that would have taken place while the client was young.

Concentration. A variety of conditions may impair a client's concentration. Anxiety, depression, organic mental disorder, and preoccupation with hallucinations will all affect the client's ability to concentrate. The nurse can test concentration by asking the client to subtract serial 7s from 100, a simple test that nevertheless requires concentration and cognitive capacity. Having clients repeat an increasingly difficult series of numbers is another way to test for concentration.

Abstract thinking. The ability to deal with concepts is a measure of cognitive functioning. Can clients explain the similarities among an apple, a pear, and a plum? Are the meanings of simple proverbs (A rolling stone gathers no moss; a bird in the hand is worth two in the bush) understood?

Intellectual functioning. The ability to measure intelligence accurately during the mental status examination is fraught with difficulty. However, the nurse can estimate intellectual function by comparing the client's fund of information and vocabulary to the client's cultural and educational background. Information and vocabulary are good indicators of underlying intelligence because they are relatively unaffected by any but the most severe psychiatric disorders, and they may be helpful in distinguishing mentally retarded adults (whose fund of information and vocabulary are poor) from those with mild or moderate dementia (whose fund of information and vocabulary are relatively good). The nurse often can estimate the client's fund of information and vocabulary during the interview. If uncertainty persists, the interviewer can ask the client to name the last five Presidents, five large cities in the United States, how many days in a week, and the number of eggs in a dozen. The nurse tests vocabulary by asking the client to give the meaning of a series of words or to use each word in a sentence. The words should be increasingly difficult.

Impulse control

Impulse control is the ability to think through one's actions and their consequences. Impulse control assessment is critical in ascertaining the client's awareness of socially appropriate behavior and in measuring the client's potential danger to self and others (Kaplan & Sadock, 1994). The nurse estimates impulse control from the psychiatric history and from the suicide/homicide assessment.

Judgment and insight

The nurse can often assess whether a client's judgment is impaired during the interview from the client's account of recent decisions. If this is not definitive, nurses should give the client some hypothetical situations and ask what the client would do. Examples of situations include:

- "You are sitting in a movie theater and you see a small fire start in one of the empty seats near you. No one else seems to notice. What do you do?"

- "You find a stamped, addressed envelope on the street. What would you do?"

Insight is the extent to which the client understands the origins, nature, and mechanisms of attitudes and behaviors. The degree of insight can usually be ascertained during the psychiatric interview. Clients who are puzzled by their situation or blame their difficulty entirely on external sources usually lack insight.

Reliability

The mental status examination ends with an estimate of the client's reliability and capacity to report information accurately. If serious question arises about the reliability of the information presented by the client, the nurse may have to verify the information through previous medical records or by interviewing family members or other significant people in the client's network.

Physical assessment

Clients with psychiatric illnesses are likely to have coexisting physical illnesses (Maricle et al., 1987; Hall et al., 1982) that go undiagnosed during outpatient psychiatric treatment (Koran, Sox, & Marton, 1989). A study of the prevalence of physical disorders among outpatients treated in Colorado's public mental health system revealed that 46% had physical conditions or laboratory test results warranting further medical evaluation. The study identified previously undiagnosed physical health problems in 20% of the screened clients (Bartsch, Shern, & Feinberg, 1990). A medical history, brief physical examination, and standard laboratory battery should be performed on all clients new to the mental health system.

Assessment of function

The ability to participate successfully in interpersonal relationships, function within a family or social group, perform useful work, maintain an independent existence, or attend to basic needs for food, shelter, and self-care is important in the assessment of clients living in the community. The most commonly used instrument for measuring functional status is the Global Assessment of Functioning (GAF) scale, which measures psychological, social, and occupational functioning on a scale that ranges from 100 (optimal functioning) to 0 (Endicott, Spitzer, & Fleiss, 1976). Because this instrument attempts to measure three aspects of functioning with one score, it is difficult to measure change in any one of these aspects independent of the other two. However, this scale is widely used and has the advantage of brevity. The scale is part of the multiaxial *DSM-IV* diagnosis and is found in Appendix C.

The Specific Level of Functioning (SLOF) assessment scale is a more detailed assessment instrument that measures directly observable behavioral functioning and daily living skills. This multidimensional rating instrument consists of 43 behavioral items that are scored on a five-point Likert-type scale. Items are grouped into six areas: physical functioning; personal care skills; interpersonal relationships; social acceptability; community living activities; and work skills. An additional item—a global "other"—gives the rater an opportunity to indicate areas of functioning not covered by the instrument that may be important for a particular client. Following this free response question is an item designed to capture the degree of confidence raters place on their own judgment, and an item encouraging raters to share the assessment with clients (Schneider & Struening, 1983). The SLOF scale is presented in Appendix D.

Diagnostic tools

Diagnostic and Statistical Manual of Mental Disorders (DSM)

Unlike in a hospital, where medical diagnosis is almost always under the purview of physicians, the diagnosis of a client's condition according to *DSM-IV* criteria is often the task of a mental health professional charged with primary responsibility for client assessment. Therefore mental health nurses must be familiar with the purpose and organization of the manual. For quick reference,

the classification of *DSM-IV* diagnoses is in Appendix A.

History of the Diagnostic and Statistical Manual of Mental Disorders

The first *Diagnostic and Statistical Manual of Mental Disorders* was published in 1951. It was influenced by the dramatic changes that had taken place in American psychiatry after World War II. During the war, psychiatrists observed that some men who had seemed emotionally stable would become psychotic after prolonged exposure to battle or after short exposure to particularly horrendous conditions. These observations led psychiatrists to think about mental illness in new ways. Observable environmental effects on the personality structure led to thinking that combined Freud's theory of personality and intrapsychic conflict with the more pragmatic and environmentally oriented mental hygiene movement, resulting in a psychosocial model of mental illness (Wilson, 1993). This new model made the following assumptions:

1. The boundary between mental wellness and mental illness is fluid; normal people can become ill if exposed to severe trauma.
2. Mental illness is conceived along a continuum of severity that extends from neurosis to borderline conditions to psychosis.
3. A mixture of noxious environment and psychic conflict causes mental illness.
4. The mechanisms by which mental illness emerges in the individual are psychologically mediated.

Although this model brought attention to the long-neglected influence of the environment on people's psychological well-being and laid the foundation for the community mental health movement of the 1960s, it had some severe drawbacks. If, as Menninger (1963) stated, mental illnesses were essentially the same in quality and differed only quantitatively, how is it possible to diagnose mental illness or communicate among professionals about clients in a common language?

Concern that the psychosocial model was impeding research and moving psychiatry away from its medical roots led to a call from a growing number of psychiatrists for explicit, descriptive, and rule-driven diagnostic criteria.

The publication of the *DSM-III* in 1980 was a landmark in the modern history of descriptive psychiatry. It provided a reliable diagnostic system to identify individuals with specific mental disorders based on readily observable psychiatric symptoms. Because it was descriptive in nature, it did not contain information about the causes of the various mental disorders unless the causes had been established and were readily accepted. The third edition was revised slightly in 1987 (*DSM-III-R*), and the fourth and latest edition was published in 1994 (*DSM-IV*). The manual is widely accepted as the standard for diagnosis of mental disorders and is used extensively for medical record keeping, for facilitating data collection and retrieval, and for reporting diagnostic data to third parties. The Health Care Financing Administration (HCFA) has mandated the use of these diagnoses for purposes of reimbursement for the Medicare system. Private insurers have followed suit, and almost all insurance companies currently require a *DSM* diagnosis for reimbursement.

Organization of the manual

DSM-IV disorders are grouped into 16 major diagnostic classes according to their shared phenomenological features (except for the Adjustment Disorders, which are grouped based on their common etiology). *DSM-IV* systematically describes each disorder, provides definitions and discussions of subtypes of the disorder, provides guidelines for recording it, and lists clinical features often associated with it. The manual also describes associated laboratory findings; associated physical examination findings; specific cultural, age, and gender features; prevalence; typical course of the illness; data on the frequency of the disorder among first-degree biological relatives; and assistance in making a differential diagnosis.

Multiaxial assessment

An important feature of the manual is a multiaxial assessment of the client's condition. Each axis refers to a different domain of information that may help the clinician plan treatment and predict outcome. Five axes are included in the assessment:

Axis I is used for reporting all disorders or conditions except personality disorders and mental retardation.

Axis II is used for reporting personality disorders and mental retardation.

Axis III is used for reporting current general medical conditions that are potentially relevant to the understanding or management of the individual's mental condition.

Axis IV is used for reporting psychosocial and environmental problems that may affect the diagnosis, treatment, and prognosis of mental disorders.

Axis V is used for reporting the clinician's judgment of the individual's overall level of functioning, using the Global Assessment of Functioning (GAF) scale (see Appendix C for the scale and instructions for its use).

A form developed by the authors of the *DSM-IV* for reporting a multiaxial assessment is reproduced in Figure 7-1. The following case example illustrates a multiaxial evaluation.

Case example

Michael is a 40-year-old single man who lives with his parents and is training to be a salesman in the insurance firm where he has worked for 20 years as an administrative assistant. He was referred to the psychiatric clinic by a cardiologist who could not find an organic basis for symptoms of cardiac distress such as palpitations, lightheadedness, chest pain, and diaphoresis. During the initial interview, Michael revealed that he had recently broken off an engagement to a woman his parents disapproved of. He was angry with his parents for interfering and felt their real motivation was to keep him at home with them. However, he also stated that they had more experience than he did and "probably knew best." He also

The following is offered as one possibility for reporting multiaxial evaluations. In some settings, this form may be used exactly as is; in other settings, the form may be adapted to satisfy special needs.

AXIS I: *Clinical Disorders*
            Other Conditions That May Be a Focus of Clinical Attention
Diagnostic code   *DSM-IV* name

— — —.— —   _____

— — —.— —   _____

— — —.— —   _____

AXIS II: *Personality Disorders*
             Mental Retardation
Diagnostic code   *DSM-IV* name

— — —.— —   _____

— — —.— —   _____

AXIS III: *General Medical Conditions*
ICD-9-CM code   ICD-9-CM name

— — —.— —   _____

— — —.— —   _____

— — —.— —   _____

AXIS IV: *Psychosocial and Environmental Problems*
Check:
☐   **Problems with primary support group.** *Specify:* _____
☐   **Problems related to the social environment.** *Specify:* _____
☐   **Educational problems.** *Specify:* _____
☐   **Occupational problems.** *Specify:* _____
☐   **Housing problems.** *Specify:* _____
☐   **Economic problems.** *Specify:* _____
☐   **Problems with access to health care services.** *Specify:* _____
☐   **Problems related to interaction with the legal system or crime.** *Specify:* _____
☐   **Other psychosocial and environmental problems.** *Specify:* _____

AXIS V: *Global Assessment of Functioning Scale Score:*   — — —
                            Time frame: _____

Figure 7-1.   *DSM-IV* form for multiaxial assessment.
(From *Diagnostic and Statistical Manual of Mental Disorders* (4th Ed.)(p. 34), by the American Psychiatric Association, 1994, Washington, DC: American Psychiatric Association.)

disclosed his unhappiness with his decision to enter the sales training program at his company, which he had done at the urging of his former fiancée. He feared that he didn't have the personality to be a salesman and felt anxious about the uncertainty of an income based on sales commissions. He felt trapped by his decision because he had resigned from his previous position with the company and would be facing unemployment if he were unable to complete the sales training program. He expressed anger at his former fiancée for "pushing" him into this decision and anger at himself for allowing others to make decisions for him.

Michael's symptoms are typical of panic attacks. Because he doesn't associate the attacks with particular situations or places, he doesn't demonstrate an agoraphobic component to the attacks.

His pattern of allowing others to make decisions for him and his reluctance to rely on his own judgment and abilities are severe enough to justify a diagnosis of dependent personality disorder. Michael's *DSM-IV* diagnosis would be as follows:

Axis I 300.01 Panic Disorder Without Agoraphobia

Axis II 301.6 Dependent Personality Disorder

Axis III None

Axis IV Threat of job loss

Axis V GAF 45 (current)

The *DSM-IV* contains more than 800 pages of text explaining diagnostic and coding procedures and has become the most common method by which mental health disciplines communicate. It is therefore essential that mental health professionals become familiar with this manual.

Several scales commonly used to aid diagnosis are included in the Appendixes. The Brief Psychiatric Rating scale (Overall & Gorham, 1962) (Appendix E) rates the severity of psychiatric symptoms after a brief unstructured interview. It also is useful to assess the effects of psychiatric treatment (Carmin & Ownby, 1994). The Hamilton Depression Rating scale (Hamilton, 1960) (Appendix F) measures the severity of depressive symptoms. The Global Assessment of Functioning (GAF) scale (Appendix C) measures psychological, social, and occupational functioning.

Nursing diagnosis

Although the *DSM-IV* is a useful diagnostic tool, it is less helpful in determining the type and intensity of treatment necessary to help a client in distress. In response to this, the nursing profession has developed a compendium of behaviorally based treatment descriptors. These descriptors, endorsed by the North American Nursing Diagnosis Association (NANDA), represent the first organized effort to systematically catalog client behaviors and link them to treatment intervention and outcome (Goodwin, Brown, & Deitz, 1992). The earlier case example can illustrate the differences in approach between diagnosis according to the *DSM-IV* and according to NANDA guidelines.

DSM-IV diagnostic criteria for panic disorder without agoraphobia (Axis I)

Recurrent unexpected panic attacks.

At least one of the attacks has been followed by 1 month (or more) of one (or more) of the following:

- Persistent concern about having additional attacks
- Worry about the implications of the attack or its consequences (e.g., losing control, having a heart attack, "going crazy")
- A significant change in behavior related to the attacks

Selected NANDA nursing diagnoses for panic disorder without agoraphobia

- Coping, ineffectual individual
- Fear (of possible loss of job)
- Anxiety (severe)

DSM-IV diagnostic criteria for dependent personality disorder (Axis II)

Pervasive and excessive need to be taken care of that leads to submissive and clinging behavior and fears of separation, beginning by early childhood and present in a variety of contexts, as indicated by five (or more) of the following:

- Difficulty making everyday decisions without an excessive amount of advice and reassurance from others
- Needs others to assume responsibility for most major areas of his or her life
- Has difficulty expressing disagreement with others because of fear of loss of support or approval (Do not include realistic fears of retribution)
- Has difficulty initiating projects or doing things on his or her own because of a lack of self-confidence in judgment of abilities rather than a lack of motivation or energy
- Goes to excessive length to obtain nurturance and support from others to the point of volunteering to do things that are unpleasant
- Feels uncomfortable or helpless when alone because of exaggerated fear of being unable to care for himself or herself

Selected NANDA nursing diagnoses for dependent personality disorder

- Decisional conflict
- Chronic low self-esteem
- Powerlessness (severe)
- Coping, ineffective individual
- Social interaction, impaired

The comparison of *DSM-IV* diagnosis with NANDA diagnosis illustrates the descriptive classification of symptom sets in medical diagnosis and the emphasis on behavioral alterations and coping deficits in nursing diagnosis.

FAMILY ASSESSMENT

Although it is always beneficial to understand a client's family history, it is especially important for the mental health nurse in the community. In the hospital the patient is (at least temporarily) separated from the family and attention is directed toward individual psychopathology. In the community mental health setting, however, nurses will often work closely with families. A family that has a severely and persistently mentally ill member, a family with a child recently diagnosed with attention deficit disorder, a family in which child abuse or neglect is suspected, a family with a history of domestic violence, and a family coping with a member who has Alzheimer's disease are examples of the types of families and problems that mental health nurses encounter in the community. Knowledge of the family's emotional system can be a powerful tool in organizing assessment data and planning treatment interventions.

Family theorists have many perspectives about the ways in which families organize and function, and derive assessment techniques from these theoretical perspectives. This section will use Natural Systems Theory (Bowen, 1971) as the theoretical framework for making a family assessment. This will allow for clarity and specificity in a limited amount of space.

Some key components of Natural Systems Theory include the following:

- An individual's emotional system is related to the emotional system to which he or she is connected.
- Understanding the stressors in a family system provides information on symptom development.
- All family emotional systems have a degree of chronic anxiety.
- Real or anticipated events create acute anxiety in a family's emotional system.
- Families have varying abilities to adapt to anxiety without one or more members becoming symptomatic. This variability in adaptation explains why some families become symptomatic in reaction to events that to other families appear only mildly stressful, and why some families experience many traumatic events with no breakdown in coping abilities.
- Families use relationship mechanisms to bind anxiety (Box 7-4). Anxiety binding mechanisms are physical, emotional, or social actions that express the adaptation required for anxiety relief in the system.
- The degree of emotional separation from the extended family will affect the nuclear family's anxiety.

Box 7-4. Anxiety binding patterns of relationships

Marital conflict Neither partner gives in or is capable of an adaptive role; the self of each is focused on the other. As each issue is addressed, new ones arise.

Dysfunction in a spouse The usual give-and-take adaptiveness between marriage partners becomes intense and fixed, resulting in decreased functioning in one and overfunctioning in the other. A moderate increase in stress triggers the more compromised spouse into physical, emotional, or social dysfunction.

Impairment of one or more children The family's emotional energy focuses on a child, providing parents a way to maintain their own emotional equilibrium.

The family genogram

Data collection through the development of a family genogram is an economical method of obtaining a picture of a family's emotional system (Figure 7-2). When completed, the genogram allows a variety of facts to be read at a glance. The nurse collects data for the genogram from the client or from one or more family members. The goal is to factually describe three generations of family members, including information on each member's functions, through objective data on education, work, births, deaths, mental or physical illnesses, drug and alcohol abuse, and criminal activities.

To draw the genogram, begin with the nuclear family and note the birth date and death of each member. Dates are important because symptoms may appear in family members without apparent cause. For example, a child may begin to act out on the anniversary of the death of a significant family member. Obtain specific information on the function of each family member. For example, if a family member is described as a heavy drinker, try to obtain information on how much and how often the person drinks, a description of behavior while drinking, whether the person has sought treatment, and if so, whether it was effective. Inquire into what effect that person's behavior had on the rest of the family. The school and work history of each family member provides important clues to the level of adaptation of the family system.

Basic questions to address when developing a family genogram include:

- What is the symptom? Which family member or family relationship is symptomatic? Symptoms are often reflected in psychiatric diagnoses such as depression and schizophrenia.
- Has symptom development been influenced by an overload of stressful events or by a low level of adaptiveness?
- What is the symptomatic person's immediate relationship system (usually the nuclear family)?
- What are the patterns of emotional functioning in the nuclear family?

The diagram of a family with low levels of adaptiveness will tend to have more members with psychological, social, or physical problems. Level of adaptiveness reflects a multigenerational process and is not a judgment on the value of the family or its members.

When assessing a symptomatic client, obtain information not only about the onset of symptoms but also about any unusual events that occurred in the family system at the time. If the client has relapsed, look closely at family events in the past 6 to 12 months. Ask "why now?"

If the client is chronically mentally ill, assess family members' understanding of the illness. Does the family have realistic expectations of the client? Does anyone in the family overfunction for the client? Can that family member be worked with to be less "helpful"? Aiding the family to understand mental illness and its impact on other family members will reduce family anxiety, always a goal of treatment.

The role of the nurse in family assessment

When nurses engage one or more family members, they become part of the family's emotional system. Therefore one nursing goal is to communicate thoughts and observations of family interactions to the family while remaining emotionally neutral and nonreactive. If the nurse "takes sides" in thoughts, words, or actions, certain family members may become calmer but others become more anxious.

Family members should be encouraged to focus on themselves, what they do as individuals to maintain problems, and what they can do as individuals to solve family problems. It is often useful to identify the family member with the greatest ability to remain calm and work closely with that person to solve the problem.

The nurse can be useful to the family as a calm, neutral person who can help reduce anxiety. Anxiety reduction will relieve symptoms and make it more likely that the family can begin to function more effectively.

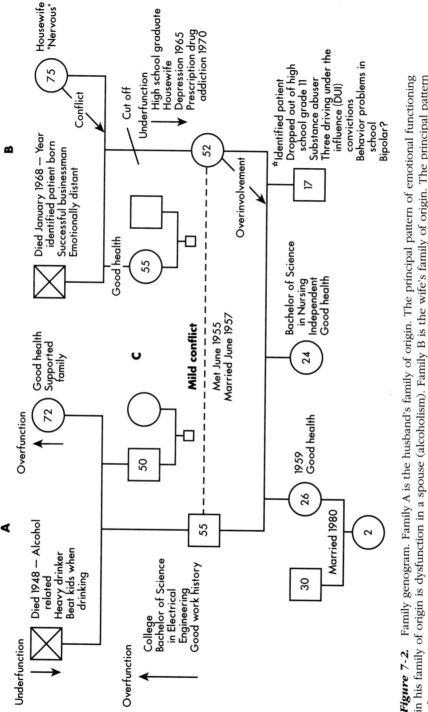

Figure 7-2. Family genogram. Family A is the husband's family of origin. The principal pattern of emotional functioning in his family of origin is dysfunction in a spouse (alcoholism). Family B is the wife's family of origin. The principal pattern of emotional functioning in her family of origin is projection to a child. Principal pattern of functioning in C (nuclear family) is dysfunction in a spouse, projection to a child, and marital conflict. Date to note: 1968—death of grandfather, birth of son. Most members doing okay, with some symptoms and some cut off. Fairly good adaptation.

SUMMARY

Careful client assessment is the cornerstone of treatment planning and intervention. This chapter has presented various techniques and rating scales for assessing the mental health of individual clients and families in the community. Techniques for assessing communities are presented in Chapter 5, Levels of Prevention. Different philosophical and theoretical perspectives have their own assessment techniques and criteria, and can be found in literature focused on these perspectives.

REFERENCES

American Nurses Association. (1994). *A statement on psychiatric-mental health clinical nursing practice and standards of psychiatric-mental health clinical nursing practice*. Washington, DC: Author.

Bartsch, D., Shern, D., & Feinberg, L. (1990). Screening CMHC outpatients for physical illness. *Hospital and Community Psychiatry, 41,* 786-790.

Bowen, M. (1971). Multigenerational process. In J. Haley (Ed.), *Changing families*. New York: Grune and Stratton.

Carmin, C., & Ownby, R. (1994). The relationship between discharge readiness inventory scales and the brief psychiatric rating scale. *Hospital and Community Psychiatry, 45,* 248-252.

Endicott, J., Spitzer, R., & Fleiss, J. (1976). The global assessment scale: a procedure for measuring the overall severity of psychiatric disturbances. *Archives of General Psychiatry, 33,* 766-771.

Goodwin, M., Brown, J., & Deitz, P. (1992). *Managing managed care, a mental health practitioner's survival guide*. Washington, DC: American Psychiatric Press.

Hall, R., Beresford, T., Gardner, E., et al. (1982). The medical care of psychiatric patients. *Hospital and Community Psychiatry, 33,* 25-34.

Hamilton, M. (1960). A rating scale for depression. *Journal of Neurology, Neurosurgery and Psychiatry, 23,* 56-62.

Kaplan, H., & Sadock, B. (1994). *Synopsis of psychiatry* (7th ed.). Baltimore, MD: Williams and Wilkins.

Keltner, N. (1995). Mood disorders. In N. Keltner, L. Schwecke, & C. Bostrom (Eds.), *Psychiatric nursing* (2nd ed.)(p. 408). St. Louis: Mosby.

Koran, L., Sox, H., & Marton, K. (1989). Medical evaluation of psychiatric patients. I. Results in a state mental health system. *Archives of General Psychiatry, 46,* 733-740.

Maricle, R., Hoffman, W., Bloom, J., et al. (1987). The prevalence and significance of medical illness among chronically mentally ill outpatients. *Community Mental Health Journal, 23,* 81-90.

Menninger, K. (1963). *The vital balance*. New York: Viking Press.

Overall, J., & Gorham, D. (1962). The brief psychiatric rating scale. *Psychological Reports, 10,* 799-812.

Schneider, L., & Struening, E. (1983). SLOF: a behavioral rating scale for assessing the mentally ill. *Social Work Research and Abstracts, 9-21.*

Tarasoff v. Regents of the University of California, 118 Cal. Rptr. 129, 529 P.2d 553(1974); on reh'g 17 Cal. 3d 425; 131 Cal. Rptr. 14, 551 P.2d 334 (1976).

Wilson, M. (1993). *DSM-III* and the transformation of American psychiatry. *American Journal of Psychiatry, 150,* 399-410.

Chapter 8

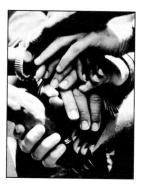

Crisis Stabilization

Donna C. Aguilera

The Chinese characters that represent the word *crisis* mean both "danger" and "opportunity." Crisis is dangerous because it threatens to overwhelm individuals and families; it may even result in suicide or a psychotic break. However, crisis also is an opportunity because during times of crisis people are most receptive to help in learning new or more adaptive methods to cope with stressful life problems. The positive outcome of a psychological crisis can be either emotional growth or emotional equilibrium. Prompt recognition of a crisis-causing situation may not only prevent the development of serious long-term disability but also allow new coping patterns to emerge that can help people function with a higher level of emotional equilibrium than before the crisis.

Most people live in a state of emotional equilibrium, a state of balance. No matter what stresses they encounter, they strive to maintain balance to be comfortable and to function. When a stress becomes so great or a problem so difficult that the usual problem-solving skills do not work, the balance of equilibrium becomes upset. As people face a problem they cannot solve, tension and anxiety increase, and eventually people cease to function. This is a crisis. People in crisis must either find a means to solve the problem or adapt to nonsolution. In either case a new state of equilibrium will develop; it may be better or worse insofar as positive mental health is concerned. The outcome of crisis depends heavily on the kinds of support people receive from those on whom they usually depend to lend understanding and emotional support.

HISTORICAL DEVELOPMENT

The origin of modern crisis intervention dates back to the work of Eric Lindemann and his colleagues after the Coconut Grove fire in Boston on November 28, 1942. In what was at that time the worst single-building fire in the country's history, 493 people perished when flames swept through the crowded Coconut Grove nightclub. Lindemann and others from Massachusetts General Hospital played an active role in helping survivors who had lost loved ones in the disaster. His clinical report (Lindemann, 1944) on the psychological symptoms of the survivors became the cornerstone for subsequent theorizing on the grief process, a series of stages through which a mourner progresses on the way toward accepting and resolving loss. Lindemann came to believe that clergy and other community caretakers could play a critical role in helping bereaved people negotiate the mourning process and thereby head off later psychological difficulties. This concept was furthered with the establishment in 1948 of the Wellesley Human Relations Service in Boston, one of the first community mental health services noted for its focus on short-term therapy in the context of preventive psychiatry.

Lindemann (1956) sought to develop approaches that would contribute to the maintenance of good mental health and the prevention of emotional disorganization on a community-wide level. He studied bereavement reactions in a search for social events or situations that were predictably followed by emotional disturbances in a significant portion of the population. In his study of bereavement reactions among the survivors of those killed in the Coconut Grove nightclub fire, he described both brief and abnormally prolonged reactions that occurred in individuals as a result of the loss of a significant person in their lives.

In his experiences working with grief reactions, Lindemann concluded that a conceptual frame of reference constructed around the concept of emotional crisis (as exemplified by bereavement reactions) might be profitable for the investigation and development of preventive efforts. Certain inevitable events in the course of the life cycle of every individual can be potentially hazardous (for example, bereavement, the birth of a child, and marriage). Lindemann postulated that in each of these situations emotional strain is

generated, stress is experienced, and a series of adaptive mechanisms occur that lead either to mastery of the new situation or to failure with more or less permanent impairment of function. Although such situations create stress for all people exposed to them, they become crises for individuals who by personality, previous experience, or other factors are especially vulnerable to stress and whose emotional resources are taxed beyond their usual adaptive resources.

Lindemann's theoretical frame of reference led to the development of crisis intervention techniques, and in 1946 he and Caplan established a community-wide mental health program in the Harvard area—the Wellesley Project.

According to Caplan (1961), the most important factors in mental health are the state of the ego, the stage of its maturity, and the quality of its structure. Assessment of the ego's state is based on three main areas:

1. The capacity of the person to withstand stress and anxiety and maintain ego equilibrium
2. The degree of reality recognized and faced in solving problems
3. The repertoire of effective coping mechanisms people employ to maintain balance in their biopsychosocial fields.

Caplan believes that all the elements comprising the emotional milieu of the person must be assessed in an approach to preventive mental health. The material, physical, and social demands of reality, and the needs, instincts, and impulses of the individual, are all important behavioral determinants. As a result of his work in Israel in 1948 and his later experiences in Massachusetts with Lindemann and with the Community Mental Health Program at Harvard University, he developed the concept of the importance of crisis periods in individual and group development (Caplan, 1951).

Caplan asserts that a crisis occurs "when a person faces an obstacle to important life goals that is, for a time, insurmountable through the utilization of customary methods of problem solving. A period of disorganization ensues, a period of upset, during which many abortive attempts at solution are made" (Caplan, 1961). The individual lives in a state of emotional equilibrium, with the goal always to return to or to maintain that state. When customary problem-solving techniques cannot meet the daily problems of living, the balance or equilibrium is upset. The individual must either solve the problem or adapt to nonsolution. Inner tension increases and there are signs of anxiety and disorganization of function, resulting in a protracted period of emotional upset. Caplan refers to this period as a "crisis." The outcome is governed by the kind of interactions that take place during the crisis period between the individual and the key figures in his or her emotional milieu.

EVOLUTION OF COMMUNITY PSYCHIATRY

After World War II the general public's increasing awareness and acceptance of the high incidence of psychiatric problems in the population resulted in changes in attitudes and demands for community action. The discovery and use of psychotropic drugs were important steps forward, creating opportunities for open wards and rehabilitation of hospitalized patients in their home milieus.

It would be incorrect to assume that all these factors merged spontaneously, creating a successful, structured cure for mental illness. Rather, it was a slow process of trial and error. Widely different programs—each striving to meet problems involving different cultures, interests, knowledge, and skills—communicated and worked with other programs that had similar goals. Disciplines once separated in their goals recognized their interdependence in attaining mutually recognized goals. New and allied disciplines developed, roles changed and expanded, tasks were diffused, and lines between disciplines became more flexible.

In 1967 crisis intervention replaced emergency detention at San Francisco General Hospital. On the psychiatric units interdisciplinary teams whose primary goal was to reestablish the independent functioning of clients as soon as possible were established. In a follow-up study Decker and Stubblebine (1972) concluded that the San Francisco crisis intervention program achieved the anticipated reduction in psychiatric inpatient treatment.

In the early 1970s the Bronx Mental Health Center (Centro de Hygiene Mental del Bronx) (Morales, 1971) was created for crisis interventions for Spanish-speaking people of low socioeconomic status; it was staffed by Spanish-speaking psychiatrists.

At about the same time suburban churches in Montreal, Canada, offered brief crisis intervention services on an experimental basis (Lecker et al., 1971). The goal of the programs was to reach families undergoing a variety of stresses by using walk-in clinics. The clinics facilitated service delivery to a population at risk, unreachable by other means, and at an early point in a life crisis.

The first crisis hot line was started at Children's Hospital in Los Angeles in 1968. Hot lines and youth crisis centers have been developed in recognition of the failure of traditional approaches to make contacts among adolescents. Twenty-four hour crisis telephones, free counseling with a minimum of red tape, walk-in service, and young people serving as volunteer staff in such services continue to be attractive to youth.

Trends such as these are being repeated around the country as community mental health programs recognize the value of providing primary and secondary prevention services unique to the needs of their clients. The need also is being recognized for more services for clients who require continuing support and rehabilitation after resolution of the immediate crisis. The major concern of community mental health centers is no longer discerning what services are appropriate for potential clients. It is not even recruiting clients for services. Instead, centers are facing the problem of obtaining an adequate supply of human resources to meet demands for services, and of obtaining the funds to pay for services. Professionals and nonprofessionals alike have been recruited and trained to fill the gap between supply and demand. This has led to the deprofessionalization of many mental health functions previously considered the sole domain of the professional. Role boundaries have been diffused as the needs of clients and their communities have become the determining factors of the appropriateness of services.

PARADIGM OF CRISIS INTERVENTION

According to Caplan (1964), a crisis has four developmental phases:

1. An initial rise in tension as the stimulus continues and discomfort is felt.
2. A lack of success in coping as the stimulus continues and more discomfort is felt.
3. A further increase in tension that acts as a powerful internal stimulus to mobilize internal and external resources. In this stage emergency problem-solving mechanisms are tried. The person may redefine the problem or feel resignation and give up certain aspects of the goal as unattainable.
4. If the problem continues and can be neither solved nor avoided, tension increases and major disorganization occurs.

When a stressful event occurs, certain recognized balancing factors can produce a return to equilibrium. These factors include perception of the event, available situational supports, and coping mechanisms, as shown in Figure 8-1. The upper portion of the figure illustrates the "normal" initial reaction of an individual to a stressful event. A stressful event is seldom so clearly defined that its source can be immediately determined. Internalized changes occur in tandem with the externally provoked stress; as a result some events may cause a strong emotional response in one person, and leave another apparently unaffected. Much is determined by the presence or absence of factors that can produce a return to equilibrium.

In column *A* of Figure 8-1, balancing factors are operating and crisis is avoided. However, in col-
umn *B* the absence of one or more of these balancing factors may block resolution of the problem, increase disequilibrium, and precipitate crisis.

Figure 8-2 demonstrates the use of the paradigm for presentation of subsequent case studies. It serves as a guideline to help the reader focus on problem areas. It presents the cases of two people affected by the same stressful event. One resolved the problem and avoided crisis; the other did not.

Balancing factors affecting equilibrium

Between the perceived effects of a stressful situation and the resolution of the problem are three recognized balancing factors that may determine the state of equilibrium: perception of the event, available situational supports, and coping mechanisms. Strengths or weaknesses in any one of these factors can be directly related to the onset of crisis or to its resolution.

Why do some people go into crisis and others do not? This is illustrated in Figure 8-2 by the cases of two men, Mr. A and Mr. B. Both men have possible symptoms of cancer and have been told of the need for diagnostic tests. Mr. A is upset but does not go into crisis, but Mr. B does go into crisis. Why does Mr. A react one way and Mr. B another? What "things" in their lives make the difference?

Perception of the event

Cognition, or the subjective meaning of a stressful event plays a major role in determining the nature and degree of coping behaviors. Differences in cognition in terms of the event's threat to an important life goal or value account for large differences in coping behaviors. The concept of "cognitive style" (Cropley & Field, 1969) suggests uniqueness in the way people take in, process, and use information from the environment.

Cognitive styles (characteristic modes for organizing perceptual and intellectual activities) play an important role in determining an individual's coping response to daily life stresses. According to Inkeles (1966), cognitive style helps set limits on information seeking in stress situations. It also strongly influences perceptions of others, inter-

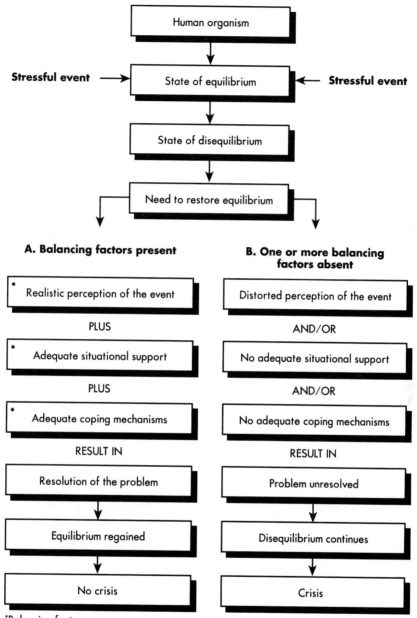

Figure 8-1. Paradigm: the effect of balancing factors in a stressful event.
(From *Crisis Intervention: Theory and Methodology* (7th ed.), by D. C. Aguilera, 1994,
St. Louis: Mosby.)

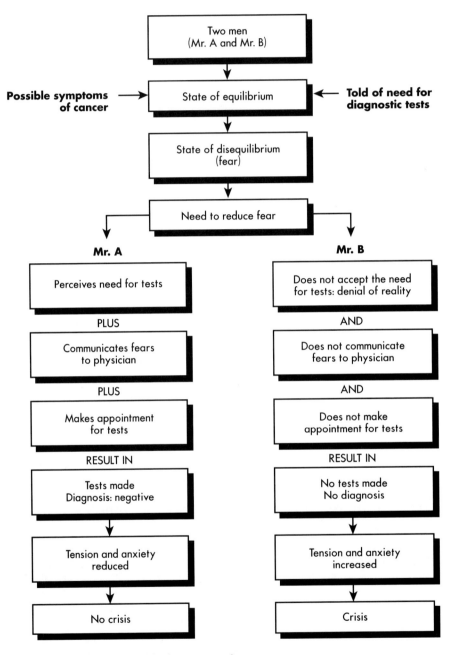

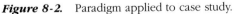

Figure 8-2.   Paradigm applied to case study.
(From *Crisis Intervention: Theory and Methodology* (7th ed.), by D. C. Aguilera, 1994, St. Louis: Mosby.)

personal relationships, and responses to various types of psychiatric treatment. For example, in stressful situations a person whose cognitive style is "field-dependent" depends on external objects in the environment for orientation to reality. This type of individual tends to use repression and denial as coping mechanisms. In contrast, the "field-independent" person prefers intellectualization as a defense mode. If the event is perceived realistically, the relationship between the event and feelings of stress is recognized. Problem solving can be appropriately oriented toward reduction of tension, and successful solution of the stressful situation is more probable.

Lazarus (1966) focused on the importance of the mediating cognitive process (appraisal) to determine the various coping methods people use. This approach recognizes that coping behaviors always represent an interaction between the individual and the environment, and that the environmental demands of each situation initiate, form, and limit coping activities that may be required in the interaction. As a result people engage in widely diverse behavioral and intrapsychic activities to meet actual or anticipated threats. Appraisal, in this context, is an ongoing perceptual process by which a potentially harmful event is distinguished from a potentially beneficial or irrelevant event in a person's life.

When a threatening situation occurs, a primary appraisal is made to judge the perceived outcome of the event in relation to the person's future goals and values. A secondary appraisal then occurs in which the person perceives the range of coping alternatives available to master the threat or achieve a beneficial outcome. As the person selects and initiates coping activities, feedback cues from changing internal and external environments lead to ongoing reappraisals or changes in original perception. As a result of the appraisal process, coping behaviors are never static. They change constantly in quality and degree as the person receives new information and cues during reappraisal activities. New coping responses may occur whenever new significance is attached to a situation.

If, in the appraisal process, the outcome is judged too overwhelming or too difficult to be dealt with through available coping skills, an individual is more likely to resort to use of intrapsychic defense mechanisms to repress or distort the reality of the situation. An appraisal of a potentially successful outcome, however, is more likely to lead to the use of direct action modes of coping such as attack, flight, or compromise. If the perception of the event is distorted, the relationship between the event and resulting feelings of stress may not be recognized. Thus attempts to solve the problem are ineffective and tension is not reduced.

What does the event mean to the individual? How will it affect the future? Does the person look at it realistically or distort its meaning? In the example, Mr. A perceived the need for diagnostic tests; his perception of the event was realistic. Mr. B was unable to accept the need for tests to confirm the cancer's presence; his perception was distorted, and he used denial.

Situational supports

Human beings are social by nature and depend on others in their environment to supply them with reflected appraisals of their own intrinsic and extrinsic values. In establishing life patterns, certain appraisals are more significant than others because they tend to reinforce the perception the individual has of himself or herself.

Dependency relationships may be more readily established with those whose appraisals protect the individual against feelings of insecurity and with those who reinforce feelings of ego integrity. These meaningful relationships with others provide a person with nurturance and support, resources vital for coping with a wide variety of stressors. Social isolation, whatever its cause, denies a person social interactions and opportunities to develop meaningful relationships. Sudden or unexpected social isolation results in the loss of usual resource supports. With these lacking, a person is much more vulnerable to daily living stressors. Loss, threatened loss, or feelings of inadequacy in a supportive relationship also may leave a person vulnerable. Confrontation with a stressful situation combined with a lack of situational support may lead to disequilibrium and possible crisis.

Appraisal of self varies across ages, sexes, and roles. The belief system that forms the basis of self-concept and self-esteem develops out of experiences with significant others in a person's life. Although self-esteem is fairly static within a certain range, it fluctuates according to internal and external environmental variables that impinge on it at specific times and in specific situations. To achieve and maintain a sense of value and self-worth, a person must feel loved by others and capable of achieving an ideal self—one that is strong, capable, good, and loving.

When self-esteem is low or when a situation is perceived as particularly threatening, the person is strongly in need of support and seeks out people from whom positive reflective appraisals of self-worth and ability to achieve can be obtained. The lower the self-esteem or the greater the threat, the greater the need to seek situational support. Conversely, people avoid or withdraw from contacts with those they perceive as threatening to self-esteem, whether the threat is real or imagined. Any potentially stressful situation can produce self-doubt about how one is perceived by others, the kind of impression being made, and real or imagined inadequacies that might be disclosed (Mechanic, 1974).

The success or failure of a coping behavior is always strongly influenced by the social context in which it occurs. The environmental variable most centrally identified is the person's significant others. From them, a person learns to seek advice and support in solving daily problems in living. Confidence in being liked and respected by these peers is based on past testing and reaffirmation of their expected supportive responses.

Any perceived failure to obtain adequate support to meet psychosocial needs may provoke or compound a stressful situation. Negative support can be equally detrimental to a person's self-esteem.

Situational supports are those persons who are available in the environment who can be depended on to help solve a problem. In the example provided in Figure 8-2, Mr. A talked to his physician and told him of his fear of having cancer. He asked about the tests that would be conducted and what would be done if the tests revealed he had cancer. He talked with his wife and children about the possibility of having cancer. He received reassurance from his family and his physician. He had strong support during this stressful event. Mr. B did not feel close enough to his physician to discuss his fears about the possibility of having cancer, and he did not talk to his family or friends about his symptoms. His denial made him isolate himself. He did not have anyone to turn to for help; therefore he felt overwhelmed and alone.

Coping mechanisms

Through the process of daily living, people learn many methods to cope with anxiety and reduce tension. Life-styles are developed around patterns of response that have been established to cope with stressful situations. These life-styles are highly individual and necessary to protect and maintain equilibrium.

The early work of Cannon (1929; Cannon, 1939) provided a basis for later systematic research on the effects of stress on people. According to Cannon's "fight or flight" theory, reactions of acute anxiety (similar to those of fear) ready the individual physiologically to meet real or imagined threats to self. From his studies of homeostasis, Cannon described the mechanisms whereby people and animals maintain steady life states, with the goal always to return to such states after conditions force a temporary departure.

Over the years it has been common to find the term *coping* used interchangeably with such similar concepts as adaptation, defense, mastery, and adjustment. Coping activities take a wide variety of forms, including all the diverse behaviors that people engage in to meet actual or anticipated challenges. In psychological stress theory the term *coping* emphasizes various strategies used, consciously or unconsciously, to deal with stress and tensions arising from perceived threats to psychological integrity. It is not synonymous with mastery over problematical life situations; rather, it is the process of attempting to solve them (Lazarus, 1966).

Coleman (1950) defined coping as an adjustive reaction made in response to actual or imagined stress to maintain psychological integrity. According to this concept, human beings respond to stress by attack, flight, or compromise reactions. These reactions are complicated by various ego-defense mechanisms whenever the stress becomes ego-involved.

Attack reactions usually attempt to remove or overcome obstacles perceived as causing stress. They may be primarily constructive or destructive in nature. Flight, withdrawal, or fear reactions may be as simple as physically removing the threat from the environment (such as putting out a fire) or removing oneself from the threatening situation (running away from the fire). They also may involve much more complex psychological maneuvering, depending on the extent of the threat and the possibilities for escape.

Compromise or substitution reactions occur when attack or flight from the threatening situation is considered impossible. This method is most commonly used in problem solving and includes accepting substitute goals or changing internal values and standards.

Masserman (1946) demonstrated that, in situations of extended frustration, individuals find it increasingly possible to accept substitute goals. This acceptance often involves rationalization, a defense mechanism whereby "half a loaf" does indeed soon appear to be "better than none."

Tension-reducing mechanisms can be overt or covert and can be consciously or unconsciously activated. They have been classified into such behavioral responses as aggression, regression, withdrawal, and repression. The selection of a response is based on tension-reducing actions that successfully relieved anxiety and reduced

tension in similar situations in the past. Through repetition the response may pass from conscious awareness during its learning phase to a habitual reaction as a learned behavior. In many instances individuals may not be aware of how, let alone why, they react to stress in given situations. Except for having vague feelings of discomfort, the individual may not notice the rise and consequent fall in tension. When a novel stress-producing event arises and learned coping mechanisms are ineffective, discomfort is felt on a conscious level. The need to "do something" becomes the focus of activity, narrowing perception of all other life activities.

Normally defense mechanisms are used constructively in the process of coping. This is particularly evident whenever the danger of becoming psychologically overwhelmed is present. Most defense mechanisms are important for survival. None are pathological unless they interfere with coping, such as if they are used to deny, falsify, or distort perceptions of reality.

According to Bandura et al. (1977), the strength of an individual's conviction of effectiveness in overcoming or mastering a problematical situation determines whether coping behavior is even attempted in the first place. People fear and avoid stressful, threatening situations that they believe exceed their ability to cope. They behave with assurance in situations they judge themselves able to manage and in which they expect eventual success. The perceived ability to master can influence the choice of coping behaviors and the level of persistence after a coping mechanism is chosen.

Available coping mechanisms are those that people usually use when they have a problem. They may sit down and try to think the problem out or talk it over with a friend. Some cry out their frustrations or try to get rid of their feelings of anger and hostility by swearing, kicking a chair, or slamming a door. Others may get into verbal battles with friends. Some may react by temporarily withdrawing from the situation in order to reassess the problem. These are just a few of the many coping methods people use to relieve tension and anxiety when faced with a problem. Each has been used at some time in the developmental past of the individual, has been found effective in maintaining emotional stability, and has become part of his or her life-style in meeting and dealing with the stresses of daily living.

Continuing with the example provided in Figure 8-2, the reader notes that Mr. A made an appointment for the tests recommended by his physician. The tests were conducted; the diagnosis was negative for cancer. His tension and anxiety were reduced, equilibrium was restored, and he did not have a crisis. Mr. B withdrew; he had no coping skills. He did not make an appointment for the needed tests, no tests were conducted, he had no definitive diagnosis, and his tension and anxiety increased. Unable to solve the problem or to function, Mr. B went into crisis.

Balancing factors that affect equilibrium were illustrated in Figure 8-2. Mr. A had a realistic perception of events and returned to his original state of equilibrium; he did not have a crisis. Mr. B had a distorted perception of events, used denial, remained in a state of disequilibrium, and went into crisis.

What if Mr. A's tests had been positive instead of negative? Figure 8-3 presents a new paradigm of comparative cases and introduces Mr. C, whose balancing factors are identical to Mr. A's, with one exception: Mr. C had the diagnostic tests for cancer and his results were positive. His tension and anxiety increased, and he had surgery that successfully removed the cancer. He did not have a crisis. The balancing factor that made the difference was his realistic perception of the event. The relationship between the event and his feelings of stress was recognized. His problem solving was appropriately oriented toward reducing tension, and his stressful situation was resolved successfully.

The minimum therapeutic goal of crisis intervention is psychological resolution of the individual's immediate crisis and restoration to at least the level of functioning that existed before the crisis period. A maximum goal is improvement in functioning above the precrisis level.

Caplan (1964) emphasizes that crises are characteristically self-limiting and last from 4 to 6 weeks. This time is a transitional period, offering both the danger of increased psychological vulnerability and the opportunity for personal growth. In any particular situation the outcome may depend to a significant degree on the ready availability of appropriate help. On this basis the length of time for intervention is from 4 to 6 weeks, with the mode being 4 weeks (Jacobson, 1965). Because time is at a premium, a therapeutic climate is generated that commands the concentrated attention of both therapist and client. A goal-oriented sense of commitment develops in sharp contrast to the more modest pace of traditional treatment modes.

CATEGORIES OF CRISIS INTERVENTION

Jacobson, Strickler, and Morley (1968; Jacobson 1980) divide crisis intervention into two major categories: generic and individual.

Generic approach

A major proposition of the generic approach is that most crises produce certain recognized patterns of behavior. In addition to Lindemann's (1944) studies of bereavement that have already been described, other studies of generic patterns of response to stressful situations have been reported. Kaplan and Mason (1960) and Caplan (1964) studied the effect the premature birth of a baby had on the mother and identified four phases or tasks she must work through to ensure healthy adaptation to the experience. Janis (1958) suggests several hypotheses concerning the psychological stress of impending surgery and the patterns of emotional response that follow a diagnosis of chronic illness. Rapoport (1963) defines three subphases of marriage during which unusual stress could precipitate crises. These are only a few of the broad research studies in this field.

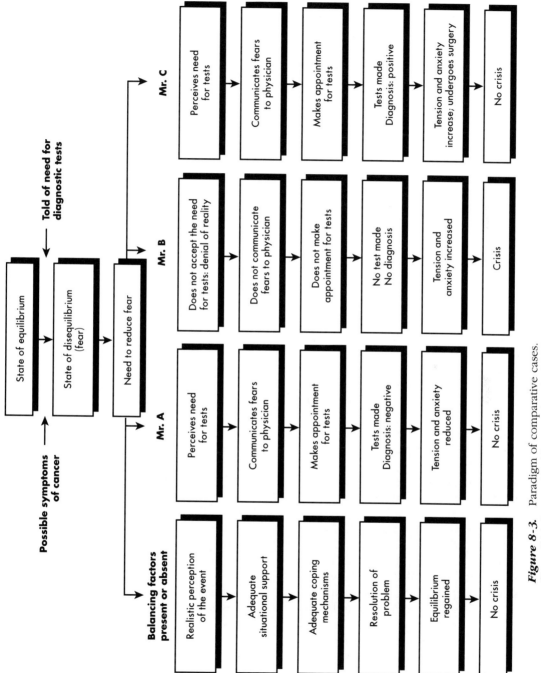

Figure 8-3. Paradigm of comparative cases.
(From *Crisis Intervention: Theory and Methodology* (7th ed.), by D. C. Aguilera, 1994, St. Louis: Mosby.)

The generic approach focuses on the characteristic course of the crisis rather than on the psychodynamics of each individual in crisis. A treatment plan is directed toward an adaptive resolution of the crisis. Specific interventions are designed for all members of a given group rather than for the unique differences of one individual. Recognition of these behavioral patterns is an important aspect of preventive mental health.

Tyhurst (1957) suggests that knowledge of behavior patterns that occur during transitional states in which there is intense or sudden change from one life situation to another might provide an empirical basis for the management of these states and the prevention of subsequent mental illness. He cites as examples studies of individual responses to community disaster, migration, and retirement from employment.

Jacobson et al. (1968) state that generic approaches to crisis intervention emphasize:

Direct encouragement of adaptive behavior, general support, environmental manipulation and anticipatory guidance. . . . In brief, the generic approach emphasizes (1) specific situational and maturational events occurring to significant population groups, (2) intervention oriented to crisis related to these specific events, and (3) intervention carried out by non–mental health professionals.

The generic approach is a feasible mode of intervention that can be learned and implemented by nonpsychiatric physicians, nurses, social workers, and others. It does not require knowledge of the intrapsychic and interpersonal processes of an individual in crisis.

Individual approach

The individual approach differs from the generic approach in its emphasis on professional assessment of the interpersonal and intrapsychic processes of the person in crisis. It is used in selected cases, usually those that do not respond to the generic approach. Intervention is planned to meet the unique needs of the individual in crisis and to reach a solution for the particular situations and circumstances that precipitated the crisis.

Unlike in extended psychotherapy, the individual approach deals relatively little with the developmental past of the client. Past information is seen as relevant only for the clues it can provide that may result in a better understanding of the present crisis situation. Emphasis is placed on the immediate causes for disturbed equilibrium and on the processes necessary to regain a precrisis or better level of functioning.

Jacobson et al. (1968) cite the inclusion of family members or other important persons in the process of the client's crisis resolution as another area of differentiation from most individual psychotherapy modalities. Jacobson views the individual approach as emphasizing the need for greater depth of understanding of the biopsychosocial process, providing intervention oriented to the client's unique situation, and mandating that intervention be carried out only by mental health professionals.

Morley, Messick, and Aguilera (1967) recommend several attitudes that are important adjuncts to individual approach techniques. These attitudes compose the general philosophical orientation necessary for the full effectiveness of the therapist.

1. It is essential that the therapist view the work being done not as a "second-best" approach but as the treatment of choice with persons in crisis.
2. Accurate assessment of the presenting problem, not a thorough diagnostic evaluation, is essential to an effective intervention.
3. Both the therapist and the client should keep in mind throughout their contacts that the treatment is sharply time-limited and should persistently direct their energies toward resolution of the presenting problem.
4. Dealing with material not directly related to the crisis has no place in an intervention of this kind.
5. The therapist must be willing to take an active and sometimes directive role in the intervention. The relatively slow-paced approach of more traditional treatment is inappropriate in this type of therapy.

6. Maximum flexibility of approach is encouraged. Such diverse techniques as serving as a resource person or information giver and taking an active role in established liaison with other helping resources are often appropriate in particular situations.

7. The goal toward which the therapist strives is explicit. Energy is directed entirely toward returning the individual to (at least) a precrisis level of functioning.

STEPS IN CRISIS INTERVENTION

There are certain specific steps involved in the technique of crisis intervention (Morley et al., 1967). Although each cannot be placed in a clearly defined category, typical interventions pass through the following sequence of phases.

Assessment

Assessment of clients and their problems is the first phase. It requires the therapist to use active focusing techniques to obtain an accurate assessment of the precipitating event and the resulting crisis that brought the client to seek professional help. One of the most important parts of the assessment is to find out whether the person is suicidal or homicidal. Questions must be direct and specific: Is the client planning to kill himself or herself or someone else? How? When? The therapist must assess the seriousness of the threat. Is the person merely thinking about suicide or has he or she selected a method? Is it a lethal method—a loaded gun? Has the client picked out a tall building or bridge to jump from? Can the client tell the therapist when the suicide will occur (for example, after the children are asleep)?

If the threat does not seem too imminent, the person is accepted for crisis therapy. If the intent is clear and details are specific and carefully planned, hospitalization and psychiatric evaluation are arranged to protect the person or others in the community. The first hour may be spent entirely on assessing circumstances directly related to the immediate crisis situation.

The first therapy session is directed toward discovering what the crisis-precipitating event was and what factors are affecting the person's ability to solve problems. It is important that both therapist and client be able to define a situation clearly before taking action to change it. Questions such as "What do I need to know?" and "What must be done?" are asked during assessment. The more specifically the problem can be defined, the more likely it is that the "correct" answer will be found.

Clues are investigated to explore the problem or situation. The therapist asks questions and uses observational skills to obtain factual knowledge about the problem area. It is important to know what has happened within the immediate situation. How the individual has coped in past situations may affect present behavior. Observations are made to determine level of anxiety, expressive movements, emotional tone, verbal responses, and attitudinal changes. It is important to remember that the therapist's task is to focus on the immediate problem. There is neither time nor need to go into the client's history in depth.

One of the therapist's first questions usually is "Why did you come for help today?" The therapist should emphasize the word *today*. Sometimes clients will try to avoid stating why they came by saying, "I've been planning to come for some time." The therapist reply should be, "Yes, but what happened that made you come in today?" Other questions to ask are "What happened in your life that is different? When did it happen?"

In crises the precipitating event usually occurs 10 to 14 days before the individual seeks help. However, sometimes the event happened the day or night before. It could be almost anything: threat of divorce, discovery of extramarital relations, finding out that a son or daughter is taking drugs, loss of boyfriend or girlfriend, loss of job or status, or an unwanted pregnancy.

The next area on which to focus is the individual's perception of the event: What does it mean? What will be its effect on the future? Does the client see the event realistically or distort its meaning?

The client is then questioned about available situational supports: Whom in the environment can the therapist find to support the person? With whom does the client live? Who is his or her best friend? Whom does he or she trust? Is there a family member to whom the client feels particularly close? Crisis intervention is sharply time-limited, and the more people involved in helping the person, the better. If others are involved and familiar with the problem, they can continue to give support when therapy is completed.

The next area of focus is the person's usual response to a problem that seems unsolvable. What are the client's coping skills? Has anything like this ever happened before? How does the client usually abate tension, anxiety, or depression? Has the same method been tried this time? If not, why not, if it usually works? If the usual method was tried and did not work, why did it not work? What does the client feel would reduce symptoms of stress? The client may remember methods of coping with anxiety that have not been used in years. One man recalled that he used to "work off tensions" by playing the piano for a few hours, and the therapist suggested he try this method again. Because he did not have a piano, he rented one; by the next session his anxiety had been reduced enough to enable him to begin problem solving.

Planning therapeutic intervention

After identifying the precipitating event and the factors influencing the individual's state of disequilibrium, the therapist plans the method of intervention. Determination must be made as to how the crisis has disrupted the individual's life. Can the client go to work? Go to school? Keep house? Care for his or her family? Are these activities being affected? These are the areas to examine for the degree of disruption. How is the client's disequilibrium affecting others in his or her life? How does the wife (or husband, boyfriend, girlfriend, roommate, or family) feel about this problem? What do they think the client should do? Are they upset?

This determination is essentially a search process during which data are collected. It requires the use of cognitive abilities and recollection of past events for information relevant to the present situation. The last phase of this step is a thinking process in which alternatives are considered and evaluated against past experience and knowledge and in the context of the present situation. Tentative theories are advanced about why the problem exists. This step requires theoretical knowledge and anticipation of more than one answer. In the study of behavior it is important to address causal relationships. Clues observed in environmental conditions are examined and related to theories of psychosocial behavior to suggest reasons for the individual's disturbed equilibrium.

Intervention

In the third step intervention is initiated. The therapist and client take action with the expectation that if the planned action is taken, an expected result will occur.

After the necessary information is collected, the problem-solving process is used to initiate the intervention. The nature of intervention techniques depends on the preexisting skills, creativity, and flexibility of the therapist. Morley suggests some of the following techniques, which he has found useful:

- **Helping clients gain an intellectual understanding of the crisis.** Often clients see no relationship between a hazardous situation occurring in life and the extreme discomfort and disequilibrium they experience. The therapist can use a direct approach here, explaining to the client the relationship between the crisis and the precipitating event.
- **Helping clients bring into the open feelings to which they may not have access.** Frequently clients suppress feelings such as anger or other inadmissible emotions toward someone they "should love or honor." This suppression also may entail denial of grief, feelings of guilt, or failure to complete the mourning process after bereavement. An imme-

diate goal of intervention is to reduce tension by providing means for the individual to recognize these feelings and bring them into the open. It is sometimes necessary to produce emotional catharsis and reduce immobilizing tension.

- **Exploring coping mechanisms.** This approach requires assisting the person to examine alternate ways of coping. If for some reason behaviors used in the past for successfully reducing anxiety have not been tried, the possibility of their use in the present situation is explored. New coping methods are sought, and frequently the client devises highly original coping methods.

- **Reopening the social world.** If the crisis has been precipitated by the loss of someone significant to the person's life, introducing new people to fill the void can be highly effective. It is particularly effective if supports and gratifications provided in the past by the "lost" person can be experienced to a similar degree from new relationships.

Resolution of the crisis and anticipatory planning

Resolution of the crisis and anticipatory planning are the last phases. The therapist reinforces adaptive coping mechanisms that the individual has used successfully to reduce tension and anxiety. As coping abilities increase and positive changes occur, they allow the person to reexperience and reconfirm the progress made. The therapist gives assistance as needed in making realistic plans for the future, and discusses with the client ways in which the present experience may help in coping with future crises.

SUMMARY

The goal of crisis intervention is the resolution of immediate crises. Its focus is on the present, its goal is the restoration of the individual to a precrisis level of functioning or possibly to a higher level of functioning. The therapist's role is direct, suppressive, and active. Techniques are varied, limited only by the flexibility and creativity of the therapist. Some of these techniques include helping the individual gain an intellectual understanding of the crisis, assisting the individual in bringing feelings into the open, exploring past and present coping mechanisms, finding and using situational supports, and assisting the client with anticipatory planning to reduce the possibility of future crises. This type of therapy is indicated when a person (or family) suddenly loses the ability to cope with a life situation. The average length of treatment is from one to six sessions. The cost of therapy depends on the geographical region.

REFERENCES

Aguilera, D. (1994). *Crisis intervention: Theory and methodology* (7th ed.). St. Louis: Mosby.

Bandura, A., et al. (1977). Cognitive processes mediating behavioral change. *Journal of Personality and Social Psychology, 35,* 125.

Cannon, W. B. (1929). *Bodily changes in pain, hunger, fear, and rage.* New York: D. Appleton.

Cannon, W. B. (1939). *The wisdom of the body* (2nd ed.). New York: W. W. Norton.

Caplan, G. (1961). *An approach to community mental health.* New York: Grune & Stratton.

Caplan, G. (1964). *Principles of preventive psychiatry.* New York: Basic Books.

Caplan, G. (1951). A public health approach to child psychiatry. *Mental Health, 35,* 235.

Coleman, J. C. (1950). *Abnormal psychology and modern life.* Chicago: Scott, Foresman.

Cropley, A., & Field, T. (1969). Achievement in science and intellectual style. *Journal of Applied Psychology, 53,* 132.

Decker, J. B., & Stubblebine, J. M. (1972). Crisis intervention and prevention of psychiatric disability: A follow-up study. *American Journal of Psychiatry, 129,* 101.

Inkeles, A. (1966). Social structure and the socialization of competence. *Harvard Educational Review, 36,* 265-283.

Jacobson, G. (1980). Crisis theory. *New Directions for Mental Health Services, 6,* 1.

Jacobson, G. (1965). Crisis theory and treatment strategy: some sociocultural and psychodynamic considerations. *Journal of Nervous and Mental Disease, 141,* 209.

Jacobson, G., Strickler, M., & Morley, W. E. (1968). Generic and individual approaches to crisis intervention. *American Journal of Public Health, 58,* 339.

Janis, I. L. (1958). *Psychological stress, psychoanalytical and behavioral studies of surgical patients*. New York: John Wiley & Sons.

Kaplan, D. M., & Mason, E. A. (1960). Maternal reactions to premature birth viewed as an acute emotional disorder. *American Journal of Orthopsychiatry, 30,* 539.

Lazarus, R. S. (1966). *Psychological stress and the coping process*. New York: McGraw-Hill.

Lecker, S., et al. (1971). Brief interventions: A pilot walk-in clinic in suburban churches. *Canadian Psychiatric Association Journal, 16,* 141.

Lindemann, E. (1956). The meaning of crisis in individual and family. *Teachers College Record, 57,* 310.

Lindemann, E. (1944). Symptomatology and management of acute grief. *American Journal of Psychiatry, 101,* 101-148.

Masserman, J. H. (1946). *Principles of dynamic psychology*. Philadelphia: W. B. Saunders.

Mechanic, D. (1974). Social structure and personal adaptation: Some neglected dimensions. In G. V. Coehlo, et al. (Eds.), *Coping and adaptation*. New York: Basic Books.

Morales, H. M. (1971). Bronx mental health center, NY state division. *Bronx Bulletin, 13,* 6.

Morley, W. E., Messick, J. M., & Aguilera, D. C. (1967). Crisis: Paradigms of intervention. *Journal of Psychiatric Nursing, 5,* 538.

Rapoport, R. (1963). Normal crises, family structure, and mental health. *Family Process, 2,* 68.

Tyhurst, J. A. (1957, April 15-17). Role of transition states—including disasters—in mental illness. Paper presented at Symposium on Preventive and Social Psychiatry, sponsored by Walter Reed Institute of Research, Walter Reed Medical Center, and National Research Council. Washington, DC: U.S. Government Printing Office.

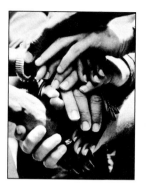

Chapter 9

Supportive Psychotherapy

Nancy K. Worley

Those of us with a psychiatric disability can recover if given the chance. We have a right to recovery. If we periodically fail in our efforts to achieve this, then let us fail. But we must be given the opportunity to succeed as well. Don't let the mental health system fail us by its entrenched and hopeless view of our potential for recovery, thus further stereotyping the mentally ill and incorrectly convincing us of the futility of our situation. Instead, we must all learn that with rewarding interpersonal contact we clients can change, that we can contribute and that we can recover (Leete, 1993).

Rockland (1993), in a review article on supportive psychotherapy, noted the renewed interest in this treatment modality over the past few years. Some of the factors that have contributed to this interest include the remedicalization of psychiatry, with a concomitant concentration on biological factors in mental illness and a decreasing interest in long-term psychodynamic treatment; the increased financial constraints that reward focused problem-solving interventions; and the growing number of persons with serious mental illness who are being treated in community settings.

Novalis, Rojcewicz, and Peele (1993) define supportive psychotherapy as therapy in which the therapist plays an active and directive role in helping clients improve their social functioning and coping skills. The emphasis is on improving behavior and subjective feeling, rather than achieving insight or self-understanding. Supportive psychotherapy is an eclectic form of psychotherapy that uses empirically based techniques. It does not depend on any specific overriding concept or theory, but rather incorporates the work of many theorists to understand how people change. The supportive psychotherapy described in this chapter should not be confused with psychodynamically oriented supportive psychotherapy, in which support of ego functions is the primary concern (Rockland, 1993). Although psychodynamic theory is used where appropriate, the clini-

---

Box 9-1. Supportive psychotherapy

Clinical focuses

The theraputic alliance
Self-esteem
Subjective mental distress

Interventions

Reassurance
Positive regard
Support of the client's strengths and coping
   skills
Assistance with situational problems
Assertive outreach
Encouragement of treatment compliance

Goals

Achieving maximum possible independence
   from psychiatric illness

---

cal focuses, interventions, and goals of supportive psychotherapy are client centered, client driven, and symptom focused (Box 9-1). The care orientation of supportive psychotherapy is very consistent with the values and assumptions of nursing, whose primary mode of intervention has always been interpersonal supportive relationships.

THE THERAPEUTIC ALLIANCE

In supportive therapy the therapeutic alliance is paramount. Although the therapeutic alliance is a vehicle for exchange of information between therapist and client, the relationship itself provides therapeutic benefits in other nonspecific ways. The nonspecificity hypothesis of psychotherapeutic change holds that these nonspecific relational elements both cultivate an expectation of change and foster that change (Novalis et al., 1993). Nonspecific factors that foster the therapeutic alliance were originally discussed by Frank (1975) and later elaborated by Mosher and Burti (1992):

- **Healing context.** Clients perceive the therapist as helping or providing the context in which they can help themselves.

- **Confiding relationship with the therapist.** Clients perceive the therapist as always attentive to their needs; the focus of the relationship is on client goals and strategies for accomplishing these goals.

- **Plausible causal explanation.** A plausible causal explanation is a conceptual schema or explanatory model that provides a rationale for the client's illness and treatment. The shared understanding that evolves from this aspect of the process facilitates the development of the positive collaborative relationship that must underlie successful intervention strategies.

- **Positive expectations from the therapist.** An optimistic problem-solving approach on the part of the therapist generates positive expectations for the client. Hope and optimism displayed by the therapist can be critical for beginning to raise the client's morale.

- **Provision of success experiences.** The helping process should be one in which the client is given the opportunity to solve problems, overcome obstacles, and accomplish goals. Even the mastery of small tasks enhances self-esteem.

In the beginning the therapist must actively support the development of the therapeutic alliance. This support requires a regard for the client as an independent human being and a willingness to support the client's healing resources. Support also involves mutuality; the therapist and the client must be in agreement about the goals of the alliance.

COMMUNICATION TECHNIQUES

A therapeutic atmosphere is nurtured through communication; communication is the foundation on which therapy is built. The following communication techniques are basic tools nurses can use to build the therapeutic alliance.

Empathic listening

The most basic yet difficult communication technique to master is empathic listening. It requires the ability to attend closely to what the client says and to let the client know the therapist is listening. Some specific listening skills are nonverbal, such as leaning forward as the client speaks, keeping good eye contact, and not appearing distracted. Other empathic communication techniques include paraphrasing or restatement, which involves the reformulation of the client's remarks in the therapist's words. Paraphrasing is not mere repetition of what the client has said, but rather mirrors the essence of what the client feels and thinks while speaking (Moursund, 1993). Paraphrases summarize whole units of client behavior and mirror the essence of the client's thoughts, feelings, and actions. Paraphrasing also gives the client the opportunity to correct any wrong impressions the therapist might have about what was said.

Case example

John is discussing a conversation he had with his wife the previous evening. His company is being restructured and he is concerned that his job might not be secure. He shared this information with his wife and asked her to be particularly careful with expenses over the next few months so that they might have some financial reserve if he became unemployed. He describes a heated argument that ensued as his wife objected to the enforced budgeting. As he spoke of his anger and disappointment at her reaction, his eyes filled with tears.

A paraphrase of John's communication would take into consideration his words as well as the affect expressed. The therapist might respond by saying, "It sounds as though you are angry with your wife, but also sad about her lack of support."

Perception checks

If the therapist continues by saying, "I get the impression that her reaction has made you anxious about how supportive she will be if you actually do lose your job," he or she is moving beyond paraphrasing to checking the perception of what the client might be thinking and feeling. Perception checks are important communication techniques because they reassure the client that the therapist is really listening and they allow the client to correct any inaccurate impressions the therapist might have about what has been said in the therapy session.

Summaries

Summaries gather the main points that have been discussed so that they can be reviewed, discussed, and confirmed or corrected. The therapist should include the main themes discussed (*content*) and the emotional tone (*affect*). Summaries should always be done toward the close of the session; they can be used to focus on a particular issue or to close a discussion and move on to something else (Rockland, 1993).

Self-disclosure

Statements about the therapist's own feelings, thoughts, or behaviors, clearly labeled to separate them from the thoughts, feelings, and behaviors of the client, can be powerful therapeutic tools when used judiciously. Self-disclosure demonstrates that the therapist also has feelings, needs, and imperfections, and serves as a model of personal openness for the client. It tells the client that sharing here-and-now feelings and reactions is acceptable and invites the client to do the same. Honest responses to the client's behavior also will help the client begin to see the therapy sessions as a microcosm of the real world. The reactions of the therapist are likely to be similar to the reactions the client engenders in social situations. The therapy session is an excellent place for the client to learn and practice more socially acceptable behaviors. The sharing of honest responses allows the client to view the therapist as a real person and invites the client to become a genuine partner in the therapeutic relationship.

DEPENDENCY ISSUES

The emphasis on the relationship between the therapist and the client in supportive therapy has led to controversy about the boundaries of the therapeutic alliance. Psychodynamically oriented clinicians believe that maintaining distance in the relationship defuses transference and counter-transference issues and helps negate dependency. Novalis et al. (1993) minimize this concern about dependency by arguing that all dependency is not harmful dependency, that dependency may be the vehicle by which the client learns the meaning of trust, and that dependency provides a model for future trusting relationships. They also point out that dependency may be unavoidable and permanent in clients who have a chronic and severe mental illness and who will require indefinite support. According to Montgomery and Webster (1994), comfort and caring are avoided by some therapists who fear encouraging the client's inherent dependency. The irony of this stance is that the diagnosis of mental illness and the mystery surrounding its treatment create the client's dependency on therapists for a cure. Moursund (1993) suspects that most therapists fall between the extremes of encouraging and discouraging dependency, and instead perceive dependency as common but not inevitable, more useful for some clients and less so for others.

SELF-ESTEEM

Persons with major mental illnesses, whether chronic or acute, commonly suffer from loss of self-esteem. Self-esteem can be defined as an individual's personal estimation of worth; the individual makes this estimation by analyzing how well his or her behavior conforms to his or her self-ideal (Stuart, 1995). Enhancing self-esteem is therefore an important clinical focus in supportive psychotherapy. The North American Nursing Diagnosis Association (NANDA) lists three diagnoses that include dysfunctional self-esteem patterns: Self-Esteem Disturbance, Chronic Low Self-Esteem, and Situational Low Self-Esteem (Gordon, 1994).

Most traditional models of psychotherapy assume that successful treatment will indirectly modify a client's low self-esteem. However, cognitive-behavioral therapists view self-esteem

as a central component of personality that affects and is affected by almost any psychological difficulty (Bednar, Wells, & VandenBos, 1991). Cognitive therapy is based on the theory that thoughts and attitudes have a major impact on feelings and behaviors. Chronic low self-esteem occurs during times of stress; clients spend a disproportionate amount of time thinking gloomy or unpleasant thoughts about themselves, their world, and their future. Interventions focus on changing these perceptions by testing their accuracy, developing rational alternatives, and identifying and modifying maladaptive thoughts and feelings. Cognitive theory and therapy techniques are important parts of the armament of supportive psychotherapy. Psychiatric nurses unfamiliar with cognitive therapy might want to read the original work in the field by Aaron Beck, which is directed toward a professional audience (1976; Beck, Rush, & Shaw, 1979), and the work of David Burns (1990), which is directed toward a lay audience.

SUBJECTIVE MENTAL DISTRESS

Clients suffering from mental disorders report a great deal of mental anguish related to their illness. These symptoms, which are often disabling, may be quite different depending on the illness. Therefore it is necessary to consider the most common major mental illnesses separately.

Schizophrenia

Symptom management and prevention of psychotic relapse are major treatment concerns in schizophrenia. Available information supports an etiological model of fluctuating stressors and moderators that influence the level of psychotic symptoms in clients with schizophrenia (O'Conner, 1994). Figure 9-1 depicts the relationships among stressors, moderators, and psychotic symptoms. The most troublesome symptoms for clients with schizophrenia are hallucinations and delusions. Helping the client respond effectively to these symptoms is a major component of supportive psychotherapy.

Stressors

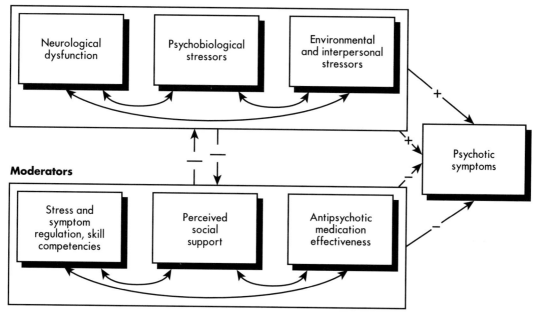

Moderators

Figure 9-1. Effects of stressors and moderators on each other and on psychotic symptoms. Straight lines denote causal relationships; curved lines denote correlations without a specified causal direction.

(From "A Vulnerability-Stress Framework for Evaluating Clinical Interventions in Schizophrenia," by F. O'Conner, 1994, *Image: The Journal of Nursing Scholarship, 26,* 231-237.)

Hallucinations

Intervention techniques used with clients who are experiencing hallucinations have changed over time. Psychoanalytical theory held that hallucinations were an expression of unconscious material, and therefore much effort was spent on interpreting the hallucinations. As behavioral techniques gained acceptance, ignoring hallucinations became an accepted technique, the rationale being that paying attention to hallucinations merely reinforces them. The current thinking is that it is more important to investigate the circumstances under which the hallucinations occur than to interpret their content. It is accepted by many theorists that hallucinations are reactions to perceived assaults on the client's self-esteem. Exploring with the client the circumstances that precede

the hallucinations will help in the planning of interventions. It also will help the client place the experience in context and thus diminish its frightening nature.

Ignoring hallucinations is no longer a commonly used technique, partly because it is difficult to foster a therapeutic alliance with a client under such circumstances and partly because certain hallucinations (particularly command hallucinations) require careful evaluation. However, once the therapeutic alliance has been established, there may be times when it is therapeutically sound to deemphasize hallucinations in order to work on other issues.

Hallucinations have a wide range of intensities; not all clients will experience the same intensity, and many clients will experience different levels

Table 9-1. Levels of intensity of hallucinations

LEVEL	CHARACTERISTICS	OBSERVABLE CLIENT BEHAVIORS
Level I: Comforting **Moderate level of anxiety** Hallucination is generally pleasant.	The hallucinator experiences intense emotions, such as anxiety, loneliness, guilt, and fear, and tries to focus on comforting thoughts to relieve anxiety. The individual recognizes that thoughts and sensory experiences are within conscious control if anxiety is managed. **Nonpsychotic.**	Grinning or laughter that seems inappropriate Moving lips without making any sounds Rapid eye movements Slowed verbal responses as if preoccupied Silent and preoccupied
Level II: Condemning **Severe level of anxiety** Hallucination generally becomes repulsive.	Sensory experience of any of the identified senses is repulsive and frightening. The hallucinator begins to feel a loss of control and may attempt to distance self from the perceived source. Individual may feel embarrassed by the sensory experience and withdraw from others. **Nonpsychotic.**	Increased autonomic nervous system signs of anxiety such as increased heart rate, respiration, and blood pressure Attention span begins to narrow Preoccupied with sensory experience and may lose ability to differentiate hallucination from reality
Level III: Controlling **Severe level of anxiety** Sensory experiences become omnipotent.	Hallucinator gives up trying to combat the experience and gives in to it. Content of hallucination may become appealing. Individual may experience loneliness if sensory experience ends. **Psychotic.**	Directions given by the hallucination will be followed, rather than objected to Difficulty relating to others Attention span of only a few seconds or minutes Physical symptoms of severe anxiety such as perspiring, tremors, inability to follow directions
Level IV: Conquering **Panic level of anxiety** Hallucination generally becomes elaborate and interwoven with delusions.	Sensory experiences may become threatening if individual doesn't follow commands. Hallucinations may last for hours or days if there is no therapeutic intervention. **Psychotic.**	Terror-stricken behaviors such as panic Strong potential for suicide or homicide Physical activity that reflects content of hallucination such as violence, agitation, withdrawal, or catatonia Unable to respond to complex directions Unable to respond to more than one person

Modified from "Neurobiological Responses in Schizophrenia and Psychotic Disorders," by M. Moller, & M. Murphy, in *Principles and Practice of Psychiatric Nursing* (5th ed.) (p. 498), by G. Stuart and S. Sundeen, 1995, St. Louis: Mosby.

of severity throughout their illness. Table 9-1 depicts the various levels of intensity of hallucinations and observable behaviors at each stage. It is important to assess the intensity of hallucinations to plan the most appropriate intervention. Clients who are experiencing hallucinations that provoke intense anxiety may need to be assessed for hospitalization to ensure their safety and that of others.

Delusions

Overly active and acute senses and an impaired ability to interpret incoming stimuli and thoughts are believed to be the major neurological causes of delusions in clients with schizophrenia. Some clients have fixed delusions that are firmly held over long periods of time, often in the absence of other overtly psychotic symptoms and behaviors. It is as therapeutically unwise to confront these "encapsulated" or circumscribed delusional systems as it is to accept them. Mild skepticism is probably the best therapeutic tool. The majority of delusional clients will experience delusions only as part of an acute exacerbation of their illness. Sacks, Carpenter, and Strauss (1974) first described the three specific phases of delusions. These phases and the appropriate interventions for them change as the client recovers. Table 9-2 summarizes the three phases of delusions and therapeutic ways to respond to them.

Mood disorders

Although the most bothersome symptoms for clients with schizophrenia involve severe cognitive and perceptual disorders, clients with mood disorders suffer primarily from affective disturbances. The most disabling of the mood disorders are major depression and bipolar disorder. The symptoms of these two major mood disorders cause quite different kinds of mental distress for clients.

Major depression

Clients with a major depressive disorder report numerous affective, cognitive, physiological, and behavioral symptoms. However, the subjective symptoms that cause the most distress to these clients cluster around feelings of hopelessness, helplessness, and loss of self-esteem. These feelings are interconnected; positive change in one of these feelings will engender change in the others. For example, the client who is helped to feel less hopeless also will feel less helpless and will usually have an increase in self-esteem. In turn, other physiological, affective, and behavioral symptoms of depression will decrease.

Supportive psychotherapy, with its emphasis on the client-therapist relationship, can play a vital role in the instillation of hope in depressed clients. Miller (1992) characterizes hope as follows:

> Anticipation of a continued good state, or a release from a perceived entrapment. The anticipation may or may not be founded on concrete, real world evidence. Hope is the anticipation of a future which is good and is based upon mutuality (relationships with others); a sense of personal competence, coping ability, psychological well being, purpose and meaning in life, as well as a sense of the possible.

Kirkpatrick et al. (1995) reported on a qualitative study in which therapists identified hope-instilling strategies. These included the therapeutic alliance, facilitating success, connecting the client to successful role models, managing the illness, and educating the client and the community about the nature of mental illness. The most frequently mentioned benefits were the positive effects of the client-therapist relationship.

Bipolar disorder

Acute mania almost always requires hospitalization. Supportive psychotherapy can contribute to the treatment of acute mania in the hospital and the continued treatment of the client's bipolar disorder in the community (Novalis et al., 1993). Although the symptoms of schizophrenia and major depression cause subjective distress for clients and motivate them to seek help, the symptoms of acute mania provide considerable pleasure for the client. This pleasure can reinforce

Table 9-2. Delusional phases and therapeutic responses

PHASE	RESPONSE
Delusional phase Client has full belief in the delusions	Mild questioning or skepticism
Double awareness phase Delusions coexist with more accurate reality testing	Begin to confront the delusion Offer consensual validation for elements of truth in the delusion
Nondelusional phase No delusions or only residuals of the delusion exist	Explore the process of delusion formation

denial and interfere with the client's willingness to participate in therapy.

Supportive psychotherapy during the manic stage of the illness will primarily consist of developing a consistent approach, and setting firm limits within therapy and protective limits outside the therapy session for the client and those in the client's immediate environment. When the client is hospitalized, frequent staff meetings will need to be held to plan limit setting and to obtain consistent compliance from staff members regarding those limits. If the client lives with his or her family or has frequent contact with it, the therapist should work closely with family members to help them consistently set limits on client behavior. After the acute phase has passed, clients with bipolar disorder can benefit from the maintenance of a supportive therapeutic relationship. Bipolar disorder is a long-term disorder that manifests in different ways at different times. Knowledge gained over the course of a client's illness can aid in the identification of new episodes (American Psychiatric Association, 1994).

Traditional thinking regarding bipolar disorder was that episodes of mania were followed by episodes of remission that were essentially symptom free. Novalis et al. (1993) argue that for many clients suffering from bipolar disorder, a chronic residue of mania manifests in denial of the possibility of recurrence of the illness and in the

justification of destructive behavior that took place during acute episodes of mania. Amaranth (1994) wrote movingly of her battle with severe bipolar disorder and the struggles she had with delusions and social dysfunction during the times she was considered to be in remission. She cautions that telling clients that they are in remission when they are only in partial remission impedes further recovery; she suggests instead that clients be assisted in moving past residual symptoms.

Kahn (1990) emphasizes a number of therapeutic issues deriving from bipolar disorder that would benefit from ongoing supportive therapy. These include:

- Interruption of developmental tasks by the illness, including the formation of relationships outside the family and career progression
- Inability to discriminate normal moods from abnormal moods and the subsequent tendency to fear strong emotions
- Demoralization from fear of recurrence
- Guilt concerning destructive acts carried out during acute mania
- Concern about genetic transmission
- Loss of self-esteem and a sense of control over one's life

The therapist can provide education, guidance, and reassurance in most of these areas, and through the therapeutic alliance work with the client to prevent a recurrence of mania.

INTERVENTIONS

Reassurance, positive regard, and support of the client's strengths and coping skills have been discussed in the previous sections of this chapter. Other supportive psychotherapy interventions include assistance with situational problems, assertive outreach, and encouragement of treatment compliance.

Assistance with situational problems

Although there is general agreement that the major mental illnesses discussed in this chapter have a strong biological component, research has shown a relationship between symptoms and psychosocial factors that influences the course and outcome of these illnesses. New approaches to treatment have arisen from attempts to better understand this relationship. The stress-vulnerability model postulates that certain people have a biological vulnerability to stress. The breakdown of coping ability in response to stress and in the absence of social supports causes vulnerability to evolve into disorder (O'Conner, 1994; Wasylenki, 1992). Medication seems to have some effect on biological vulnerability by raising the threshold for the appearance of symptoms related to stress (Ventura et al., 1992). Intervention into the stress side of the stress-vulnerability equation necessitates the discovery of the client's particular stressors and of ways to moderate them.

A variety of environmental and interpersonal stressors have been implicated in symptom exacerbation, including stressful life events (Ventura et al., 1989), an over-stimulating or under-stimulating environment, and criticism and unrealistic expectations from families and others in the client's social network (Leff & Vaughn, 1987). The therapist can play a pivotal role in the reduction of these stressors by encouraging positive family and peer support and by collaborating with clients to help them learn personally effective strategies to prevent and counteract stress and symptoms.

Family support

Mobilizing positive family support for the client is particularly important if the client lives at home or has frequent contact with family members. The use of supportive family counseling, including information and education about the client's illness, and the perception of the family as basically healthy will usually aid the therapist in establishing a warm and supportive relationship with the family. Table 9-3 illustrates the mutual benefits for the therapist, the family, and ultimately the client in this partnership.

Peer support

Peers can help clients reduce stress by providing social support and encouragement. As a reference group, they can promote norms of consistent medication use, avoidance of illicit drugs and alcohol, and assistance in symptom monitoring (O'Conner, 1994). The therapist should be familiar with peer support groups in the community and encourage the client to participate in peer support activities. See Chapter 3, Family and Consumer Movements, for more detailed information on peer groups.

Assertive outreach

The supportive psychotherapist will sometimes need to work with other mental health workers and outside agencies. Although controversy has arisen in mental health as to whether the therapist also should be the client's case manager, the reality is that in most mental health systems these two functions have remained separate. However, the supportive psychotherapist will find situations in which it is therapeutically beneficial to work with the client on issues that might ordinarily be considered within the realm of case management. For example, a client told her therapist that after a 4-hour wait at the welfare office, she was told that she didn't have the proper documentation to file for welfare benefits. The client was so upset by

Table 9-3. Benefits from therapist-family interaction

THERAPIST CAN:	FAMILY CAN:
Address the family's problems and agenda Educate family about the disease and reduce self-blaming behaviors of family Help family monitor compliance and prevent relapse Make services and support available in times of crisis Assist the family and client in developing social skills, thereby reducing the family's social dysfunction Link family to support groups and help them reestablish their own social networks Give the family an overall picture of the comprehensive needs and corresponding services for the client	Provide the therapist with a longitudinal picture of the illness Learn appropriate behavioral strategies with client that lower intrafamilial stress and relapse Alert therapist to noncompliance and early symptoms of relapse Provide support to client to avert crisis hospitalization Assist client with daily living tasks, including transportation of client to clinic if necessary Reduce overinvolvement with client, fostering independence Serve as an advocate for improved services, even in areas where the therapist cannot be effective

Modified from *Clinical Manual of Supportive Psychotherapy* (p. 318), by P. Novalis, S. Rojcewicz, & R. Peele, 1993, Washington, DC: American Psychiatric Press.

this that she is now concerned that she didn't pay attention to the instructions of the benefits counselor. The therapist calls the welfare office and obtains a list of the necessary documentation.

Conversely, case managers need to know many of the skills and techniques of supportive psychotherapy in order to establish a therapeutic alliance with their clients. In a study by Goering and Stylianos (1988), clients were asked to comment on the helpful aspects of working with case managers. Clients' comments included "finally having someone there for me," "being accepted," and "being understood." Many commented on how special and rare the relationships that had developed were, compared to their usual experience with mental health professionals.

Assertive outreach to the client is another aspect of supportive psychotherapy that distinguishes it from other forms of psychotherapy. A telephone call reminder the day before a scheduled appointment should be common practice. Every effort should be made to contact a client who has missed a scheduled appointment. This kind of outreach conveys to clients their thera-

pist's caring and concern about their welfare, and helps maintain the therapeutic alliance.

Encouragement of treatment compliance

It is becoming more common for both clients and practitioners to object to the use of the term *compliance* when speaking of treatment planning. Corrigan, Liberman, and Engel (1990) point out that the term perpetuates the misconception that adherence to a treatment plan derives primarily from the client's motivation or resistance and that the clinician is powerless to affect the client's behavior. If compliance is reframed as the collaboration between the client and clinician as partners in the treatment regimen, adherence to treatment is likely to improve.

Adherence to medication treatment regimens by clients with major mental illnesses has been notoriously poor (Axelrod & Wetzler, 1989). Investigations of psychosocial programs have revealed drop-out rates of 18% to 40% (Van Dam-Baggen & Kraaimaat, 1986; Sultan & Johnson, 1985). A comprehensive review of barriers to treatment adherence revealed that difficulties existed in the domains of treatment techniques, client characteristics, family characteristics, therapist-client relationships, and treatment delivery systems (Corrigan et al., 1990). Because a supportive psychotherapist can help ameliorate many of these difficulties, a brief review of these barriers and techniques for overcoming them follows.

Barriers related to treatment techniques

Medication side effects. The majority of clients with serious mental illness take psychotropic medications. Side effects of these medications range from those that are annoying (dry mouth, blurred vision, and sedation) to those that cause severe distress (dystonia, akinesia, akathisia, dysphoria, and tardive dyskinesia). The therapist can assist the client in adhering to medication regimens by encouraging the client to report side effects and by listening carefully to these reports. Medication side effects can be minimized by carefully titrating medications and by using anticholinergic agents to reduce extrapyramidal symptoms. (See Chapter 13, Medication Management, for detailed information on drug dosages and side effects.)

Psychosocial treatment. The side effects of psychosocial treatment have not been as well studied as the side effects of medications. However, the high drop-out rate from these programs suggests that attention needs to be paid to titrating the "dosage" of these treatment modalities. It is important to match the level of intensity of these programs with the cognitive abilities and level of functioning of the client. Psychosocial programs that are geared below the client's capacity to perform will usually result in boredom and dropping out of treatment. Conversely, prolonged and intensive rehabilitation sessions can cause exacerbation of symptoms. Therapists can teach clients to monitor their symptoms and can aid clients in finding psychosocial programs that best match their level of functioning.

Complex treatment regimens. Clients are often treated with a variety of medications, each

of which may have a different daily dosage schedule. Shortened hospital stays have decreased the amount of time nursing staff can devote to teaching patients about medication schedules, and few hospitals engage in self-medication education programs before patient discharge. Consequently, patients who may still be cognitively disorganized and anxious about their ability to make the transition from hospital to community are sent home with several prescriptions with few instructions other than to get the prescriptions filled at their pharmacy. The supportive psychotherapist can give great assistance to the client in this situation by helping the client write out a daily dosage schedule and by suggesting that the schedule be displayed in a prominent place. A few minutes of each therapy session might be devoted to checking with the client about adherence to the medication schedule. Psychosocial and behavioral therapy programs often have complicated schedules and tasks the client is expected to perform outside program hours. The therapist can support the client engaged in these programs by careful listening, by encouraging the client to continue, by offering help in clarifying "homework" assignments, and by praising accomplishments.

Barriers related to client characteristics

Cognitive disorganization, psychotic symptoms, lack of insight, and denial of illness are all barriers to adherence to treatment programs. Cognitive disorganization can be partially compensated for by written instructions, by giving instructions in small steps, by frequent repetition, and by having the client repeat the instructions. (See Table 17-1 in Chapter 17, Community Mental Health Centers, for a detailed explanation of cognitive deficits in schizophrenia and ways to aid clients in overcoming them.)

Delusions and thought disorders make it difficult for clients to have insight into the ramifications of their illnesses. Remission of these symptoms often leads clients to stop taking their medications. Therapists can be extremely helpful to clients, particularly during times of remission, by educating them about the nature of their illness, including symptoms and treatment.

The client's denial of a mental illness is a common and difficult issue faced by all therapists. Understanding the stigma that society still places on those who are mentally ill will help the therapist to empathize with the client's predicament. However, continued denial will often lead to nonadherence to treatment and will decrease the chances of learning from experience and thus preventing recurrences. Therefore, after establishing a working alliance with the client, the therapist should gently begin to point out the correlation between stopping a medication regimen and the return of symptoms. Some clients are helped to overcome denial by the analogy of mental illness to other chronic diseases such as diabetes, in which the problem is physiological and needs to be treated on a long-term basis with medication. This kind of comparison also helps the client to more readily understand the need to monitor symptoms and to accept that the disease is at least partially in the client's control.

Barriers related to family characteristics

Approximately two thirds of clients with a severe and persistent mental illness live with their families (Hatfield & Lefley, 1993). Family reactions to the mental illness of a family member range from overconcern to anxiety and confusion to detachment and indifference. Because families have a great impact on the client's ability to cope successfully with illness, it is vital for the therapist to establish a working alliance with family members and to support them in coping with the client's illness. (See Chapter 3, Family and Consumer Movements, for detailed information on working with families.)

Barriers related to the therapist-client relationship

Several studies have focused on the therapist's attitudes toward working with clients who have a severe and persistent mental illness. Mirabi, Weinman, and Magnetti (1985), in a study of therapist attitudes toward working with clients with severe and persistent mental illnesses, found that 85% believed this client population was not a preferred one to treat. Many of the respondents agreed that most therapists avoid contact with these clients and try to refer them elsewhere for treatment. Packer et al. (1994) conducted a survey of psychiatric residents' attitudes toward clients with chronic mental illness and found that residents reported many negative attitudes toward this client population. Only 29% moderately or strongly agreed that working with this population leads to high job satisfaction. Eighty-nine percent thought that an ambitious psychiatrist would not work with this population, and 80% agreed that psychiatrists who did so were not very academic. Ninety-one percent of the residents moderately or strongly agreed that such clients cannot form a therapeutic alliance.

The fact that therapists find working with clients who have a chronic mental illness frustrating, hopeless, unrewarding, and lacking in professional status has been a major barrier to forming the kinds of relationships that encourage clients to adhere to treatment plans. Efforts are underway to change these attitudes through education and practicum experiences with severely and persistently mentally ill clients. One of the most hopeful signs of change has been the renewed interest in collaboration between state mental health departments and universities (Wilson, 1992; Douglas et al., 1994).

To build a genuine therapeutic alliance, therapists need to foster genuine collaboration with clients and decrease paternalistic and authoritarian attitudes (Corrigan et al., 1990). In the California Well-Being Project, a survey of 331 clients in the state system revealed that 57% reported being told that they were resistant, rebellious, or mentally ill when they disagreed with the opinions or advice of mental health professionals. Fifty-six percent believed that mental health professionals only infrequently listened to them or considered what they had to say valid and important (Campbell, 1989).

Barriers related to treatment delivery systems

Clients' negative feelings about the mental health system can have a profound effect on treatment adherence. Some clients complain of being required to attend day treatment programs that offer little in the way of rehabilitation; poorly staffed and disorganized vocational training, indifferent clinicians, and long waits for scheduled appointments also were sources of frustration (Hatfield & Lefley, 1993; Corrigan et al., 1990).

ACHIEVING MAXIMUM POSSIBLE INDEPENDENCE FROM PSYCHIATRIC ILLNESS

The goals of supportive psychotherapy are to aid clients in learning how to cope with their symptoms and manage their illness, develop interpersonal skills, and cope with the demands of everyday living. Hogarty et al. (1991), Hamera et al. (1992), and O'Conner (1994) have all explored strategies to regulate symptoms without medication through activities that affect both stressors and moderators of stress. Supportive interventions include ongoing encouragement to use symptom monitoring skills and assistance with problem solving and empathic communication (O'Conner, 1994). Medication management skills can be taught to clients, enabling them to monitor the effects of medications on a daily basis and to report side effects or early warning signs of relapse (Eckman, Liberman, & Phipps, 1990). By endowing clients with information, skills, and knowledge and establishing a genuine interpersonal collaboration, supportive psychotherapists can be pivotal in helping clients achieve the best possible quality of life.

SUMMARY

It is important to take into consideration the massive changes that have taken place in the mental health system in recent years in order to put supportive psychotherapy in perspective. The movement toward the community treatment of persons with mental illness has resulted in large numbers of clients being treated primarily in outpatient settings, and in a search for more cost-effective and efficient ways to treat those clients. Advances in understanding the biology and chemistry of the brain have resulted in the use of psychopharmacology as the most common treatment modality for people with major mental illnesses. However, because pharmacology alone cannot overcome the individual and social deficits caused by these illnesses, case management, brief therapy, goal-oriented and practical problem-solving strategies, and rehabilitation programs have all emerged in a relatively brief time as adjunct treatment modalities. In the rush to implement these new treatment modalities, interest in individual supportive psychotherapy waned. However, because of poor adherence to treatment regimens and the emergence of the stress-vulnerability model that posits that dysfunction is related to environmental stress, new interest in supportive psychotherapy has emerged (Wasylenki, 1992; Zahniser, Coursey, & Hershberger, 1991; Rockland, 1993).

A warm and genuine therapeutic alliance between the therapist and the client, in which the two work in collaboration to reduce mental distress, raise self-esteem, and develop strategies to reduce stress and increase adherence to treatment, can result in the client obtaining the maximum possible independence from psychiatric illness. Such an outcome will result in satisfaction for both client and the clinician.

REFERENCES

Amaranth, E. (1994). On alleged "remission" from severe bipolar disorder. *Hospital and Community Psychiatry, 45,* 967-968.

American Psychiatric Association. (1994). New APA practice guidelines provide help to clinicians in the treatment of bipolar disorder. *Hospital and Community Psychiatry, 45,* 1152-1153.

Axelrod, S., & Wetzler, S. (1989). Factors associated with better compliance with psychiatric aftercare. *Hospital and Community Psychiatry, 40,* 397-401.

Beck, A. (1976). *Cognitive therapy and the emotional disorders*. New York: International Universities Press.

Beck, A., Rush, A., & Shaw, B. (1979). *Cognitive therapy of depression: A treatment manual*. New York: Guilford Press.

Bednar, R., Wells, M., & VandenBos, G. (1991). Self-esteem: A concept of renewed clinical relevance. *Hospital and Community Psychiatry, 42,* 123-125.

Burns, D. (1990). *The feeling good handbook*. New York: The Penguin Group.

Campbell, J. (1989). The well-being project: Mental health clients speak for themselves. In California Department of Mental Health (Ed.), *In pursuit of wellness* (Vol. 6). Sacramento: The California Network of Mental Health Clients.

Corrigan, P., Liberman, R., & Engel, J. (1990). From noncompliance to collaboration in the treatment of schizophrenia. *Hospital and Community Psychiatry, 41,* 1203-1211.

Douglas, E., Faulkner, L., Talbott, J., Robinowitz, C., et al. (1994). A ten-year update of administrative relationships between state hospitals and academic psychiatry departments. *Hospital and Community Psychiatry, 45,* 1113-1116.

Eckman, T., Liberman, R., & Phipps, C. (1990). Teaching medication management skills to schizophrenic patients. *Journal of Clinical Psychopharmacology, 10,* 33-38.

Frank, J. (1975). General psychotherapy: The restoration of morale. In D. Freeman, & J. Dyrud (Eds.), *American handbook of psychiatry* (2nd ed.) (Vol. 5) (pp. 117-132). New York: Basic Books.

Goering, P., & Stylianos, S. (1988). Exploring the helping relationship between the schizophrenic client and rehabilitation therapist. *American Journal of Orthopsychiatry, 58,* 271-279.

Gordon, M. (1994). *Nursing diagnosis, process and application* (3rd ed.). St. Louis: Mosby.

Hamera, E., Peterson, K., Young, L., & Schaumloffel, M. (1992). Symptom monitoring in schizophrenia: Potential for enhancing self-care. *Archives of Psychiatric Nursing, 6,* 324-330.

Hatfield, A., & Lefley, H. (1993). *Surviving mental illness*. New York: The Guilford Press.

Hogarty, G., Anderson, C., Reiss, D., & Kornblith, S. (1991). Family psychoeducation, social skills training, and maintenance chemotherapy in the aftercare treatment of schizophrenia. II. Two-year effects of a controlled study on relapse and adjustment. *Archives of General Psychiatry, 48,* 340-347.

Kahn, D. (1990). The psychotherapy of mania. *Psychiatric Clinics of North America, 13,* 229-240.

Kirkpatrick, H., Landeen, J., Byrne, C., Woodside, H., et al. (1995). Hope and schizophrenia: Clinicians identify hope-instilling strategies. *Journal of Psychosocial Nursing and Mental Health Services, 33,* 15-19.

Leete, E. (1993). The interpersonal environment: A consumer's personal recollection. In A. B. Hatfield, & H. P. Lefley (Eds.), *Surviving mental illness*. New York: The Guilford Press.

Leff, J., & Vaughn, C. (1987). Expressed emotion. *Hospital and Community Psychiatry, 38,* 1117-1118.

Miller, J. (1992). *Coping with chronic illness: Overcoming powerlessness* (2nd ed.). Philadelphia: F. A. Davis.

Mirabi, M., Weinman, M., & Magnetti, S. (1985). Professional attitudes toward the chronically mentally ill. *Hospital and Community Psychiatry, 36,* 404-405.

Moller, M., & Murphy, M. (1995). Neurobiological responses in schizophrenia and psychotic disorders. In G. Stuart, & S. Sundeen (Eds.), *Principles and practice of psychiatric nursing* (5th ed.) (p. 498). St. Louis: Mosby.

Montgomery, C., & Webster, D. (1994). Caring, curing and brief therapy: A model for the nurse psychotherapist. *Archives of Psychiatric Nursing, 8,* 291-297.

Mosher, L., & Burti, L. (1992). Relationships in rehabilitation: When technology fails. *Psychosocial Rehabilitation Journal, 15,* 11-17.

Moursund, J. (1993). *The process of counseling and therapy*. Englewood Cliffs, NJ: Prentice Hall.

Novalis, P., Rojcewicz, S., & Peele, R. (1993). *Clinical manual of supportive psychotherapy*. Washington, DC: American Psychiatric Press.

O'Conner, F. (1994). A vulnerability-stress framework for evaluating clinical interventions in schizophrenia. *Image: The Journal of Nursing Scholarship, 26,* 231-237.

Packer, S., Prendergast, P., Wasylenki, D., Toner, B., et al. (1994). Psychiatric residents' attitudes toward patients with chronic mental illness. *Hospital and Community Psychiatry, 45,* 1117-1121.

Rockland, L. (1993). A review of supportive psychotherapy, 1986-1992. *Hospital and Community Psychiatry, 44,* 1053-1060.

Sacks, M., Carpenter, W., & Strauss, J. (1974). Recovery from delusions: Three phases documented by patient's interpretation of research procedures. *Archives of General Psychiatry, 30,* 117-120.

Stuart, G. (1995). Self-concept responses and dissociative disorders. In G. Stuart, & S. Sundeen (Eds.), *Principles and practice of psychiatric nursing* (5th ed.) (p. 379). St. Louis: Mosby.

Sultan, F., & Johnson, P. (1985). Characteristics of dropouts, remainers, and refusers at a psychosocial rehabilitation program for the chronically mentally disabled. *Journal of Psychology, 119,* 175-183.

Van Dam-Baggen, R., & Kraaimaat, F. (1986). A group social skills training program with psychiatric patients:

Outcome, dropout rate and prediction. *Behaviour Research and Therapy, 24,* 161-169.

Ventura, J., Nuechterlein, K., Hardesty, J., & Gitlin, M. (1992). Life events and schizophrenic relapse after withdrawal of medication. *British Journal of Psychiatry, 161,* 615-620.

Ventura, J., Nuechterlein, K., Lukoff, D., & Hardesty, J. (1989). A prospective study of stressful life events and schizophrenic relapse. *Journal of Abnormal Psychology, 98,* 407-411.

Wasylenki, D. (1992). Psychotherapy of schizophrenia revisited. *Hospital and Community Psychiatry, 43,* 123-127.

Wilson, W. (1992). Psychiatric education in the state hospital: A current approach. *Community Mental Health Journal, 28,* 51-59.

Zahniser, J., Coursey, R., & Hershberger, K. (1991). Individual psychotherapy with schizophrenic outpatients in the public mental health system. *Hospital and Community Psychiatry, 42,* 906-913.

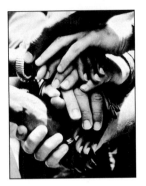

Chapter 10

Case Management

Nancy K. Worley

The complexities of providing and coordinating services in the community for people with serious mental illness require a great deal of organizational work. For the most part, community services are decentralized, with each agency specializing in a particular service. Duplication and overlap of services adds to the difficulty of obtaining coherent and comprehensive community care. For example, a client's financial support may come from the Department of Health and Human Services, Social Security, Aid to Families with Dependent Children (AFDC), or the Department of Public Welfare, depending on the client's work history, family makeup, and local regulations. The local housing authority may provide housing if the client can live independently and is financially eligible. Many community mental health centers provide supervised housing for clients who meet eligibility criteria. A client can often obtain free general medical care from the community health clinic, but a client who meets

eligibility criteria for Medicaid and acquires a Medicaid card has vastly increased options for obtaining general health care. Clients obtain mental health care from community mental health centers, psychiatric hospital outpatient clinics, clinicians in private practice, psychiatric emergency units, and a variety of other providers. However, for a client with severe mental illness to successfully negotiate this maze of services, entitlements, and eligibility criteria is difficult. This complex delivery system for mental health care originates from the deinstitutionalization movement of the 1960s and 1970s.

RESULTS OF DEINSTITUTIONALIZATION

Since the early 1960s, deinstitutionalization (the relocation of clients from state hospitals to the community) has been a mental health system priority. For deinstitutionalization to occur, a dual policy was necessary: a dramatic reduction in the number of patients already in state hospitals through discharge and discouragement of admission of new patients through diversion to other services. The reduction in the state hospital populations from nearly 600,000 patients in 1955 to fewer than 110,000 in 1995 indicates that deinstitutionalization has been at least partially successful (Mechanic, 1992). The integration into the community of former patients and those who had been diverted from state hospitals was more problematic. An underestimation of the community resources needed to serve the complex needs of this heterogeneous population, coupled with an uncoordinated and fragmented service system and community resistance, had unfortunate consequences. Among them was a startling increase in homelessness among people with mental illness (Mosher & Burti, 1994), increases in state hospital readmission rates, a quality of life in the community often worse than that experienced in the state hospital, high unemployment rates (Mechanic, 1987), and an increased burden on families (Clark, 1994).

COMMUNITY SUPPORT SYSTEMS

By the 1980s, mental health care providers realized that mentally disabled people needed help negotiating the complex service system and assistance in lobbying for needed but unavailable services. The National Institute of Mental Health (NIMH), responding to the distress of deinstitutionalized persons, their families, and the mental health professionals who worked with them, began providing technical and financial assistance to states to develop community support systems (CSSs).

Components of a community support system include the following:

- Identification of a target population and outreach to offer appropriate services to participants
- Assistance in applying for entitlements
- Crisis stabilization services
- Psychosocial rehabilitation services

- Supportive services including supportive living and working arrangements
- Medical and mental health care
- Support to families, friends, and community members
- Involvement of concerned community members in planning and offering housing or job opportunities
- Protection of client rights
- Case management to ensure continuous availability of appropriate services

Emergence of case management

From the NIMH definition of a community support system, a new mental health care provider—the case manager—emerged as the care provider responsible for ensuring the provision of a proper range of services to each client. Case management comprises all activities aimed at linking the service system to the client and coordinating the various service components to achieve a successful outcome. Case management includes problem solving to ensure continuity of services and overcome problems of rigid systems, fragmented services, misuse of certain facilities, and inaccessibility.

TARGET GROUPS
Heavy users

Mental health case management is almost exclusively a tertiary (rehabilitative) preventive effort aimed at clients who have a history of serious mental illness. Like all preventive efforts, priority is given to people most in need of case management services. These include people who use mental health services heavily, especially state hospital and community inpatient services and community mental health, emergency, and crisis services. Priority also is given to people with severe mental illness who may not use mental health services but who use other community services. Examples of the latter group include the following:

- Homeless people with mental illness
- Children and families at high risk

- Criminal offenders with mental illness
- Individuals with a dual diagnosis of mental illness and substance abuse

The rationale for targeting "heavy users" of services comes from research indicating that a comparatively small proportion of people with severe mental illness use a disproportionate amount of services (Rothbard, Hadley, & Schinnar, 1989; Surles & McGurrin, 1987). Targeting "heavy users" allows investigation of the reasons for high service use. Community options may not have been available for heavy users, or they may be using services ineffectively and inappropriately. Whatever the reason the goal of targeting case management services to these clients is to decrease their use of services and thus make more services available to people not in a high-priority group. Specific outcome goals for heavy user groups include the following:

- Increased community tenure, measured by a reduction in the number of admissions to psychiatric hospitals and number of days of hospitalization and reduced use of emergency services
- Decreased frequency of crisis situations
- Increased independence in living arrangements
- Increased involvement in vocational activities
- Enhanced social support networks including families, peers, and support systems in the community
- Achievement of client-initiated goals

FUNCTIONS OF CASE MANAGEMENT

Case managers attempt to make the service system responsive to the needs of each client. Although no definition of case management is universally accepted, most case management literature includes the following criteria (Harris & Bergman, 1988; Intagliata, 1982; Levine & Fleming, 1985; Suber, 1994):

- Identification and outreach
- Assessment
- Service planning and linkage with needed services
- Monitoring of service delivery
- Advocacy

Identification and outreach

A comprehensive delivery system must have strategies to locate potential clients, inform them of available services, and ensure access to these services. Establishing and maintaining close working relationships with potential referral sources, such as public and community hospitals, community mental health centers, and social service agencies, is essential to meeting these goals. Some case management agencies specialize in working with particular target populations such as homeless people or people with a dual diagnosis of mental illness and substance abuse. These case managers establish contacts with potential clients in homeless shelters, soup kitchens, drug treatment centers, and emergency facilities (Worley, 1995). Improvements in computer information systems have made identifying heavy users of mental health services possible through paid claims data from Medicaid and Medicare.

Assessment

Thorough assessment of a client's strengths and deficits is required for an effective service plan. Assessments should consider all aspects of a person's life, including psychological, emotional, financial, medical, educational, vocational, social, and residential needs. The knowledge and skills needed for comprehensive assessment are generally beyond the ability of one case manager and require a multidisciplinary approach. According to Moxley (1989) the assessment process attempts to identify the following:

- The extent and nature of client needs
- The capacity of the client to address these needs
- The capacity of the client's social network to address these needs
- The capacity of the service system network to address these needs

This assessment strategy facilitates an important goal of case management—the client's active involvement in the process. The client is a good source of needs identification; an interview with the client should thus be a priority in data collection. Because direct observation of the client's living situation aids the case manager in assessment and planning, the interview should occur in the client's home. If possible the client's significant others should be invited to contribute information that may be useful in the needs assessment. The review of hospital records and conversations with previous service providers provides a more complete picture of the client's situation. A useful guide for ensuring that all aspects of the assessment process are completed is provided in Table 10-1.

Measuring functional status

Traditional diagnostic systems have limited use in assessing needs and planning interventions for clients with chronic mental illness. This realization has resulted in attempts to develop standardized instruments that measure the many

Table 10-1. The structure of case management assessment

	DIMENSIONS OF ASSESSMENT			
	IDENTIFICATION OF CLIENT NEEDS	**ASSESSMENT OF SELF-CARE**	**ASSESSMENT OF MUTUAL CARE**	**ASSESSMENT OF PROFESSIONAL CARE**
Organizing concepts	Unmet needs	Client functioning	Social networks and social support	Formal human services
Basic units of assessment	Income	Physical functioning	Social network structure	Resource inventory
	Housing and shelter	Cognitive functioning	Social network interaction	Availability
	Employment and vocation	Emotional functioning	Emotional support	Adequacy
	Physical health	Behavioral functioning	Instrumental support	Appropriateness
	Mental health		Material support	Acceptability
	Social and interpersonal			Accessibility
	Recreation and leisure			
	Activities of daily living			
	Transportation			
	Legal			
	Education			
Process of assessment	Review with client and professional the needs of the client in key areas of daily living	Match needs with client functional areas to assess whether client can fulfill own needs	Match needs with mutual care resources to assess whether social network can fulfill client's needs	Match needs with professional care resources to assess whether formal services can fulfill client's needs.

Modified from *The Practice of Case Management* (p. 57), by D. Moxley, 1989, Newbury Park, CA: Sage Publications.

life dimensions affected by a mental illness, from the ability to perform basic activities of daily living to the complex cognitive and affective processes that influence interpersonal relationships.

The most commonly used instrument for measuring functional status is the Global Assessment of Functioning (GAF) scale (Endicott et al., 1976), which is found in Appendix C. This instrument measures psychological, social, and occupational functioning on a single scale; it is a useful overall measure but lacks specificity and is difficult to use to measure any one aspect independent of the other two. The Specific Level of Functioning (SLOF) scale is a more detailed instrument that measures the client's level of skill in activities of daily living and occupational, interpersonal, and behavioral functioning (Schneider & Struening, 1983) (see Appendix D).

The use of standardized instruments in case management's assessment process has become quite common. They ensure no aspect of client functioning is overlooked and provide a readily available basis for evaluation of the service plan.

Service planning and linkage with needed services

A comprehensive service plan guides all case management activities with a client. Therefore nurses must formulate service plans carefully with extensive client and family involvement. The overall goal of the service plan is to assist people with mental illness to live in the community. It is developed based on needs identified during the assessment process and requires the participation of the client, the client's social network, and professional care resources. It should clearly state treatment objectives and specific actions that will be taken to meet them. According to Moxley (1989) the major components of the plan include the following:

- Specification of problem areas to be addressed
- Identification of goals
- Identification of the service and supports needed to achieve goals

- Identification of the people or agencies who will undertake specific activities to achieve the objectives of the plan
- Specification of a timeline for the completion of each objective
- Identification of changes expected to result from the completion of each objective

Monitoring of service delivery

Monitoring is the core of case management and perhaps the most difficult component to implement successfully (Worley, Drago, & Hadley, 1990). The monitoring function of case management serves two basic purposes. It ensures that the objectives of the service plan are being met and provides the information necessary for ongoing plan evaluation. The case manager assists the client in obtaining the services specified in the service plan. Because the needs of people with chronic mental illness are usually complex and require the services of many agencies, the case manager must be a coordinator and facilitator. Case managers frequently engage in "boundary spanning" across agencies, organizations, and systems to gather client information, negotiate resources, obtain accountability for service delivery, and monitor and evaluate the outcome of services (Moxley, 1989). Periodic review of the client's progress with each service provider is one of the case manager's duties. The case manager uses information gained from these contacts in periodic reviews of the entire service plan.

Advocacy

Helping people receive all available services and influencing providers to improve existing services and develop new ones also are important case manager functions. *Client level advocacy* refers to helping clients overcome barriers that keep them from getting the services or entitlements they need to live successfully in the community. *Systems level advocacy* refers to bringing attention to service system deficits that affect large numbers of clients. Although this kind of advocacy is usually beyond the scope or influence of an individual case manager, it is an appropriate activity for citizen groups. The National Alliance for the Mentally Ill (NAMI) and local mental health associations have become powerful voices for change in the care and treatment of people with mental illness.

MODELS OF CASE MANAGEMENT

The concept of case management has been used to define functions ranging from therapy to service integration, training ranging from minimal to professional, and organizational roles ranging from advocate to gatekeeper (Mechanic, 1993). Since the inception of case management in the early 1980s, debate has focused on whether it is primarily a clinical or an administrative process.

Service broker model

Service brokerage is a term most commonly used by those who regard case management as primarily administrative. Under this model the case manager assists clients in accessing housing, therapy, health care, finances, vocational and social skills training, and employment. This model stresses practical help in obtaining needed services. Service brokers require strong advocacy and vigorous outreach skills as they attempt to find services to meet the special needs and interests of clients (Worley, 1991).

Clinical model

Proponents of the clinical case management model view the forging of a relationship between the client and the case manager, the ongoing availability of the case manager as a role model for healthy behaviors, and the active intervention of the case manager in the client's daily life as primary tasks (Kanter, 1989). Lamb (1980), an early proponent of clinical case management, argues that the client's primary therapist should be the client's case manager because case management is the duty of a conscientious therapist.

The philosophical differences between the service broker and clinical case management models essentially translate into a debate about the education, skills, and experience needed to fulfill the

case management role effectively (Worley, 1991). Those who favor a service broker case management model tend to focus on the managerial functions of the role. Their primary interest is linking clients with needed services. Familiarity with community services and an ability to negotiate bureaucratic barriers are essential skills in this type of case management. Those who favor the clinical case management model argue for the importance of the relationship between the client and the case manager and hold that case management is a new mental health practice modality requiring a wide range of clinical skills.

Intensive model

A relatively new case management model that combines the best features of service brokerage and clinical case management and emphasizes outreach to clients in their natural settings is intensive (or assertive) case management. Primary features of this model include high staff-to-client ratios with caseloads no larger than 10 to 15 clients for each case manager, 24-hour responsibility for clients, and assertive outreach and treatment in the community. Because this case management model is labor intensive and thus more costly than traditional models, it is usually reserved for clients who have great difficulty adjusting to their illnesses, a poor record of community tenure, and a record of hospitalizations and visits to psychiatric emergency facilities. Table 10-2 illustrates the characteristic activities, goals, and staffing patterns of the various case management models.

CASE MANAGEMENT MODEL PROGRAMS
Service broker model

The Texas Statewide Case Management Program is an example of the service broker model. This program seeks to ensure that clients receive services rather than to provide services directly. Its goal is to improve the services delivered to people with mental illness or mental retardation. Local mental health authorities—community mental health centers or state hospital outreach

Table 10-2. Case management models

	CHARACTERISTIC ACTIVITIES	PRIMARY SERVICE GOALS	STAFFING	PRIMARY EVALUATION INDICATORS
Service broker	Offering of assistance to clients in accessing housing, therapy, health, finances and money management, entitlement, employment, education, and legal services	Increases client's access to full range of necessary services, acts as advocate for client	Most often social workers or mental health workers (non-MD), master's level supervisors	Level of client's access and use of full range of human services Level of client's quality of life Level of advocacy for client's unmet needs or special interests
Clinical case manager	Initial phase: engagement, assessment, planning Environmental interventions: linkage with community resources, consultation with families and other caregivers, maintenance and expansion of social networks, collaboration with physicians and hospitals, advocacy Client interventions: intermittent individual psychotherapy, training in independent living skills, psychoeducation Client environment interventions: crisis intervention, monitoring	Assists clients in adjusting to every aspect of their community environment, both formal and informal; promotes continuity of care in cooperation with psychiatrists	Probably social worker (MA), psychologist, or psychiatric nurse, all of whom must receive special training in clinical case management skills	Continuity of care Client resourcefulness Level of advocacy for client Degree of collaboration with physicians and hospitals
Intensive case manager	Predominately in the community, daily contact with client, staff-to-client ratio of 1:10, team on call 24 hours	Maintains client's independence to the extent possible, anticipates and prevents crises, maintains medication schedules, addresses problems in living	Nurses, psychiatrists, and social workers, with nurses more common in this model because of emphasis on medication management	Community tenure, improvement or maintenance of level of functioning, change in service utilization patterns

programs—provide case management services. The program has 77 local units and 500 supervisors and case managers and serves more than 11,000 clients (Robinson & Toff-Bergman, 1990). Service broker case management models tend to have higher client-to-staff ratios and a greater mix of clients with acute and chronic conditions in each caseload.

Clinical model

Community Connections in Washington, DC, is the best-known example of the clinical case management model. Because an important aspect of clinical case management is the relationship between the case manager and the client, individual case management is the organizational mode used, and much effort is expended on making a good match between case manager and client. Case management is a clinical process, a mode of therapy in itself. Emphasis thus shifts from the managerial functions of case management onto functions that make case management a potential vehicle for intrapsychic growth (Harris & Bergman, 1988).

Intensive model

Intensive case management for people with chronic mental illness can be traced to an innovative program that began in Wisconsin in the early 1970s called the *Training in Community Living (TCL)* program. The TCL program continues today. All intensive case management programs now in existence for severely and persistently mentally ill clients are variations of this pioneering program developed by Stein and Test (Stein & Test, 1985). The following description of the beginnings of this revolutionary program is quoted directly from Stein (1992):

In brief, the program was implemented by mental hospital ward staff who were transplanted to the community. Staff coverage was available twenty-four hours a day, seven days a week. Patient programs were individually tailored and were based primarily on an assessment of the patient's coping skill deficits and requirements for community living. Most treatment took place in vivo: in patients' homes, neigh-

borhoods, and places of work. More specifically, staff members on the scene in patients' homes and neighborhoods taught and assisted them in daily living activities such as laundry upkeep, shopping, cooking, restaurant use, grooming, budgeting and use of transportation. In addition, patients were given intensive assistance in finding a job or sheltered workshop placement, and the staff then continued their daily contact with patients and patients' supervisors or employers to help resolve on-the-job problems. Staff guided patients in the constructive use of leisure time, and in the development of effective social skills.... They capitalized on patients' strengths rather than focusing on pathology. Also, providing support to patients, patients' families and community members was a key function of the staff. The program was "assertive": if a patient did not show up for work, a staff member immediately went to the patient's home to help with any problem that was interfering.

Evaluation of the first 14 months of the TCL program showed that clients had a hospital readmission rate of less than 10% compared with a control group readmission rate of 60%. Other significant differences favoring the TCL group over the control group included improvements in symptoms and social relationships, higher rates of employment, and greater subjective satisfaction with life (Stein & Test, 1985).

Although the TCL program was a startling departure from the traditional methods of providing care to people with mental illness, the program also was a carefully controlled research project. The combination of new technology with a well-designed evaluation was responsible for the program becoming the prototype for the assertive or intensive case management initiatives that followed.

The original TCL model has been replicated under names such as *Continuous Treatment Teams (CTTs)*, *Program for Assertive Community Treatment (PACT)*, and *intensive case management (ICM)*. Each model provides a full range of medical, psychosocial, and rehabilitative services by a community-based team that operates 24 hours a day, 7 days a week. A recent survey of assertive community treatment programs in the United States (Deci et al., 1995) revealed that teams shared a common caseload in 45% of the programs, case managers had a mean caseload of 16.5 clients, and 71% of the programs provided services 24 hours a day. In 88% of the programs a psychiatrist was a team member, and in 88%, a nurse was a team member. Approximately 75% of all services were delivered in the community, and 55% of the programs reported that client services were directly provided by program staff and were not brokered.

ROLE OF THE NURSE
Service broker model

As a result of a federal government mandate stating that "all persons with serious and persistent mental illness who are eligible for publicly funded mental health services must receive case management services" (Pub. L. No. 99-660), thousands of case managers have been hired and trained over the past decade. A scarcity of funds to comply with this mandate has led to the widespread use of paraprofessionals to provide direct services to clients (Dill, 1987). The majority of these case managers operate under the service broker case management model.

The most common staffing configuration in this model is for a mental health professional with a graduate degree in one of the core mental health professions to supervise 5 to 10 case managers who have individual caseloads. Nurses bring several advantages to this supervisory role. Supervision of paraprofessional staff is an integral part of the training of professional nurses in hospital settings; nurses can transfer these acquired skills to the case management supervisory role. Moreover, nurses are familiar with the nursing process of assessment, planning, implementation, and evaluation that closely parallels the stages in the case management process. Nursing's holistic approach, which emphasizes the integration of knowledge about the biological, emotional, social, and spiritual needs of the client, prepares nurses particularly well to supervise direct care staff who must attend to the complex needs of the chronically mentally ill client.

Using the advanced practice psychiatric nurse as a consultant in service broker case management is cost effective (Worley, 1991). Paraprofessional direct care workers have limited knowledge about proper nutrition, side effects of psychotropic medications, and rudimentary health screening. Nurse consultants can serve as educators and role models for case management staff, thereby expanding the knowledge and expertise of the entire case management team. Increasing the awareness of case managers about the physical health care needs of their clients is particularly important because an increased incidence and prevalence of physical illnesses among people with chronic mental illness has been well documented (McCarrick et al, 1986; Hall et al, 1982). However, nearly half of these physical health problems go undiscovered during outpatient psychiatric treatment (Koran et al, 1989; Maricle, Hoffman, & Bloom, 1987). The use of psychotropic medications is widespread among people with chronic mental illness. Direct care workers who have frequent contact with clients can be instrumental in encouraging medication regimen compliance. Nurse consultants can educate case managers to understand the purposes of these medications and recognize their side effects.

Although the use of psychiatric nurse consultants in case management teams is not widespread, the following example illustrates the many roles and functions a nurse consultant can serve on a case management team.

Case example

As part of the continuing effort to move the locus of care for people with chronic mental illness to the community, the public mental hospital that served a major city in the eastern United States was closed. Although this hospital had housed as many as 7500 patients at one time, it had been in the process of deinstitutionalization for many years and at the time of closure had a population of approximately 350 patients. A case management agency consisting of nine case management teams was developed for the care of former patients in the community. These case management teams were staffed by state hospital employees who were educated for this new role. Most case managers were former psychiatric technicians or nurse's aides. The team leaders who served as coordinators and supervisors were trained social workers with master's degrees. Several psychiatrists provided part-time coverage. Psychiatric nurses were hired as consultants to each of the nine teams to supplement the limited time available from the psychiatrists. Nurse consultants performed health screenings as part of a comprehensive assessment and assisted staff in creating treatment plans that included attention to the physical health care needs, nutrition, and self-care limitations of the clients. They also facilitated communication between psychiatrists and case managers. They worked closely with the staff to implement and monitor treatment plans. They assisted case managers in obtaining appropriate medical care for clients when necessary, helped the case manager develop a strategy for working with clients who were noncompliant with medications, deescalated crisis situations, and expedited admissions to hospitals when necessary. Their expert knowledge of the health care delivery system and legal rights of clients allowed them to facilitate the advocacy role of the case manager (Worley, 1990).

In addition to helping case managers carry out their case management functions, nurse consultants have proved invaluable in expanding the knowledge base of the agency staff. Formal and informal education on psychopharmacology, psychiatric diagnosis, health problems, AIDS prevention, and many other health-related subjects has increased the case managers' competence and confidence as they work with difficult clients in a complex service delivery environment. The following case example illustrates the nurse's role in the service broker model.

Case example*

David is a 34-year-old African-American man with a diagnosis of mental retardation and undif-

---

*Courtesy Andrea Macfadden, Philadelphia, Pennsylvania.

ferentiated schizophrenia who resides in a boarding home. During a team meeting, David's case manager reported that during the past week, David had become increasingly agitated, pacing the dayroom of the boarding home and talking to himself. The case manager was concerned that David might be experiencing side effects from his neuroleptic medications and asked the nurse consultant for advice. The nurse consultant assessed David's medication records, which showed that he had been on the same medication at the same dosage for several years and that his symptoms had remained stable. The nurse consultant went to the boarding home to further assess the situation. After interviewing David and the boarding house staff, the consultant discovered that the furniture had been rearranged in the dayroom to accommodate a new Ping-Pong table. In the rearrangement the chair in which David spent much of his time watching television had been moved to another location. This change had apparently disturbed an important routine in David's life and contributed to his recent decompensation. After the room was modified slightly to accommodate David's chair, his mental status improved remarkably without any change in his medications.

Clinical model

Clinical case management includes three therapeutic tasks:

1. The forging of a relationship between the client and case manager
2. The assigning of a case manager as a model for healthy behavior and a potential object for identification
3. The active intervening of the case manager in the client's daily life to structure an environment that will be tolerable to the client and tolerant of the client's symptomatic behavior

Because clinical case management is essentially an expansion of the traditional psychotherapist role, clinical case managers usually have advanced degrees in a core mental health discipline. Advanced practice nurses are well qualified to assume the role of primary therapist. Indeed, with their educational preparation in the biological and social sciences, advanced practice psychiatric nurses bring unique skills to the primary therapist role. The ability to distinguish functional illness from organic illness and to skillfully monitor medication is advantageous to the primary therapist. Except in three states (Alabama, Illinois, and Oklahoma), advanced practice nurses can prescribe and monitor medications for their clients. In some states only certified nurse practitioners are eligible for prescriptive privileges, but in others, legislation includes both nurse practitioners and clinical nurse specialists (Pearson, 1995).

Intensive model

Of intensive case management teams, 88% have a psychiatric nurse as an integral member according to a recent national survey of this case management type (Deci et al., 1995). Intensive case management differs from the other types (service broker and clinical) in that most treatment, rehabilitation, and case management functions are provided by a treatment team composed of specialists in vocational rehabilitation, occupational therapy, nursing, social work, and psychiatry (Robinson & Toff-Bergman, 1990). The treatment team provides clinical interventions such as supportive psychotherapy, crisis intervention, and medication management; client and family education on symptom management, medication monitoring, and coping skills; and encouragement toward vocational and recreational activities. The team brokers links to services that it cannot provide directly, such as supportive housing and vocational training.

Psychiatric nurses bring valuable skills to intensive case management. Because intensive case management requires a more clinical approach to needs assessment, a formal diagnostic component is included in the initial assessment, which consists of a mental status examination and complete psychiatric history. These clinical skills are an integral part of the education of psychiatric nurses and are included in the standards of psychiatric-mental health clinical practice (ANA, 1994). In keeping with the clinical approach of most intensive case management programs, a central focus of treatment is on psychopharmacological intervention. This includes careful monitoring of the clinical efficacy, side effects, and compliance of prescribed medications. Because noncompliance with medication regimens may lead to relapse and as many as one third of clients on medication regimens are noncompliant (Chen, 1991), team members often deliver and monitor medication use daily with some clients. Psychiatric nurses play a major role in this aspect of treatment because clients often require education regarding the necessity of compliance. Side effects from neuroleptic medications are common and a major cause of medication noncompliance. Helping clients relate the actions of psychotropic medications to control of psychiatric symptoms can improve compliance and help clients tolerate uncomfortable side effects (Hellwig, 1993).

Client and family education are essential components of intensive case management programs. Very often, clients and their family members will have little understanding of symptoms, psychotropic medications, etiology, and precipitating events. Knowledge of diagnosis, prognosis, and the expected course of the illness is often limited or faulty (Lefley, 1987). Psychiatric nurses, who have traditionally been responsible for patient and family education in the hospital, can readily transfer these skills to the community setting and help implement this vital component of the treatment plan.

Nurses play a vital role in the case management of chronically mentally ill clients. In the service broker model the supervisory and consultative skills of psychiatric nurses are paramount. In the clinical case management model, advanced practice psychiatric nurses use their skills in psychotherapy and medication management in direct client care. In the intensive case management model, psychiatric nurses have proved valuable as client and family educators, skilled assessors and diagnosticians, and prescribers and monitors of medications.

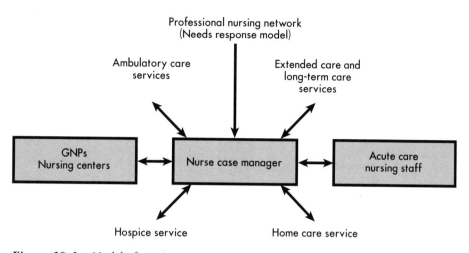

Figure 10-1. Model of nursing case management.
(Modified from "Professional Nursing Case Management Improves Quality, Access and Costs," by R. Ethridge and C. Lamb, 1989, *Nursing Management, 20,* 30-35.)

A NURSING CASE MANAGEMENT MODEL

One of the most cost-effective and integrated systems of nursing case management was developed at Carondelet Saint Mary's Hospital and Health Center in Tucson, Arizona (Cohen & Cesta, 1993). Called the *Nursing Network,* the system is made up of a number of components, including acute inpatient, extended, home hospice, and ambulatory care. Client movement across these services is coordinated by the professional nurse case manager (PNCM), who is organizationally located at the hub of these services (Figure 10-1). Each PNCM carries an active caseload of approximately 40 clients—10 in the acute care setting and 30 in the community. Referrals to the PNCM are made from the community or acute care setting. The PNCM is responsible for collaborating with the multidisciplinary health care team and community agencies to facilitate the achievement of agreed-on health care outcomes and evaluate progress toward goal attainment. One unique aspect of the Nursing Network is that a PNCM follows the progress of the client and family throughout hospitalization and into the community (Ethridge & Lamb, 1989). Data showed reduc-

tions in length of stay for acutely and chronically ill clients (Ethridge, 1991).

SUMMARY

Over the past decade, case management has gained recognition as a major method to promote and provide service delivery to people with severe mental illness and to achieve continuity of care. Case managers are the fixed point of responsibility in a decentralized and complex service system. Diverse models and organizational structures for case management have emerged.

Case management presents challenges and opportunities for psychiatric-mental health nurses in direct care, consultation, supervision, and administration.

REFERENCES

American Nurses Association. (1994). *A statement on psychiatric-mental health clinical nursing practice and standards of psychiatric-mental health clinical nursing practice.* Washington, DC: Author.

Chen, A. (1991). Noncompliance in community psychiatry: A review of clinical interventions. *Hospital and Community Psychiatry, 42,* 282-287.

Clark, R. (1994). Family costs associated with severe mental illness and substance abuse. *Hospital and Community Psychiatry, 45,* 808-813.

Cohen, E., & Cesta, T. (1993). *Nursing case management: From concept to evaluation.* St. Louis: Mosby.

Deci, P., Santos, A., Hiott, D., Schoenwald, S., & Dias, J. (1995). Dissemination of assertive community treatment programs. *Psychiatric Services, 46,* 676-683.

Dill, A. (1987). Issues in case management for the chronically mentally ill. In D. Mechanic (Ed.), *Improving mental health services: What the social sciences can tell us* (New Directions for Mental Health Services, No. 36) (pp. 61-70). San Francisco: Jossey-Bass.

Endicott, J., Spitzer, R., Fleiss, J., & Cohen, J. (1976). The global assessment scale—a procedure for measuring overall severity of psychiatric disturbance. *Archives of General Psychiatry, 33,* 766-771.

Ethridge, P. (1991). A nursing HMO: Carondelet St. Mary's experience. *Nursing Management, 22,* 22-27.

Ethridge, P., & Lamb, G. (1989). Professional nursing case management improves quality, access and costs. *Nursing Management, 20,* 30-35.

Hall, R., Beresford, T., Gardner, E., & Popkin, M. (1982). The medical care of psychiatric patients. *Hospital and Community Psychiatry, 31,* 463-472.

Harris, M., & Bergman, H. (1988). Clinical case management for the chronically mentally ill: A conceptual analysis. In M. Harris, & L. Bachrach (Eds.), *Clinical case management* (New Directions for Mental Health Services, No. 40) (pp. 5-13). San Francisco: Jossey-Bass.

Hellwig, K. (1993). Psychiatric home care nursing: Managing patients in the community setting. *Journal of Psychosocial Nursing and Mental Health Services, 31,* 21-24.

Intagliata, J. (1982). Improving the quality of community care for the chronically mentally disabled: The role of case management. *Schizophrenia Bulletin, 8,* 655-674.

Kanter, J. (1989). Clinical case management: Definitions, principles, components. *Hospital and Community Psychiatry, 40,* 361-368.

Koran, L., Sox, H., Marton, K., et al. (1989). Medical evaluation of psychiatric patients, I: Results in a state mental health system. *Archives of General Psychiatry, 46,* 733-740.

Lamb, R. (1980). Therapist-case managers: More than brokers of service. *Hospital and Community Psychiatry, 31,* 762-764.

Lefley, H. (1987). The family's response to mental illness in a relative. In A.B. Hatfield (Ed.), *Families of the mentally ill: Meeting the challenges* (New Directions for Mental Health Services, No. 34) (pp. 3-21). San Francisco: Jossey-Bass.

Levine, I., & Fleming, M. (1985). *Human resource development: Issues in case management.* College Park, MD: Center for Resource Development.

Maricle, R., Hoffman, W., & Bloom, J. (1987). The prevalence and significance of medical illness among chronically mentally ill outpatients. *Community Mental Health Journal, 23,* 81-90.

McCarrick, A., Manderscheid, R., Bertolluci, D., Goldman H., et al. (1986). Chronic medical problems in the chronically mentally ill. *Hospital and Community Psychiatry, 37,* 289-291.

Mechanic, D. (1987). Evolution of mental health services and areas for change. In D. Mechanic (Ed.), *Improving mental health services: What the social sciences can tell us* (New Directions for Mental Health Services, No. 36) (pp. 3-13). San Francisco: Jossey-Bass.

Mechanic, D. (1992). Managed care for the seriously mentally ill [Editorial]. *American Journal of Public Health, 82,* 788-798.

Mechanic, D. (1993). Mental health services in the context of health insurance reform. *Milbank Quarterly, 71,* 349-364.

Mosher, L., & Burti, L. (1994). *Community mental health, a practical guide.* New York: W.W. Norton & Company.

Moxley, D. (1989). *The practice of case management.* Newbury Park, CA: Sage Publications.

Pearson, L. (1995). Annual update on how each state stands on legislative issues affecting advanced nursing practice. *Nurse Practitioner, 20,* (1).

Robinson, G., & Toff-Bergman, (1990). *Choices in case management: Current knowledge and practice for mental health programs* (pp. 16-35). Washington, DC: Mental Health Policy Center.

Rothbard, A., Hadley, T., & Schinnar, A.(1989). The Philadelphia capitation plan for mental health services. *Hospital and Community Psychiatry, 40,* 356-358.

Schneider, L., & Struening, E. (1983). SLOF: A behavioral scale for assessing the mentally ill. *Social Work Research & Abstracts, 19,* 9-21.

State Mental Health Services Plan Act, P. L. 99-660, Title V.

Stein, L. (1992). Innovating against the current. In L. Stein (Ed.), *Innovative community mental health programs* (New Directions for Mental Health Services, No. 56). San Francisco: Jossey-Bass.

Stein, L., & Test, M. (1985). *The training in community living model: A decade of experience* (New Directions for Mental Health Service, No. 26). San Francisco: Jossey-Bass.

Suber, R. (1994). An approach to care. In R.W. Suber (Ed.), *Clinical case management, a guide to comprehensive treatment of severe mental illness* (pp. 3-20). Newbury Park, CA: Sage Publications.

Surles, R., & McGurrin, M. (1987). Increased use of psychiatric emergency services by young chronic mentally ill patients. *Hospital and Community Psychiatry, 38,* 401-405.

Worley, N. (1990). Case managers facilitate the closing of Philadelphia State Hospital through community treatment teams. *Case Management Advisor, 1,* 74-76.

Worley, N. (1991). Born in the USA. *Nursing Times, 32,* 32-34.

Worley, N. (1995). Community psychiatric nursing care. In G. Stuart, & S. Sundeen (Eds.), *Principles and practice of psychiatric nursing* (5th ed.) (pp. 831-839). St. Louis: Mosby.

Worley, N., Drago, L., & Hadley, T. (1990). Improving the physical health-mental health interface for the chronically mentally ill: Could nurse case managers make a difference? *Archives of Psychiatric Nursing, 4,* 108-113.

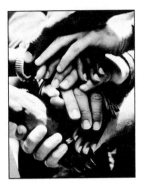

Chapter 11

Psychoeducation

Carol A. Williams

*P*sychoeducation is defined in this chapter as a program of didactic and experiential learning offered in individual, group, or family contexts and directed at a variety of educational and psychosocial goals. These goals include understanding the illness, its course, and its treatment; recognizing and managing early symptoms and signs of exacerbation of illness; and developing effective lifestyle behaviors to reduce stress and promote mentally healthy coping.

Psychoeducation is a relatively new phenomenon in mental health treatment, having emerged as a major force in psychiatric treatment in the mid 1980s. Yet, education is inherent in psychotherapy and a critical component of other approaches to psychiatric treatment (Goldman, 1988; Williams, 1989). Nevertheless, controversy persists regarding what term should be used to designate education for people with mental illness and their families. Moller and Wer (1989), for example, provide education for seriously mentally ill people

and their families that meets the definition of psychoeducation used in this chapter. However, they consider the term "psychoeducation" prejudicial and do not use it. Similarly, Goldman (1988) expresses concern about the misuse of the term and suggests it be restricted to educational programs provided to clients. He argues that using the term to describe education provided to families implies that the family is ill and needs treatment. Possible misunderstanding of the meaning of the term is an important issue consistent with concerns voiced by other commentators (Hatfield, 1986; Hatfield & Lefley, 1987). Nevertheless, the term seems well established and restricting its use may no longer be possible.

Before the emergence of psychoeducational approaches, dominant theories of the origin of mental illness assigned responsibility to families. Consequently, family therapy approaches were developed to treat family pathology. Such approaches resulted in tension between families and mental health professionals. Families who wanted support and guidance from mental health professionals were placed on the defensive and frequently put in a "patient" role by the mental health system's tendency to redefine the mental health problem as a family system problem and then treat the family as a whole. Residual recognition of this problem is reflected in Goldman's (1988) concern regarding the application of the term *psychoeducation* to family education about a member's mental illness.

Several factors contributed to the emergence and growth of psychoeducational models, including deinstitutionalization, problems with maintaining people with serious mental illness in the community, the emergence of the National Alliance for the Mentally Ill (NAMI) as an advocacy force for people with mental illness, and a considerable body of research supporting the efficacy of psychoeducation as an approach to psychiatric treatment (Falloon, 1990; Falloon et al., 1985; Glick, 1992; Glick et al., 1994; Haas et al., 1988; Hogarty et al., 1991; Kane, DiMartino, & Jiminez, 1990).

LEVELS OF PREVENTION

Psychoeducation evolved largely as a way to help families manage seriously mentally ill family members after discharge in an effort to reduce the frequency of rehospitalization. Consequently, much early literature on psychoeducation was directed at the tertiary level of prevention although some addressed all three levels of prevention. For example, in psychoeducational interventions that focus on the family as a group at risk of succumbing to stress associated with caregiving, efforts to strengthen the family include elements of primary prevention. Furthermore, a family psychoeducational approach recognizes the vulnerability of minor children of mentally ill parents and provides interventions to this high-risk group at the primary prevention level. Newly diagnosed clients and their families may initially be involved in psychoeducation to provide immediate treat-

ment and support as part of secondary prevention. From the beginning of psychoeducational treatment, however, the goals are to enable client and family to cope better in the future, recognize and manage future symptoms, and avoid rehospitalization, all tertiary prevention goals.

TARGET GROUPS

Psychoeducation is most effective when the illness is long term and requires life-style adjustment to prevent recurrences. Groups with whom psychoeducation has been used most frequently include newly diagnosed clients and their families, people at risk for rehospitalization, and families coping with problems in the home.

Newly diagnosed clients and their families

Clients and families undergo a tumultuous emotional experience as they come to terms with a diagnosis of serious mental illness and its implications. For some clients a diagnosis such as schizophrenia implies a whole new identity and shift in life-style and life expectations. For family members it may mean giving up lifelong expectations and goals. Psychoeducation with newly diagnosed clients requires sensitive recognition of the ongoing struggle of the client and family to come to terms with the illness. This type of life shift involves a grief process, and working through grief usually includes a stage of denial. Families may rationalize and normalize the changes occurring in the mentally ill family member, attributing unusual behavior to normal adolescent turmoil, for example. Leff and Vaughn (1985) interviewed families who claimed they had never been told their family member's diagnosis of schizophrenia. When Leff and Vaughn talked with the health care provider and the client, they discovered that in fact family members had been told, but were not able to "hear" it at that time. Similarly, people in a stage of denial (whether clients or families) may not be ready to learn about the illness or its treatment. A variety of threats may motivate denial, including fear of stigma or loss of control, identity, or role (Understanding Denial, 1993). Main, Gerace, and Camilleri (1993) content analyzed 11 interviews of adult siblings of people with schizophrenia. They found considerable variation in family information-seeking patterns. They identified families who did not seek information and families who withheld information from the mental health team. They considered the former group of families in denial. The latter families realized the importance of the information, so they were not in denial, but they elected to hide what they knew. Main et al. (1993) recommend that mental health professionals consider the family's readiness to receive information. It is of course possible that parents do not share all they know about the illness with the client's siblings, but this finding and Main et al.'s recommendation are consistent with Johnson's (1990) suggestions regarding the grief process and the theory that the client and family need to grieve for the lost self and its possibilities (Hatfield & Lefley, 1993).

Clients at risk of rehospitalization

People at greatest risk of rehospitalization are those who have been admitted frequently in the past. For some clients and families, rehospitalization becomes a way of coping. Families of people with psychiatric illness experience considerable stress, feelings of burden, and sometimes dangerous escalations of family conflict (Johnson, 1990; Maurin & Boyd, 1990). Psychoeducation can provide families with techniques for managing their own stress and the behavioral problems manifested by their ill family member.

People in certain diagnostic groups are particularly susceptible to recurrences of illness and readmission. These groups include people with diagnoses of schizophrenia, bipolar disorder, and substance abuse who must develop long-term ways of coping with their illness. Thus client and family psychoeducation is an important way to help them learn to live with their disorders. The psychoeducational approach may be general and include clients and families with many different

illnesses (Bernheim & Lehman, 1985) or it may be specifically developed for a particular diagnostic group (Anderson, Reiss, & Hogarty, 1986).

Families coping with problems in the home

Although estimates vary, a majority of clients return to their families after discharge (Johnson, 1990), and families are increasingly expected to assume responsibility for the community management of their mentally ill family members. Most assume this role with no preparation and often in great isolation (Hatfield & Lefley, 1987). Mental health professions have been late in recognizing the need to provide appropriate preparation to these families. Nurses develop care plans for the management of behavioral problems of patients while they are in the hospital; it is a natural extension of this activity to share behavior management strategies with families at the time of discharge. Community mental health nurses can then continue this activity by collaborating with the family in monitoring progress and revising plans as appropriate to the client's progress. Collaboration with the family can thus be an integral part of the psychoeducational program or an adjunct to it.

INTERVENTIONS
Models of psychoeducation

Intervention models can be classified by mode (individual, group, or family), conceptual emphasis, and diagnostic emphasis. The categories are not independent, so it is possible for a psychoeducational program to address any combination of psychoeducational modes, conceptual approaches, or diagnostic emphases. The categories also are not exhaustive. Thus it is possible to address other diagnostic groups or use other conceptual frameworks besides those identified in the model.

Several models of psychoeducation have been developed that reflect different conceptual emphases such as vulnerability and cognitive, behavioral, and social skills. Figure 11-1 depicts catego-

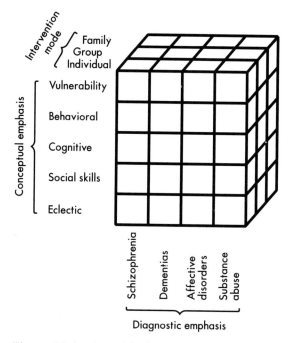

Figure 11-1. A model of psychoeducational approaches.

ries of psychoeducational intervention modes and conceptual and diagnostic emphases, using a cubic model. Nursing models of psychoeducation fit within or overlap these broad categories of psychoeducational programs. They will be discussed separately but related to other models as appropriate.

Intervention mode

Individual. Individual approaches to psychoeducation have been used with seriously mentally ill inpatients (Holmes et al., 1994; Williams, 1989) and with a comparison group in a study of the effects of behavioral family therapy (Falloon et al., 1985). Anderson et al. (1986) work with patients during hospitalization while concurrently beginning to establish rapport with the rest of the family. Most psychoeducational models are focused on the family or group rather than on the

individual client. However, a need for individual approaches to education within the larger context of the therapeutic relationship will probably continue (Williams, 1989). Nevertheless, formal approaches to psychoeducation at the individual level are probably too expensive to implement widely. In Falloon et al.'s (1985) study, behavioral family therapy using a psychoeducational model was more effective and economical than an intensive individual treatment that also included psychoeducation.

Group. Group approaches to psychoeducation are used frequently in inpatient and outpatient settings. Groups are a common approach to the presentation and discussion of didactic content and are particularly common with psychoeducation directed at depression (Maynard, 1993). Huddleston (1992), however, described a psychoeducational group for people with schizophrenia and their families that was offered in conjunction with a clinic for antipsychotic medications.

Family. Individual family psychoeducation and multiple family therapy (essentially a group of families) have been common approaches to psychoeducation. These family sessions may or may not include the mentally ill member depending on the orientation of the professionals involved and sometimes on the condition of the family member. Multiple family approaches were found more effective than individual family approaches (McFarlane et al., 1993).

Conceptual emphasis

Vulnerability. Although the terms *stress-diathesis model* and *stress-vulnerability model* are sometimes used interchangeably to describe mental illness (particularly schizophrenia), Yank, Bentley, and Hargrove (1993) distinguish their meanings. The *stress-diathesis model* refers to a genetically determined diathesis that interacts with developmental stressors to cause schizophrenia (Rosenthal, 1963; Yank et al., 1993). The stress-vulnerability model integrates etiological theories based on genetics, the structure and functioning of the brain, physiological and psychological development, and early experience and training (Yank et al., 1993). The concept of vulnerability subsumes factors that contribute to the development of schizophrenia and interact with stress to create a threshold for symptoms of the illness. This model asserts that the likelihood of symptoms can be lessened by reducing stress or promoting coping skills to decrease the impact of stressors.

Cognitive. The cognitive approach is used widely in the treatment of depression and therefore fits naturally with a cognitive approach to psychoeducation with depressed people. This model posits that disturbed thought content and processes contribute to mental illness. The most widely known of the cognitive psychoeducational approaches is one developed by Lewinsohn, Breckenridge, and Teri (1984) that uses a structured group approach. Green (1993) proposes that the research foundation on information processing deficits in schizophrenia is now sufficient to warrant remediation of cognitive deficits. Tryssenaar and Goldberg (1994) reported successful cognitive training to ameliorate attention deficits in a young adult with chronic schizophrenia. Attention was improved, and the client gained functioning in living, social, and work situations. It can be anticipated that cognitive remediation will increasingly be incorporated into psychoeducation for clients with schizophrenia.

Behavioral. Behavioral approaches to psychoeducation are manifested in the work of Falloon et al. (1985), who use a multidimensional behavioral approach to family psychoeducation. This approach emphasizes the development of selected skills including assertiveness, problem solving, and communication. In addition, specific behaviors are targeted for change and are used to measure progress. Families are helped to use the skills and monitor their effectiveness over time.

Social skills. Several models of rehabilitation and psychosocial skill development have been reported. An early model, Social Skills Training (SST), was developed by Anthony (1979). SST uses a behavioral approach to improve coping skills and role performance and decrease anticipatory anxiety through rehearsal of social skills (Liberman et al., 1986). SST was compared with a holistic health treatment (10 hours a week for 9 weeks) for inpatients with a diagnosis of schizophrenia. At 2-year follow-up, patients who received SST had half the rehospitalization rate and greater improvements in ratings of negativism and overall psychopathology compared with a control group (Liberman, Mueser, & Wallace, 1986). Mann et al. (1993) described a Social Skills Training program for schizophrenic inpatients that is coordinated by nurses. Some program components are offered to all patients and some are used more selectively. Content related to basic social skills is easily integrated into a variety of other approaches to psychoeducation. Groups meet daily for 30 to 45 minutes, five to seven times a week, and consist of four to six patients and two staff. Less emphasis is placed on the disease, its treatment, and symptom monitoring than in other psychoeducational models; instead the model emphasizes the development of functional skills.

Eclectic. An eclectic approach integrates two or more conceptual approaches. The Bernheim and Lehman (1985) approach can be considered eclectic. It integrates a variety of theories and presents them in a general model suitable for people with a variety of mental illnesses.

Diagnostic emphasis

Psychoeducational programs vary somewhat according to the diagnostic group or groups for whom they are developed. Some programs are developed to meet the needs of a diverse client population and thus are necessarily general. Bernheim and Lehman (1985) developed one such general model. Their book on this program is still an excellent resource on psychoeducation and on the development of a general program. Other resources fit certain diagnostic groups particularly well and are cited when relevant even though they may no longer be current.

Schizophrenia. Anderson et al. (1986) developed a comprehensive approach to psychoeducation for people with schizophrenia and their families. The hallmark of this approach is its slow, steady pace and emphasis on giving the client time to heal. Williams (1989) presented a model for nursing psychoeducation for clients with schizophrenia including a detailed content outline that is still relevant.

Literature suitable for families is available in local libraries and bookstores. Torrey (1995) specifically addresses schizophrenia; however, books on mental illness in the family by Hatfield and Lefley (1987, 1990, 1993) are generally useful for all major mental illnesses. In addition, the National Alliance for the Mentally Ill (NAMI), an advocacy organization for the families and friends of people with mental illness, publishes relevant literature. Affiliated organizations are available in every state and in many communities. NAMI's toll-free help number is 800-950-6264.

Affective disorders. Bipolar disorders are often incorporated within general approaches to psychoeducation including those presented by Bernheim and Lehman (1985) and the nursing model proposed by Holmes et al. (1994). Van Gent (1991), however, proposes a psychoeducational program for partners of people with bipolar disorders of manic type. Maynard (1993) proposes an outline for topical sessions for depressed women and Lewinsohn et al. (1984) propose a formal course for other depressed clients. Daley, Bowler, and Cahalane (1992) described a modification of the Anderson (1986) model for clients with affective illness and their families. Glick et al. (1993) reported that psychoeducational family therapy during inpatient treatment was particularly effec-

tive at discharge and 6 months after discharge for female clients and clients with chronic schizophrenia and bipolar disorder. Literature described in the section on schizophrenia is applicable to the major affective disorders as is the information concerning NAMI.

Substance abuse. The psychoeducational model is a relative newcomer to substance abuse treatment, but it seems likely to become an important approach. Treatment programs based on the principles of Alcoholics Anonymous already include important educational elements but have often not adequately addressed basic life and coping skills. La Salvia (1993) describes a psychoeducational program that aims to promote ego functions and repair deficits in the life skills of substance abusers. Rawson et al. (1993) report on three relapse prevention models that use psychoeducation to treat substance abuse. All three models use a combined cognitive and behavioral approach and focus on identifying situations with high risk of relapse, providing techniques of drug monitoring, and promoting development of coping skills and new life-style behaviors. Psychoeducational programs for people with dual diagnoses of mental illness and substance abuse also are emerging (Rosenthal et al., 1992; Ryglewicz, 1991) as are other services for people with dual diagnoses. Literature addressing problems associated with substance abuse in the family is available in local libraries and bookstores (O'Neill & O'Neill, 1992). However, psychoeducational programs for this population are just developing, and there are currently few resources dealing with broad psychoeducational issues; the existing literature is more likely to focus on such topics as codependency.

Dementia. In the early stages of illness psychoeducational approaches can be used for people with dementia, and reports suggest some success in cognitive training for this group. However, the group that will benefit most from psychoeducation as the disease advances is the family, particularly when it is in a caregiving role. Family caregivers of people with dementia experience great stress as they provide physical and emotional care to declining family members. Nurses may be in the position of providing support and psychoeducational services to this group whether they work within a mental health or community health system. The nursing role is particularly important in working with people with dementia. The problems families confront in this situation are nursing problems associated with activities of daily living and behavioral management. For example, families need nursing information on how to develop a home environment that reduces disorientation and confusion. Gallagher-Thompson and Devries (1994) teach relaxation and assertiveness techniques for caregivers of clients with dementia to use in stressful situations. Hinkle (1991) describes a group approach to working with elderly people and their caregivers that focuses on supportive interaction, medication monitoring, and a behavioral approach to problem solving. Many times, however, caregivers of people with dementia cannot get to groups. Home visits for individual family psychoeducation may be more effective in this situation. A variety of resources is available in libraries and bookstores that can be useful in developing programs for this population and can be recommended to families (Cohen & Eisdorfer, 1987, 1993; Konek, 1991; Ronch, 1993). The Alzheimer's Disease and Related Disorders Association (ADRDA) is a national organization concerned with research, education, and advocacy for this group. It can provide information or referrals to local self-help groups (800-621-0379). (See Chapter 27, Elderly Persons with Mental Illness, for additional information on working with the caregivers of clients with dementia.)

Functions of psychoeducation

Psychoeducation has many purposes and functions. Although the most obvious function is the transfer of information and the development of skills, most psychoeducational programs also accomplish other tasks and goals.

Assessment, triage, coordination, and referral

The assessment, triage, coordination, and referral aspects of psychoeducational programs are not always obvious but probably always occur to some extent. Anderson et al. (1986) describe patient assessment and coordination with the treatment team during the hospitalization period. They suggest beginning work concurrently with the family while the patient's readiness to join in the family work is assessed.

Emotional catharsis and support

Newly diagnosed clients need to come to grips with their illness, and families need to work through feelings related to the illness. A new diagnosis of major psychiatric illness presents a crisis for the family and the client. Typically, families engage in a variety of normalizing behaviors to rationalize and explain their ill family member's behavior. Denial, emotional turmoil, blaming behavior, grief, and feelings of guilt are typical responses (Bernheim & Lehman, 1985). Psychoeducational programs need to allow time for the expression of these feelings without forgetting their educational purpose and moving to a therapy model.

Development of support network

Family psychoeducation is often offered within a multiple family therapy framework in which several families meet together. These programs provide the nucleus of a new support network. Sometimes families of people with mental illness have withdrawn from social connections as they attempt to cope with their family members. Meeting and listening to other families allow them to begin to realize that they are not alone, to share solutions to problems, and to develop bonds with a new network of people who share their problems. People who receive their psychoeducational programs in a multiple family group format do better than those who participate in an individual family program (McFarlane et al., 1993).

Client psychoeducation also provides opportunities for sharing in a group, but in this case an assessment must be made of the client's readiness for group activity. Although clients seem to respond well to small group education, they do not always respond well in larger, more didactic settings. A major problem experienced by people with schizophrenia is the difficulty of screening stimuli; just as clients and families need help to recognize and work with this difficulty through reduction of excessive emotional stimulation, professional staff need to bear this difficulty in mind as they develop therapeutic programs for these clients.

Information sharing

As implied in the name, psychoeducation necessarily involves considerable sharing of information about the illness and its management. An element of information sharing within the client-family relationship is less obvious but is critical to the success of psychoeducation. Families who have lived with and struggled to manage their family members at home provide a great deal of information about the client's functioning in the community, activities that do and do not help, and the client's response to medication and other treatment. Families have often resented mental health professionals for their lack of respect for the family, its interest, and its potential contribution. Family psychoeducation recognizes families as important allies in the treatment of the client and requires that the professional form a different relationship with the family than the traditional one. The program typically includes information about the disease process to give the client and family a conceptual framework with which to understand it. The information shared may vary according to the professional's background or psychoeducational approach. For example, Anderson et al. (1986) use a stress-diathesis model that emphasizes brain dysfunction and the client's difficulty in screening incoming stimuli to explain schizophrenia and the resulting need to reduce emotional expression in the environment.

Skill development

A variety of skills are taught within psychoeducational models. Specific skills dealt with in each program vary with the target population, goals and conceptual framework, and needs of the group. A generic educational program, such as that developed by Bernheim and Lehman (1985) to meet the needs of diverse populations, will develop a very different set of skills than one targeted to the needs of a specific population or family. Nevertheless, common skill foci include assertiveness training, problem solving skills, activities of daily living, cognitive training, communication skills, and stress management techniques. Techniques for teaching these skills are widely reported in the nursing literature and can be assimilated within a psychoeducational program. A program of problem-solving lessons, graduated by level of complexity, is described by Mann et al. (1993) and would be useful in a psychoeducational program for people with serious mental illnesses. Although designed for inpatients it could easily be adapted for community clients.

Linking with community and other resources.

Families of people with mental illness have often become alienated from their communities and friends. Preoccupation with the problem in the family, feelings that others will not understand, and feelings of guilt and shame interact to support and sustain this isolation. Psychoeducational programs provide opportunities to renew community linkages. Multiple family groups and workshops provide a forum for the exchange of information and ideas with other families, which can reduce the sense of isolation and reinforce the understanding that problems are shared. Representatives of the National Alliance for the Mentally Ill, self-help groups for clients, the Alzheimer's Association, and other organizations appropriate to a particular group are often involved in the psychoeducational program. Representatives of self-help groups provide a useful perspective on the illness, negotiating the mental health system, and problems in the client's or family's role, a perspective mental health professionals can only attempt to capture. Furthermore, these organizations provide the client and family with a natural group to move into as they become ready for advocacy roles. The family, for example, often has to give up some degree of direct involvement with the client as the client develops social, work, or residential linkages outside the home. Moving into an advocacy role within the National Alliance for the Mentally Ill allows a family member to use some of the same energies to improve conditions for people with mental illness generally.

Medication education

Education regarding medication is virtually universal in psychoeducational programs for people with serious and persistent mental illness who need to integrate effective and continuing medication use into their life-styles. Information about medication also is an important component of psychoeducation for the families of these clients. Families may discourage clients from taking their medications if they do not understand the role of medication in the management of illness. Families and clients may decide there is no further need for medication when symptoms resolve. Medication education is sometimes offered as the only educational program in inpatient settings. In isolation, medication education cannot be considered psychoeducation, but it is always a critical component of any psychoeducational program. Clients need to understand their medications, their importance, and their risks; how to recognize common side effects; why medications need to be continued after symptoms abate; and how to work with the health provider to arrive at an optimal dosage. Ziel and Pesut (1994) discuss issues related to informed consent for neuroleptic medication. When medications carry the risk of tardive dyskinesia, ongoing and adequate education regarding medication, its risks, and its benefits is needed. Discussion of medications can be integrated into the psychoeducational program for clients and families.

Symptom monitoring and self-management

At the heart of psychoeducational programs is the notion that clients and families can learn to understand the illness, identify early or prodromal symptoms, and act to prevent exacerbation of symptoms. This notion has been discussed in different terms by different people. For example, Heinrichs, Cohen, and Carpenter (1985) discuss helping patients develop "early insight." More commonly the concepts of self-monitoring, self-control, or self-regulation have been used. Several instruments have been used to assist symptom monitoring. One developed by nurses is the Moller-Murphy Symptom Management Assessment Tool (MM-SMAT) (Murphy & Moller, 1993), which identifies triggers of psychiatric symptoms and symptom management techniques. Categories of symptom management include distraction, fighting back, help seeking, attempts to feel better, isolation, and escape-oriented strategies. The MM-SMAT can be completed by clients and families and used to guide the psychoeducational process. A problem with many clients who are frequently readmitted (and with some families of these clients) is that they can identify symptoms requiring hospitalization but tend to overlook earlier signs of increasing tension (Holmes et al., 1994). One goal of psychoeducation needs to be to encourage clients to notice symptoms at an earlier stage when less radical intervention is needed. Hamera et al. (1992) conducted a descriptive study of 51 clients of a mental health center's community support program who had diagnoses of schizophrenia to identify the indicators of illness reported by clients in interviews. They classified these as anxiety-based, depressive, or psychotic. Although the authors do not indicate this, clients who identify anxiety-based rather than psychotic indicators may be identifying symptoms at an earlier and more easily modifiable stage.

General health promotion

Good general health is critical to mental health; clients should understand the need to maintain regular patterns of rest, nutrition, exercise, and general health care because these are important in themselves and also because they leave the body in optimal condition to withstand stress.

Current and anticipated research

Typically, psychoeducational programs use specific research findings to emphasize various points. For example, research related to brain structure and function in schizophrenia may be used to discuss the genetic and biological aspects of the illness. Pratt and Gill (1990) describe a more unusual approach to sharing research with chronically mentally ill clients. Clients and staff read, and then meet weekly to discuss, research literature from professional journals concerned with mental illness and psychiatric treatment. Helping clients and families understand the status of research related to mental illness has several benefits:

- It provides a scientific foundation for the information provided.
- It helps clarify unanswered questions for which future research is needed.
- It leaves open the possibility for new and more positive answers to client and family questions in the future, which provides an element of hope.
- It helps families understand the importance of advocacy to raise funds for research on the problems of people with mental illness.

MODEL PROGRAMS

Figure 11-2 illustrates the relationships among elements in a psychoeducational model. As depicted in the model, client, family, and staff variables influence the psychoeducational approach directly; client and family outcomes are influenced directly by client and family variables and indirectly by psychoeducation. Client and family outcomes interact.

Staff variables that influence the psychoeducational approach include discipline, clinical and life experience, conceptual framework, and various

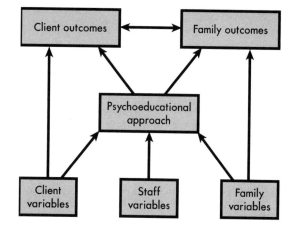

Figure 11-2. A model of the relationships of psychoeducation and client and family outcomes.

system issues such as staffing adequacy, caseload, and supervisory support.

Client variables include demographic characteristics, diagnosis, psychiatric history, clinical symptoms, ego strengths, social skills, and relational history.

Family variables include the role of the client in the family, other life demands and responsibilities, caregiving history, experience of burden, number of involved family members, the family's overall physical and emotional health, time involved in caregiving, and patterns of emotional expression.

Home visits

Home visits have been used in psychoeducational models reported from other mental health disciplines (Falloon et al., 1985); however, nursing's long history of home visiting makes this approach a particularly good fit for the nursing profession. Home visits by nurses have been reported intermittently in the treatment of clients with mental illness for many years. For example, Davis, Dinitz, and Passamanick (1972) reported on the successful use of public health nurses to provide home care to clients with psychiatric illness, with support from psychiatric staff. In this project public health nursing care was used as an alternative to hospitalization. With the advent of community care and the continuing search for cost effectiveness, home visits to people with psychiatric illness are again becoming common. Psychoeducational models can be incorporated into intensive case management approaches by nurses and others.

Recently, Brooker et al. (1994) reported on the successful training of community psychiatric nurses in England to provide psychosocial interventions (including psychoeducation) to families caring for a member with schizophrenia. These nurses provided support to 34 families who were followed for 12 months. Clients demonstrated significant improvement in both positive and negative symptoms of schizophrenia and improvement in social functioning at 12 months. Relatives had more knowledge about medication and less emotional distress than members of a control group who received delayed intervention. With relation to the model in Figure 11-1, home visiting involves individual and family work; and the most likely diagnostic groups are people with schizophrenia, bipolar disorder, and dementia. Any conceptual approach may be used.

Group approach for depressed women

Maynard (1993) proposed a 10-week psychoeducational program for 8 to 10 depressed women. The goals of the program were to help the clients recognize the importance of social factors; learn about the development and symptoms of depression; identify and correct self-defeating thoughts; develop coping and assertiveness skills; and learn about goal setting, personal health, and methods of increasing self-esteem. Groups focus on group, knowledge, and skill development. Maynard's approach uses a group mode and a primarily cognitive and behavioral conceptual emphasis and emphasizes depression. It is even more specialized by addressing only depressed women.

Short-term psychoeducation for seriously ill inpatients

Kane et al. (1990) described a comparison of state hospital inpatients with a *DSMIII-R* diagnosis of schizophrenia or affective disorder, a family member able to participate in care, and face-to-face contact between the patient and family at least once a week. Of the 104 patients who met criteria, 37 families agreed to participate. The study used a quasiexperimental, nonequivalent comparison group design. Groups had between five and eight family members with 24 relatives assigned to psychoeducational groups and 25 to support groups. The groups met for four sessions of about 2 hours each. Falloon's model was used as a guide for psychoeducation. The support groups used a lay self-help model. Knowledge about mental illness, perceived social support, distress and inability to cope with problems, depression, intolerance of ambiguity, and satisfaction with group experience were measured. Analysis of covariance was used to examine differences. Only depression and satisfaction with group differed significantly and in the direction predicted. Kane's model uses a family mode of intervention and a behavioral conceptual emphasis and focuses on schizophrenia.

Nursing model of psychoeducation for patients and families

Williams (1989) and Holmes et al. (1994) describe nursing models that use individual and combined individual and family approaches respectively with seriously ill psychiatric patients. In the program model described by Holmes et al., clinical nurse specialists assess patients and families, develop goals with patients and families, provide psychoeducation, and promote continuity of treatment between the outpatient and inpatient setting. Protocols for the program are presented in Box 11-1, and a brief outline of educational topics for patients and families is presented in Table 11-1. Williams' (1989) model uses an individual mode of intervention, focuses on schizophrenia, and uses an eclectic framework including vulnerability and ego psychological concepts. Holmes et al. (1994) modified Williams' conceptual framework and applied it to individual and family modes of intervention with clients with schizophrenia, schizoaffective disorder, and bipolar disorder.

Box 11-1. Nursing psychoeducational protocols in the combined individual and family approach

1. Screening for eligibility and obtaining informed consent

Patient participation
Patient identification of family member to participate
Family member consent

2. Background information retrieved from record

Days hospitalized previous 12 months
Number of hospitalizations last 12 months
First hospitalization
Record of clinic visits since last hospitalization
Psychiatric diagnoses
Nursing diagnoses
Medication history
Other medical problems

3. Clinical assessment of patient

Patient understanding of illness
Patient perception of reason for hospitalization
Patient recognition of signs of impending illness
Things patient has found helped with symptoms
Patient attitudes toward illness and treatment
Nursing diagnoses
Psychiatric symptoms (Problem Appraisal Scale)
Patient goals
Patient social and leisure activities

4. Family member interview (when consent to participate)

Family member's perception of reason for hospitalization
Family member's identification of signs of impending illness
Things family member has found helped with symptoms
Family member's goals for patient's treatment
Hours per week family member spends with patient
Family attitudes toward patient
Perception and expectation of social and leisure activities

5. CNS* synthesizes data and carries out psychoeducational plan

Generates mutual goals for psychoeducation, considering perspectives of patient, family, and CNS's assessment
Develops and carries out individual plan for psychoeducation for patient and family as indicated by patient and family needs

6. Discharge planning and follow-up

Interdisciplinary discharge planning
Contacts with aftercare staff regarding discharge
Telephone communication with CNS as needed
12-month post-discharge measurement

Modified from "Nursing Model of Psychoeducation for the Seriously Mentally Ill," by H. Holmes, J. Ziemba, T. Evans, & C. A. Williams, 1994, *Issues in Mental Health Nursing, 15,* 92.
*Clinical nurse specialist.

Table 11-1.   Topical outline for patient and family psychoeducation*

BOTH PATIENTS AND FAMILY	PATIENTS	FAMILY
Understanding nature of illness, etiology, and treatment	Monitoring stress, balancing stimulation with caution about adding stressors	Maintaining simple, structured, consistent environment
Discovering relationship of illness and stress	Self-regulating specific symptoms of illness	Managing specific behavioral problems
Identifying early symptoms of acute episodes of illness	Learning to understand others, empathy development	Realizing importance of low-key, noncritical attitude and communication
Understanding medications, their purpose and importance	Developing social and leisure skills, balancing with constructive activity	Including the patient in activities
Learning from aftercare visits, using staff for consultation on problems	Learning to live with stigma, taking part in self-help groups for the mentally ill	Understanding importance of developing own life
Honing communication and problem-solving skills		Taking part in support groups for families, advocacy for mentally ill

Modified from "Nursing Model of Psychoeducation for the Seriously Mentally Ill," by H. Holmes, J. Ziemba, T. Evans, & C. A. Williams, 1994, *Issues in Mental Health Nursing, 15,* 93.
*Education is tailored to the needs of individual patients and families, but includes information in these areas when appropriate.

ROLE OF THE NURSE
Educational responsibilities of nurses

Nurses have fundamental responsibilities for the education of their clients. This responsibility is recognized in the nurse practice acts of most states and in the American Nurses Association Standards of Practice for all specialties (Williams, 1989). Until fairly recently psychiatric nurses did not always assume this responsibility with inpatients, but in the last 2 decades recognition of the importance of education for this group of people, who must learn to live with disorders that affect all areas of their lives, has been growing. Many nurses are currently developing and implementing psychoeducational programs.

Levels of educational preparation for psychoeducation

All nurses have responsibilities related to psychoeducation. Responsibility may vary by educa-

tional level and experience. Anderson et al. (1986) require previous training in family therapy for the people they train to provide psychoeducation to families of people with schizophrenia. Most other authors have not addressed this issue, but literature on the topic suggests that psychoeducators come from various disciplines and educational backgrounds. Psychoeducation is ideally multidisciplinary because most programs address so many dimensions; members of all core mental health disciplines (including psychiatric-mental health nursing specialists) can contribute to the development and planning of psychoeducational programs. In addition, generalist-level psychiatric nurses and members of adjunct disciplines can assist with program implementation. Several models of psychoeducation have been developed and reported by nurses (as previously discussed); most of these are not interdisciplinary. Nurses who work in inpatient settings need to help patients prepare for their return to the community. Nurses who work in the community need to help clients maintain and manage their life situations.

Future directions

Predicting the future is always difficult, but psychoeducation seems firmly grounded with a research foundation supporting its effectiveness as an approach to treatment of serious mental illnesses. Literature review suggests psychoeducation is being widely used for a variety of other, less serious emotional problems, physical health concerns, and general problems of living. The need remains for more research to validate the extension of psychoeducational techniques from the treatment of people with serious mental illness to these other groups.

The growing trend toward psychoeducational approaches suggests that nurses will need to develop programs to meet these needs. When developing programs to fit the needs of people with serious mental illness, there are a number of models to choose from, several of which have been reviewed in this chapter. When nurses need to develop psychoeducational programs for new groups, they may have to extrapolate from existing programs or modify programs to fit issues of concern in the population of interest. Box 11-2 outlines steps that may be used in developing a new psychoeducational program.

Box 11-2. Planning a psychoeducational program

1. Identify the target population

   Specify initial assumptions about psychoeducational needs for the population
   Conduct a literature review

2. Identify the most important issues and content for this population

   Primary prevention issues
   Secondary prevention issues
   Tertiary prevention issues

3. If the literature does not identify priority issues and content areas, interview clients, families, and professionals to obtain ideas regarding needed content. If ideas are available in literature, review themes with clients, families, and other professionals to assess appropriateness of content and determine priorities

4. If not identified in initial planning, identify the disciplines to be involved in program development and specific representatives to be involved in implementation

5. Identify the goals of the program at each level of prevention

6. Select the conceptual approaches to be used

7. Identify people and organizational resources in the community appropriate to the population and selected topics

8. Determine specific plans such as timing of program, length, intervention modes to be used, and responsibility for specific content

9. Identify supportive literature

   For staff
   For clients
   For families

SUMMARY

Psychoeducational approaches are increasingly important in dealing with mental health problems. When a client has a long-term illness that requires major adaptation in life-style, the mental health system must provide information to help the client (and often the family) learn to understand the illness and manage it in a way that permits a normal life-style to the fullest extent possible.

REFERENCES

Anderson, C. M., Reiss, D. J., & Hogarty, G. E. (1986). *Schizophrenia and the family: A practitioner's guide to psychoeducation and management.* New York: Guilford Press.

Anthony, W. A. (1979). *The principles of psychiatric rehabilitation.* Amherst, MA: Human Resource Development Press.

Bernheim, K. F., & Lehman, A. F. (1985). *Working with families of the mentally ill.* New York: W. W. Norton & Company.

Brooker, C., Falloon, I. R. H., Butterworth, A., Goldberg, D., et al. (1994). The outcome of training community psychiatric nurses to deliver psychosocial intervention. *British Journal of Psychiatry, 165,* 222-230.

Cohen, D., & Eisdorfer, C. (1987). *The loss of self: A family resource for the care of Alzheimer's disease and related disorders.* New York: Penguin Books (Plume).

Cohen, D., & Eisdorfer, C. (1993). *Caring for your aging parents.* New York: G. P. Putnam's Sons.

Daley, D. C., Bowler, K., & Cahalane, H. (1992). Approaches to patient and family education with affective disorders. *Patient Education and Counseling, 19,* 163-174.

Davis, A. E., Dinitz, S., & Passamanick, B. (1972). The prevention of hospitalization in schizophrenia: Five years after an experimental program. *American Journal of Orthopsychiatry, 42,* 375-388.

Falloon, I. R. H., et al. (1985). *Family management of schizophrenia: A study of clinical, social, family, and economic benefits.* Baltimore: Johns Hopkins University Press.

Falloon, I. R. H. (1990). Behavioral family therapy with schizophrenic disorders. In M. I. Herz, S. J. Keith, & J. P. Docherty (Eds.), *Handbook of schizophrenia, Vol 4: Psychosocial treatment of schizophrenia* (pp. 135-151). Amsterdam: Elsevier.

Gallagher-Thompson, D., & Devries, H. M. (1994). "Coping with frustration" classes: Development and preliminary outcomes with women who care for relatives with dementia. *Gerontologist, 34,* 548-552.

Glick, I. D. (1992). Medication and family therapy for schizophrenia and mood disorder. *Psychopharmacology Bulletin, 28,* 223-225.

Glick, I. D., Burti, L., Okonogi, K., & Sacks, M. (1994). Effectiveness in psychiatric care III. Psychoeducation and outcome for patients with major affective disorder and their families. *British Journal of Psychiatry, 164,* 104-106.

Glick, I. D., Clarkin, J. F., Haas, G. L., & Spencer, J. H. (1993). Clinical significance of inpatient family interventions: Conclusions from a clinical trial. *Hospital and Community Psychiatry, 44,* 869-873.

Goldman, C. R. (1988). Toward a definition of psychoeducation. *Hospital and Community Psychiatry, 39,* 666-668.

Green, M. F. (1993). Cognitive remediation in schizophrenia: Is it time yet? *American Journal of Psychiatry, 150,* 178-187.

Haas, G. L., Glick, I. D., Clarkin, J. F., Spencer, J. H., Lewis, A. B., Peyser, J., DeMane, N., Good-Ellis, M., Harris, E., & Lestelle, V. (1988). Inpatient family intervention: A randomized clinical trial: Results at hospital discharge. *Archives of General Psychiatry, 45,* 217-224.

Hamera, E. K., Peterson, K. A., Young, L. M., & Schaumloffel, M. M. (1992). Symptom monitoring in schizophrenia: Potential for enhancing self-care. *Archives of Psychiatric Nursing, 6,* 324-330.

Hatfield, A. B. (1986). Semantic barriers to family and professional collaboration. *Schizophrenia Bulletin, 12,* 325-333.

Hatfield, A. B., & Lefley, H. P. (Eds.) (1987). *Families of the mentally ill: Coping and adaptation,* New York: Guilford Press.

Hatfield, A., & Lefley, H. P. (1990). *Stress, coping, and adaptation.* New York: Guilford Press.

Hatfield, A., & Lefley, H. P. (1993). *Surviving mental illness: Stress, coping, and adaptation.* New York: Guilford Press.

Heinrichs, D. W., Cohen, B. P., & Carpenter, W. T. (1985). Early insight and the management of schizophrenia decompensation. *Journal of Nervous and Mental Disease, 173,* 133-137.

Hinkle, J. S. (1991). Support group counseling for caregivers of Alzheimer's disease patients. Special issue: Group work with the aging and their caregivers. *Journal for Specialists in Group Work, 16,* 185-190.

Hogarty, G. E., Anderson, C. M., Reiss, D. J., Kornblith, S. J., Greenwald, D. P., Ulrich, R. F., & Carter, M. (1991). Family psychoeducation, social skills training, and maintenance chemotherapy in the aftercare treatment of schizophrenia. II. Two-year effects of a controlled study on relapse and adjustment. *Archives of General Psychiatry, 48,* 340-347.

Holmes, H., Ziemba, J., Evans, T., & Williams, C. A. (1994). Nursing model of psychoeducation for the seriously mentally ill. *Issues in Mental Health Nursing, 15,* 85-104.

Huddleston, J. (1992). Family and group psychoeducational approaches in the management of schizophrenia. *Clinical Nurse Specialist, 6,* 118-121.

Johnson, D. L. (1990). The family's experience of living with mental illness. In H. P. Lefley, & D. L. Johnson (Eds.), *Families as allies in treatment of the mentally ill: New directions for mental health professionals* (pp. 31-64). Washington, DC: American Psychiatric Press.

Kane, C. F., DiMartino, E., & Jiminez, M. (1990). A comparison of short-term psychoeducational and support groups for relatives coping with chronic schizophrenia. *Archives of Psychiatric Nursing, 4,* 343-353.

Konek, C. W. (1991). *Daddy-boy: A family's struggle with Alzheimer's.* St. Paul, MN: Graywolf Press.

La Salvia, T. A. (1993). Enhancing addiction treatment through psychoeducational groups. *Journal of Substance Abuse Treatment, 10,* 439-444.

Leff, J. P., & Vaughn, C. (1985). *Expressed emotion in families.* New York: Guilford Press.

Lewinsohn, P. M., Breckenridge, J. S., & Teri, L. (1984). *The coping with depression course: A psychoeducational intervention for unipolar depression.* Eugene, OR: Castalia Co.

Liberman, R. P., Massel, H. K., Mosk, M. D., & Wong, S. E. (1986). Social skills training for chronic mental patients. *Hospital and Community Psychiatry, 36,* 396-403.

Liberman, R. P., Mueser, K. T., & Wallace, C. J. (1986). Social skills training for schizophrenic individuals at risk for relapse. *American Journal of Psychiatry, 143,* 523-526.

Main, M. C., Gerace, L. M., & Camilleri, D. (1993). Information sharing concerning schizophrenia in a family member: Adult siblings' perspectives. *Archives of Psychiatric Nursing, 7,* 147-153.

Mann, N. A., Tandon, R., Butler, J., Boyd, M., Eisner, W. H., & Lewis, M. (1993). Psychosocial rehabilitation in schizophrenia: Beginnings in acute hospitalization. *Archives of Psychiatric Nursing, 7,* 154-162.

Maurin, J. T., & Boyd, C. B. (1990). Burden of mental illness on the family: A critical review. *Archives of Psychiatric Nursing, 4,* 99-107.

Maynard, C. (1993). Psychoeducational approach to depression in women. *Journal of Psychosocial Nursing and Mental Health Services, 31*(12), 9-14.

McFarlane, W. R. (1990). Can the family literature be integrated? In H. P. Lefley, & D. L. Johnson (Eds.), *Families as allies in treatment of the mentally ill: New directions for mental health professionals* (pp. 65-75). Washington, DC: American Psychiatric Press.

McFarlane, W. R., Dunne, E., Lukens, E., Newmark, M., McLaughlin-Toran, J., Deakins, S., & Horen, B. (1993). From research to clinical practice: Dissemination of New York State's family psychoeducation project. *Hospital and Community Psychiatry, 44,* 265-270.

Moller, M. D., & Wer, J. E. (1989). Simultaneous patient/family education regarding schizophrenia. *Archives of Psychiatric Nursing, 3,* 332-337.

Murphy, M. F., & Moller, M. D. (1993). Relapse management in neurobiological disorders: The Moller-Murphy Symptom Management Assessment Tool. *Archives of Psychiatric Nursing, 7,* 226-235.

O'Neill, R. B., & O'Neill, D. (1992). *How to cope with an addictive person: Living on the border of the disorder.* Minneapolis: Bethany House.

Pratt, C. W., & Gill, K. J. (1990). Sharing research knowledge to empower people who are chronically mentally ill. *Psychosocial Rehabilitation Journal, 13*(3), 75-79.

Rawson, R. A., Obert, J. L., McCann, M. J., & Marinelli-Casey, P. (1993). Relapse prevention models for substance abuse treatment. Special issue: Psychotherapy for the addictions. *Psychotherapy, 30,* 284-298.

Ronch, J. L. (1993). *Alzheimer's disease: A practical guide for families and other caregivers.* New York: Crossroad.

Rosenthal, D. (Ed.) (1963). *The Genain quadruplets.* New York: Basic Books.

Rosenthal, R. N., Hellerstein, D. J., Miner, C. R, & Christian, R. (1992). A model of integrated services for outpatient treatment of patients with comorbid schizophrenia and addictive disorders. *American Journal on Addictions, 1,* 339-348.

Ryglewicz, H. (1991). Psychoeducation for clients and families: A way in, out, and through in working with people with dual disorders. Special issue: Serving persons with dual disorders of mental illness and substance use. *Psychosocial Rehabilitation Journal, 15*(2), 79-89.

Torrey, E. F. (1995). *Surviving schizophrenia: A manual for families, consumers, and providers.* New York: Harper.

Tryssenaar, J., & Goldberg, J. (1994). Improving attention in a person with schizophrenia. *Canadian Journal of Occupational Therapy, 61,* 198-205.

Understanding denial: Fear underlies it. *NAMI Advocate, 14* (8), 9 (October 1993).

Van Gent, E. M. (1991). Psychoeducation of partners of bipolar-manic patients. *Journal of Affective Disorders 21,* 15-18.

Williams, C. A. (1989). Patient education for people with schizophrenia. *Perspectives in Psychiatric Care, 25,* 14-21.

Yank, G. R., Bentley, K. J., & Hargrove, D. S. (1993). The vulnerability-stress model of schizophrenia: Advances in psychosocial treatment. *American Journal of Orthopsychiatry, 63,* 55-69.

Ziel, S. E., & Pesut, D. J. (1994). Schizophrenia, neuroleptics, and tardive dyskinesia: Issues to consider in client decision-making. *Capsules and Comments in Psychiatric Nursing, 1*(3), 4-9.

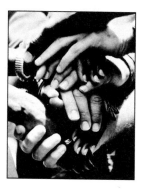

Chapter 12

Psychosocial Rehabilitation

Richard C. Baron

Psychosocial rehabilitation is perhaps best understood as a fusion of principles, programs, and practices that help people with severe mental illness lead more independent and satisfying lives in community settings. The psychosocial principles that characterize the field emphasize a belief in the potential of people with serious psychiatric disabilities and a commitment to the empowerment of the individual. A broad range of psychosocial programs use these principles to help clients respond successfully to the pragmatic demands of community life through social, residential, vocational, and educational rehabilitation services. Within these programs psychosocial practices emphasize the development of practical skills in a "real world" environment in which learning-by-doing helps people attain the goals they have established for themselves. Psychosocial rehabilitation professionals charged with fusing these principles, programs, and practices into a coherent whole are sometimes surprised at how dramatically successful they can be in offering real hope to people who otherwise would face institutional care or community abandonment.

Because of its success, psychosocial rehabilitation (PSR) has grown from a handful of small, nonprofit, private agencies in the 1960s to several thousand programs in public and private settings throughout the country today. PSR programs were once considered adjunctive to clinical treatment of people with serious mental illness, but psychosocial rehabilitation is now broadly established as a central and critical element of the service delivery system in every state in the country. Psychosocial rehabilitation practitioners, initially seen by clinicians as maverick outsiders, have established themselves as independent and well-regarded mental health professionals. Although the field continues to draw personnel from many core mental health and rehabilitation professions, psychosocial rehabilitation's commitment to quality service delivered by qualified staff is supported by its own vigorous professional association, the International Association of Psychosocial Rehabilitation Services (IAPSRS).

Rapid growth and broadening responsibilities have made a once simple and straightforward concept a bit more complex. The principles characterizing psychosocial rehabilitation have grown in number and depth, competing program models suggest varied emphases and alternate approaches, and the field's evolving practice guidelines are under continuous scrutiny. This chapter provides an overview of the PSR dynamic, examining the historic growth of the field and its underlying principles, the major service elements and program designs embraced under the expanding psychosocial rehabilitation umbrella, and the roles that psychosocial practitioners play in the care of people with serious mental illness.

PRINCIPLES OF PSYCHOSOCIAL REHABILITATION: A HISTORICAL AND CONTEMPORARY OVERVIEW

Psychosocial rehabilitation is a relatively young field whose evolution parallels the changes in the country's broader mental health service delivery system during the past 50 years. At the end of World War II the vast majority of persons with serious mental illness lived in public or private institutions; they were likely to have lived there many years, and they were more than likely to live out their lives in those same settings. However, the introduction in the 1950s of a new generation of psychotropic medications, with significant positive effects on the more active and disruptive symptoms of serious mental illness, prompted institutions to begin—slowly at first and then more vigorously—to discharge patients to community life (Goertzel & Lamb, 1971). Most discharge plans returned patients to their families, but as the pace of deinstitutionalization quickened in the early 1960s discharges were just as (or more) likely to be to boarding homes, "old age" homes, single room occupancy hotels, or worse (Allen, 1974).

Effective clinical treatment remained difficult for many clients to access outside the institutional setting (this was especially true for clients with limited incomes), and there were few rehabilitation-oriented services to help those who had difficulty adjusting to community life after what

had sometimes been 10, 20, or 30 years of regimented hospital routine. Discharged patients—whether living with their families or on their own—often felt at a loss; tremendous isolation compounded their sense of inadequacy. Slowly, small groups of former patients in New York, Philadelphia, Boston, and elsewhere, began to meet together, perhaps only once a week, to compare notes on how to survive in the community and to find a temporary antidote to their loneliness. Some groups met on their own, and others enlisted the support of volunteer or paid mental health staff.

From these modest beginnings psychosocial rehabilitation began to take shape. By the 1960s a number of professionally operated programs (for example, Fountain House in New York, Horizon House in Philadelphia, Center House in Boston, Thresholds in Chicago, Portals in Los Angeles, and Hill House in Cleveland) had grown from weekly social gatherings into rehabilitation programs that offered social support, classes in a variety of pragmatic skills areas, and vocational preparation opportunities several days a week. By the 1970s many communities supported fully staffed programs with a broad array of residential, social, vocational, and educational services. These programs in turn served as models for dozens of other nonprofit private agencies across the country (Anthony & Liberman, 1986).

By this time deinstitutionalization was on its inexorable march, and in the 1970s state after state made dramatic efforts to discharge patients from hospitals into the community. A variety of factors fueled deinstitutionalization: ongoing advances in psychopharmacology, President Kennedy's early sponsorship of (and the later proliferation of) community mental health and mental retardation centers, the rising tide of "progressive" approaches to diversity in the broader society, and perhaps most importantly the opportunity for states to minimize their financial support of state hospitals by relying on federal government support for community services. Consequently, many people with serious emotional problems and ongoing adjustment crises found themselves adrift in community settings (Stroul, 1987).

By the end of the 1970s it was clear that community mental health and mental retardation (MH-MR) centers, with their clinical emphasis on inpatient, outpatient, and partial hospitalization services, were unable to meet the needs of a growing number of people who could not find adequate housing, establish and maintain friendships, locate appropriate employment, or adequately manage their own financial or medical benefits. Psychosocial rehabilitation programs that focused on such issues proliferated. Even more importantly the psychosocial rehabilitation approach found new sponsorship; county mental health clinics, community MH-MR centers, and other organizations (including state hospitals) began to offer psychosocial rehabilitation programs to meet some of their clients' most pressing needs.

Fundamental principles

The rapid emergence of the psychosocial rehabilitation field, however, owes its success to more than the sudden presence in the community of large numbers of people with serious emotional and adjustment problems. The strength of psychosocial rehabilitation is the appeal and effectiveness of its central principles. Although no set of psychosocial principles is definitive—indeed, one of the most important characteristics of the field may be its tendency to "let a thousand flowers bloom"—a number of authors (Blankertz & Cnann, 1994; Dincin, 1994; Hughes, 1994; Rutman, 1994) have identified the core values that shaped the field's development:

- **Normalizing roles and relationships.** Psychosocial rehabilitation asserts that people with serious mental illness need not be separated from the rest of society, treated especially gently or within an especially controlling environment, or relegated to only a limited range of living circumstances, work opportunities, or social relationships. Rather it is assumed that a full range of life experiences is within their grasp.

- **Acknowledging the potential for growth.** Closely related to the concept of normalization is the belief that people with serious mental illness, despite the disabling aspects of their conditions, have a unique potential to develop skills, make personal choices, manage the illness, and achieve many goals that may have once seemed unattainable.

- **Focusing on here-and-now services.** Psychosocial rehabilitation services most often begin pragmatically (for example, by focusing on housing needs, vocational ambitions, social isolation, and financial crises) and work with clients to address their most urgent concerns but tend to leave the management of the underlying illness to clinical staff in other settings. PSR seeks to strengthen the client's ability to accept and meet the responsibilities of day-to-day life.

- **Learning-by-doing.** To address problem areas, psychosocial rehabilitation practitioners provide opportunities for problem solving within a real world environment. PSR encourages less talk about problem solving, more actual engagement in the problem itself, and an increasing tendency to avoid agency-based classes in favor of working with people in their homes, at their jobs, and in their communities.

- **Emphasizing informal and egalitarian relationships.** Psychosocial programs deemphasize formal relationships with their superior-inferior status implications and replace them with a friendlier, "first names only" approach in which more egalitarian staff-client relationships can promote both the dignity of the clients receiving services and the importance of their assuming primary responsibility for establishing the focus, tone, and pace of their rehabilitation programs.

- **Approaching community life holistically.** Psychosocial programs recognize the interrelatedness of the various domains of community life. Consequently, although PSR programs often begin with a single social, vocational, or residential focus, they soon add other elements of rehabilitation programming, recognizing that successful community living depends on simultaneously addressing needs in many arenas.

- **Blurring professional roles.** Psychosocial programs tend to blur professional distinctions. Although PSR team members recognize that each traditional mental health discipline brings a special strength to the psychosocial environment, psychiatrists, psychologists, social workers, and psychiatric nurses may nevertheless find themselves listening with genuine regard to other workers—including residential staff, job coaches, case managers, and vocational counselors—who may know their clients just as well.

Emerging principles

Over the years, psychosocial rehabilitation has grown, adding new principles to the PSR canon in an ongoing effort to sustain the field's relevance in a changing mental health environment. These principles include the following:

- **Multicultural sensitivity.** Psychosocial agencies are increasingly wrestling with the implications of their work in a multicultural society; this concern has meant ensuring that staff are representative of the communities they serve and that services are offered in a way that does not discriminate against clients from minority backgrounds. To do this, psychosocial services have grown more aware of the need to provide diversity training for their practitioners.
- **Consumer empowerment.** Similarly the emergence of a strong and effective mental health consumer movement over the past 20 years has engendered initiatives to ensure that programs provide clients the rights to which they are entitled, include consumers on advisory and policy-making boards, and consider consumers as potential staff members.
- **Recognition of the role of the family.** Psychosocial programs have in the past held the clinical perception of the family as the incubator of the client's illness and functional incapacities, but they have come a long way toward

recognizing the inaccuracy of such generalizations and the importance of family members as emotional and practical supporters (and as informal case managers) for clients receiving psychosocial services.

- **Strong focus on outcomes.** Psychosocial agencies are keenly concerned with demonstrating the impact of their services on the functional capacities and sense of satisfaction of their clients and the cost effectiveness of the services they offer. In tight economic circumstances, with budget pressure at state and federal levels, psychosocial agencies are committed to demonstrating that their services decrease the use of crisis facilities, community inpatient institutions, and state hospitals.
- **Stronger collaboration with treatment services.** Although psychosocial practitioners used to tend to dismiss clinical treatment and doubt the usefulness of medications, they are growing in appreciation for stronger collaborations (on an egalitarian basis) with clinicians, the central role of psychotropic medications in supporting clients' rehabilitation goals, and the value of accurate diagnosis, psychodynamic treatment, and medically oriented care.
- **Emphasis on recovery.** Tying many of these principles together is a gradually emerging focus on recovery. Recovery, as used in this context, does not imply that each client can attain a "cure" through psychosocial rehabilitation (although some do) but rather that psychosocial rehabilitation can help people recover a sense of hope and a degree of functional competence that permit more full and satisfying lives as members of society (Anthony, 1993).

It is not hard to imagine a younger reader or any reader new to mental health issues responding to a list of PSR principles such as the one presented in Box 12-1 with an extended yawn and the observation that such "motherhood-and-apple-pie" statements are hardly unique. Two points might be made in response. First, 30 years ago most of these principles challenged much estab-

Box 12-1. Principles of psychosocial rehabilitation

- Hope is an essential ingredient in psychosocial rehabilitation. All people have an underused capacity to learn and grow that should be developed.
- All people should be treated with respect and dignity. No one should be labeled or discriminated against based on disability, dysfunction, illness, or disease. The whole person, not the illness, is the focus of psychosocial rehabilitation.
- Multicultural diversity among psychosocial rehabilitation program staff, participants, and the community at large is appreciated as a source of strength and program enrichment. Programs take active measures to respond in ways that are considerate and respectful of diversity.
- Psychosocial rehabilitation encourages consumer self-determination and empowerment. Programs and practitioners work to expand choices, help consumers make informed choices, and understand their rights and responsibilities.
- A pluralistic approach to the development and provision of psychosocial rehabilitation services will best meet the needs of people who use these services. Assessments and interventions are individually tailored and flexible; they are available whenever needed and for as long as they are needed.
- The psychosocial rehabilitation practitioner's role is intentionally informal and participatory in activities designed to engage consumers in real world tasks and relationships. Minimizing the distance between practitioners and consumers requires promoting consumer participation in policy, administration, direct practitioner roles, service design and implementation, and evaluation.
- Psychosocial rehabilitation focuses on real world activities, providing skills and support for people to participate as fully as possible within family and community settings. Helping people pursue and retain employment and other goals that promote independence, integration, and inclusion are emphasized.
- The prevention of unnecessary hospitalization and the use of early intervention and long-term strategies to promote and stabilize community tenure are the primary goals of psychosocial rehabilitation.
- Psychosocial rehabilitation equips people with coping skills and environmental resources to support the achievement of individually determined interpersonal, social, vocational, educational, residential, and recreational goals.
- Psychosocial rehabilitation focuses on a person's strengths and values and capitalizes on abilities and interests while developing strategies to overcome or compensate for deficits that impede goal attainment.

Modified from "Evaluating Psychiatric Rehabilitation Programs," by L.E. Blankertz, 1994, *Psychiatric Rehabilitation*, 416.

lished thinking in the mental health professions; however commonplace today, they were indeed radical for their time. Second, even now consumers of mental health services commonly find themselves in treatment settings where their illness overshadows their potential, where their dignity is under continuous assault, or where stabilization rather than rehabilitation and recovery is the perceived goal. Translating broad principles into program imperatives remains the most fundamental of challenges.

PROGRAM ELEMENTS AND MODELS IN PSYCHOSOCIAL REHABILITATION

Two broad organizing principles inform a discussion of the ways in which psychosocial rehabilitation professionals deliver services. The first describes an array of program elements that a comprehensive psychosocial rehabilitation program should offer and the second describes an expanding number of complementary program models currently in use around the country.

However, before proceeding further, some terms need clarification. The term *psychosocial rehabilitation* (PSR), coined some 40 years ago and applied to both program elements and program models, is passionately clung to by some and passionately disliked by others; debate has periodically arisen over whether to change the term. Over the past decade a number of agencies and individuals have begun to prefer *psychiatric rehabilitation* as a more readily grasped and descriptive term, but considerable debate has swirled around this term as well. The unsettled nomenclature of the field is exemplified in the fact that the official journal of the International Association of Psychosocial Rehabilitation Services is entitled the *Psychiatric Rehabilitation Journal*.

No one "owns" these terms and any service provider can blithely assert that it offers psychosocial or psychiatric rehabilitation services with little regard to the principles or programs enunciated here. One is therefore well advised when seeking services from (or employment with) a program that characterizes itself as a psychosocial or psychiatric rehabilitation agency to explore whether the range of service elements and the specific model employed indeed reflect key PSR principles and approaches.

Program elements

The range of problems and issues that PSR programs respond to has expanded over the years. This brief overview is designed as a basic introduction to service components, and it should be noted that although some agencies focus on only a few service elements, others continuously add new components to their offerings. The strongest programs either provide support for or ensure clear linkages to a wide range of complementary service programs. A recurring theme in these service programs has been an ongoing shift from in-house to in vivo service delivery and from the delivery of services within a psychiatric milieu to the use of mainstream resources also available to people without serious mental illness.

Social programs

PSR agencies are valued for their responsiveness to the social isolation and loneliness felt by people with serious mental illness. Many agencies have a busy schedule of client-planned social events, educational and current events classes, psychoeducational programs, health maintenance discussions, recreational services, and purely social afternoon and evening gatherings for movies, dancing, barbecuing, and so forth. Because serious mental illness often leaves clients uncomfortable in a variety of social settings, many PSR agencies offer classroom programs and social activities that provide opportunities for them to practice social interaction, conversational techniques, and friendship. More recently, PSR practitioners have broken through their own discomfort and have begun to help clients address issues of sexuality, sexual abuse, sexual preference, and sexual safety—issues long ignored despite their universality. Social rehabilitation workers lead classes, facilitate group discussions, offer one-to-one counseling, and—because PSR principles deemphasize professional distance—model the give-and-take of friendship in their interactions with clients. Within the context of social rehabilitation, PSR workers also discuss with clients the impact of the stigma of mental illness on their lives and their responses to it (Baron, Klaczynska, & Rutman, 1980).

Residential programs

One of the most urgent needs for many clients is a safe, affordable, decent place to live and call their own. Early in the history of the field, PSR agencies started establishing group homes for clients who had no homes or chose to live independently from their families. These facilities used existing housing in the community and rigorously attempted to fashion a normal appearance and life-style for residents, but the often inappropriate size of facilities, restrictive zoning ordinances, and strong community opposition forced a reexamination of the therapeutic effectiveness of such programs. A variety of alternative formats have begun to replace large group homes: single homes for no more than eight people, a cluster of two-person or three-person apartments in a single building, scattered apartment programs, and individual support for clients in their own (or the agency's) housing arrangements. These individualized arrangements are termed *supported housing* and seek to offer the client in vivo support on site. The roles of residential workers are quite varied and may include working with one client or a group to ensure that the household is budgeting funds adequately to pay the rent; to assist in clarifying cleaning, cooking, and maintenance responsibilities and developing skills necessary to ensure their completion; and to provide the emotional support or conflict negotiation skills needed by people who may be on their own for the first time in their lives (Carling, 1994). Specialized residential programs for people who are both mentally ill and homeless or suffering from both mental illness and substance abuse disorders also are growing in number (Blankertz & Cnaan, 1994); another set of specialized residential programs provides crisis services that offer a short-term alternative to hospitalization.

Vocational programs

Many PSR programs attach considerable importance to "the work ordered day," and assign each client to one of several in-house programs that keep the agency operating (for example, clerical workshops, janitorial crews, kitchen staff, or similar operations), helping clients to appreciate their work capabilities and capacity for further growth (National Institute on Disability and Rehabilitation Research, 1992). Some agencies—in fact, a growing number of providers—operate their own businesses (for example, office cleaning operations, landscaping crews, temporary secretarial services, and franchise restaurants) to provide additional training opportunities (Granger, 1996). Increasingly agencies are seeking "transitional" or "supported" employment opportunities in which the client works a real job for real pay and receives

PSR agency support in finding and keeping the job (McGurrin, 1994). PSR practitioners in this arena may be job developers (working with employers to open job opportunities for clients); job coaches (helping clients locate jobs and prepare for interviews and working alongside clients on the job until they can gradually minimize the intensity and visibility of their support; or long-term support workers (providing ongoing counseling, problem solving, and occasionally on-site interventions to sustain the client's long-term involvement in the labor market) (Baron, 1995). Two troubling issues face PSR workers in these endeavors. First, the combination of labor market forces and client reluctance to jeopardize financial assistance and medical support from SSI and SSDI keeps many clients in entry-level, low-wage, low-benefit, and part-time jobs, and second, with nearly 75% of placements in such menial positions, motivating clients to seek more demanding and rewarding employment is difficult (Kregel et al., 1990). Nonetheless, consensus is growing on the need to prioritize employment programs in the cost-conscious years ahead.

Educational programs

Similarly, a small but growing emphasis is on helping clients return to school; many agencies offer basic education and high school equivalency programs, and a few offer "supported education" programs in which the educational equivalent of a job coach assists clients in planning for, enrolling in, and successfully completing the educational degrees they have always wanted to pursue (Danley & Mellen, 1987). PSR workers may offer educational classes, but more often they provide a link between the agency and independent educational opportunities. Such programs are important to clients not just because of their relevance to future work opportunities but also because mental illness has emerged in their lives in their late teens or early twenties and effectively cut them off from the educational advancement they might otherwise have pursued.

Activities of daily living

One of the most discouraging aspects of serious mental illness is its impact on clients' instrumental functioning; the most basic life activities are either never learned or largely unattended. Fundamentals of personal hygiene, appropriate clothing, proper nutrition and meal preparation, budgeting, and public transportation are all skills that some clients may not have developed, may have lost during long, quiet years of institutional care, or may be too unmotivated or distracted by their illness to address. PSR workers help in a variety of ways. Special classes in an agency setting, working on immediate issues within the residential program, field trips, and community events for which clients have primary responsibility are all ways in which skills are taught, rehearsed, practiced, and learned (Blackwell et al., 1993).

Case management

PSR agencies frequently link services together through case management approaches, providing a professional or paraprofessional resource to clients to define their needs, access in-house and external resources, and track client progress. Several models of case management exist: in one the case manager brokers services by helping clients define their priorities and the programs and financial resources necessary to meet them; in another the case manager links the client to services when necessary and serves as a support worker, residential counselor, job coach, or teacher as circumstances require (Stein & Test, 1978).

Other innovative service elements—helping young mothers with mental illness raise their children more successfully, helping clients start their own businesses, and supporting system advocacy initiatives—should be mentioned. However, not every client needs all these services; each brings to the PSR setting a unique blend of skills and interests, disabilities and incapacities. PSR programs function at their best when they respond to individual needs with individualized services.

Program models

PSR models have proliferated in recent years. Although the principles and program elements underlying most PSR services are similar, the way in which services are organized and the use of psychosocial rehabilitation personnel varies considerably from site to site. Part of this variation is caused by differences in funding patterns, but variation also results from the individuality associated with local leadership. Three broad models are discussed here: agency-based professional programs, consumer-run service programs, and case management programs. This categorization is arbitrary and overlapping and includes in a single category programs that may have serious reservations about one another's approaches. Nonetheless, the three categories described briefly here capture the range of experience of psychosocial programs.

Agency-based professional programs

This category dominates the PSR field; most practitioners in the field work for professional agencies (International Association of Psychosocial Rehabilitation Services, 1990). These agencies, however, have different auspices: some are private nonprofit independent facilities, others are units within private or publicly operated community mental health centers, some are smaller units within a county-operated or state-operated mental health program, and some are operated by state mental hospitals or private institutions. They draw staff from diverse academic disciplines and life experiences, operate a dizzying array of service elements, and access public and private funds in unique ways, although even well-established psychosocial agencies often remain vulnerable to economic and political changes. Professionally run agencies, however, also can adhere to one of two approaches:

- **The clubhouse model** is based primarily on how Fountain House in New York City organizes its service delivery. Members are always welcome at the clubhouse; they are encouraged but not forced to participate in the work ordered day of the agency; and they may fill a series of "transitional employment" positions (short-term, entry-level, real world jobs in the community) for as long as they like before moving on to competitive employment. Multidisciplinary staff teams work interdependently without regard for professional distinctions (Beard, Malamud, & Propst, 1982). There are currently hundreds of clubhouse programs across the country (and in several other countries), and Fountain House has recently spearheaded the establishment of the International Center for Clubhouse Development (ICCD) to generate practice guidelines and standards for this portion of the PSR community.

- **The eclectic model** embraces the greater number of agencies; it may provide a number of service elements under varying arrangements. Some agencies use a "high expectation" approach, setting specific time limits for the client's participation in the program as an inducement toward ever greater independent functioning; other agencies use a classroom learning approach, in which social skills are taught, practiced, and used within a psychoeducational model (Blackwell et al., 1993); and still other agencies combine elements of the clubhouse philosophy with both high expectation and classroom learning approaches.

The advent of managed behavioral health care, with its emphasis on lowered costs and measurable outcomes, will likely pressure PSR programs for less open-ended nonspecific program participation and for more limited and goal-specific programs in the years ahead. Such pressures may challenge the ways in which these agencies respond to client needs in the future (Bernstein & Landress, 1993).

Both types of programs have considerable variations. Some, for instance, emphasize a detailed assessment of client strengths and weaknesses, develop ongoing task statements designed to chart the client's rehabilitation, and monitor the client's progress (Anthony, Cohen, & Cohen, 1983). Other agencies permit clients to participate informally in various program activities and move forward (or backward) at their own pace. Some agencies rely on the strength of the therapeutic alliance between a staff member and a client to sustain rehabilitative momentum and other programs rely on the agency's group milieu or the effectiveness of multidisciplinary staff teams to engage and motivate the client (Stein & Test, 1975). For all these programs, however, psychosocial rehabilitation at its core offers the client an accepting and hopeful environment in which to develop and try out the skills necessary to achieve a more independent and satisfying life.

Consumer-run service programs

One of the more encouraging by-products of the recent emphasis on consumer empowerment has been the degree to which consumers of mental health services have demonstrated that they can provide psychosocial rehabilitation services themselves. A growing number of professionally operated PSR agencies are now willing (after many years of resistance) to hire people with mental illness for their own staffs in paraprofessional and professional positions, and in many communities consumer groups have expanded beyond their traditional advocacy and agitation roles and established their own service agencies (Deegan, 1992).

Consumer-run programs may offer a range of services. Peer support programs in which small groups meet regularly to share experiences and encouragement are perhaps the most common services offered, but the number of consumer-run drop-in centers and socialization programs, prevocational and job placement services, and housing collectives is growing. The larger and more sophisticated the operation the more likely it is to have translated basic PSR principles into operating guidelines for its programs; several consumer-run programs are currently active in psychosocial rehabilitation's larger professional community.

Staffing for consumer-run programs will vary considerably from the professional agency model; few consumer programs use nonconsumer staff. However, the consumer community has been able to staff programs with a mixture of people with professional mental health training and experience and people without professional training but with a depth of feeling and a natural capacity for the role of "helper." Several agencies across the country are now more than a decade old and have demonstrated both their effectiveness and their solidity.

Case management programs

A third PSR model draws its underlying principles from the growing literature on the effectiveness of case management approaches in meeting client needs and offers in effect a "psychosocial rehabilitation program without walls." That is, individual case managers or a multidisciplinary team of case managers meet regularly with the client but work almost entirely within a community context. Rather than work from a specific facility (for example, the clubhouse or agency), case managers spend less time in their offices and more time with clients in their homes, at their jobs, and with their families and friends within the community.

One of the best-known models, the Assertive Community Treatment (ACT) program developed by Stein and Test in Madison, Wisconsin, draws its multidisciplinary team together each morning to review caseloads and issues to be confronted that day and then dispatches team members into the community for individual work with clients (Stein & Test, 1975). Some intensive care management (ICM) programs may place less emphasis on interdisciplinary team work but will similarly eschew agency-based programs in favor of meeting clients within the community.

Both models strongly emphasize the flexibility of staff members and their willingness and capacity to manage without the support of an office interview, ongoing collegial contacts throughout the day, and support personnel. They also rely far less on the therapeutic or rehabilitative tools of the established milieu in agency-based program models but still show comparable results.

One might argue that such diversity of models does not contribute to a coherent professional identity, but the psychosocial rehabilitation movement nonetheless coalesces around common principles and program emphases for several important reasons.

First, psychosocial rehabilitation practitioners, however disparate their approaches, are in many cases the only people with an ongoing commitment to the rehabilitation work needed to help people with serious mental illness with the pragmatic concerns of everyday life. Psychosocial providers care deeply about the quality of the client's living circumstances and social life; psychosocial personnel may be the only professionals who believe the person with a long-term mental illness can and should go to work or school. Psychosocial agencies of all types persist in finding ways to teach functional independence.

Second, psychosocial professionals have growing confidence in their effectiveness. Although PSR agencies have in the past been lax in developing detailed evaluations of their program outcomes, a growing body of anecdotal evidence and program research (Bond, 1994) indicates that such programs have a significant impact on clients' lives, helping them avoid repeated hospitalizations, promoting lengthened community tenure, helping them recover lost capacities and develop new competencies, and assisting them in the often lengthy process of reestablishing meaningful and satisfying lives for themselves.

Third, the relative newness of the field holds the psychosocial rehabilitation community together. After nearly 40 years of work the field finds itself somewhere between its roots as a radical innovation and its goal of being an established professional group. It is not, as the earlier discussion suggests, a highly structured enterprise, replete with unambiguous guidelines, firm funding bases, and pristine clarity about professional roles and hierarchies. Indeed, psychosocial rehabilitation has often argued against such structures and for the flexibility to innovate and experiment in the process of discovering how best to meet the individual needs of people with serious mental illness.

PSYCHOSOCIAL REHABILITATION PRACTICES AND PRACTITIONERS

Despite the fluid and dynamic nature of psychosocial rehabilitation, in recent years a number of efforts have been made to identify specific techniques that PSR practitioners use in their work

(Danley & Mellen, 1987; Farkas, Nemec, & O'Brien, 1988; Gill & Pratt, 1992). The most recent effort, undertaken by IAPSRS in 1994, used "concept mapping" to identify competency areas that define the capacities of the skilled PSR worker (Figure 12-1).

To date, skill development among PSR practitioners has been varied; the cross-disciplinary nature of PSR program staffing has brought to the field psychiatric and psychological perspectives on clients' problems, and social work and psychiatric nursing have contributed techniques for problem solving and community caregiving.

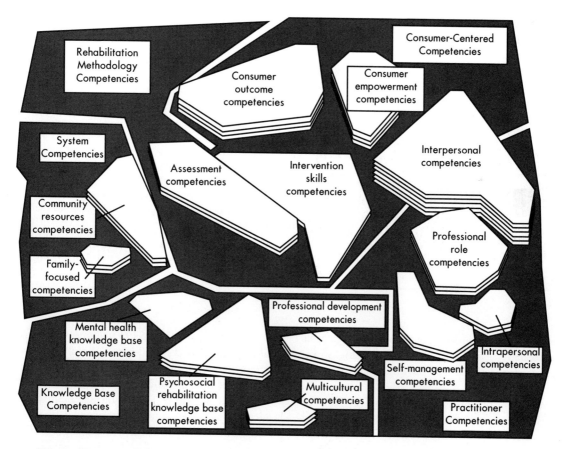

Figure 12-1. Workforce competencies for psychosocial rehabilitation workers: a concept mapping project.
(Based on the work of W.M.K. Trochim, Cornell University, and J. Cook, Thresholds National Research and Training Center on Rehabilitation and Mental Illness.)

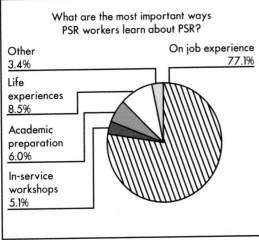

What are the most important ways
PSR workers learn about PSR?

Other
3.4%

On job experience
77.1%

Life
experiences
8.5%

Academic
preparation
6.0%

In-service
workshops
5.1%

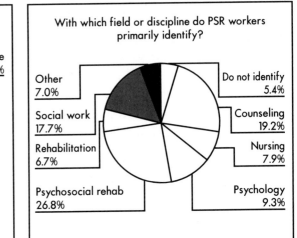

With which field or discipline do PSR workers
primarily identify?

Other
7.0%

Do not identify
5.4%

Social work
17.7%

Counseling
19.2%

Rehabilitation
6.7%

Nursing
7.9%

Psychosocial rehab
26.8%

Psychology
9.3%

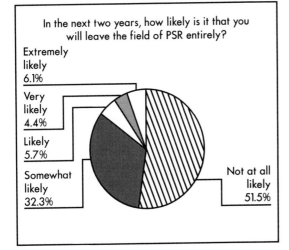

In the next two years, how likely is it that you
will leave the field of PSR entirely?

Extremely
likely
6.1%

Very
likely
4.4%

Likely
5.7%

Somewhat
likely
32.3%

Not at all
likely
51.5%

Figure 12-2. The national survey of PSR workers, 1993, a nationwide survey of PSR workers conducted by Matrix Research Institute and the International Association of Psychosocial Rehabilitation Services (IAPSRS) for the National Institute on Disability and Rehabilitation Research (NIDRR). (Modified from "Who is the PSR worker?" by L.E. Blankertz, & S. Robinson, 1995, *Psychosocial Rehabilitation Journal.*)

Occupational and recreational therapy, vocational rehabilitation, and community organizing strategies (among others) also have had an impact on PSR practices.

A variety of approaches are used in PSR settings. Group counseling and one-to-one meetings remain in broad use but so too does peer counseling, milieu therapy, classroom learning, goal attainment scaling, reinforcement therapy, and recreational programming. An array of approaches is used by different agencies, and each agency uses an eclectic mix of rehabilitation approaches.

As a consequence, PSR practitioners must have at their disposal a broad range of skills and must choose among those skills as dictated by the needs of clients and their particular circumstances. The field is, as a result, generally free of received wisdom and "preconceived routines." Although some PSR workers find this places them in an insecure and confused professional position, others welcome the freedom to use their professional judgment in responding to client needs. This give-and-take has kept the field fresh and exciting.

Efforts have been undertaken in recent years to provide a firmer practice base for new PSR workers. Liberman and his colleagues have been teaching "skills training" techniques—including description, exploration, demonstration, and practice—to strengthen practitioner competencies (Blackwell et al., 1993); at Boston University, Anthony and his colleagues teach a variety of functional assessment, goal planning, and client empowerment approaches for use with PSR clients (Anthony, 1983); and a handful of academic programs (usually in 2-year associate degree programs) provide an introduction to PSR principles, programs, and practices (Farkas & Furlong-Norman, 1995).

The vast majority of practitioners in the psychosocial rehabilitation workforce develop a knowledge base about clients and a skills base regarding PSR practice on the job (Blankertz and Robinson, 1995). The lack of degree-granting PSR programs has made it necessary for many programs to develop extensive orientation and on-the-job training programs. Although many staff members come to PSR from other mental health and rehabilitation disciplines (Blankertz & Robinson, 1995), PSR programs rarely offer discipline-specific jobs for psychiatrists, psychologists, social workers, or psychiatric nurses. Another portion of the workforce enters the field with academic training from a discipline other than mental health, and a significant percentage of people comes to PSR with only a basic education and life experience (Blankertz & Robinson, 1995). Figure 12-2 presents the results of a national survey of PSR workers that details opinions about the PSR field.

Indeed, many of the staff members who interact with clients most intensively in residential roles or as job coaches come to the field with little human services background or mental health training. PSR agencies increasingly recognize the importance of providing training through job shadowing, orientation programs, site visits, and readings to better prepare staff for PSR work.

Despite the unsettled nature of the field, recent research into the psychosocial rehabilitation workforce provides positive perspectives; most people in the PSR workforce like their jobs, enjoy the clients, agree with the fundamental principles of the field, and wish to stay in the field for the foreseeable future (Blankertz & Robinson, 1995).

SUMMARY

What then should one expect when entering the psychosocial workforce? The field is characterized by highly motivated staff, an emphasis on teamwork, a deemphasis on hierarchical staff relationships, a strong commitment to the basic principles of the field, and the flexibility to learn and innovate. It is still a young field of professional endeavor, and a major challenge in the years ahead will be to balance the need for greater professionalism (for example, standards, credentials, and accountability) with the need to maintain the creative individual responsiveness to client needs that has characterized PSR thus far.

REFERENCES

Allen, J. (1974). Psychosocial rehabilitation: A consumer's view of California's mental health care system. *Psychiatric Quarterly, 48.*

Anthony, W. A. (1983). Philosophy, treatment process, and principles of the psychiatric rehabilitation approach. *New Directions for Mental Health Services, 17.*

Anthony, W. A., Cohen, B. F., & Cohen, R. (1983). Philosophy, treatment process, and principles of the psychiatric rehabilitation approach. *New Directions for Mental Health Services, 17.*

Anthony, W. A., & Liberman, R. P. (1986). The practice of psychiatric rehabilitation: Historical, conceptual, and research base. *Schizophrenia Bulletin, 12*(4), 542-559.

Baron, R. C. (1995). The competence of practitioners providing employment services to persons with serious mental illness. *Best practices in psychosocial rehabilitation.* Columbia, MD: IAPSRS.

Baron, R. C., Klaczynska, B., & Rutman, I. D. (Eds.) (1980). *A national conference on overcoming public opposition to community care for the mentally ill: The community imperative.* Philadelphia: Horizon House Institute.

Beard, J. H., Malamud, T. J., & Propst, R. N. (1982). The Fountain House model of psychiatric rehabilitation. *Psychosocial Rehabilitation Journal, 5*(1), 47-53.

Bernstein, M. A., & Landress, H. J. (1993). Managed care 101: An overview of implications for psychosocial rehabilitation services. *Psychiatric Rehabilitation Journal, 17*(2), 5-14.

Blackwell, G., Eckman, T. A., Kuenhnel, T. G., Liberman, R. P., Vaccaro, J. V., & Wallace, C. J. (1993). Innovations in skills training for people with serious mental illness: The UCLA social and independent living skills modules. *Innovations and Research, 2*(2), 46-59.

Blankertz, L. E. (1994). Evaluating psychiatric rehabilitation programs. In L. Spaniol, M. A. Brown, L. Blankertz, et al. (Eds.), *Psychiatric rehabilitation* (pp. 416-420). Columbia, MD: IAPSRS.

Blankertz, L. E., & Cnaan, R. A. (1993). Serving the dually diagnosed homeless: Program development and intervention. *Journal of Mental Health Administration, 20*(2), 100-112.

Blankertz, L. E., & Robinson, S. (1995). Who is the PSR worker? *Psychosocial Rehabilitation Journal.*

Bond, G. R. (1994). Psychiatric rehabilitation outcome. In L. Spaniol, M. A. Brown, L. Blankertz, et al. (Eds.), *Psychiatric rehabilitation* (pp. 490-494). Columbia, MD: IAPSRS.

Carling, P. J. (1994). Supports and rehabilitation for housing and community living. In R.W. Flexer, & P. L. Solomon (Eds.), *Psychiatric rehabilitation practice* (pp. 99-118). Boston: Andover Medical Publishers.

Danley, K. S., MacDonald-Wilson, K., Nicolellis, D. L., & Sullivan, A. P. (1994). Choose-Get-Keep: A psychiatric rehabilitation approach to supported education. *Psychiatric Rehabilitation Journal, 17*(1), 55-68.

Danley, K. S., & Mellen, V. (1987). Training and personnel issues for supported employment programs which serve persons who are severely mentally ill. *Psychosocial Rehabilitation Journal, 11*(2), 87-102.

Deegan, P. E. (1992). The independent living movement and people with psychiatric disabilities: Taking back control over our own lives. *Psychosocial Rehabilitation Journal, 15*(3), 3-19.

Dincin, J. (1994). Psychiatric rehabilitation. *Schizophrenia Bulletin, 13,* 131-147.

Farkas, M. D., & Furlong-Norman, K. (1995). *Psychosocial rehabilitation training resources.* Columbia, MD: IAPSRS.

Farkas, M. D., Nemec, P. B., & O'Brien, W. F. (1988). A graduate level curriculum in psychiatric rehabilitation: Filling a need. *Psychiatric Rehabilitation Journal, 12*(2), 53-66.

Gill, K. J., & Pratt, C. W. (1992). Developing interagency in-service training. *Psychosocial Rehabilitation Journal, 16*(1), 3-12.

Goertzel, V. & Lamb, H. R. (1971). Discharged mental patients—Are they really in the community? *Archives of General Psychiatry, 24,* 29-34.

Granger, B. (1993). *A national survey of agency-sponsored entrepreneurial businesses employing individuals with long-term mental illness.* Philadelphia: Matrix Research Institute.

Hughes, R. (1994). Psychiatric rehabilitation: An essential health service for people with serious and persistent mental illness. In L. Spaniol, M. A. Brown, L. Blankertz, et al. (Eds.), *Psychiatric rehabilitation* (pp. 9-17). Columbia, MD: IAPSRS.

International Association of Psychosocial Rehabilitation Services. (1990). *Organizations providing psychosocial rehabilitation and related community support services in the United States.* Columbia, MD: Author.

Kregal, J., Schafer, M. S., Wehman, P., & West, P. (Eds.) (1990). *Emerging trends in the national supported employment initiative: A preliminary analysis of twenty-seven states. Policy and program developments in supported employment: Current strategies to promote statewide systems change.* Richmond, VA: Rehabilitation Research and Training Center.

McGurrin, M. C. (1994). An overview of the effectiveness of traditional vocational rehabilitation services in the treatment of long term mental illness. *Psychosocial Rehabilitation Journal, 17*(3), 37-54.

National Institute on Disability and Rehabilitation Research. (1992). *Strategies to secure and maintain employment for people with long-term mental illness.* Washington, DC: Author.

Rutman, I. D. (1994). What is psychiatric rehabilitation? In L. Spaniol, M. A. Brown, L. Blankertz, et al. (Eds.), *Psychiatric rehabilitation* (pp. 4-8). Columbia, MD: IAPSRS.

Stein, L. I., & Test, M. A. (1975). Training in community living: Research design and results. In L. I. Stein, & M. A. Test (Eds.), *Alternatives to mental hospital treatment.* New York: Plenum Press.

Stein, L. I., & Test, M. A. (1978). The clinical rationale for community treatment: A review of the literature. In L. I. Stein, & M. A. Test (Eds.), *Alternatives to mental hospital treatment.* New York: Plenum Press.

Stroul, B. A. (1987). *Crisis residential services in a community support system.* Rockville, MD: National Institute of Mental Health, Community Support Program.

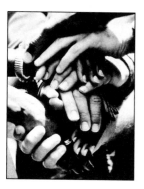

Chapter 13

Medication Management

Dan E. Harris and Norman L. Keltner

DRUGS USED TO TREAT MENTAL DISORDERS

Mental disorders are common in our society. Narrows et al. (1993) and Regier et al. (1993) indicate that 28.1% of Americans older than 17 years old will be affected by mental or addictive disorders in a given year. Accordingly the American Nurses Association (Laraia et al., 1994) has developed guidelines for psychiatric nurses who incorporate psychopharmacology in their practice (Box 13-1).

Based on the decline in public mental hospital occupancy, most mentally disordered people will come under the umbrella of community mental health services at some time. Disorders of significant societal impact and consequently of particular interest to community mental health nurses include anxiety disorders (12.6% of the adult population), depression (5% of the adult population), dementia (2.7% of the adult population), bipolar disorder (1.2% of the adult population), and schizophrenia (1.1% of the adult population) (Regier et al., 1993). Each of these disorders is thought to be caused by alterations in brain neurophysiology. Table 13-1 presents psychiatric dis-

orders and the primary neurotransmitter actions related to them. Understandably, this simplistic, "one neurotransmitter" view is only a starting point. Evolving research suggests multineurotransmitter involvement in many mental disorders.

Because psychotropic drugs theoretically restore neurophysiological balance, community mental health nurses must understand and use these agents as part of their interventions. Accordingly the following pages offer important information about the major psychopharmacological agents used to treat anxiety, depression, dementia, bipolar disorder, and schizophrenia. The reader who wishes to gain a thorough understanding of psychopharmacology is advised to consult a text dedicated to that topic.

Antipsychotics: drugs used to treat schizophrenia

Indications

Antipsychotic drugs are used primarily to treat schizophrenia and other mental disorders such as acute mania, depression with psychotic features,

---

Box 13-1. Objectives from the ANA guidelines on psychopharmacology

The psychiatric mental health nurse can:

1. Describe psychopharmacological agents based on similarities and differences
2. Discuss actions of psychopharmacological agents from global responses to cellular responses
3. Differentiate psychiatric symptoms from medication side effects
4. Apply basic principles of pharmacokinetics and pharmacodynamics
5. Identify appropriate use of psychopharmacological agents in special populations
6. Involve clients and their families
7. Identify factors that may prevent the active involvement of clients in their care
8. Describe appropriate nonpsychopharmacological interventions
9. Discuss the use of standardized rating scales
10. Demonstrate the knowledge necessary to develop psychopharmacological education and treatment plans

---

Modified from *Psychiatric Mental Health Nursing Psychopharmacology Project* (p. 42), by M. T. Laraia, L. S. Beeber, G. B. Callwood, S. Caverly, J. A. Clement, F. Gary, N. L. Keltner, M. A. Nihart, L. Scahill, S. Simmons-Alling, S. R. Stanley & S. Tally, 1994, Washington, DC: American Nurses Association.

delirium, dementia (psychotic thinking and agitation), and Tourette's syndrome (Arana & Hyman, 1991). Medically, antipsychotics provide an antiemetic effect and interrupt intractable hiccoughs.

How antipsychotics work

Schizophrenia may be caused by a relative overabundance of dopamine in the brain (Table 13-1). This theory, first put forth by Matthysse (1977), is known as the dopamine hypothesis of schizophrenia. Because antipsychotics block dopamine and are effective in the treatment of schizophrenia and because l-dopa increases dopamine and worsens schizophrenia (Yaryura-Tobias, Diamond, & Merlis, 1970), Matthysse postulated that excessive brain dopamine played a primary role in the development of schizophrenia. Current thinking views the dopamine hypothesis as too simplistic (Remington, 1993); however, the hypothesis still provides a foundation for understanding a pharmacological response to this disorder.

Time to clinical effect

Antipsychotic medications typically require 7 to 10 days for a significant reduction in symptoms. However, they can take 3 to 6 weeks or longer to achieve a full clinical effect.

Efficacy

Antipsychotic agents are effective for the treatment of schizophrenia and related psychoses for most clients. However, a substantial number of

---

Table 13-1. Neurotransmitters and related mental disorders

NEUROTRANSMITTER ACTION	RELATED MENTAL DISORDER
Increase in dopamine	Schizophrenia
Decrease in norepinephrine	Depression
Decrease in serotonin	Depression
Decrease in acetylcholine	Alzheimer's disease
Decrease in gamma-aminobutyric acid (GABA)	Anxiety

clients do not respond well. Roughly 10% to 20% of clients with schizophrenia never respond, and another 20% to 30% relapse within 2 years.

Categorizations and their clinical significance

Traditional antipsychotics. Antipsychotic drugs are technically grouped by chemical classification, a cumbersome and not particularly helpful method of classification. A more clinically relevant way of thinking about antipsychotic agents is to divide them into high-potency, moderate-

potency, and low-potency groupings (Table 13-2). High-potency drugs require a smaller dosage on a milligram to milligram basis but cause a considerably greater incidence of extrapyramidal side effects (EPSEs). Low-potency antipsychotics require a higher dosage but cause fewer EPSEs and produce a greater incidence of anticholinergic, anti-adrenergic, and sedation side effects. Because traditional antipsychotic drugs are equally effective, the choice of drug is typically based on what set of side effects is desired (for example, sedation), best tolerated, or best avoided.

Table 13-2. Major traditional antipsychotic drugs and atypical antipsychotic drugs

	DOSAGE[a]	EPSE[b]	ANTI[c]	OH[d]
TRADITIONAL ANTIPSYCHOTIC DRUGS				
High-potency antipsychotic drugs				
Fluphenazine (Prolixin)	0.5-40	XXX[e]	X[g]	X
Haloperidol (Haldol)	1-15	XXX	X	X
Thiothixene (Navane)	8-30	XXX	X	X
Trifluoperazine (Stelazine)	2-40	XXX	X	X
Moderate-potency antipsychotic drugs				
Loxapine (Loxitane)	20-250	XXX	X	XX[f]
Molindone (Moban)	15-255	XXX	X	X
Low-potency antipsychotic drugs				
Chlorpromazine (Thorazine)	30-800	XX	XX	XXX
Thioridazine (Mellaril)	150-800	X	XXX	XXX
ATYPICAL ANTIPSYCHOTIC DRUGS				
Clozapine (Clozaril)	300-900	X	XXX	XXX
Risperidone (Risperdal)	4-6	X	X	XX

[a] DOSAGE = Adult daily dosage in milligrams.
[b] EPSE = Extrapyramidal side effects.
[c] ANTI = Anticholinergic effect.
[d] OH = Orthostatic hypotension.
[e] XXX=High incidence; [f] XX= Moderate incidence; [g] X=Low incidence.

Atypical antipsychotics. The earlier discussion of high-potency and low-potency medications focused on traditional antipsychotic drugs. Because of the significant number of clients whose disorders are resistant to traditional agents, clinicians and therapists have searched for years to find a better antipsychotic. Two drugs, both substantially different from traditional agents, have been released since 1990: clozapine (Clozaril) and risperidone (Risperdal). Both drugs move beyond the "dopamine hypothesis" of traditional antipsychotics. Traditional antipsychotics block dopamine D-2 receptors (Matsubara et al., 1993). Clozapine produces a weaker blockade of D-2 receptors and a more significant blockade of D-1 and D-4 receptors (Kane, 1993). Clozapine has a greater affinity for limbic than striatal dopaminergic neurons, which accounts for the lower incidence of EPSEs associated with this drug (Keltner & Folks, 1991). Risperidone blocks both D-2 receptors and serotonin receptors (Keltner, 1995a). This unique property may be responsible for improvements observed in previously treatment-resistant clients with schizophrenia, most of whom have negative symptoms.

The atypical antipsychotics now available have a significantly better side effect profile than traditional antipsychotic medications. Clozapine and risperidone both cause fewer EPSEs than earlier antipsychotics. Additionally, risperidone has low anticholinergic properties and is not particularly sedating. Neither agent is at high risk for causing tardive dyskinesia.

Side effects

The major categories of side effects related to atypical antipsychotic drugs are EPSEs, anticholinergic side effects, and antiadrenergic side effects. (See Table 13-2 and Box 13-2 for dosage and side effect information.) EPSEs are associated with high-potency agents and include akathisia (an unbearable need to move), dystonia (muscle rigidity), akinesia (absence of movement), drug-induced parkinsonism (tremor and rigidity), and neuroleptic malignant syndrome (a potentially fa-

tal side effect manifested in hyperthermia, rigidity, and impaired breathing) (Keltner & McIntyre, 1985).

Anticholinergic effects are caused by the blockade of the cholinergic receptors. Common anticholinergic effects include dry mouth, anhidrosis, blurred vision, constipation, and urinary retention. Undiagnosed narrow-angle glaucoma in combination with an anticholinergic effect can lead to a medical emergency (Arana & Hyman, 1991). When a history of glaucoma is documented a high-potency drug should be prescribed (Arana & Hyman, 1991).

Antiadrenergic responses result from the blockade of alpha-1 receptors, which prevents vascular constriction. Orthostatic hypotension, resultant tachycardia (reflex tachycardia), and related falls are signs that result from this blockade. Other side effects associated with antipsychotic drugs include cardiac conduction problems (mostly from low-potency drugs) and hematological problems.

Side effects of clozapine and risperidone.

Agranulocytosis, a potentially life-threatening side effect, is a major concern with clozapine administration but is not associated with risperidone. Other clozapine-induced side effects include sialorrhea (excessive saliva), sedation, and a lowering of the seizure threshold. Relatively few EPSEs are associated with clozapine. Major side effects related to risperidone include hypotension, agitation, nausea, tachycardia, anxiety, and insomnia (Meltzer, 1993). Significant EPSEs and anticholinergic side effects are uncommon with risperidone (Marder & Meibach, 1994).

Interactions

Antipsychotic drugs interact with many other drugs. Drugs such as alcohol, antihistamines, anxiolytics, antidepressants, barbiturates, meperidine, and morphine—all central nervous system (CNS) depressants themselves—react in an additive fashion with antipsychotics. Other interactant agents include amphetamines, anticholinergics, benzodiazepine derivatives, beta-blockers, cimetidine,

---

Box 13-2. Major adverse responses to psychotropic drugs

Serotonin syndrome*

Caused by: A hyperserotonergic state

Offending agents: Combination of serotonin-potentiating drugs such as monoamine oxidase inhibitors (MAOIs), selective serotonin reuptake inhibitors (SSRIs), and clomipramine

Signs and symptoms:

Diaphoresis

Diarrhea

Hyperreflexia†

Mental changes

Confusion

Hypomania

Myoclonus†

Restlessness†

Shivering

Tremor

Unsteady gait†

Neuroleptic malignant syndrome

Caused by: A hypodopaminergic state

Offending agents: Antipsychotics

Signs and symptoms:

Agitation

Altered levels of consciousness

Autonomic hyperactivity‡

Electrolyte imbalance

Hyperkalemia

Hyponatremia

Metabolic acidosis

Hyperreflexia

Hyperthermia

Diaphoresis

Tachypnea

Impaired breathing

Muscular rigidity‡

Muteness

Pallor‡

Rhabdomyolosis—acute myoglobinuric renal failure

Anticholinergic side effects

Caused by: Blockade of cholinergic receptors

Offending agents: Anticholinergic drugs such as tricyclic antidepressants (TCAs), low-potency antipsychotics, and anticholinergic antiparkinsonian drugs

Signs and symptoms:

Anhidrosis

Blurred vision

Constipation

Diminished lacrimation

Dry mouth

Mydriasis

Tachycardia

Urinary hesitancy or retention

Extrapyramidal side effects

Caused by: Hypodopaminergic state

Offending agents: Typically high-potency antipsychotics

Signs and symptoms:

Akathisia

Akinesia

Dystonia

Dyskinesia§

Drug-induced parkinsonism

---

*Modified from "Serotonin Syndrome," by H. Sternbach, 1991, *American Journal of Psychiatry, 147*(6), 705-712.

†More pronounced in serotonin syndrome than in neuroleptic malignant syndrome.

‡More pronounced in neuroleptic malignant syndrome than in serotonin syndrome.

§Tardive dyskinesia is thought to be related to a dopamine hypersensitivity rather than the actual hypodopaminergic state.

guanethidine, insulin, L-dopa, lithium, phenytoin, and trazodone.

Length of trial before changing to another drug

Although individual clinicians vary in their willingness to wait for a client to respond to a certain drug, as a rule of thumb an adequate trial is 3 to 6 weeks at an effective dosage. Of course, the emphasis on short hospital stays makes evaluation of a therapeutic response more difficult. If a change in medication is indicated, the client should switch to a drug with a different chemical classification.

Implications for long-term treatment with antipsychotic agents

Many clients experience relapse even when they conscientiously adhere to their antipsychotic medication regimen. Many people who are successfully treated on a long-term maintenance basis would also be prone to relapse if medications were discontinued. Research supports the supposition that maintenance therapy decreases exacerbations of mental disorders (Arana & Hyman, 1991). The major concern associated with long-term use is tardive dyskinesia, an irreversible side effect of some antipsychotic drugs. Clinicians responsible for long-term maintenance therapy must skillfully and regularly monitor their clients for this debilitating effect. The abnormal involuntary movement scale (AIMS) is the standard instrument used to assess for tardive dyskinesia.

Organ systems vulnerable to antipsychotic drugs

The hematological system is vulnerable to antipsychotic drugs. Agranulocytosis, a condition in which the number of granulocytic leukocytes decreases, is a potentially fatal blood dyscrasia related to antipsychotic medication use. By far the greatest offender is clozapine, with a risk rate for agranulocytosis of 1% to 2%. In the past the condition produced a mortality rate of 40% among affected individuals. Currently, stringent monitoring procedures have reduced the number of agranulocytosis fatalities. A drop in the granulocyte count below 1500 per centimeter indicates a need to discontinue clozapine. Signs and symptoms of agranulocytosis include susceptibility to infection, sore throat, malaise, and bleeding.

Antidepressants: drugs used to treat depression

Reports of lifetime incidences of depression range from 6% to 17% (Kessler et al., 1994). Estimates indicate approximately 15% of people who suffer from depression eventually die by suicide (Coryell, Noyes, & Clancy, 1982). Treatment for depression requires a two-pronged approach. Studies have shown clients who receive psychotherapy or appropriate medication do better than clients who receive no treatment. However, the combination of psychotherapy and antidepressant therapy is more efficacious than either treatment by itself (Roundsville, Klerman, & Weisman, 1986).

Indications

Antidepressants are primarily indicated for major depression (Table 13-3). These drugs also are used to treat depression associated with bipolar disorder, cyclothymic disorder, obsessive-compulsive disorder, anorexia, phobia, and even schizophrenia.

How antidepressants work

To understand how antidepressants work in the brain, we must get to the heart of the biochemical theories behind depression. If depression were only a response to loss, grief, disappointment, or failure, pills would be of no value. However, if depression has a chemical component, bolstering a client's chemical defenses might alleviate the depression. The treatment of depression with psychotropic drugs is based on this latter view.

Antidepressants work by changing the neuronal chemical environment in ways that cause the neurons to work more efficiently and thus theoretically decrease the symptoms of the illness.

Table 13-3. Drugs for mood disorders: usual adult daily dosage, therapeutic plasma level, reuptake blockade, and side effect profile

AGENT	USUAL ADULT DAILY DOSAGE (mg/day)	THERAPEUTIC PLASMA LEVEL	REUPTAKE BLOCKADE		SIDE EFFECTS PROFILE			
			5-HT	Ne	ANTICHOLINERGIC	SEDATION	ORTHOSTATIC HYPOTENSION	SEXUAL DYSFUNCTION
Tricyclics								
Amitriptyline (Elavil)	100–300	110–250 ng/ml	Y	Y	+++§	+++	+++	+†
Clomipramine (Anafranil)	100–250	150–300 ng/ml	Y	Y	+++	+++	+++	+++
Desipramine (Norpramin)	100–300	125–300 ng/ml	N	Y	+	+	++‡	+
Imipramine (Tofranil)	100–300	200–350 ng/ml	Y	Y	++	++	+++	+
Nortriptyline (Pamelor)	50–200	50–150 ng/ml	Y	Y	++	++	+	+
SSRIs								
Fluoxetine (Prozac)	10–80	N/A	Y	N	0/+*	0/+	0/+	+++
Paroxetine (Paxil)	20–50	N/A	Y	N	0/+	++	0/+	+++
Sertraline (Zoloft)	50–200	N/A	Y	N	0/+	+	0/+	+++
Fluvoxamine (Luvox)	100–300	N/A	Y	N	0/+	+	0/+	+++
MAOIs								
Phenelzine (Nardil)	45–90	N/A	Inhibit monoamine oxidase		+	++	+++	++
Tranylcypromine (Parnate)	20–50	N/A			+	0/+	+++	++

Continued.

Table 13-3. Cont'd

AGENT	USUAL ADULT DAILY DOSAGE (mg/day)	THERAPEUTIC PLASMA LEVEL	REUPTAKE BLOCKADE		SIDE EFFECTS PROFILE			
			5-HT	Ne	ANTICHOLINERGIC	SEDATION	ORTHOSTATIC HYPOTENSION	SEXUAL DYSFUNCTION
Other antidepressants								
Amoxapine (Asendin)	200-600	N/A	Y	Y	+	+	+	+
Bupropion (Wellbutrin)	200-450	N/A	N	N	0/+	0/+	0/+	0/+
Nefazodone (Serzone)	300-600	N/A	Y	Y	0/+	+	0/+	0/+
Trazodone (Desyrel)	200-600	N/A	Y	N	0/+	+++	+++	+
Venlafaxine (Effexor)	75-375	N/A	Y	Y	0/+	+	0/+	+++
Mood stabilizers								
Lithium (Eskalith, Lithobid)	Acute: 1200-2400 Maintenance: 900-1200	Acute: 0.8-1.5mEq/L Maintenance: 0.6-1.2 mEq/L	N/A	N/A	Common side effects: nausea, fine hand tremor, polyuria, polydipsia			
Carbamazepine (Tegretol)	10-20 mg/kg/day	5-12 µg/ml	N/A		Common side effects: nausea, dizziness, sedation, headache, dry mouth, constipation			
Valproic acid	15-40 mg/kg/day	50-100 µg/ml	N/A		Common side effects: nausea, diarrhea, abdominal cramps, sedation, tremor			

Modified from "Review of Psychotropic Drugs," by T. Puzantian & G. L. Stimmel, 1995, January, *Retail Pharmacy News*, 13.

*0/+ = Very mild effects.

†+ = Mild effects.

‡++ = Moderate effects.

§+++ = Profound effects.

Time to clinical effect

Although the presence of antidepressants in blood serum can be detected soon after they are administered, a full clinical effect usually does not appear for 2 to 4 weeks. Maximal clinical effectiveness may take as long as 6 weeks to occur (Baer & Williams, 1992). Therefore it is important to maintain contact with clients during this time to ensure their depression does not deepen as they wait for clinical effectiveness. Paradoxically, antidepressants may energize a severely depressed person to plan and carry out a suicide attempt. Clients should therefore be encouraged to report to their primary care provider any thoughts of suicide or any deepening of depression.

Efficacy

All categories of antidepressant drugs—the tricyclics and related drugs, monoamine oxidase inhibitors, selective serotonin reuptake inhibitors, and the atypical agents—are approximately equally efficacious. Meta-analysis performed by the U.S. Department of Health and Human Services indicates practitioners can expect a response rate of roughly 50% to 60% (Depression Guideline Panel, 1993). Response rates are slightly better in some client populations.

Categories of antidepressants

Tricyclic antidepressants (TCAs) and related drugs.

The term *tricyclic* actually refers to the chemical structure of the drugs; they contain three hydrocarbon rings. Some newer drugs that have four hydrocarbon rings are more truly called tetracyclics. However, this entire group of heterocyclic drugs generally has the same efficaciousness, side effects, and clinical profiles, and for these reasons is usually classified as tricyclic by most clinicians.

HOW TCAs WORK.   TCAs work by blocking the uptake of catecholamine neurotransmitters (norepinephrine, serotonin, and dopamine) into the nerve endings from which they were released. Blocking the reuptake of these chemicals pro-longs neuron stimulation. These chemical actions begin to take place within hours of ingesting the medication, although clinical effect may not be evident for 2 weeks and full effect can take as long as 6 weeks. One possible reason for this delay is the time needed to normalize the hyposensitive receptor sites associated with depression (Baer & Williams, 1992).

SIDE EFFECTS OF TCAs.   True tricyclics and phenothiazine derivatives are structurally similar and consequently have similar side effect profiles, including sedation, orthostatic hypotension, and anticholinergic effects (Lehne et al., 1994). The side effects of the tricyclics are primarily peripheral anticholinergic side effects, orthostatic hypotension, and central nervous system effects of sedation, disorientation, delusion, confusion, hallucination, and lowering of the seizure threshold. If blood serum levels rise above the therapeutic range, a drug-induced mania or delirium can occur. Table 13-4 highlights the major side effects and nursing interventions for the TCAs.

Because TCAs do not induce euphoria and are nonaddictive they have a low abuse potential, but concern about overdose is a significant issue. Tricyclic antidepressant overdose accounts for 25% to 50% of all hospital admissions for overdose (Harsch & Holt, 1988). TCAs are especially cardiotoxic; a dosage as small as 10 times the usual daily dosage can cause acute cardiac failure and arrhythmias. TCAs are rarely prescribed for clients who have cardiac conditions. For this reason, some clinicians will initiate TCA therapy with only a 7-day supply of medication. Any client who arrives at the physician's office or the emergency room with a TCA overdose should be hospitalized immediately and monitored for cardiac status. Clients with cardiac disease should receive an electrocardiogram before initiation of therapy. Because toxic blood levels may not be much higher than therapeutic levels, levels should be monitored until clinical effect and side effects have been balanced.

Table 13-4. Side effects and nursing interventions for TCAs

SIDE EFFECTS	INTERVENTIONS
Peripheral nervous system	
Dry mouth	Advise frequent sips of water, hard candies, sugarless gum.
Mydriasis	Advise wearing sunglasses outdoors.
Diminished lacrimation	Suggest artificial tears.
Blurred vision	Caution about driving and potential for falls. Usually subsides in 1 to 2 weeks. The client should remove objects in the house that might be tripped over (for example, throw rugs and small tables).
Eye pain	Advise client to report eye pain immediately because it may indicate an acute glaucoma attack. All elderly people should be screened for glaucoma before treatment with TCAs is initiated.
Urinary hesitancy or retention	Monitor fluid intake. Client should be told to avoid putting off urinating. Running water or pouring water over the perineum can stimulate urination. Catheterization may be needed.
Constipation	Monitor fluid and food intake. Urge client to heed the urge to defecate. A high-fiber diet and large amounts of water (2500 to 3000 ml per day) are helpful.
Anhidrosis	Monitor sweating; decreased sweating can lead to increased body temperature. Adequate fluids, appropriate clothing, and sensible exercise should be stressed.
Cardiovascular effects	Avoid prescribing TCAs during the recovery phase of myocardial infarction.
Orthostatic hypotension	Advise client to assume sitting position on side of bed, wait and dangle feet for 1 full minute, then rise slowly. Clients should not stand in one position too long and should avoid hot showers and tub baths. Elderly people may require assistance at these times.
Central nervous system	
Sedation	Caution client about driving.
Delirium or mania	Discontinue the drug and call the physician.
Suicidal ideation	Observe clients closely because TCAs may increase energy for suicide.

Modified from *Psychiatric Nursing* (2nd ed.) (p. 260), by N. L. Keltner, L. H. Schwecke, & C. E. Bostrom, 1995, St. Louis: Mosby.

Some TCAs have a therapeutic window. Plasma levels above or below this "window" are less effective. Side effects typically increase at higher plasma levels (see Table 13-3).

INTERACTIONS. Drug interactions may be predicted by considering the chemical properties of TCAs and how their receptor sites may be impacted by the chemical properties of other drugs. For example, because TCAs produce neural stimulation, other drugs that act in the same manner should be avoided. Likewise, drugs that possess similar side effect profiles should be avoided to prevent an additive effect. Combining TCAs with other drugs should be done carefully and clients should be warned to avoid any over the counter medications without first consulting their primary care providers.

Interactions with monoamine oxidase inhibitors. The combination of TCAs with monoamine oxidase inhibitors (MAOIs) should be avoided because the excessive adrenergic stimulation of the cardiovascular system may lead to severe hypertension. This combination of drugs greatly potentiates the effect of catecholamines in the autonomic nervous system.

Interactions with direct-acting sympathomimetics. Epinephrine and norepinephrine are potentiated by TCAs because reuptake will be slowed, causing cardiovascular hyperstimulation.

Interactions with indirect-acting sympathomimetics. Tricyclic antidepressants decrease the response of indirect-acting sympathomimetics by blocking their uptake into the nerve terminals in which they produce their effect.

Interactions with anticholinergics. Because TCAs exert an anticholinergic effect, clients should be advised to avoid other medications that have anticholinergic properties (for example, antihistamines and certain over the counter sleep medications). An anticholinergic delirium can result from this interaction.

Interactions with central nervous system (CNS) depressants. The TCAs cause CNS depression, probably because of their blockade of central histamine receptors (Lehne et al., 1994); any concomitant use with CNS depressants would cause an additive effect.

Monoamine oxidase inhibitors. Monoamine oxidase inhibitors (MAOIs) are still in use and despite wider use of the newer agents are considered as effective as the new drugs. The main reasons MAOIs are no longer widely used are their wide-ranging dietary and drug restrictions

and the adverse reactions associated with violating those restrictions, including the possibility of a potentially fatal hypertensive crisis. Nonetheless, MAOIs are prescribed by some clinicians for cases of atypical depression. Table 13-3 lists major side effects associated with MAOIs.

HOW MAOIs WORK. Similar to the TCAS, monoamine oxidase inhibitors alter the neuronal environment by enhancing neurotransmitter availability, albeit by a different mechanism. The MAOIs inhibit monoamine oxidase, the enzyme that deactivates norepinephrine, epinephrine, and serotonin. As with other antidepressants, although MAOIs produce this chemical effect rapidly a full clinical response may not be seen for weeks. Obviously, other factors beyond the enhancement of neurotransmitter availability are at work for both TCAs and MAOIs. Those factors can be reviewed in pharmacology texts.

SIDE EFFECTS OF MAOIs. The MAOIs cause direct CNS stimulation and can produce anxiety, agitation, hypomania, and mania. Many clients report increased appetite and weight gain. Other adverse effects include drowsiness, dizziness, rash, peripheral edema, and the anticholinergic effects of constipation, dry mouth, urinary retention, and transient impotence. Orthostatic hypotension frequently occurs, especially in clients with preexisting hypertension.

The most serious adverse consequence of MAOI therapy is the possibility a food-drug or drug-drug interaction will induce a potentially fatal hypertensive crisis (Box 13-3, Table 13-5). Hypertensive crisis is characterized by increased blood pressure, headache, heart palpitations, nausea, vomiting, neck stiffness, fever, and mydriasis or other visual disturbance (Baer & Williams, 1992). Clients should avoid foods rich in tyramine, an amino acid precursor to dopamine, norepinephrine, and epinephrine. Additional dietary tyramine can produce a synaptic flooding of catecholamine into the peripheral nervous system, causing a hypertensive crisis. Clients should be

---

Box 13-3. Tyramine-rich foods to avoid with MAOIs

Alcoholic beverages

Beer and ale
Chianti and sherry wine

Dairy products

Cheese: cheddar, blue, Brie, mozzarella
Sour cream
Yogurt

Fruits and vegetables

Avocados
Bananas
Fava beans
Canned figs

Meats

Bologna
Chicken liver
Fish, dried
Liver
Pickled herring
Salami
Sausage

Other foods

Caffeinated coffee, cola, tea (large amounts)
Chocolate
Licorice
Soy sauce
Yeast
Meat tenderizer

Modified from *Psychiatric nursing* (2nd ed.) (p. 267), by N. L. Keltner, L. H. Schwecke, & C. E. Bostrom, 1995, St. Louis: Mosby.

Table 13-5. Significant drug interactions with MAOIs

DRUGS	EFFECT OF INTERACTION
Anticholinergic drugs	Compound anticholinergic response
Anesthetics (general)	Deepen CNS depression
Antihypertensives (diuretics, beta-blockers, hydralazine)	Cause hypotension
CNS depressants	Intensify CNS depression
Guanethidine, methyldopa, reserpine	Produce severe hypertension
Sympathomimetics (mixed and indirect acting): amphetamines, methylphenidate, dopamine, phenylpropanolamine (in many over the counter hay fever, cold, and diet medications)	Precipitate hypertensive crisis, cardiac stimulation, arrhythmias, cerebrovascular hemorrhage
Sympathomimetics (direct acting): epinephrine, norepinephrine, isoproterenol; less likely to cause problems	Cause same effects as above but theoretically should not produce as severe a reaction
Tricyclic antidepressants	Cause same effects as above
SSRIs	Can be fatal and this combination should be avoided

Modified from *Psychiatric nursing* (2nd ed.) (p. 266), by N. L. Keltner, L. H. Schwecke, & C. E. Bostrom, 1995, St. Louis: Mosby.

educated about tyramine-rich foods and should be assessed for willingness to restrict themselves to the correct diet.

DRUG INTERACTIONS. MAOIs should not be used with other drugs that cause hypertension, including mixed-acting or indirect-acting sympathomimetics. Drugs to avoid include over the counter cold medications, weight loss aids, stimulants, and prescription drugs such as amphetamines and methylphenidate (Ritalin). Similarly, clients should avoid street stimulants such as cocaine and "crack," which when combined with MAOIs can prove fatal.

Also to be avoided are TCAs and SSRIs. A potentially fatal consequence of this combination, serotonin syndrome, has recently been recognized in the literature. This syndrome may result in neurological excitement, seizures, and extreme hyperpyrexia (Baer & Williams, 1992). Meperidine (Demerol) is to be avoided during MAOI therapy because of the possibility of neurological excitation, hypertension, high fever, and coma. Fatalities from serotonin syndrome have been reported. Clients should avoid using meperidine for 2 weeks after MAOIs have been discontinued. Hypoglycemic agents used with MAOIs may cause pronounced hypoglycemia because of the prolonged effect of the agents in the body in the presence of MAOIs.

Selective serotonin reuptake inhibitors (SSRIs).

Since its introduction in 1985, fluoxetine (Prozac) has become the most widely prescribed antidepressant in the United States. (See Table 13-3 for information about SSRIs.) Fluoxetine was the first of the SSRIs which are strongly selective in preventing the reuptake of serotonin at the presynaptic nerve ending. In the last few years SSRIs have become the most widely reported antidepressants in the lay media, probably because of their widespread use. At first hailed as wonder drugs, then vilified as mind-altering chemicals capable of turning the most mild-mannered person into a killer or suicide victim,

these agents have experienced wide swings in public and professional opinion. Scientific evidence supports neither extreme. What is confirmed about SSRIs is that for the first time a unique class of drugs has become available that has far fewer and less serious side effects than any previously known antidepressants. This has resulted in more clinicians feeling comfortable with prescribing an antidepressant. Fluoxetine and the newer drug fluvoxamine (Luvox) are used to treat obsessive-compulsive disorder; fluoxetine also has been used investigationally with clients with eating disorders.

HOW SSRIs WORK. As the name implies, SSRIs act by selectively preventing the reuptake of serotonin into the presynaptic neuron thus prolonging its bioavailability to the neural conduction process. SSRIs have no effect on dopamine or norepinephrine. SSRIs are not potent antagonists of cholinergic, histaminergic, or alpha-adrenergic receptors and thus tend to produce CNS stimulation rather than sedation.

SIDE EFFECTS OF SSRIs. Because SSRIs do not block cholinergic, histaminergic, or alphaadrenergic receptors, they produce few of the annoying side effects associated with TCAs and MAOIs. Their manageable side effect profile has contributed to their widespread use. However, a few troublesome side effects have been reported, including nausea, constipation, diarrhea, loose stools, and weight loss. CNS side effects include headache, dizziness, tremors, nervousness, decreased libido, and inhibited orgasm. Sexual inhibition (occurring in as many as 20% to 30% of clients taking SSRIs) has caused many clients to take these drugs inconsistently. The new antidepressants nefazodone and bupropion are often prescribed for these clients. Cardiovascular side effects are uncommon; SSRIs are usually well tolerated by elderly clients.

INTERACTIONS. Selective serotonin reuptake inhibitors and monoamine oxidase inhibitors in

Box 13-4. Serotonin syndrome

Serotonin syndrome, a recently recognized phenomenon, is a potentially lethal consequence of combining serotonin-enhancing psychotropic drugs such as SSRI + MAOI, MAOI + L-tryptophan, and clomipramine (Anafranil) + MAOI.

Clients suffering from the serotonin syndrome experience hyperreflexia, hyperthermia, myoclonus, and other symptoms suggestive of the better-known neuroleptic malignant syndrome (NMS). Keltner and Harris report the case of a woman who, after taking one dose of sertraline (100 mg), became unconscious, hyperthermic (108° F), and myoclonic, and died within a few days. The client, who had been taking an MAOI, went to her general practitioner with complaints of depression. She was prescribed the SSRI and did not wait the required 14 days before initiating therapy with sertraline.

Nurses should be aware of the following:

1. MAOIs and SSRIs should not be given concomitantly.
2. A period of 14 days is required between stopping an MAOI and starting an SSRI.
3. A period of 5 weeks is required between stopping the SSRI fluoxetine (Prozac) and starting an MAOI.
4. MAOIs and clomipramine (Anafranil) should not be given concomitantly.

Modified from "Serotonin Syndrome: A Case of Fatal SSRI/MAOI Interaction," by N. L. Keltner and C. Harris, 1994, *Perspectives in Psychiatric Care, 30*(4), 26-31.

combination can produce the lethal serotonin syndrome (see Box 13-2 and Box 13-4) (Keltner & Harris, 1994; Sternbach, 1991). A 5-week interval is recommended between discontinuing an SSRI and initiating an MAOI medication. The SSRI drug fluoxetine can elevate the plasma levels of tricyclic antidepressants and lithium. These combinations should be prescribed cautiously.

Length of trial

A clinical lag time of as long as 2 to 4 weeks may elapse before any improvement in symptoms is seen. Therefore there should be a reasonable trial of the selected antidepressant before switching to another drug. If a client has not responded at all or only minimally in 6 weeks, the clinician must reassess the diagnosis and adequacy of treatment (Depression Guideline Panel, 1993). Some treatment failures are caused by subtherapeutic dosage. The TCAs and SSRIs are considered drugs of choice for antidepressant therapy. Choice of a specific drug depends on client variables such as age, symptoms, and side effect profile (Depression Guideline Panel, 1993). For example, if a client has trouble sleeping, a medication with a side effect of drowsiness may be desirable and should be prescribed at bedtime. On the other hand, if a client seems overly somnolent an SSRI might be tried first with a view toward boosting CNS alertness.

How long should antidepressants be given: maintenance treatment

The Depression Guideline Panel (1993) recommends medication treatment continue for at least 4 months after the remission of symptoms. For clients who have previously experienced long periods of depression, treatment should continue for as long as 9 months. If clients have experienced repeated periods of depression in their lives, even longer trials may be indicated.

Atypical antidepressants

Bupropion (Wellbutrin) is a unique antidepressant similar in chemical structure to amphetamines (Lehne et al., 1994). Similar to amphetamines it has stimulant effects and suppresses appetite. Bupropion has none of the anticholinergic effects associated with the TCAs. Clinical effects take 1 to 3 weeks. The most common side effects are dry mouth, weight loss, and dizziness. A slight tremor and insomnia or agitation also can occur.

Venlafaxine (Effexor) is a newer drug (introduced in 1994) that is chemically different from the drugs previously mentioned (Cunningham et al., 1994). It inhibits the reuptake of both serotonin and norepinephrine, and to a lesser extent dopamine (Keltner, 1995b). It produces a low incidence of anticholinergic side effects. The most common side effect is nausea. Other side effects include drowsiness, dry mouth, dizziness, constipation, nervous agitation, and anorexia.

Nefazodone (Serzone), the newest antidepressant on the market, is structurally related to trazodone and is a moderately potent inhibitor of serotonin reuptake (Goldberg, 1995). It is effective in the treatment of moderate to severe major depression. The most common side effects associated with nefazodone include nausea, weakness, headache, dizziness, dry mouth, constipation, and light-headedness (Goldberg, 1995). It differs from other SSRIs because it does not produce significant sexually inhibitory side effects and has a normalizing effect on sleep (Goldberg, 1995).

Antimanic agents: drugs used to treat bipolar disorder

Nearly two million Americans suffer from bipolar disorder (Depression Guideline Panel, 1993). This illness, previously called manic depression, is known for the disabling polarity of moods suffered by its victims. Mood swings most often occur over a period of weeks to months. These mood swings are characterized by periods of depression, despondency, guilt, and suicidal thoughts in the depressive part of the illness and euphoria, hyperactivity, grandiosity, racing thoughts, and pressured speech on the high or manic side. This lability of affect is disruptive to the client's work and family life, often causing the deterioration and dissolution of these relationships.

Indications

Lithium therapy is indicated for the mania of bipolar disorder and cyclothymic disorder (another disruptive mood swing disorder with somewhat less severe symptoms). Lithium also is used as an adjunctive agent in the treatment of psycho-sis, depression, obsessive-compulsive disorder, and cocaine abuse. (See Table 13-3 for side effects and variables related to mood stabilizers.)

How lithium works

Lithium is a naturally occurring salt and an element of the periodic table. It has been prescribed for mania since 1970 in the United States and for a decade before that in Europe. The exact mechanism of action of lithium is not known. Lithium is thought to compromise the ability of neurons to release, activate, or respond to neurotransmitters by substituting itself for the sodium ions in the cell. Lithium is well absorbed by the intestine, and peak plasma levels are reached in 1 to 4 hours. About 95% of lithium is excreted through the kidneys unmetabolized. Its half-life is about 24 hours. Most commonly prescribed as lithium carbonate (Li_2CO_3) in 300 mg capsules and tablets, it also is available in extended-release form in 450 mg capsules (Lithobid). Dosing usually begins with 300 mg three times a day or 450 mg twice a day for the extended-release capsules. The chief benefit of the extended-release capsule is that a sustained release may promote a more steady blood level thus eliminating some distracting side effects that occur most frequently with blood levels greater than 1.5 mEq/L. Lithium also is available in a liquid concentrate form (lithium citrate).

Time to clinical effect

Clinical efficacy may take 1 to 3 weeks even though blood levels are achieved rapidly. For this reason antipsychotics or benzodiazepine derivatives may be used together with lithium until the drug begins to take effect (Lehne et al., 1994). Blood levels of 0.6 mEq/L to 1.2 mEq/L are considered therapeutic. Within this range the clinician should find the level at which symptom containment is maximized and the side effect profile is minimized. Toxic effects appear at levels above 1.5 mEq/L in some clients and in almost all clients at levels above 2.0 mEq/L.

Efficacy

Lithium has proven effective in 70% to 80% of clients in a manic or hypomanic state within 1 to 2 weeks (Baer & Williams, 1992). It has proven particularly useful in reducing symptoms such as elation, grandiosity, flight of ideas, irritability, and anxiety. Relapse occurs in as many as 90% of clients who discontinue medication and in as many as 40% of clients who continue medication (Baer & Williams, 1992).

Side effects

Lithium's side effects are linked primarily to blood serum levels. The higher the levels, the greater the likelihood of side effects and toxic effects. Side effects can occur within the therapeutic range of 0.5 mEq/L to 1.2 mEq/L but are more frequent at the higher end of the range. Central nervous system side effects include headache, drowsiness, hand tremor, twitching, ataxia, seizure, slurred speech, restlessness, confusion, stupor, memory loss, and clonic movements. Peripheral side effects include dry mouth, anorexia, nausea, vomiting, diarrhea, hypertension, leukocytosis, blurred vision, hypothyroidism, hyponatremia, and muscle weakness.

At levels between 1.5 mEq/L and 2.0 mEq/L, diarrhea, gastric upset, drowsiness, and weakness may be seen. At levels from 2 mEq/L to 3 mEq/L giddiness, ataxia, slurred speech, blurred vision, tinnitus, blackout, fasciculation, and incontinence may occur. Medication should be stopped immediately and the physician notified for any serum level over 1.5 mEq/L. At levels higher than 3 mEq/L multisystem failure, seizures, vascular collapse, and coma are possible.

Because lithium replaces sodium in the body, these two elements have a converse relationship in body fluids. When dietary sodium levels increase, serum levels of lithium decrease because of the replacement of lithium by sodium. When the body's sodium levels decrease, lithium levels will increase. Therefore if the body loses sodium through a salt-restricted diet, excessive sweating, diarrhea, or vomiting, lithium levels will increase.

Because therapeutic levels of lithium are not much lower than toxic levels, the clinician must emphasize maintenance of a balanced diet and avoidance of activities likely to cause excessive sweating. For this reason, clinicians and nurses should question clients about their fluid intake history if lithium is becoming less effective. Likewise, questions regarding physical activities, vomiting, or diarrhea are warranted if symptoms indicative of an increased serum lithium level (including increased side effects) are present.

Interactions

The most significant drug interactions are those that occur with nonsteroidal antiinflamatory drugs and thiazide diuretics. Both categories of drugs increase serum levels of lithium and can provoke toxicity. Other drug interactions include increased clearance time for sodium bicarbonate, acetazolamide, mannitol, and aminophylline. Theophyllines and urinary alkalinizers can decrease the effects of lithium. Use with carbamazepine can cause neurotoxic effects.

The angiotensin-converting enzyme (ACE) inhibitors may produce a threefold to fourfold increase in serum lithium levels that could prove fatal. Although lithium is often used with either benzodiazepine derivatives or antipsychotics until a clinical effect is achieved, lithium can cause neurotoxicity when combined with haloperidol. Lithium also may increase the incidence of extrapyramidal side effects.

How long can lithium be given?

Lithium therapy is a long-term approach to symptom management that for some clients may entail a lifetime of taking lithium because of the chronic nature of bipolar disorder. Clients who continue taking lithium for 2 years can reduce their incidence of relapse by 50% (Baer & Williams, 1992). Lithium therapy often continues for 3 to 6 months after a manic episode and is then tapered off. Serum levels are usually tested monthly, but some compliant, long-term clients may require blood work only once or twice a year (Varcarolis, 1994).

Organ systems vulnerable to lithium

Lithium is not considered toxic to any specific organ system except when given in overdose quantities or if a system is already compromised (Groleau, 1994). Nonetheless, many clinicians closely monitor kidney function because renal injury has occurred (Morton, Sonne, & Lydiard, 1993).

Peripheral nervous system. A common side effect of lithium is fine hand tremor that may subside as the client stabilizes on medication. It is more bothersome when the client is under stress or is fatigued (Lehne et al., 1994). If manic symptoms are well controlled but the hand tremor is becoming more significant, reducing the dosage of lithium or spreading the doses more evenly throughout the day may reduce the tremor. If dosage manipulation is ineffective, tremor may be reduced with a beta-blocking agent such as propranolol (Inderal) (Keltner & Folks, 1993).

Thyroid. Long-term lithium use can cause enlargment of the thyroid gland (goiter). Usually benign, lithium-induced goiter may sometimes be associated with hypothyroidism. Withdrawal of lithium will usually reverse thyroid hypertrophy. Blood serum levels of thyroid hormones (T3 and T4) and thyroid-stimulating hormone (TSH) should be obtained before treatment and once a year thereafter (Lehne et al., 1994).

Renal. Chronic administration of lithium has been associated with degenerative changes in the kidney although, as mentioned earlier, lithium is not considered toxic to any organ. The risk may be minimized by keeping dosages as low as possible and avoiding long-term therapy when possible (Groleau, 1994). Kidney function should be assessed before initiation of therapy and once a year thereafter.

Polyuria occurs in 50% to 70% of clients taking lithium. Frank diabetes insipidus may occur in some clients and result in a urinary output of as much as 9 liters a day (Morton et al., 1993). Lithium antagonizes the effects of antidiuretic hor-

mone, thereby increasing urination (Morton et al., 1993). Clients should be instructed to maintain adequate fluid intake by drinking 8 to 12 glasses of water a day. Clients who notice excessive dry mouth need to drink more water. Clients' complaints of polyuria, nocturia, and thirst are often given as reasons why they are no longer compliant with their medication schedule. Lithium-induced polyuria has been shown to improve with a thiazide diuretic (Keltner & Folks, 1993). The cause of this paradoxical effect is not completely understood. However, because thiazide diuretics increase plasma levels of lithium, a dosage reduction may be necessary.

Use in pregnancy. Lithium therapy is contraindicated during pregnancy because of its teratogenic effects. An approximate 11% incidence of birth defects, usually malformations of the heart, has been noted with lithium use continued through the first trimester (Lehne et al., 1994). If antimania treatment is essential during this time, treatment with thioridazine, carbamazepine, or valproate may be helpful (Keltner & Folks, 1993). However, these drugs carry unknown risks. Lithium dosages should be reduced by as much as 50% before delivery to reduce the risk of neonatal intoxication (Cohen, 1989). Likewise, lithium therapy should be avoided during breastfeeding because it is excreted in breast milk and may cause toxicity in the infant.

Alternatives to lithium for lithium-resistant clients

Lithium helps the majority of clients who use it, but for some the side effects may become intolerable. Also, for some clients (20% to 30%) the therapeutic results may be inadequate enough to warrant an investigation of alternative mood stabilizers (Calabrese et al., 1993). Carbamazepine (Tegretol) and valproic acid (Depakene) are often considered when lithium therapy must be discontinued. Both are primarily known as antiepileptic drugs but have been shown to have a mood stabilizing effect for both depression and mania.

Carbamazepine. Carbamazepine is chemically related to the tricyclic antidepressants. Clients with a rapidly cycling bipolar disorder may actually respond better to carbamazepine than to lithium. It also has a better side effect profile than lithium. It carries an FDA pregnancy category C rating, indicating that it can be given during pregnancy. Carbamazepine has been used in combination with lithium to good effect. Blood serum levels and clinical effects are used to determine dosage. The initial dosage is usually 200 mg twice a day (for adults), increasing by weekly intervals at 200 mg per day, with dosages to be evenly divided three or four times a day. Therapeutic blood levels are 4 µg/mL to 12 µg/ml. Fatal blood dyscrasias have been reported but the absolute incidence is low (about 1 in 50,000).

Valproic acid. Valproic acid (Depakene) also is known primarily as an antiseizure drug but has been used successfully as an alternative to lithium therapy. It has recently received Food and Drug Administration approval as an antimanic drug. Studies show it can help control manic episodes and can be used prophylactically against recurrent episodes of mania and depression. Dosing is initiated at 300 mg to 500 mg per day and may gradually increase to between 750 mg and 3000 mg per day in divided doses. Valproic acid alters gamma-aminobutyric acid (GABA), a major inhibitory neurotransmitter.

Antianxiety agents

Anxiety is a universal experience, but for some it can become a life-altering disability. When anxiety interferes with work and family functioning or keeps the client from experiencing a normal life, treatment is necessary. Usually treatment includes counseling for management of psychosocial stressors and medication for the relief of nervous, behavioral, or somatic discomfort. Treatment based on changes in behavior, nutrition, activity, and attitude may be the most important and long-lasting approach to the alleviation of anxiety. However, such changes come slowly. When anxiety affects life and work, medication may be necessary. Medication may be continued until counseling, new cognitive skills, and changes in behavior are sufficient to control anxiety without medication.

Indications

Benzodiazepine derivatives are frequently prescribed for anxiety, but SSRIs are becoming the drugs of choice for many clinicians because they produce fewer side effects and a decreased tendency to abuse. Benzodiazepine derivatives are emphasized in this section because SSRIs have already been described (Table 13-6).

Before the clinician can prescribe treatment for anxiety, etiology factors and severity must be assessed. Anxiety is generally classified as organic in origin, symptomatic of a major mental disorder (for example, depression, schizophrenia, or mania), situational, generalized anxiety disorder, or panic disorder (Dubin & Weiss, 1991). Chemical intervention (using antianxiety agents) plays a prominent role in the treatment of the latter three conditions.

Anxiety related to a medical condition (organic anxiety syndrome) is characterized by prominent recurrent anxiety attacks unrelated to psychosocial factors. In clients over 40 years old who exhibit mild hypertension, tachycardia, sweating, and tremors, organic anxiety syndrome may be suspected. Some prescription drugs such as antidepressants, antipsychotics, benzodiazepine derivatives, aminophylline, steroids, digoxin, beta-blockers, sympathomimetics, anticholinergics, and salicylates also can cause "organic" anxiety. When organic anxiety syndrome is suspected, the client should be referred to a primary care provider. Another common underlying cause of anxiety is drug or alcohol abuse and withdrawal. In such cases the client must be given a firm recommendation to participate in a detoxification or rehabilitation program. Antianxiety drugs should not be the initial treatment for organic anxiety syndrome because the underlying medical condition must first be evaluated and treated.

When anxiety is related to a major mental illness, it must be treated in conjunction with the psychotropic medications already prescribed for

Table 13-6. Antianxiety agents: daily adult dosage range, onset, and half-life

AGENT	DAILY ADULT DOSAGE RANGE (mg per day)	ONSET	HALF-LIFE
Benzodiazepine derivatives			
Alprazolam (Xanax)	0.75-4.0	Fast	Intermediate
Chlordiazepoxide (Librium)	15-60	Fast	Long
Clonazepam (Klonopin)	1-6	Moderate	Long
Diazepam (Valium)	2-40	Very fast	Long
Lorazepam (Ativan)	0.5-10.0	Fast	Short
Oxazepam (Serax)	30-120	Slow	Short
Others			
Buspirone (BuSpar)	15-60	0.5-1.5 hours	N/A

Modified from "Review of Psychotropic Drugs," by T. Puzantian & G. L. Stimmel, 1995, January, *Retail Pharmacy News,* 11.

that disorder. Often treating the primary mental illness effectively eliminates the need for an anxiolytic. If a benzodiazepine derivative is required it should be used carefully because of its abuse potential and cumulative central nervous system (CNS) depressant effects. For example, benzodiazepine derivatives can be prescribed for clients with major depression along with their antidepressant medications. However, these clients will require careful supervision, particularly those individuals with a history of chemical abuse or suicidal behavior.

Three conditions for which antianxiety drugs (particularly benzodiazepine derivatives) are specifically prescribed are situational crisis, generalized anxiety disorder, and panic disorder. In a situational crisis the client may experience normal responses to a severe stressor (for example, a death in the family, divorce, financial reversal, or legal problem). Benzodiazepine derivatives can be beneficial in helping the client cope with these crises. Occasionally anxiety occurs in anticipation of a stressor such as surgery, marriage, a new job, or even public speaking. This type of anxiety (including stage fright) is often treated with 10 mg to 20 mg of the beta-blocker propranolol (Inderal) (sometimes in conjunction with a benzodiazepine

derivative) 1 hour before the feared event to reduce autonomic symptoms of perspiration, dry mouth, and palpitations.

Generalized anxiety disorder (GAD) is characterized by unrealistic, excessive anxiety and worry about two or more life circumstances. Diagnosis is made when at least three of the following symptoms are present: hypervigilance, poor concentration, sleeping problems, muscle tension, and autonomic hyperactivity (including palpitations, tachycardia, sweating, and clammy hands). Benzodiazepine derivatives are frequently prescribed for GAD.

The third type of anxiety problem for which medications are used is panic disorder. Panic disorders create a subjective feeling of impending doom, loss of control, "going crazy," or even heart attack. Benzodiazepine derivatives (alprazolam and clonazepam), tricyclics (imipramine and desipramine), and SSRIs have all been used successfully in this disorder. All three conditions—situational crisis, GAD, and panic disorder—may be treated using benzodiazepine derivatives or SSRIs as first-line antianxiety medications. However, obsessive-compulsive disorder is most often treated with the antidepressant clomipramine (Anafranil) or with SSRIs and not with benzodiazepine derivatives.

How benzodiazepine derivatives work

Benzodiazepine derivatives potentiate the actions of gamma-aminobutyric acid (GABA), an inhibitory neurotransmitter found throughout the central nervous system. Because benzodiazepine derivatives are not direct GABA agonists but act by amplifying the actions of endogenous GABA rather than by directly mimicking GABA, CNS depression is limited. For this reason benzodiazepine derivatives are safer than barbiturates (drugs that can directly mimic GABA and have played a role in many accidental and purposeful overdoses).

Benzodiazepine derivatives induce a general quieting of the central nervous system, causing some drowsiness and muscle relaxation. In fact, hypnotic benzodiazepine derivatives also are the most commonly prescribed medications to relieve insomnia. The anxiolytic and hypnotic benzodiazepine derivatives differ mainly in their onset times and half-lives.

Time to clinical effect

Generally the benzodiazepine derivatives take effect very quickly and have varying half-lives.

Efficacy

Though safer than barbiturates, benzodiazepine derivatives are considered equally efficacious and are often prescribed for the treatment of anxiety. All benzodiazepine derivatives reduce anxiety; however, some are marketed specifically as anxiolytics and others are marketed as hypnotics. The distinction between these purposes is based on their respective half-lives and subsequent length of action. The anticonvulsant benzodiazepine derivative clonazepam (Klonopin) also has been widely prescribed for anxiety and may induce less disinhibition than that associated with the other benzodiazepine derivatives.

Abuse potential. Benzodiazepine derivatives, although safer and less habit forming than barbiturates, nevertheless have abuse potential. Abusers seek the drowsy, unconcerned feeling or the disinhibition euphoria associated with these drugs. When prescribed appropriately, neither of these effects is particularly prominent. Clients who experiment with drugs or have histories of chemical abuse, however, may find higher dosages are a quick way to leave anxiety and the concerns of life far behind. This misuse creates two problems: (1) the client fails to learn to handle anxiety; and (2) the client develops new difficulties, abuse, and dependence. Physiological dependence may develop in 3 months for benzodiazepine derivatives used regularly in therapeutic dosages. It can occur much more quickly when clients overmedicate themselves.

Obviously benzodiazepine derivatives should not be used carelessly or without regard for their abuse potential. They should be reserved for clients who require immediate anxiety relief and who have no history of chemical dependency. It also should be noted that although benzodiazepine derivatives have not been implicated in successful suicides when used alone, they can contribute to a lethal suicide plan when added to other CNS depressants such as alcohol, barbiturates, or narcotics. Clients should be warned to avoid alcoholic beverages and to consult with their physician or nurse practitioner before combining benzodiazepine derivatives with pain medications or cold preparations.

Side effects

The most common side effects of benzodiazepine derivatives are drowsiness, fatigue, and ataxia. Slowing of reflexes and cognitive abilities occurs as well. With long-term use, depression and confusion may be experienced, especially by elderly clients. Peripheral nervous system side effects include occasional constipation, double vision, hypotension, and incontinence or urinary retention. Benzodiazepine derivatives may exacerbate narrow-angle glaucoma.

If a client becomes more nervous after having used benzodiazepine derivatives successfully, the nurse should suspect dependence. Tolerance, a need for higher levels of medication, is a primary sign of dependence. If a client does become dependent, the medication must be withdrawn slowly, not "cold turkey." Systematic detoxification is necessary to avoid a withdrawal syndrome. Withdrawal symptoms can include agitation, tremor, irritability, insomnia, sweating, vomiting, and grand mal seizures. As a rule of thumb, the body experiences the opposite of the sought-after effect during withdrawal—instead of calmness and relaxation, agitation and increased CNS irritability occur. This is an important point to ponder because this CNS irritability and agitation can be mistaken for a return of anxiety.

Interactions

Benzodiazepine derivatives are much safer than all previous antianxiety medications, but they are still CNS depressants. As such, they can produce dangerous CNS depression when mixed with other CNS depressants such as narcotics, antipsychotics, MAOIs, and even over the counter antihistamines. Clients should be warned not to drink alcoholic beverages, take pain medication, or use cold preparations without consulting their care providers.

Alternatives to benzodiazepine derivatives

Nonbenzodiazepines. A nonbenzodiazepine anxiolytic from the chemical group of azapirones that is gaining acceptance is buspirone (BuSpar). Buspirone does not influence the GABA system, but instead acts as a serotonin agonist. Buspirone is considered the first purely antianxiety agent to be developed. Much of the interest in this drug is caused by its lack of sedative properties and absence of CNS depression. Buspirone does not potentiate the effects of other CNS depressants nor does it produce dependence, tolerance, or withdrawal. Buspirone appears to have a particular potential for the client with a history of substance abuse problems.

Buspirone effectively provides relief from anxiety after 7 to 10 days of treatment. It reaches its maximal therapeutic potential after about 3 to 4 weeks. Dosing is usually two to three times daily. Brief treatment with other anxiolytics may be necessary for the first week and a half until buspirone begins to take effect. Buspirone has been used adjunctively with atypical antidepressants.

Buspirone is a very safe drug. No deaths from overdose have been reported. However, adverse effects have been reported when coadministered with haloperidol, monoamine oxidase inhibitors, and cimetidine.

Beta-blockers. The beta-blocker propranolol (Inderal), though less effective than the benzodiazepine derivatives, has been used to interrupt the physiological effects of anxiety (including sweating, dry mouth, and tachycardia), particularly for episodic anxiety such as stage fright. It does not produce dependence. Side effects are usually brief and mild; however, light-headedness, bradycardia, and heart block can occur.

Tricyclic antidepressants. Clomipramine (Anafranil) is a tricyclic antidepressant used to treat obsessive-compulsive disorder. It has proven effective at doses of 100 mg to 150 mg per day. Major problems associated with long-term use are dental problems related to dry mouth. The nurse should warn clients about this effect and encourage them to engage in frequent oral hygiene.

Imipramine (Tofranil), at a dose of 150 mg per day or higher, has proven effective in the treatment of panic attacks. Other tricyclics used in the treatment of anxiety disorder include desipramine (Norpramin) and amitriptyline (Elavil). Trazodone (Desyrel) has been used to treat the anxiety associated with cocaine withdrawal. Sedation is its significant side effect and therefore it is often used for clients with anxiety, particularly elderly clients, to facilitate sleep. Priapism is a significant issue associated with trazodone and should be monitored.

Drugs for the treatment of dementia: tacrine

The only approved drug for the treatment of Alzheimer's disease at this time is tacrine (Cognex). Several other agents are currently under investigation and some will probably receive approval for marketing in the near future. To date, research seems to indicate that tacrine and placebo are equally effective.

Indications

Tacrine is indicated for the treatment of mild to moderate dementia related to Alzheimer's disease (Box 13-5).

How tacrine works

Tacrine is a cholinesterase inhibitor. As can be noted in Table 13-1, Alzheimer's disease is related to a decrease in the availability of acetylcholine in the brain. Cholinesterase is the enzyme that metabolizes acetylcholine; a drug that could inhibit that metabolism has the potential to increase brain acetylcholine levels (Keltner, 1994). In principle this is exactly how tacrine works.

Time to clinical effect

If improvement in cognitive function is to occur with tacrine, it will usually do so within 6 weeks (Deglin & Vallerand, 1995).

Box 13-5. Tacrine: dosage, pharmacokinetics, and contraindications

Dosage: 10 mg four times a day (40 mg per day) for 6 weeks, then increase to 20 mg four times a day (80 mg per day) if alanine amino-transferase (ALT) levels have not increased significantly. Maximum dosage is 40 mg four times a day (160 mg per day).

Half-life: 2 to 4 hours.

Metabolism: Tacrine is metabolized in the liver.

Absorption: Rapidly absorbed, but with limited bioavailability.

Contraindications: Hypersensitivity to cholinomimetics; active liver disease; untreated gastric or duodenal ulcers, and mechanical obstructions of the intestine or urinary tract.

Efficacy

The efficacy of tacrine is debatable. Early reports were glowing. Summers et al. (1986) published the first article about tacrine to draw much attention. They found tacrine very beneficial. One client returned to her part-time job, one played golf again, and a third resumed her role as a homemaker (Small, 1992). However, since those earlier reports, a number of less optimistic reports also have been published. The opinion among many clinicians today is that tacrine may help a few clients with Alzheimer's disease (perhaps 10% to 20%) to slow down the disease process for a while. For most victims of Alzheimer's disease, however, tacrine seems to offer little if any respite.

Side effects

The most common side effect (30%) associated with tacrine is an elevation in serum transaminase levels most particularly in alanine aminotransferase (ALT). Liver toxicity occurs at this same frequency. ALT levels should be monitored weekly for the first 18 weeks of treatment, then at 3-month intervals unless a change in dosage or elevated ALTs occur. If a change in dosage occurs, weekly monitoring should be resumed for at least 3 weeks (Parke-Davis, 1993). ALT levels greater than three times the upper limit of normal require a downward dosage adjustment. ALT levels five times the upper limit of normal necessitate discontinuation of the drug (Deglin & Vallerand, 1995).

A second major group of side effects stems from tacrine's cholinomimetic properties. Cholinergic side effects include vasodilation, which can result in flushing, hypotension, and a rise in skin temperature; diaphoresis; cardiovascular vagotonic effect (bradycardia); increased gastric acid secretion, which can lead to gastrointestinal bleeding; increased salivation; bronchial constriction; intestinal cramping and diarrhea; increased micturition; increased tearing; and miosis (Parke-Davis, 1993). Many of these side effects can effectively be reversed with an anticholinergic drug such as atropine.

Other adverse effects include nausea and vomiting (20%), gastrointestinal bleeding, anorexia, dizziness, and headache.

Interactions

Major interactions with tacrine are relatively few. Theophylline blood levels increase when given with tacrine; thus it is recommended that theophylline dosage be reduced by 50% in this combination (Parke-Davis, 1993). Tacrine serum levels increase by 40% when coadministration with cimetidine occurs. Tacrine potentiates succinylcholine-cased paralysis. Tacrine, related to its propensity to increase gastric secretions, should be cautiously coadministered with nonsteroidal antiinflammatory drugs (NSAIDs) because of a potential for ulcers and gastrointestinal bleeding. Finally, tacrine can have an additive effect if given concomitantly with other cholinergics.

If tacrine is given with food, absorption is decreased causing a 30% to 40% reduction in plasma levels.

How long should tacrine be given to a client?

Presumably, once initiated, tacrine will be given to a client as long as an observable decline or stabilization in cognitive deterioration is noted. Of course, ALT levels violating the parameters noted previously or a lack of therapeutic benefit would require discontinuance of the drug.

Organs systems vulnerable to tacrine

The hepatic system is most at risk with tacrine use. The protocols of ALT monitoring previously mentioned will assist the clinician in preventing liver failure.

PSYCHOPHARMACOLOGICAL ISSUES IN COMMUNITY MENTAL HEALTH

The community health nurse works with the client, the client's family, and others significant to the client's life situation. The nurse is sensitive to include all appropriate parties in decision making and goal setting. Many issues confront the community mental health nurse in the quest to help the client and family attain optimal mental health. Frequently encountered issues of particular importance include compliance, teaching, use during pregnancy, and prescriptive authority. A summary of those issues follows.

Compliance to the drug regimen

Noncompliance to medication regimens is a serious problem for many psychiatric clients that causes great concern for clinicians and families (Forman, 1993). The term noncompliance in the context of community mental health describes the act of not adhering to the prescribed course of drug treatment. Technically this definition can be stretched to include any straying away from the "five rights" of medication administration for any of several reasons. More often, however, noncompliance refers to an intentional refusal to take medications as prescribed. The consequences of noncompliance can include reemergence of symptoms, regression, socially incorrect behavior, and violent and aggressive outbursts. Causes of noncompliance include lack of accessibility, lack of finances, or illness-related issues.

Accessibility issues

Some clients lack the wherewithal to secure medications. Whether because of relative geographical isolation (with a concomitant unavailability of transportation), objective geographical isolation (such as living in a rural area), physical disability, or lack of an adequate support network, clients can be noncompliant related to inability to obtain psychotropic agents. Problem solving with the client and family is the first step to resolving this problem.

Financial issues

Prescribed medications can be a financial burden, particularly for people living on fixed incomes. Some clients do not obtain medications because of cost. Even in situations in which the client or family contributes a relatively small "co-payment," it is prudent for the nurse to consider the impact of that contribution on finances. The timeworn adage, "When we say 'yes' to one thing, we are saying 'no' to something else," can be applied to the person with limited resources. A recommended problem-solving approach includes exploring what things the client will have to say "no" to (whether frivolous or essential) in order to pay for medications.

Illness-related issues

Many clients are noncompliant because of their illness. Kelly and Scott (1990) indicate that as many as 46% of inpatients and 35% to 65% of outpatients are noncompliant. Nurses have been socialized to believe that noncompliance is related to knowledge deficits that can be remedied through education. Lund and Frank (1991) refute this reasoning and find clients offer many reasons for not taking medications:

1. Medications are not needed
2. Clinicians are conspiring against them
3. Side effects are too severe
4. Medications are "making them worse"
5. Medications are ineffective

All except the second reason are correct at times. For example, 30% of clients with bipolar disorder either fail to respond to lithium or cannot tolerate its side effects (Harrow et al., 1990), 10% to 20% of clients with schizophrenia are never helped by traditional antipsychotics, and another 20% to 30% relapse within 2 years of treatment.

Noncompliant behaviors can be countered somewhat successfully by rapport building and by more effective teaching. Two other available routes of administration can reduce noncompliant behaviors. Liquid medications can prevent the "cheeking" of medications; injection of long-acting depot medications is effective for other noncompliant behaviors.

Teaching issues

Today people are encouraged to be responsible for their own health care. Responsibility begins with information. For many psychiatric clients this information will be provided in the context of the nurse-client relationship.

Psychiatric clients seem particularly ill informed about their medications. Macpherson et al. (1993) found that 92% of the psychiatric clients they studied demonstrated no understanding of their drug therapy. Yet when understanding occurs, side effects decrease (Brown, Wright, & Christen, 1990).

Clarity

The clarity of information is crucial. Clients come with different levels of education (from illiterate to PhD), with different abilities to listen, and at different points in the recovery process. Additionally, communication can be impeded by perceptual barriers (for example, past experiences coloring current situations), semantic barriers (for example, the nurse slipping into jargon), and transmission barriers when information is communicated serially (for example, when nurses attempt to teach something they do not clearly understand) (Pringle, Jennings, & Longnecker, 1988). Because teaching psychopharmacology is difficult, the nurse should be selective when deciding on the content to be taught.

Brevity

Teaching efforts should be brief. Listening is hard work. Internal thought processes associated with some mental disorders make the listening process even more difficult. The sessions should be brief, to the point, and relevant to the client. It is important to avoid overloading clients with more information than they can handle.

Balance

Keltner (1985) described balance as a key component of the psychotherapeutic management model. In teaching about medication, balance simply means weighing the client's need to know against information overload. Information overload can lead to decreased learning and perhaps more importantly can result in unwarranted apprehension. The latter point is of particular significance in highly suggestible clients. The nurse should teach "patients about what effects are visible, what can be felt, and what the possibilities are of becoming drug-dependent" (Keltner, Schwecke, & Bostrom, 1995).

Use during pregnancy

Psychotropic drug use during pregnancy or while breastfeeding should be carefully monitored. The Food and Drug Administration (FDA) has established the following pregnancy categories for medications:

A: No risk to fetus based on human studies

B: No evidence of risk to fetus based on animal and human studies; not as conclusive as "A"

C: Potential risk

D: Evidence of fetal harm; may be used if benefit outweighs risk

X: Contraindicated during pregnancy

Antipsychotics

Antipsychotics pose few risks for the fetus; however, during the first trimester these drugs should be avoided if possible. Most antipsychotic drugs fall under FDA pregnancy category C.

Antidepressants

Tricyclic antidepressants are typically placed in FDA category B or C. During pregnancy agents with lower anticholinergic properties should be used. Tricyclic use should be tapered off before delivery to avoid transient perinatal toxicity (Cohen, 1989).

Monoamine oxidase inhibitors are placed in category C. They should be given during pregnancy only when anticipated results justify the potential risk.

Selective serotonin reuptake inhibitors are pregnancy category B drugs.

Antimanic agents

Lithium is known to cause birth defects. If the mother's condition necessitates treatment in the first trimester, carbamazepine (FDA category C) may be a beneficial substitute. If lithium is prescribed in the second and third semesters the dosage should be reduced by 50% (Cohen, 1989). Lithium is a category D drug, as is valproic acid.

Antianxiety agents

Benzodiazepine derivatives have the potential to cause birth defects if prescribed during the first trimester (Shlafer, 1993). Benzodiazepine derivatives also are excreted in breast milk and may cause sedation, lethargy, poor feeding habits, weight loss, and altered liver function in the infant (Shlafer, 1993). Most benzodiazepine derivatives are category C or D drugs, and clients should be made aware of their possible risks. A few fall under category X indicating their unequivocal contraindication during pregnancy.

Tacrine

Tacrine is used exclusively among women beyond the childbearing age.

Prescriptive authority

Most states now grant prescriptive authority to nurse practitioners. States vary on what educational preparation is required for psychiatric nurses to prescribe. In some states psychiatric nurses with advanced education are given prescriptive authority without having a formal nurse practitioner background; in others a nurse practitioner certificate is needed. Within the large domain of prescriptive privilege, actual ability to prescribe varies greatly from state to state. Only a few states have legal provision for "substitutive" privilege, which allows the nurse to prescribe independent of a physician. Practitioners in most states still have a defined relationship to a physician or what is termed "complementary" privilege. As larger numbers of community mental health nurses gain prescriptive authority, clients will have greater access to psychotropic agents and will be more carefully monitored for side effects and efficacy.

SUMMARY

The development of psychotropic drugs was a key factor in the community mental health movement. Public and professional confidence in these agents bolstered the morale of people willing to fight for a change in treatment site from hospital to the community. Because psychotropic drugs are such a major component of community mental health care, nurses play a crucial role in assessment, prescription, monitoring, and evaluation.

REFERENCES

Arana, G. W., & Hyman, S. E. (1991). *Handbook of psychiatric drug therapy.* Boston: Little, Brown, and Company.

Baer, C. L., & Williams, B. R. (1992). *Clinical pharmacology and nursing* (2nd ed.) Springhouse, PA: Springhouse Corporation.

Brown, C. S., Wright, R. G., & Christen, D. B. (1990). Risk management for extrapyramidal symptoms. *Quality Assurance Review Bulletin, 17,* 116-122.

Calabrese, J. R., Woyshville, M. J., Kimmel, S. E., & Rapport, D. J. (1993). Brief report: Predictors of valproate response in bipolar rapid cycling. *Journal of Clinical Psychopharmacology, 13*(4), 280-283.

Cohen, L. S. (1989). Psychotropic drug use in pregnancy. *Hospital and Community Psychiatry, 40,* 566-568.

Coryell, W. R., Noyes, R., & Clancy, J. (1982). Excess mortality in panic disorder: A comparison with primary unipolar depression. *Archives of General Psychiatry, 39,* 701-703.

Cunningham, L. A., Borison, R. L., Carman, J. S., Crowder, J. E., Diamond, B. I., et al. (1994). A comparison of venlafaxine, trazodone, and placebo in major depression. *Journal of Clinical Psychopharmacology, 14(2),* 99-106.

Deglin J. H., & Vallerand, A. H. (1995). *Davis's drug guide for nurses.* Philadelphia: F. A. Davis.

Depression Guideline Panel. (1993). *Depression in primary care: Volume 2. Treatment of major depression, clinical practice guidelines* (AHCPR Publication No. 93-0551). Rockville, MD: U.S. Department of Health and Human Services.

Dubin, W. R., & Weiss, K. J. (1991). *Handbook of psychiatric emergencies.* Springhouse, PA: Springhouse Corporation.

Forman, L. (1993). Medication: Reasons and interventions for noncompliance. *Journal of Psychosocial Nursing and Mental Health Services, 31*(10), 23-25.

Goldberg R. J. (1995). Nefazodone: a novel antidepressant. *Psychiatric Services, 46*(11), 1113-1114.

Groleau, G. (1994). Lithium toxicity. *Emergency Medicine Clinics of North America, 12*(2), 511-531.

Harsch H. H., & Holt R. E. (1988). Use of antidepressants in attempted suicide. *Hospital and Community Psychiatry, 39,* 990-993.

Harrow, M., Goldberg, J., Grossman, L., & Meltzer, H. (1990). Outcome in manic disorders: A naturalistic follow-up study. *Archives of General Psychiatry, 47,* 665-671.

Kane, J. (1993). Newer antipsychotic drugs: A review of their pharmacology and therapeutic potential. *Drugs, 46,* 585-593.

Kelly, G. R., & Scott, J. E. (1990). Medication compliance and health education among outpatients with chronic mental disorders. *Medical Care, 28,* 1181-1185.

Keltner, N. L. (1985). Psychotherapeutic management: A model for nursing practice. *Perspectives in Psychiatric Care, 23*(4), 125-130.

Keltner, N. L. (1994). Tacrine: A pharmacological approach to Alzheimer's disease. *Journal of Psychosocial Nursing and Mental Health Services, 32*(3), 37-39.

Keltner, N. L. (1995a). Risperidone. The search for a better antipsychotic. *Perspectives in Psychiatric Care, 31*(1), 30-33.

Keltner, N. L. (1995b). Venlafaxine: A novel antidepressant. *Journal of Psychosocial Nursing and Mental Health Services, 33*(1), 51-53.

Keltner, N. L., & Folks, D. (1991). Clozapine: Miracle or mirage? *Perspectives in Psychiatric Care, 27*(1), 35-36.

Keltner, N. L., & Folks, D. (1993). *Psychotropic drugs.* St. Louis: Mosby.

Keltner, N. L., & Harris, C. P. (1994). Serotonin syndrome: A case of fatal SSRI/MAOI interaction. *Perspectives in Psychiatric Care, 30*(4), 26-31.

Keltner, N. L., & McIntyre, C. (1985). Neuroleptic malignant syndrome. *Journal of Neurosurgical Nursing, 17,* 363-366.

Keltner, N. L., Schwecke, L., & Bostrom, C. (1995). *Psychiatric nursing* (2nd ed.). St. Louis: Mosby.

Kessler, R. C., McGonagle, K. A., Shanyang, Z., Nelson, C. B., Hughes, M., Eshleman, S., Wittchen, H. U., & Kendler, K. S. (1994). Lifetime and 12-month prevalence of *DSM-IIIR* psychiatric disorders in the United States. *Archives of General Psychiatry, 51*(1), 8-19.

Laraia, M. T, Beeber, L. S., Callwood, G. B., Caverly S., Clement, J. A., Gary, F., Keltner, N. L., Nihart, M. A., Scahill, L., Simmons-Alling, S., Stanley, S. R., & Tally, S. (1994). *Psychiatric mental health nursing psychopharmacology project.* Washington, DC: American Nurses Association.

Lehne, R. A., Moore, L. A., Crosby, L. J., & Hamilton, D. B. (1994). *Pharmacology for nursing care* (2nd ed.). Philadelphia: W. B. Saunders.

Lund, V. E., & Frank, D. I. (1991). Helping the medicine go down. *Journal of Psychosocial Nursing and Mental Health Services, 29*(7), 6-9.

Macpherson, R., et al. (1993). Long-term psychiatric patients' understanding of neuroleptic medication. *Hospital and Community Psychiatry, 44*(1), 71-73.

Marder, S., & Meibach, R. (1994). Risperidone in the treatment of schizophrenia. *American Journal of Psychiatry, 151,* 825-835.

Matsubara, S., Matsubara, R., Kusumi, I., Kogama, T., & Yamashita, I. (1993). Dopamine D-1, D-2 and serotonin-2 receptor occupation by typical and atypical antipsychotic drugs in vivo. *Journal of Pharmacology and Experimental Therapeutics, 2* (65), 498-508.

Matthysse, S. (1977). The role of dopamine in schizophrenia. In E. Usdin, D. Hamburg, & J. Barchas (Eds.), *Neuroregulators and psychiatric disorders* (pp. 3-13). New York: Oxford University Press.

Meltzer, H. (1993). New drugs for the treatment of schizophrenia. *Psychiatric Clinics of North America, 16,* 365-385.

Morton, W. A., Sonne, S. C., & Lydiard, R. B. (1993). Lithium side effects in the medically ill. *International Journal of Psychiatry, 23(4),* 357-382.

Narrows, W. E., Regier, D. A., Rae, D. S., Manderschied R. W., & Locke, B. Z. (1993). Use of services by persons with mental and addictive disorders: Findings from the NIMH epidemiologic catchment area program. *Archives of General Psychiatry, 50,* 95-107.

Parke-Davis Company. (1993). Cognex treatment IND investigator's brochure. Morris Plains, NJ: Author.

Pringle, C. D., Jennings, D. F., & Longnecker, J. G. (1988). *Managing organizations: Functions and behaviors.* Columbus, OH: Merrill Publishing Company.

Puzantian, T., & Stimmel, G. L. (1995, January). Review of psychotropic drugs. *Retail Pharmacy News,* 11, 13.

Regier, D. A., Narrow, W. E., Rae, D. S., Manderschied, R. W., Locke, B. Z., & Goodwin, F. K. (1993). The de facto U.S. mental and addictive disorders service system: Epidemiologic catchment area prospective 1-year prevalance rates of disorders and services. *Archives of General Psychiatry, 50,* 85-94.

Remington, G. (1993). Clinical considerations in the use of risperidone. *Canadian Journal of Psychiatry, 38*(Supp. 3), S96-S100.

Roundsville, B. J., Klerman, G. L., & Weisman, M. N. (1986). Do psychotherapy and psychopharmacology for depression conflict? *Archives of General Psychiatry, 38,* 24.

Shlafer, M. (1993). *The nurse, pharmacology, and drug therapy: A prototype approach.* Redwood City, CA: Addison-Wesley Publishing.

Small, G. W. (1992). Tacrine for treating Alzheimer's disease. *Journal of the American Medication Association, 268*(18): 2564-2565.

Sternbach, H. (1991) The serotonin syndrome. *American Journal of Psychiatry, 147,* 705-712.

Summers, W. K., Majovski, L. V., Marsh, G. M., Tachiki, K., & Kling, A. (1986). Oral tetrahydroaminoacridine in long-term treatment of senile dementia. *New England Journal of Medicine, 315*(20),1241-1245.

Varcarolis, E. M. (1994). *Foundations of psychiatric nursing* (2nd ed.). Philadelphia: W. B. Saunders.

Yaryura-Tobias, Y., Diamond, B., & Merlis, S. (1970). The actions of L-dopa on schizophrenic patients (a preliminary report). *Current Therapeutic Research, 12,* 528-531.

Unit 5

Community Settings

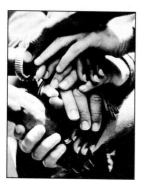

Chapter 14

Home Care

Karen Hellwig

DEVELOPMENT AND GROWTH OF HOME CARE

Community-based mental health nursing services date back to the early 1900s (Osborne & Thomas, 1991). Many factors contributed to the growth of the home health care industry and the development of psychiatric home care nursing as an area of specialization. Public Law 89:97, an amendment to the Social Security Act of 1965, mandated Medicare reimbursement for home care services for a large percentage of the population. Medicare is the most commonly held health insurance in the United States today (Delong, 1994). Medicare is funded by Social Security taxes and is available primarily to people who contributed to Social Security while employed. Medicare beneficiaries must be over 65 years old, younger than 65 but disabled for 2 years, or diagnosed with permanent kidney failure and receiving dialysis.

The advent of diagnosis-related groups (DRGs) in 1983 resulted in a major shift in Medicare payment for acute health care providers. Before 1983 hospitals received retrospective payment for services. After 1983 prospective payment was instituted. Instead of paying hospitals based on bills submitted after the patient's discharge, Medicare now pays hospitals a fixed amount based on the patient's diagnosis. Hospitals are thus rewarded for treating and discharging patients as quickly as possible. They are penalized if patients remain hospitalized too long or are readmitted within a short period of time for the same DRG diagnosis. Private insurance companies follow a similar payment system. This major realignment in payment contributed to the growth of the home care industry. Between 1980 and 1985 the number of Medicare-certified home health agencies more than doubled from 2924 to 5983. As of May, 1994, 7521 Medicare-certified home health agencies were in operation (National Association for Home Care, 1994).

Hospitals soon recognized that client management in the home helped prevent readmission. Patients, who usually prefer to be at home, could be discharged sooner with the expectation that home care personnel and the physician would provide follow-up to keep the client stable. The hospital discharge planner became more actively involved with home care liaison nurses in the role of providing continuity of care for the client at home.

Another factor contributing to the growth of home health care was a 1987 lawsuit brought against the Health Care Financing Administration (HCFA), which distributes Medicare funding. The suit, brought by a coalition of U.S. Congress members, consumer groups, and the National Association for Home Care, challenged the HCFA's increasing paperwork and unreliable payment policies. The suit resulted in the National Association for Home Care's participation in rewriting Medicare home health payment policies. It also resulted in a proliferation of home care agencies (National Association for Home Care, 1994).

Finally, growth in the home health care industry was boosted by financial trends and technological advances. Hospital downsizing has exacerbated the trend of discharging patients as soon as they are stabilized. Hospitals are increasingly becoming trauma and intensive care centers. Health care personnel who are finding their jobs eliminated are looking to the home care field where jobs are more plentiful. The increasing abundance of managed care plans with their emphasis on cost containment has forced health care to be more outpatient and community focused. A projected comparison of 1994 charges for hospital, skilled nursing facility, and home health care indicated home health charges of $83 per visit were indeed a bargain compared with hospital charges of $1756 per day and skilled nursing facility charges of $284 per day (National Association for Home Care, 1994). Technological advances have simplified many types of medical equipment to the point that clients and caregivers can manage them in the home. For instance, blood sugar monitors and feeding pumps can be easily operated by lay people after instruction from health care personnel.

EMERGENCE OF PSYCHIATRIC HOME CARE

The growing field of home health care has recently expanded to include psychiatric home care, which was formally acknowledged as a reimbursable service by HCFA in 1979 (Pelletier, 1988). Although psychiatric facilities are exempt from DRG payment, the trend in psychiatric inpatient treatment has been to decrease length of stay. It is estimated that 70% (1.2 million to 2 million) of all seriously mentally ill people live in the community (Esser & Lacey, 1989); psychiatric home care is emerging as a viable, cost-effective alternative to hospitalization for this population.

Eligibility for psychiatric home care

Medicare and Medicaid will reimburse for psychiatric home care visits if clients meet the necessary criteria. The client must be homebound, the care must be a "medical necessity," and the client must require intermittent (not continuous) skilled nursing care. Homebound status includes medical conditions that impair mobility and psychiatric disabilities such as agoraphobia, paranoia, or generalized anxiety about new situations. Private insurance companies generally do not require homebound status for payment. Common *Diagnostic and Statistical Manual of Mental Disorders* (*DSM-IV*) Axis I diagnoses that Medicare and Medicaid will reimburse include psychosis, schizophrenia, major depression, and bipolar disorder (American Psychiatric Association, 1994). Personality disorders are not reimbursable as primary diagnoses but their coexistence with Axis I diagnoses is frequent and therefore indirectly reimbursable.

Clients are generally certified for home care for 2-month periods. They can be discharged during or at the end of the certification period or recertified if they continue to need skilled nursing care (that is, if they have not stabilized, continue to have knowledge deficits, or are on injectable psychotropic medications such as fluphenazine decanoate or haloperidol decanoate). Medicare does not require preauthorization for home care; however, Medicaid and most private insurance companies do require preauthorization and will grant a specific number of home visits for each discipline. Clients are usually visited one to three times a week during the certification period.

ROLE OF THE PSYCHIATRIC HOME CARE NURSE

Assisting adaptation to the community

Psychiatric home care nurses play a pivotal role in helping clients adapt to the community setting whether it be their own home, the home of a relative or friend, a board and care facility, or a retirement home. Clients with major mental illnesses are particularly vulnerable to alterations in routine, and nurses must be sensitive to behavioral changes that indicate the client is decompensating physically or psychiatrically. Nurses can arrange for more intense community treatment or rehospitalization. Such foresight may result in a shorter acute hospitalization, and nurses can then resume their support in assisting the client's readjustment to community living.

Collaboration with the home health care team

Autonomy balanced with collaboration is the hallmark of psychiatric home care nursing. The psychiatric home care team consists primarily of the client's physician and psychiatric nurse, but the team also may include occupational, physical, or speech therapists, home health aides, and social workers, depending on the client's treatment needs. The team collaborates to design, implement, and monitor the treatment plan. According to Medicare regulations, clients with a primary psychiatric diagnosis must have a psychiatrist's signature on the treatment plan and a psychiatric nurse must manage the client's nursing care. Psychiatric nursing assessments can be ordered by nonpsychiatric physicians. However, if a physician other than a psychiatrist signs the treatment plan the primary diagnosis must be medical rather than psychiatric to qualify for Medicare reimbursement. In that case the psychiatric nurse manages the

client's care or may share management duties with a medical home care nurse. Physicians rely on the nurse's expertise in assessing and intervening with both psychiatric and medical problems. This requires that nurses be knowledgeable and confident in their skills. The nurse implements the nursing process autonomously in the home. At the same time the nurse must collaborate with the physician, who is required by home care regulations to authorize nursing and other home care personnel visits and provide the focus of care. Changes in treatment plan, medications, or frequency of visits require supplemental orders signed by a physician.

The following case example illustrates the importance of collaboration between the psychiatric home care nurse and the physician.

Case example

A woman who was diagnosed with bipolar disorder expressed to her home care nurse feelings of hopelessness regarding her future. On further assessment, she admitted to suicidal ideation that was becoming increasingly pervasive. She had not mentioned these feelings to her psychiatrist. After assessing the degree of suicidal ideation the nurse coordinated a treatment plan with the psychiatrist that included increased nursing visits, implementation of a no-suicide contract with the client, and development of a plan for her future. Ultimately the plan was successful in reducing the client's depressive and suicidal symptoms (Hellwig, 1993).

Another example of successful collaboration between a psychiatric home care nurse and a physician involved initiating clozapine (Clozaril) treatment for a client with schizoaffective disorder. The nurse coordinated laboratory follow-up of blood work for agranulocytosis and the pharmacy filling of weekly clozapine orders. She handled client assessment and education regarding response to and side effects of clozapine as the client was weaned off previous psychotropic medications. The psychiatric nurse and the psychiatrist conferred weekly on the medication management of this client.

The psychiatric home care nurse and psychiatrist have much to teach and learn from each other concerning the scope of practice, medication actions and responses, and behavioral management. The nurse can greatly benefit from physician input regarding the biochemical aspects of mental illness and medication actions, interactions, and side effects. Medication orders and changes can be facilitated by nurses who share with physicians their observations of client behaviors and responses to medications. Nurses can educate physicians regarding the client's living situation and nursing approaches to management of behavioral problems.

The psychiatric home care nurse is in a unique position to act as liaison between the client and the many physicians who provide medical and psychiatric care. The nurse needs to discuss the client's medications, treatment, and interventions with the client's physicians not only to apprise them of the "total picture" but also to interpret medical treatment plans to the client.

Acquiring skills and knowledge

Psychiatric home care nurses must demonstrate sensitivity and versatility in assessing and intervening with psychiatric behaviors and problems. They must be alert to nuances in client behaviors and adapt the treatment plan to meet the client's needs. Nurses who provide psychiatric home care must have an intensive and extensive psychiatric knowledge base that includes psychopathology, psychopharmacology, neurobiology, neurochemistry, and the ways in which medical and physical problems can be influenced by and can influence psychiatric impairments. In addition, they must be knowledgeable about management of medical problems. This knowledge comes from literature, conferences, and experience. However, it is the clients themselves along with their caregivers who are the best teachers regarding mental illness, effects of medications, and behavioral management in the home.

PSYCHIATRIC INTERVENTIONS IN THE HOME

Assessing factors in the home

Many nursing interventions in the home care setting are the same as in the acute or outpatient setting. However, in this case the nurse is a guest in the client's home and as such is operating on the client's "turf." The client has the right to refuse treatment and refuse the nurse admittance into the home. By receiving nursing care in the home the client experiences a sense of comfort and control often lacking in the acute or outpatient environment, and the nurse has a unique opportunity to assess factors in the home that may impinge on the client's ability to cope. The nurse can assess the influence of family, friends, the physical environment, and the client's financial resources.

Developing trust

Nurses who provide psychiatric home care must adapt to a variety of situations and use many different social skills. They must display genuine caring for their clients, even those who present with undesirable or bizarre behaviors. They must develop trust with clients, their families and friends, and sometimes even their pets. They must maintain a tolerant and nondefensive posture and attitude to allay the fears of paranoid and hostile clients. Sometimes psychiatric home care nurses need to be persuasive and convincing just to be allowed into the home. A socioeconomic chasm may exist between the nurse and the client, the client's caregivers, or family members. It is not uncommon to enter a home that is infested with vermin, cluttered, or dirty, or a home whose moral, religious, or cultural values are antithetical to those of the nurse. It is imperative that the nurse demonstrate an unbiased attitude and be cognizant of the clients' surroundings from their point of view. The nurse must determine if client behaviors are normal expressions of cultural, religious, or moral values or manifestations of psychopathology.

Clients and caregivers often enjoy being hospitable to the home care nurse. They may offer refreshments or even gifts. How the nurse accepts or rejects these offers can nurture or impair the therapeutic relationship. Learning what is appropriate social etiquette in each situation is a skill all nurses must develop. They must be aware of their own comfort levels and biases as well as the meaning of the offer and its acceptance or rejection to the client.

Safety issues

Safety in the home is a key issue in home care and must be addressed according to Medicare and Medicaid regulations. The nurse should examine the client's living environment for possible hazards such as frayed electrical cords, slippery floor surfaces, use of stove burners for heating the home, or unsafe use of or lack of knowledge about equipment such as oxygen tanks or walkers. The nurse also determines the client's mental status and ability to safely manage medications, treatments, and activities of daily living. The home safety assessment and the client's mental status must be written on the HCFA Form 485 (see item numbers 15 and 19 on Figure 14-1). Instructing the client and caregiver regarding home safety is an important part of the nurse's role. The nurse's ability to view the client within a social and physical context contributes to the development of a workable, realistic treatment plan.

In addition to client safety issues, home health care nurses must seriously consider their own safety. Nurses who travel in the community need to employ common safety sense. Being aware of the environment and activities on the street and taking precautions such as locking doors and not leaving the car if the area looks dangerous will decrease the likelihood of threats or injury. Nurses should call ahead to the client as a courtesy and to alert the client to the impending visit.

Once in the home the nurse must be sensitive to client behaviors that might pose a risk to nurse or client safety. Clients who are managed in the home are generally stabilized on psychotropic medications and thus less likely to be threatening than acutely ill clients. However, medication non-compliance, lack of medication efficacy, or worsening psychopathology can predispose the client to psychiatric relapse in the home. Clients may become increasingly paranoid, agitated, and hostile and may even threaten the nurse. It is critical that the nurse project an air of calm, fearless, nonthreatening support. By using quiet, simple words and by not invading the client's private space, nurses can deescalate the client's threatening behaviors. Nurses have a duty to protect themselves and the client. Calling for emergency assistance, notifying the client's physician, and assisting with rehospitalization may all be necessary nursing actions.

Clarifying relationship parameters

The nurse must clarify the parameters of the nurse-client relationship by educating the client and caregiver regarding the nurse's role, the reasons for the visits, and the expected length of time the client will be receiving home care services. This presentation of expectations helps create a therapeutic nurse-client alliance and models straightforward communication, an area that psychiatric clients often have difficulty developing.

Boundary issues must be recognized and addressed in the home care setting. Psychotherapeutic issues such as transference and countertransference can arise between nurse and client. Countertransference can result in a therapeutic impasse by neutralizing the nurse's ability to identify and intervene with the client's relationship issues. Psychiatric home care nurses should have a forum (with a supervisor or psychiatric team) for discussion and clarification of these issues. They may use this forum to obtain input regarding management of complex and manipulative behaviors, validate therapeutic nursing interventions, and express personal feelings. Because the therapeutic alliance is so crucial to the success of home care, psychiatric home care nurses usually manage their own caseloads of clients. The intense involvement between nurse and client may continue for years if the client is receiving injectable psychotropic medications. Nurses must use their "therapeutic selves" while maintaining a professional relationship. Objective input from supervisors and peers can help prevent boundary diffusion, burnout, and codependency. Management of clients with dual diagnoses in particular requires a team approach to treatment.

Using humor

Humor can be an effective communication tool, decreasing tension and lowering barriers to a trusting relationship. It can help clients express emotions and develop insight. For example, during administration of the Mini-Mental State Exam, one bipolar client's response to the question, "What state are we in?" was "The state of happiness!" Both nurse and client enjoyed a tension-relieving laugh after that statement. During another visit the nurse commented on the lovely fruit sitting on the client's kitchen table. The client responded, "My husband gave them to me. He knows I'm such a fruitcake!" Again the nurse's enjoyment of the client's humor encouraged their therapeutic relationship. Moreover, it demonstrated the client's growing insight into her mental illness, which she had been denying. One nurse used humor to encourage expression of emotions and develop a closer bond with a client diagnosed with paranoid schizophrenia. When leaving the client's apartment the nurse would jokingly say, "Now, don't get into trouble." The client would respond with a giggle, "Don't **you** get into trouble—I don't have money to bail you out of jail!" (Hellwig, 1993).

Using touch

The therapeutic nurse-client alliance can be further encouraged through the judicious use of touch. Mentally ill people are typically outcasts in society and as such are shunned physically and emotionally (Hellwig, 1993):

A hug can be more therapeutic to psychiatric clients who hunger for care than eloquent words of reassurance. Even paranoid clients can learn to trust and appreciate the positive feelings that a caring touch can communicate.

Client and caregiver education

Focusing on the emotional and learning needs of caregivers or significant others is an essential aspect of the psychiatric home care treatment plan. The psychiatric home care nurse needs to mobilize resources around the client to maximize the client's potential to stabilize and cope. The nurse often teaches appropriate techniques and strategies to people who care for the client. For example, nurses should instruct caregivers that going for walks with depressed clients may prevent many of the physical sequelae of immobility such as constipation, anorexia, and pressure ulcers. In addition to teaching, the home care nurse may need to nurture the caregiver. The nurse can encourage the caregiver to talk about concerns, anxiety, and frustrations. Taking the time to listen to caregivers validates their concerns and opens the door to further discussion of how to cope with these feelings so they will be able to continue providing client care.

Client education regarding psychopathology and the relationship of medications to emotional stability is an important element of the psychiatric home care nurse's role. Approximately two thirds of repeat hospitalizations can be traced to medication noncompliance (Esser & Lacey, 1989). Clarification of instructions about medications can help prevent relapse and rehospitalization. Even clients who have been taking the same medications for years may not have received instructions about their medications or may have forgotten them. The nurse must monitor medication compliance at each home visit. Clients need reinforcement of the necessity of compliance because side effects range from annoying to incapacitating and life threatening. Working with clients to manage side effects such as dry mouth and constipation helps maintain compliance. Helping clients and caregivers understand the relationship of medications to psychiatric symptom relief and management can improve compliance and make side effects more tolerable.

Availing the client of community resources that provide activities, intellectual stimulation, socialization, and support also is part of client and caregiver education. The National Alliance for the Mentally Ill (NAMI) and other support groups are excellent resources to assist clients and families with reinforcement of positive behavior and provide a forum for dealing with feelings regarding mental illness. *Surviving Schizophrenia: A Family Manual* (Torrey, 1988) and *Mental Illness: A Homecare Guide* (Esser & Lacey, 1989) are valuable references that provide insight into mental illness and how to manage dysfunctional behaviors.

Managing geropsychiatric problems

Elderly people with psychiatric symptoms are becoming a more common focus for psychiatric home care. Dementia may result in or complicate psychiatric symptoms in elderly people. Medicare will pay for clients and caregivers to be instructed in the care of chronic disabling diseases such as Alzheimer's disease or multiinfarct dementia. However, Medicare will not reimburse for long-term management of such clients unless they have concomitant physical problems such as decubitus ulcers or require Foley catheters. The focus of the psychiatric home care nurse with clients who have both dementia and mental illness is to assist clients and caregivers in managing aggressive and unsafe behaviors and dealing with feelings of anger, loss, and grief that often accompany these conditions.

Developing and implementing the treatment plan

Client or caregiver involvement in the development of the treatment plan is imperative. Joint plan development gives clients control over their care and increases the chances they will achieve the plan's goals. The resulting empowerment can improve self-esteem and increase the likelihood that the client will achieve goals such as medication compliance after home care discharge. The treatment plan focuses on improving the client's ability to manage activities of daily living. It involves assessing behaviors, developing goals, planning and implementing interventions, and evaluating goal achievement. If the client is too disabled (mentally or physically) to work with the nurse in developing the treatment plan the nurse should involve the caregivers.

The psychiatric nursing treatment plan is developed by the nurse in conjunction with the physician. It is documented according to a prescribed formula determined by HCFA. The physician must sign the treatment plan within 20 working days of the start of client care. One such psychiatric treatment plan (Figure 14-1) was developed for the following case example.

Case example

M.J. was an 84-year-old white woman who lived with her dog in a duplex she owned. She became increasingly withdrawn and eventually bedridden because of severe depression. She had a history of coronary artery disease, chronic obstructive pulmonary disease, and hypertension. A case manager referred her to the home care agency for psychiatric evaluation. The psychiatric home care nurse found her in a hospital bed in her dining room. All drapes were drawn. M.J. was constipated, had lost several pounds, was not taking her antihypertensive medication, complained of insomnia, and was suspicious, negative, and "cantankerous."

The nurse's initial approach was to develop a therapeutic bond with M.J. by sitting on her bed, gently eliciting her concerns, and encouraging her to express her feelings. Because M.J.'s concern was her discomfort from constipation the nurse obtained an order for enema, administered it, and began instructing her in a bowel regimen. She also instructed M.J. regarding the importance of taking her antihypertensive medications to manage her elevated blood pressure. She explained the ramifications of uncontrolled hypertension. She obtained an order for a home health aide to assist M.J. in bathing and for a social worker to assist with community resources. The nurse encouraged her to walk by walking with her. She discussed with M.J. how activity relates to the relief of constipation and insomnia, appetite stimulation, and alleviation of depressive symptoms. She also

Home Health Certification and Plan of Treatment

1. Patient's H1 Claim No.	2. SOC Date	3. Certification Period	4. Medical Record No.	5. Provider No.
	121692	From: 121692 To: 021693		

6. Patient's Name and Address

7. Provider's Name and Address.

8. Date of Birth:	9. Sex ☐ M ☒ F

10. Medications: Dose/Frequency/Route (N)ew (C)hanged

Papaverine Hydrochloride 50 mg bid po (N)
Atarax 25 mg bid po (N)
Prozac 20 mg qam po (N)
Corzide i tab bid po (N)

11. ICD-9-CM	Principal Diagnosis	Date
263.9	Protein-Cal Malnutr NOS	121692

12. ICD-9-CM	Surgical Procedure	Date
N/A		

13. ICD-9-CM	Other Pertinent Diagnoses	Date
276.5	Hypovolemia	121692
311	Depressive Disorder Nec	120192
496	Chr Airway Obstruct Nec	010187
401.9	Hypertension NOS (487)	010182

14. DME and Supplies
wheelchair, walker, cane

15. Safety Measures Safe home environment with clear pathways

16. Nutritional Req. Regular diet; Ensure (487)

17. Allergies: No Known Allergies

18.A. Functional Limitations

1 ☐ Amputation
2 ☒ Bowel/Bladder (Incontinence)
3 ☐ Contracture
4 ☐ Hearing
5 ☐ Paralysis
6 ☒ Endurance
7 ☒ Ambulation
8 ☐ Speech
9 ☐ Legally Blind
A ☐ Dyspnea With Minimal Exertion
B ☐ Other (Specify)

18.B. Activities Permitted

1 ☐ Complete Bedrest
2 ☐ Bedrest BRP
3 ☒ Up As Tolerated
4 ☐ Transfer Bed/Chair
5 ☐ Exercises Prescribed
6 ☐ Partial Weight Bearing
7 ☐ Independent At Home
8 ☐ Crutches
9 ☒ Cane
A ☒ Wheelchair
B ☒ Walker
C ☒ No Restrictions
D ☐ Other (Specify)

19. Mental Status:
1 ☒ Oriented
2 ☐ Comatose
3 ☒ Forgetful
4 ☒ Depressed
5 ☐ Disoriented
6 ☐ Lethargic
7 ☐ Agitated
8 ☐ Other

20. Prognosis:
1 ☐ Poor
2 ☐ Guarded
3 ☒ Fair
4 ☐ Good
5 ☐ Excellent

21. Orders for Discipline and Treatments (Specify Amount/Frequency/Duration)

SN 2 x w x 6 Skilled nursing observation/assessment of: vital signs related to dehydration, unstable blood pressure, temperature status, cardiac status, pulmonary status, response to medication regimen, GI/bowel status, nutrition/hydration status, emotional status, coping skills; teach/train patient/caregiver in: administration/side effects of new/changed/complex medication regime, preparation/compliance with increased calorie, Ensure/Ensure Plus 1-3 cans qd prn decreased oral intake diet, bowel program: increase bulk and fluids; instruct in s/s psychiatric crisis & actions. Skilled nursing to perform: provide emotional support, assist in developing coping skills for depression, insomnia

Aide 3 x w x 1
2 x w x 2 personal care and hygiene assistance   (487)

22. Goals/Rehabilitation Potential/Discharge Plans

Rehab potential fair for stated goals
D/c home with caregiver assistance and MD follow-up
Pt/PCGs will demonstrate knowledge of health care teaching
Pt/PCGs will be knowledgeable in: s/s CP, psychiatric crisis & actions   (487)

23. Verbal Start of Care and Nurse's Signature and Date Where Applicable:

24. Physician's Name and Address	25. Date HHA Received Signed POT	26. I ☐ certify ☐ recertify that the above home health services are required and are authorized by me with a written plan for treatment which will be periodically reviewed by me. This patient is under my care, is confined to his home, and is in need of intermittent skilled nursing care and/or physical or speech therapy or has been furnished home health services based on such a need and no longer has a need for such care or therapy, but continues to need occupational therapy.
27. Attending Physician's Signature (Required on 485 Kept on File in Medical Records of HHA)	**Date Signed**	

Form HCFA-485 (U4) (4-87)   PROVIDER

Figure 14–1. Home health certification and plan of treatment form.
(Courtesy Home Health Care Agency of California, Torrance, CA.)

Department of Health and Human Services
Health Care Financing Administration

Form Approved
OMB No. 0938-0357

Addendum to: ☒ Plan of Treatment ☐ Medical Update

1. Patient's H1 Claim No.	2. SOC Date	3. Certification Period	4. Medical Record No.	5. Provider No.
	121692	From: 121692 To: 021693		

6. Patient's Name	7. Provider's Name

8. Item No.	
13	414.9 Chr Ischemic Hrt Dis NOS 010182
16	Supplement 1-3 cans/Day prn decreased oral intake; no fluid restriction
21	MSS Daily x 1 Skilled assessment of social/emotional factors that interfere with patient/PCG/families adjustment to the illness, counseling for care planning and decision making; evaluate home environment—assist with development of in-home care system, arrange for social, financial, and environmental support services to ensure provisions for continuation of the care plan, crisis intervention needed for: reaction/adjustment to problems related to patient's illness
22	Patient will attain optimal level of functioning/independence Pt's physiological condition will be stabilized Pt/PCGs to identify long-term needs Pt/PCG to receive counseling to improve their adjustment to the pt's illness Pt/PCG to become knowledgeable in coping with depression Pt. will receive assistance with ADL management/personal hygiene

9. Signature of Physician — 10. Date

11. Optional Name/Signature of Nurse/Therapist — 12. Date

Form HCFA-485 (U4) (4-87) PROVIDER

Figure 14–1. For legend, see opposite page.

obtained an order from the physician for fluoxe-tine (Prozac). Because M.J.'s tenant was helping her with marketing and errands the nurse instructed her and her neighbor about the need for nutritious foods and liquid meal supplements such as Ensure. Throughout this process the nurse focused on M.J.'s emotional needs. By working with the nurse to achieve the goals of the jointly developed treatment plan, M.J.'s depression decreased. When she was discharged from home care after 2 months, she was having regular bowel movements, had gained 10 pounds, had improved sleep patterns, and was bathing daily and cleaning her home. She was compliant with her medications and expressed confidence in her ability to cope with depression in the future.

Documentation of the need for skilled nursing care, goals, and interventions is critical for payment of psychiatric home care visits. Table 14-1 describes treatment plans for commonly encountered psychiatric behaviors in home care clients.

Table 14-1. Nursing treatment plans for frequently encountered behaviors in psychiatric home care clients

BEHAVIORS	NANDA DIAGNOSIS	OUTCOMES	INTERVENTIONS
History of medication noncompliance	Knowledge deficit regarding medication regimen	Client or caregiver will state medication action, schedule, dosage, and side effects	Instruct client or caregiver in medication regimen
	Medication noncompliance	Client or caregiver will demonstrate medication compliance	Monitor compliance each visit by counting pills, check medication box, ask client or caregiver about compliance
History of recurrent hospitalizations	Knowledge deficit regarding signs and symptoms of psychiatric decompensation	Client or caregiver will identify signs and symptoms of psychiatric decompensation	Instruct client or caregiver in signs and symptoms of psychiatric decompensation
Laughs inappropriately	Sensory-perceptual alteration	Client will state decrease in hallucinations	Assess behaviors every visit
Stares into space Talks to self			Reorient to reality Assess precipitating factors Develop and reinforce coping mechanisms—ignoring, changing environment, saying "no" to voices Assess for suicidal ideation
Delusional	Altered thought process	Client will make reality-based statements	Assess behaviors every visit Assess precipitating factors Don't reinforce delusions Develop and reinforce coping mechanisms—relaxation techniques, redirection of focus

Table 14-1—Cont'd

BEHAVIORS	NANDA DIAGNOSIS	OUTCOMES	INTERVENTIONS
Poor relationships with family or caregiver	Ineffective family coping	Client and caregiver will state improved relationships	Involve client and caregiver in developing care plan Encourage discussion between client and caregiver about communication, relationship, feelings about illness, coping skills when client or caregiver is upset Encourage expression of client and caregiver feelings about relationship
Increasing withdrawal	Potential for self-directed violence	Client will state coping mechanisms when suicidal	Assess for suicidal ideation—when client is suicidal, assess method and strength of feelings
Expressions of worthlessness No hope about the future Suicidal ideation		Client will not harm self	Assist client in developing coping mechanisms Contract with client to not harm self Instruct caregivers in providing for and monitoring client safety and reporting to physician if increased suicidal ideation occurs Report to physician Instruct client to call 911 if suicidal
Manipulative behaviors Splitting behaviors	Ineffective individual coping	Client will express needs directly	Clarify requests Don't "side" with client Instruct client in expressing needs directly Don't reinforce attention-seeking behaviors
Angry outbursts	Potential for injury to self or others	Client will express anger without injury to self or others	Discuss with client precipitating causes and coping skills to manage anger

Continued

Table 14-1—Cont'd

BEHAVIORS	NANDA DIAGNOSIS	OUTCOMES	INTERVENTIONS
Difficulty managing anger Hyperactivity			Instruct client in ways of relieving anger—assertion, increasing physical activity, counting to 10
Verbal expression of loss of control over living situation or treatment Withdrawal behaviors	Powerlessness	Client will state increased sense of control over situation	Involve client in development of treatment plan and goals Encourage client's expression of feelings of powerlessness Identify areas client has control or no control over Give client choices
Expressions of depression	Hopelessness	Client will state feeling hopeful	Encourage client's expression of grief or depressed feelings
Excessive grieving behaviors or lack of grieving behaviors	Dysfunctional grieving	Client will state resolution of depression or grief	Encourage development of coping skills for depressed feelings or grieving—increased physical activity, sharing feelings with others
Withdrawal behaviors	Social isolation	Client will increase social activities	Encourage social activities and use of community resources Assess for suicidal ideation
Self-deprecating statements	Low self-esteem	Client will state increased self-esteem	Instruct client in assertiveness skills and diversional activities Encourage positive self-worth statements
Decreased activity of daily living (ADL) management	Self-care deficit	Client or caregiver will manage ADL	Assess for physical immobility Instruct client and caregiver in mobility and ADL management—walking, bathing, adequate food and fluid intake

REIMBURSEMENT

Medicare and Medicaid

In 1994 home care expenses amounted to 3% ($23.7 billion) of national health care expenditures (National Association for Home Care, 1994). As of 1992 Medicare accounted for 37.8% of the payment for home care, Medicaid accounted for 24.7%, private insurance 5.5%, out of pocket 31.4%, and other sources 0.6%. Medicare insurance is divided into Part A and Part B. Home care benefits are an entitlement under Medicare Part A. Services and supplies are 100% reimbursable to the home care agency if they are ordered by the physician and medically necessary. Allowable durable medical equipment is reimbursable at 80% after a $100 deductible under Medicare Part B. Medicare reimbursement is managed through fiscal intermediaries such as Blue Cross and Blue Shield and other private insurance companies. Home health care billings are closely scrutinized and psychiatric home care justification is becoming more demanding and specific. Thus the documentation of skilled nursing needs and client or caregiver knowledge deficits and interventions is crucial for payment.

Managed care and private insurance

Managed care plans and private insurance companies require prior authorization for visits. This is not a requirement for Medicare. Home care agencies negotiate rates with managed care plans and private insurance companies for home care services. Health maintenance organizations may offer home care benefits for their enrollees or may contract with private home care agencies for these services. Visits to a skilled nursing facility are not reimbursable because such facilities are expected to provide skilled nursing care.

SUMMARY

Psychiatric home care nursing is still in its infancy but the focus in health care will undoubtedly continue to move toward community man-agement of medical and psychiatric problems. The growing geriatric population, which requires more health care than the younger generation, will further contribute to the need for an increase in long-term care and home care, and the home health care field will continue to expand. Estimates placed home care market growth at an annual rate of 10% between 1986 and 1991. It is estimated to grow at a rate of 12% annually from 1991 to 1996 (National Association for Home Care, 1994). This rapid growth will expand the need for more nurses, including psychiatric home care nurses. Community studies are needed to validate the efficacy of psychiatric home care in the reduction of recidivism.

Nurturing distressed clients in the community requires combining problem-solving skills with a sensitive and caring approach. It provides the opportunity to develop rewarding relationships with clients who otherwise might decompensate earlier and return to the hospital sooner and sicker. The psychiatric home care nurse can play a significant role in maintaining psychiatric clients in the community setting where many prefer to remain (Hellwig, 1993).

The rapidly changing health care arena has stimulated the growth of psychiatric home care. Medicare, as the primary payer, has specific criteria for justification of psychiatric home care nursing services. Psychiatric nurses provide a variety of skills and interventions uniquely suited to the homebound client. They are confronted with managing psychiatric and medical problems in the home. Providing nursing care for clients in the home is a rewarding challenge and adventure for psychiatric home care nurses.

REFERENCES

American Psychiatric Association. (1994). *Diagnostic and statistical manual of mental disorders* (4th ed.). Washington, DC: Author.

Delong, M. (1994). A healthcare professional's guide to medicare plans. *Nurseweek, 7,* 16-17.

Esser, A., & Lacey, S. (1989). *Mental illness: A homecare guide.* New York: John Wiley & Sons.

Hellwig, K. (1993). Psychiatric home care nursing: Managing clients in the community setting. *Journal of Psychosocial Nursing and Mental Health Services, 31,* 21-24.

National Association for Home Care. (1994). *Basic statistics about home care 1994.* Washington, DC: Author.

Pelletier, L. (1988). Psychiatric home care. *Journal of Psychosocial Nursing and Mental Health Services, 3,* 22-27.

Torrey, E. (1988). *Surviving schizophrenia: A family manual.* New York: Harper & Row.

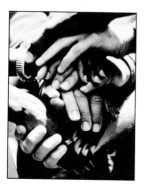

Chapter 15

Managed Behavioral Health Services

Cynthia D. Zubritsky

HISTORY AND BASIC CONCEPTS

Over the past 15 years health care costs in the United States have risen at an alarming rate. These costs have been passed on to private employers, citizens, and government programs at all levels through higher insurance prices and higher taxes to support government health care programs. Changes in the health care field are occurring in an effort to control rising health care expenditures through management of the use of services. The rapid development of managed care has changed the way health care, including mental health care and substance abuse treatment, is provided.

Most health insurance plans regardless of their form now have managed care components. *Managed care* is a generic term that includes a wide variety of practices designed to regulate the use of health care (Applebaum, 1993; Dorwart, 1990; Tischler, 1990; Zimet, 1989). The term *managed care* is somewhat misleading; a more accurate term would be *managed use of care*. The care

provided by health care practitioners has not changed, only the delivery, coordination, and use of that care. Falik (1991a) has found that mental health care and substance abuse treatment services are frequently managed within larger managed care networks.

This chapter will introduce the background and basic issues and concepts related to managed care generally and behavioral managed care specifically and will suggest the implications of managed care for community mental health nursing.

ECONOMICS OF HEALTH CARE

Health care has long been a major industry in the United States but its recent rapid growth has outstripped the growth of many traditional manufacturing and consumer product industries. During the 20-year period from 1975 through 1995, health care spending increased at a rate of more than 10% per year, more than twice the rate of inflation (Broskowski, 1991). During the same period, employers and other health care purchasers experienced significant increases in their health care expenditures with a more than 20% increase in 1990 alone (England & Vaccaro, 1991). For employers, health care expenditures amounted to approximately 10% of total payroll costs or an average of more than $3200 per employee. Total spending for health care in the United States in 1992 amounted to more than $800 billion—more than 12% of the gross national product.

Insuring health care as a method of payment began early in the 20th century. This method of paying for health care through third-party reimbursement has evolved into today's three-tiered health insurance system: tax-supported care for poor people (Medicaid) and elderly people (Medicare), tax-supported care for people with no third-party reimbursement (state, county, and city hospitals and clinics), and private insurance or private pay.

When health care costs began to escalate in the early 1980s, managed care was introduced as a way to control costs. The first generation of managed care sought to control medical costs for employers and insurers by controlling the price paid for various procedures through the implementation of diagnosis-related groups (DRGs). The second generation of managed care evolved with the development of procedures to ensure access to and use of services. The managed care process is currently in its third generation of development and quality and outcome measures have been added to the process. The coming generation will focus on personal and community health as companies invest in prevention to further reduce costs.

In the public arena, Medicaid has begun to use managed health care services to reduce costs for public programs. Medicaid is the largest government-funded health care program for the poor, with the federal government and the states sharing program costs. Reflecting national increases in health care costs, Medicaid has grown at a rate of about 10% per year throughout the 1980s with a sharp increase beginning in 1989 (U.S. General Accounting Office, 1993). For the federal fiscal year 1992 to 1993, state and federal spending on Medicaid topped $119 billion, a 29% increase from the previous year. The states alone spent more than $60 billion on Medicaid in 1992. The average state currently spends approximately 15% of its budget on Medicaid and with increases are pushing these expenditures upward. With costs rising so quickly, states are looking for new methods to control health care expenditures.

MANAGED CARE ORGANIZATIONAL MODELS

New models for financing and delivering health care are evolving rapidly, often combining elements of health care delivery organizational forms such as traditional health insurance, health maintenance organizations, and preferred provider organizations. Almost all new health care models include some managed care components (Task Force on Managed Health Care, 1991). Even public health insurance programs such as Medicare and Medicaid are using managed care models (Hadley & Langwell, 1991). Landress and Berstein (1993) project that managed care will soon control or influence 90% of all health care benefits. Models currently in use include the health maintenance organizations, preferred provider organizations, employee assistance programs, and managed care processes such as utilization review and case management.

Health maintenance organizations

Health maintenance organizations (HMOs), the oldest model of managed health care, are organized single systems of health care providers that offer a full range of services to an enrolled population (U.S. Bureau of the Census, 1992). An enrollment process identifies participating individuals as members (Bennet, 1992). HMOs receive a predetermined amount of money based on the number of enrollees and in return are responsible for health care for all enrollees. Generally HMOs assume responsibility for all medical care and expenses for participants. If the cost of the care provided to an enrollee exceeds the predetermined payment the HMO absorbs the additional expense (its "risk"). An HMO can be an independent company or can be sponsored by an insurance company, employer, hospital, union, or government agency (Landress & Berstein, 1993). The U.S. Bureau of the Census (1992) identifies three classes of HMOs: groups, independent practice associations, and open-ended HMOs. The "group" category is divided into three types: "pure" group practice, staff model systems, and network systems.

HMOs typically limit annual mental health care benefits while often offering unlimited physical health care. The HMO Act of 1973 (Freeman & Trabin, 1994) promoted and set minimal standards for HMO development. These standards included minimum mental health benefits of 20 emergency and crisis intervention outpatient visits per year. The Act expanded mental health and substance abuse benefits for some prepaid plans at a time when these benefit offerings by indemnity plans were minimal. This narrow mental healthcare benefit prevented many HMOs from developing sophisticated behavioral health management capabilities. Peterson (1992) reported that the average HMO limits inpatient mental health care to 32 hospital days per year and outpatient mental health care to 22 visits per year.

Capitated and "carve-out" models

There are two types of HMOs: those that have a capitated system and those that have a "carve out." To most behavioral health professionals, the word *capitation* has come to represent the assumption of all fiscal risk and the provision of all behavioral health care services for a specific population. However, the word *capitation* actually refers to payment using a "per-person" payment plan. In behavioral health there are three types of capitation:

- **Administrative Services Only (ASO) Capitation Fee.**   Under this payment arrangement a provider is paid a fixed fee per person per month for administrating the behavioral health benefit plan. Under ASO arrangements the HMO is "at risk" for administrative services such as preadmission certification, case management, treatment planning, reporting, eligibility determination, fee negotiation, and claims payment. The payer retains the risk for the cost of treatment.

- **ASO Capitation Fee With Risk Sharing.** Under this capitation arrangement the provider is paid a per-member per-month administrative fee. The provider and the payer set a target for treatment costs or utilization. The provider receives a bonus if costs remain below the target but pays a "rebate" or penalty to the payer if the target is exceeded.

- **Full Risk Capitation.**   The provider organization is paid a per-member per-month fee that generally includes all administrative costs and treatment services costs. In this arrangement the provider assumes all fiscal risk for behavioral health care benefits while the payer's liability is limited to the monthly capitation payment.

Another method of funding mental health and substance abuse services is to "carve out" these services from a total package of health care services. In a carve-out model, behavioral health services are separated from general health services and provided through a separate behavioral health care provider; carve-out arrangements exist in both private and public sector systems (Falik, 1991b). Several public sector mental health and substance abuse programs currently use the carve-out model (McFarland, 1994) to offer behavioral healthcare services to their Medicaid populations. States using public carve-out programs include California, New York, Pennsylvania, Rhode Island, and Utah.

Managed mental health care organizations

A new type of managed care organization, the managed mental health care organization (MMHCO), has emerged to deliver mental health care and substance abuse treatment services. Such organizations provide comprehensive inpatient and outpatient services, including substance abuse treatment, using a variety of reimbursement techniques. MMHCOs contract with employers, unions, insurers, and HMOs to manage all aspects of behavioral health care benefits provided in their plans. Specific mental health services are covered and paid for on a per-person prepaid or capitated basis.

Typically MMHCOs are service brokers, developing organized networks of local providers. Providers within the MMHCO's network are paid for services rendered on a negotiated fee-for-service basis. Precertification and concurrent review methods are used by MMHCOs.

Managed care models for Medicaid recipients are currently being tested in most states. These models use various cost containment methods including mandatory enrollment in health maintenance or preferred provider organizations, full and partial capitated rates, and case management. States obtain federal approval for Medicaid waivers that require Medicaid recipients to join HMOs or preferred provider organizations or to participate in other forms of managed medical care. In 1993 nearly 4 million Medicaid recipients were enrolled in managed care programs in 36 states, representing about 12% of all Medicaid recipients (U.S. General Accounting Office, 1993).

Preferred provider organizations

A preferred provider organization (PPO) is a formal network of doctors and hospitals that contracts with employer groups and other insurers to provide an identified range of health care services to enrolled participants. The PPO can negotiate discounts or reduced fees for its services as part of the negotiated enrollment. Enrollees must use providers within the PPO network or risk having the provider not pay for services.

PPOs give enrollees greater freedom of choice of providers than HMOs. The advantage of participating in a PPO for a health care provider is an increased number of clients in exchange for a reduced fee for services (Hirshfeld, 1990).

Employee assistance managed behavioral health care programs

Employee assistance programs (EAPs) are work-site based and are designed to assist in the early identification and resolution of employee productivity problems associated with pressing personal concerns (Feldman, 1994). EAPs began as occupational health services for alcoholism treatment in the 1950s. They initially focused on early intervention for alcohol and drug abuse but gradually expanded their service offerings. Two of the most beneficial aspects of such programs are employees' easy access to them and their provision of appropriate referral in a sometimes daunting behavioral health care system. EAPs have created an informal network of trusted providers and developed criteria and procedures for directing clients to the most appropriate care.

Managed care is now performing many of these rapid access, evaluation, and triage functions. With the advent of managed behavioral health care, EAPs are reevaluating their roles. Some EAP vendors have expanded their services and evolved into managed care companies themselves while others have maintained their traditional roles. Thus there now is a range of types of EAPs. Some EAPs provide services internally to a corporation through counselor employees or externally through a contracted EAP vendor. In either case EAPs typically offer services such as employee education and outreach in wellness and illness prevention; early detection, evaluation, and referral services; management training and consulting; critical incident stress debriefing; responses to drug testing requirements; post-treatment workplace reintegration; legal and financial counseling; and child care and elder care.

During the late 1980s several internal corporate EAPs branched into broader managed care functions. Under such arrangements employers carve out behavioral health care benefits to the EAP and the EAP in turn performs network development and management functions, case management and utilization review, and similar operations that are typically the domain of the carve out vendor. EAP-managed behavioral health care programs have survived because they offer employers the opportunity to have a benefit program and delivery system specifically tailored to their needs.

Utilization review

Medical necessity reviews and case management reviews (known as utilization management or utilization reviews (URs)) (Falik, 1991b; Hodgkin, 1992; Tischler, 1990) began in the 1970s. Early benefit authorization programs used telephone interviews for preadmission and concurrent reviews for hospital admissions and inpatient stays. UR companies typically did not have a contractual agreement with the hospital but made authorization a requirement for reimbursement. The focus was almost exclusively on disability and medical-surgical cases. A UR team typically comprised a staff of registered nurse reviewers supervised by physicians. Reviewers used criteria based on diagnosis-specific statistical norms for hospital length of stay.

UR companies modified their procedures and criteria to include psychiatric and substance abuse disorders in the early 1980s. The Civilian Health and Medical Program of the Uniformed Services (CHAMPUS) gave significant impetus to utilization review. It contracted with the American Psychiatric Association and the American Psychological Association to develop and implement standards for retrospective peer review. CHAMPUS then contracted for telephone-based UR through several vendors. This UR model is now standard practice within managed health care review.

MANAGED BEHAVIORAL HEALTH CARE

Managed behavioral health care has developed as a way to find alternatives to psychiatric hospitalization within a framework of provider accountability, performance, and quality, critical values that must be included in any mental health and substance abuse treatment system. These programs are characterized by management teams devoted exclusively to mental health and substance abuse issues; mental health care management personnel specially credentialed under the supervision of board-certified psychiatrists; specifically developed mental health and substance abuse treatment criteria for level of care assignment and case management that address medical necessity and appropriateness; and specialized behavioral group, staff model, and PPO networks that provide a continuum of care, access to a full range of services, and negotiated discounts (Feldman, 1994). Other distinguishing features include continuous quality improvement programs, specialized behavioral information systems, outcome management systems, clinical practice guidelines, and provider network management systems (Freeman & Trabin, 1994). As an increasing number of state and local mental health and substance abuse authorities divest themselves of service responsibilities, they are adopting managed care practices to ensure that costs are controlled and consumers have appropriate, necessary, and essential services provided within a framework of choice, responsiveness, involvement, and quality. Mental health and substance abuse treatment dollars (especially public ones) are extremely limited and may become even more scarce as more conservative fiscal policies are adopted. Efforts to achieve cost effectiveness will dominate the concerns of mental health and substance abuse care providers in the next decade.

Expenditures for behavioral health care

Behavioral health care is a component of managed health care that encompasses treatment for alcohol and drug abuse (substance abuse) and mental health conditions. About 10% of all health care expenditures are for behavioral health care (Oss, 1994). In 1990 almost $54 billion was spent on behavioral health treatment: $42.4 billion on mental health services, $3 billion on drug addiction treatment, and $8.5 billion on alcohol addiction treatment. Of this almost $54 billion, $22.2 billion was paid through private insurance funds, $9.5 billion through Medicaid, $15.9 billion through state and local governments, and the balance through Veterans' Affairs, Medicare, and other federal sources (Oss, 1994). In 1990 35 million uninsured Americans sought health care through a myriad of government-sponsored services; 16% of them had a serious mental health or substance abuse problem. The most frequently paid behavioral health care benefits were for inpatient services. Private insurance plans spend 60% of their behavioral health care budget on inpatient services; Medicaid spends 65%. States that direct public sector behavioral health care services spend 59% of their behavioral health care budgets on hospitalization.

Public sector behavioral health service per capita expenditures far exceed private insurance expenditures. Behavioral health care spending for people with private insurance in 1990 was $138 per person. Behavioral health care spending for people with no insurance was $575 per person, 90% of which was for behavioral health services for people with serious and persistent mental illness.

Cost control techniques in the public sector

Restrictions on choice of provider. Consumers can obtain services only from providers enrolled in an approved provider network. A penalty is imposed if the insured person obtains services from providers who are not in the network. The penalty can range from a higher copayment to full payment by the client.

Limit on visits or days. Most insurance plans cap the amount of benefits that can be received by placing limits on the number of outpatient visits or inpatient days that can be provided in a year or even over the life of the policy. Behavioral health care benefits are traditionally much smaller than physical health benefits.

Medical necessity reviews. Authorization is usually required based on the medical necessity of treatment before mental health services can begin. Once services are authorized an ongoing review of the necessity of continuing services may occur.

Case management. Case management is typically assigned to clients who require costly, long-term interventions. The case manager coordinates services, finds treatment alternatives to costly inpatient treatment, and participates in discharge planning (Hodgkin, 1992; Landress & Berstein, 1993).

Data are in conflict about whether behavioral health care costs are rising significantly faster than general health care costs. It has been reported that costs for mental health benefits increased at more than twice the annual rate of increase for other health benefits in 1988 (Falik, 1991a) and that employers' costs for behavioral health care have risen faster than other medical costs (Broskowski, 1991), with reported increases as great as 60% per year (England & Vaccaro, 1991). However, evidence also indicates that behavioral health care's share of total health care costs has remained relatively constant at 12% to 14% over the past 20 years (Oss, 1994). Regardless of conflicting fiscal analyses a major portion of behavioral health care costs is directly attributable to inpatient psychiatric hospitalization (England & Vaccaro, 1991).

The significant growth in the number of inpatient psychiatric programs during the mid and late 1980s contributed to the rapid increase in behavioral health care expenditures. This growth can be attributed to many factors including aggressive behavioral health marketing campaigns that helped fill inpatient beds with behavioral health referrals at a time when the number of filled hospital medical-surgical beds was declining, few early mental health intervention programs, few substance abuse prevention programs, few outpatient and community-based care alternatives, a national reduction of stigma on mental illness, and an increase in the use and abuse of alcohol and drugs (Broskowski, 1991). Consequently, large for-profit "chains" of specialty psychiatric and chemical dependency hospitals proliferated. Between 1979 and 1986 the number of inpatient psychiatric treatment facilities grew by 40% (Berlant, Trabin, & Anderson, 1994). Concomitantly, increased inpatient psychiatric costs have been the driving force behind increases in behavioral health care expenditures. Although approximately 70% of all mental health care expenditures are for psychiatric hospitalization, only 7% of all behavioral health care patients account for these expenditures. Furthermore, fewer than 50% of inpatient admissions account for more than 80% of all costs (Broskowski, 1991).

LEGAL AND REGULATORY ISSUES

Many states have passed legislation regulating managed care practices including certification requirements that mandate minimum qualifications for reviewers and provisions for appeal of reviewers' decisions (American Medical Association, 1990; Freudenheim, 1991).

New initiatives and developments among accrediting organizations also seek to provide a source of managed care accountability. Examples of accrediting organizations include the Utilization Review Accreditation Commission (URAC), the Joint Commission on Accreditation of Health Care Organizations (JCAHO), and the National Committee on Quality Assurance (NCQA). As accreditation by one or more of these organizations becomes a prerequisite for bidding on certain contracts, accountability standards will have more influence. Each of these organizations has specific initiatives underway concerning accreditation of behavioral health management organizations. These and other factors will affect future forms of managed care.

Clinical issues

In a managed care system clinicians are not always able to provide or obtain care that they consider necessary for clients. If a reviewer for the organization managing the insurer's mental health care benefits concludes that recommended care is not medically necessary, coverage may be denied despite the client's not having exhausted all benefits (Hall & Anderson, 1992). Although mental health professionals have always had to deal with limited benefits, denial of coverage has until now not been a problem for clients.

Standards of care

Early data suggest that the introduction of managed care has led to modifications in professional standards with marked shifts from inpatient to outpatient treatment (Thompson, Burns, Goldman, & Smith, 1992) and reductions in the number of outpatient sessions per episode of treatment (Norquist & Wells, 1991). As the approaches to mental health treatment reflected in these data become widely practiced, professions and courts will likely recognize them as legitimate alternative standards of care (Hall, 1989; Hirshfeld, 1990).

Quality control measures related to outcome management include the development and use of practice guidelines. Delivery systems that use research-based practice guidelines and continuously improve on those guidelines through outcome research will be more likely to deliver consistent high-quality care. Some organizations use outcome data to develop and refine practice guidelines.

Outcome measures and program evaluation

Providers in organized care systems reimbursed on a capitated basis have an economic incentive to undertreat. A capitated system means that monthly receivables are constant and therefore profits can be increased only through cost controls, which may result in less treatment or inappropriate treatment for consumers of behavioral health care services. The health care system must build in checks and balances so this incentive does not overwhelm long-term incentives to provide quality services. Cost control may result in barriers to access to services with a concurrent increase in waiting lists and ineffective treatment.

Two important balances to offset this trend within the system would be to adequately fund behavioral health care benefits and services and find ways to measure and reinforce standards for accessibility, appropriateness, quality, and effectiveness of treatment (such as through "report card" delivery system performance indicators) (Freeman & Trabin, 1994). These report cards would be based on predetermined performance objectives that measure domains such as effectiveness, efficiency, appropriateness, accessibility, capacity, and use.

IMPLICATIONS FOR COMMUNITY NURSING

Behavioral managed care is quickly becoming a major force in mental health and substance abuse service delivery in both the public and private sectors. This change in the service delivery system will have a major impact on the education and skills needed for effectiveness in community human services organizations. Although traditional skills in therapy, rehabilitation, and administration will still be valued, additional skills including case management, familiarity with short-term therapy modalities such as cognitive therapy, and the ability to work in interdisciplinary teams will be highly valued.

Nurses will continue to be valued within the managed care environment for many reasons. As licensing and regulatory agencies develop standards for managed health care, licensed professional workers will provide a central focus for a staff model. Managed care companies will value professionals such as nurses who understand both a traditional medical model and a community model of delivering care.

SUMMARY

The rapid development of managed care in all its forms—HMOs, preferred provider organizations, utilization review, and case management—has changed the way health care is provided and administered in the United States. More attention is being paid to the cost effectiveness of services, treatment guidelines, and ongoing outside review of treatment plans.

Managed care represents a shift in national values. Health care spending has reasonable limits, and employers, the government, and individual people are reaching the limits of their resources. Management of health care use is in its infancy; models currently in place will be modified and changed as the needs and limits of health care are realized. Behavioral health care's greatest challenge will be to fit within the new paradigm and still provide cost-efficient, treatment-effective services.

REFERENCES

American Medical Association. (1990). Utilization review. *State Health Legislation Report, 18*(2), 30-35.

Applebaum, P.S. (1993). Legal liability and managed care. *American Psychologist, 48*(3), 251-257.

Bennett, M.J. (1992). The managed care setting as a framework for clinical practice. In J.L. Feldman, & R.J. Fitzpatrick (Eds.), *Managed mental health care.* Washington, DC: American Psychiatric Press.

Berlant, J., Trabin, T., & Anderson, D. (1994). The value of mental health and chemical dependency benefits: More than meets the eye. In E. Sullivan (Ed.), *Driving down health care costs: Strategies and solutions.* Frederick, MD: Panel Publishers.

Broskowski, A. (1991). Current mental health care environments: Why managed care is necessary. *Professional Psychology: Research and Practice, 22*(1), 6-14.

Dorwart, R. A. (1990). Managed mental health care: Myths and realities in the 1990s. *Hospital and Community Psychiatry, 41*(10), 1087-1091.

England, M. J., & Vaccaro, V. A. (1991). New systems to manage mental care [Commentary]. *Health Affairs, 10*(4), 129-137.

Falik, M. (1991b). Harnessing the potential of managed care. *Policy in Perspective,* January, Washington, DC: Mental Health Policy Resource Center.

Falik, M. (1991a). Health maintenance organization's mental health benefits—separate and unequal. *Policy in Perspective* January, Washington, DC: Mental Health Policy Resource Center.

Freeman, M., & Trabin, T. (1994). Managed behavioral healthcare: History, models, key issues, and future course. Washington, DC: U.S. Department of Health and Human Services, Substance Abuse and Mental Health Services Administration.

Freudenheim, M. (1991, February 13). Doctors press states to curb reviews of procedures costs. *New York Times,* pp. D1, D9.

Hadley, J. P., & Langwell, K. (1991). Managed care in the United States: Promises,evidence to date and future directions. *Health Policy, 19,* 91-118.

Hall, M. A. (1989). The malpractice standard under health care cost containment. *Law, Medicine, and Health Care, 17,* 347-355.

Hall, M. A., & Anderson, G. F. (1992). Health insurers' assessment of medical necessity. *University of Pennsylvania Law Review, 140,* 1637-1712.

Hirshfeld, E. B. (1990). Economic considerations in treatment decisions and the standard of care in medical malpractice litigation. *Journal of the American Medical Association, 264,* 2004-2012.

Hodgkin, D. (1992). The impact of private utilization management on psychiatric care: A review of the literature. *Journal of Mental Health Administration,* 19(2), 143-157.

Landress, H., & Berstein, M. (1993). Managed care 101: An overview and implications for psychosocial rehabilitation services. *Psychosocial Rehabilitation Journal,* 17(2), 5-14.

McFarland, M. D. (1994). Health maintenance organizations and persons with severe mental illness. *Community Mental Health Journal,* 30 (3), 221-241.

Norquist, G. S., & Wells, K. B. (1991). How do HMOs reduce outpatient mental health care costs? *American Journal of Psychiatry, 148,* 96-101.

Oss, M. (1994). Integrated delivery systems: Issues & considerations. *Open Minds,* 8(8), 6-8.

Peterson, M.S. (1992). *National survey of mental health, alcohol, and drug abuse treatment in HMOs: 1989 chartbook.* Excelsior, Minn: InterStudy Center for Managed Care Research.

Task Force on Managed Health Care, Board of Health Professions. (1991). *Report to the Commission on Health Care for All Virginians.* Richmond, VA: Virginia Department of Health Professions.

Thompson, J. W., Burns, B. J., Goldman, H. H., & Smith, J. (1992). Initial level of care and clinical status in a managed mental health program. *Hospital and Community Psychiatry, 43,* 599-603.

Tischler, G.L. (1990). Utilization management of mental health services by private third parties. *American Journal of Psychiatry,* 130: 913-916.

U.S. Bureau of the Census. (1992). *Statistical abstract of the United States: 1992* (112th ed.). Washington, DC: U.S. Government Printing Office.

U.S. General Accounting Office. (1993). *Medicaid: States turn to managed care.* Washington, DC: U.S. Government Printing Office.

Zimet, C.N. (1989). The mental health care revolution, will psychology survive? *American Psychologist,* 44(4), 703-708.

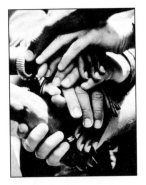

Chapter 16

Schools

Nancy K. Worley and V. Jann Owens

SCHOOL-BASED CLINICS

At least 500 school-based clinics are in operation in middle schools and high schools across the United States (Dryfoos, 1994). For about half of all enrolled students school-based clinics provide the sole or primary source of health care (McCord et al., 1993). Models for school-based health care that have been most successful have four features (Robert Wood Johnson Foundation, 1993):

1. They are located in the schools
2. They are operated by health professionals
3. They provide comprehensive services
4. They are funded by other sources than the school

The benefits of each of these features are discussed in the following sections.

Located in the schools

School-based health care increases children's access to health care. Of all schoolchildren in the United States, 20% to 25% live in poverty. However, these figures become more dismaying when percentages are categorized by racial and ethnic groups. Of all African-Americans under 18 years old, 44% live in poverty; the figure is 38% for Hispanics under 18 years old (U.S. Bureau of the Census, 1990). A substantial number of these poor children lack access to basic health care because of low family income or lack of health insurance. Medicaid, the largest insurance program for poor people, covers only a small portion of low-income families; many others do not fit into the special categories the program was designed to serve (National Center for Health Statistics, 1991). Families that do have Medicaid coverage may still find access to care restricted because physicians are hesitant to accept the lower fees and cumbersome paperwork attendant with Medicaid reimbursement. Many poor children come from single-parent families in which the custodial parent holds a full-time job and can ill afford to take time off from work for anything less than a medical emergency. For all these reasons, health care in schools increases access especially for children living in poverty.

Schools also offer convenient care provided by staff familiar with the children and sensitive to the unique needs of children and adolescents. Health professionals in schools can be instrumental in altering the risk-taking behaviors that have become common in recent years among school-age children.

Operated by health professionals

Many schools have responded to budget difficulties by hiring fewer nurses and using health aides or volunteers to provide immunizations and health and vision screenings (Adams, 1992). Professional organizations recommend a ratio of one nurse for every 750 students (American Nurses Association, 1983). So few schools meet this recommended nurse/student ratio that Igoe and Speer (1992) assert that a ratio of one nurse to every 1500 students is more realistic; however, even this goal has yet to be achieved in many school districts. In many school districts one or two nurses make up the total school health team, with an assignment of three to five schools each. Under these circumstances nurses are often unable to provide quality care and are limited to providing screenings and taking care of emergencies. Education on health promotion and disease prevention is either provided by teachers or not taught at all. School health environmental services that ideally should be provided by school nurses are delegated to maintenance and building personnel or principals. As the health needs of students become more complex and the level of care delivered in schools increases, the need grows for school health programs to be managed by health professionals who are knowledgeable about the clinical aspects of care. However, a 1986 national survey of school nurse supervisors revealed that only 60% of school nurses were supervised by a registered professional nurse. Other school nurse supervisors were school administrators, health and physical education teachers, psychologists, and counselors (Igoe & Campos, 1991). The in-

creasing popularity of school-based health centers may change the traditional responsibilities of the school nurse. The evaluation of several school-based health center demonstration projects (Kornguth, 1990) indicated that nurse practitioners with appropriate physician consultation provide excellent health care, reduce unnecessary referrals, and decrease the amount of time away from school for students whose only alternative source of health care is a public clinic where waiting time is lengthy.

Provide comprehensive services

School-based clinics are tailored to the needs and resources of the communities they serve. The majority of clinics are committed to the principle of comprehensive care and usually offer a full spectrum of services with a strong educational component (Kirby, Waszak, & Ziegler, 1991). The three core components of a comprehensive school health program are health services, health education, and environmental health.

Health services

Screenings. Traditionally schools have scheduled screenings for vision, speech, and hearing problems, dental disease, growth abnormalities, tuberculosis, pediculosis, and immunization compliance. Some schools, particularly in poor inner city neighborhoods, also screen for nutrition problems, sickle cell anemia, and evidence of lead poisoning. School systems that recognize the role of the school health program as the primary provider of care for underserved students have expanded the scope of screenings. Screening for psychosocial and developmental problems has become more common as the number of medically underserved children increases. Box 16-1 provides an outline of a comprehensive approach to biopsychosocial screening.

Primary health care. A growing number of students need to obtain primary health care services in school. This type of care includes a health history, physical examination, simple laboratory

---

Box 16-1. HEADS: A comprehensive biopsychosocial screening approach

H Screening for problems in the **home** that affect children's health
E **Education** and eating disorders
A **Accidents,** appetite, and activities
D **Drug** abuse
S **Sex** and suicide

---

tests, and diagnosis and treatment of minor health problems. The American School Health Association recommends that mental health programs be made available in the schools (American Medical Association, 1990b); some nurses who are primary care providers work exclusively with students experiencing emotional disorders.

Health education

During the past decade health education has been closely identified with the health promotion movement (Igoe & Speer, 1992). However, health-promoting activities rest on assumptions about individual potential that may be incongruent with the resources available to many families. The socioeconomic status of a population influences many facets of life; for example, poverty is associated with poor nutrition, substandard housing, a disruptive social environment, and lack of education. It also is the leading predictor of poor health among children (Zill & Rogers, 1988). When family resources are lacking, meeting the needs of the family assumes greater importance than enhancing individual coping abilities or well-being. Thus basic needs are likely to override health promotion concerns in at-risk families. Limited parental involvement in health promotion activities and preventive health care may influence adolescents to develop health care values that are not prevention focused. However, students are in school 6 hours a day and during that time health profes-

sionals can influence student values about healthy life-styles. School nurses and teachers can model healthy life-styles. Health fairs can combine entertainment with health promotion activities. Health promotion strategies such as Life Skills Training (LST) can promote the development of coping skills that increase students' ability to function competently in social situations and reduce the motivation to participate in drinking, smoking, and other destructive life-style choices.

Parents in low-income areas can be encouraged to participate in school-based health programs if the programs are well designed and sensitive to the social environments in which many disadvantaged families live (Dryfoos, 1994). Most successful school-based health programs have an advisory council that includes parents as members. The Yale Child Study Center project described later in this chapter hired parents at minimum wage to act as classroom aides. In Los Angeles, where no money was available to hire aides from the community, vouchers for food markets and free child care were used to compensate people for their services (Dryfoos, 1994).

Environmental health

The third component of the school health program is environmental health—physical and psychosocial. Inspecting for asbestos and lead paints, monitoring the safe use of toxic chemicals in science and art classrooms, and reducing risk of injury in classrooms, hallways, and playgrounds are all activities that affect environmental health.

The psychosocial factors that contribute to a healthy school environment have received little attention until recently, when escalating violence in schools, high drop-out rates, and a lack of parental involvement drew attention to this aspect of the school environment. Comer (1988) argues that schools, instead of focusing heavily on teachers' credentials and test scores, must promote development and learning by building supportive bonds that draw together children, parents, and schools. In 1968 Comer and his colleagues from the Yale University Child Study Center implemented a project that sought to improve the psychosocial environment of two inner city grade schools in New Haven, Connecticut. A total of 650 pupils, 99% of whom were African-American, attended the two schools. Almost all of the students were poor; 70% came from families receiving Aid to Families with Dependent Children (AFDC). At the beginning of the project the children were ranked near the bottom in achievement and attendance among the 33 schools in the city. One rationale for the intervention was that current educational reforms de-emphasize interpersonal factors and focus instead on instruction and curriculum. Such approaches assume that all children come from mainstream backgrounds and arrive at school equally well prepared to perform. However, children from poor or marginal families are likely to enter school unprepared. Children may begin school without having learned such social skills as negotiation and compromise. They may come with underdeveloped or substandard language skills but still be expected to be prepared to read in school. Behaviors that are considered survival skills in poor neighborhoods, such as fighting back when provoked, are counterproductive in the classroom environment. The hierarchical and authoritarian structure of most schools makes it difficult for underprepared students to gain the skills and experience necessary to fulfill the expectations of the school. Such students quickly become labeled as unmotivated, stupid, or incorrigible, and are often punished or suspended from school. Parents perceive these problems as personal failures or as evidence of animosity and rejection, lose hope and confidence, and become less supportive of the school. The result is a high degree of mutual distrust between the home and school.

The members of the New Haven team realized that little progress could be made to help the children achieve without fostering positive interactions between the parents and the school. Therefore a governance and management team was created in each school led by the principal and elected parents and teachers, a mental health specialist, and a member of the nonprofessional support staff. The teams negotiated over issues ranging from the school's academic and social programs to changes in school procedures that seemed to engender behavioral problems. A number of parents were paid minimum wage to serve as classroom assistants. Parents and staff sponsored activities such as potluck suppers, book fairs, and graduation ceremonies. These activities fostered good relations between staff and parents. As a result, the school climate and student behavior improved and more parents attended school activities. Parents and teachers devised a curriculum of social skills and subjects the children would need to know to operate successfully in mainstream society. The children learned how to write thank-you notes and invitations, how to serve as hosts, how to write checks, and how to plan school events such as concerts and talent shows.

The intervention program produced significant academic gains. By 1984, without any change in the socioeconomic makeup of the schools, pupils in the fourth grade in these schools ranked third and fourth highest on the Iowa Test of Basic Skills in the entire New Haven school system. By the early 1980s attendance rates, which had been among the lowest in the school system, were first and second in the city. There have been no serious behavior problems in either school for more than a decade. The program has since been implemented in more than 165 schools around the country.

Funded by other sources

The final feature of successful models of school-based care is that they should not depend on the school system for financial support. Schools encounter financial difficulties with even the most basic school health programs. Therefore if a community's school-age population is to benefit from using the school setting as a primary health center, the responsibility of organizing, financing, and delivering services must be shared with other health systems including community, state, and federal systems (Igoe & Speer, 1992).

TARGET GROUPS

Medically underserved

By 1991 more than 14 million children (22% of all children) in the United States lived below the poverty line, the highest number and rate since 1965 (Dryfoos, 1994). The relationships between low-income environments and health outcomes are complex but striking. A number of child health indicators (mortality rates, health ratings, and measures of illness and injury) show substantial disparities in the health status of children from different socioeconomic segments of American society (Rogers & Bianchi, 1992). African American and Hispanic children, especially those in inner city and rural areas, are less healthy on average than nonminority children. Most children in households headed by women are poor. For children in African-American families headed by women in which the mother is single, under 30 years old, and did not complete high school, the poverty rate is 92.8% (Miller, Fine, & Adams-Taylor, 1989).

Medically underserved individuals are often oriented toward illness care rather than health care or health maintenance (Uphold & Graham, 1993).

The health of disadvantaged young people is an important issue addressed by federal efforts to reduce the socioeconomic stratification of health care. In 1985 the Secretary's Task Force on Black and Minority Health issued recommendations to reduce inequalities in the health of racial and ethnic minorities in the United States. One recommendation urged that the Department of Health and Human Services "should continue to investigate, develop, and implement innovative models for delivery and financing of health services" (Report of the Secretary's Task Force on Black and Minority Health, 1985). The American Medical Society, the Society for Adolescent Medicine, and the American Academy of Pediatrics have established access to care as a current priority (Fisher et al., 1992).

Adolescents

Despite immunization laws, improved immunization rates, and improved sanitation, optimal health has not been achieved in adolescent populations. In fact, over the past 30 years adolescents have been the only age group in the country whose health status has not improved (Robert Wood Johnson Foundation, 1993). Teenagers are natural risk takers and many live in an environment in which risk taking can be dangerous. Add poverty, sexually transmitted disease, and violence to this scenario and one has a population at risk for many interrelated problems.

Because adolescents spend a significant number of their formative years in school and their lives revolve around friends and school, schools have unique opportunities to address adolescent health needs. Adolescents explore adult roles, social identity, interpersonal skills, and patterns of behavior and values from which their adult lifestyles will evolve. Adolescence is a period of experimentation with smoking, alcohol and drugs, fad diets, reckless driving, and sex (Jessor, 1993). To manage their major developmental needs and experiment with new behaviors, adolescents must possess many functional skills. Developing the skills necessary to practice health-promoting activities involves clarifying of values and adding new skills to the adolescent's existing repertoire of skills. Decision making, problem solving, communication, and consumer skills are but some of the complex abilities and strategies adolescents must develop to enjoy a healthy life-style.

Adolescents are not emotionally, socially, or financially equipped to manage their health needs independently. If they come from families at risk or neighborhoods where conditions of poverty, limited education, and few opportunities for social interaction in the community exist, they are at risk for developing potentially harmful health habits. Without intervention these young people risk developing physical and mental health problems that will impede their ability to complete school or become productive citizens and effective parents to their own children.

Two recent national surveys eliciting adolescents' self-reported knowledge, beliefs, and health behavior reported similar findings. The first was a two-phase longitudinal evaluation of seven consolidated physical and mental health services for 2787 high-risk young people funded by the Robert Wood Johnson Foundation. This study investigated directly the association between social and health behaviors in an effort to understand how socialization during adolescence influences life-style (Robert Wood Johnson Foundation, 1993). Life-style was defined as a general way of living based on the interaction of environmental conditions and subjective forces that shape individual patterns of behavior. The Foundation reported that adolescent life-style is a process of socialization into adult norms that includes developing both healthful and harmful behaviors. Social activities, peer influence, and religious activities were noted as factors that could facilitate the adoption of healthful or harmful behaviors.

The second study was a national survey of 11,419 eighth and tenth graders to assess their knowledge of critical adolescent health concerns: injury prevention, substance use, suicide, violence, nutrition, sexually transmitted diseases, and consumer skills. Findings of this study indicated that a significant proportion of adolescents place themselves at risk of serious injury, believe having sex is acceptable, believe their parents need not be informed if they are treated for sexually transmitted diseases, have been involved in at least one physical fight in a year's time, and have tried cigarettes, alcohol, or marijuana (Centers for Disease Control, 1989).

African-American adolescents, especially those living in urban working-class neighborhoods, pose an even greater challenge than other adolescents because they are at greater risk for unprotected sexual intercourse, school failure, delinquency, pregnancy, and substance abuse than their white middle class counterparts (Dryfoos, 1990).

These findings indicate that traditional medical care, which emphasizes the diagnosis and treatment of acute, episodic physical illness, is inadequate to address the multidimensional, preventable health problems that are currently most prevalent. Medical care should be augmented by holistic nursing services that provide social support through the therapeutic nursing relationship (with individuals and in groups) to reduce behavioral risks, redefine normative social and health behavior, and enhance self-competence to increase self-esteem.

Dryfoos (1994) characterizes adolescent pregnancy, drug use, violence, and depression as the "new morbidities" that threaten the future of today's children. A short synopsis of the scope of these problems and some successful interventions follows.

Adolescent pregnancy

The United States leads all other developed nations in rates of teenage pregnancy, abortion, and childbearing. The most striking contrast is among the youngest adolescents. American teenagers under 15 years old are at least five times as likely to give birth than teenagers in any other country for which data are available (Hayes, 1987). Among adolescents 15 to 17 years old, the percentage of births to unmarried mothers increased from 43% in 1970 to 73% in 1986. In this age group, 6 out of 10 births to whites and 9 out of 10 births to African-Americans were to unmarried mothers. In 1988 more than one third of subsequent births to teenage mothers occurred within 18 months of a previous birth (National Center for Health Statistics, 1988).

The consequences of becoming an unmarried teenage mother are serious for both mother and child. Teenage mothers are disproportionately poor and dependent on public assistance. Teen mothers complete fewer years of school and are less likely to earn a high school diploma or attend college than their counterparts who delay motherhood until their 20s (Sullivan, Brooks-Gunn, & Schwarz, 1992). Pregnant teenagers younger than 15 years old are at risk for increased complications of pregnancy such as eclampsia, anemia, and cesarean sections (Dryfoos, 1990). Children of adolescent mothers have a vastly increased chance of growing up in poverty, scoring lower in academic achievement, and being socially impaired (Furstenberg, Brooks-Gunn, & Morgan, 1987).

Few issues cause more intense debate than the issue of what constitutes effective solutions to the problem of teenage pregnancy. Moral, political, and social conflicts have continued to make it difficult to reach agreement on the best approaches. Largely educational programs that attempt to increase knowledge about the physiology of reproduction, the risks of pregnancy, and sexually transmitted diseases are the least controversial and are available in most high schools. However, no evidence indicates that educational programs alone make an impact on the level of adolescent sexual activity or teen pregnancy (Zabin, 1992). School-based or school-linked reproductive health services offering contraceptive services, treatment of sexually transmitted diseases, and pregnancy testing have shown they can reduce pregnancy rates (Zabin, Hirsch, & Smith, 1986). However, this option is the most controversial of all services offered by school-based clinics; many clinics, in order to be allowed to open and serve the other health needs of students, have had to forego contraceptive services. Nevertheless, all schools can offer programs that enlarge future opportunities for adolescents and discourage high-risk behaviors. Education, job opportunities, mentors, and role models may open new vistas and encourage the delay of parenthood.

Violence

Violence is a major adolescent health problem and a leading cause of adolescent death in the United States. Homicide is endemic in urban areas with low socioeconomic indicators and is the leading cause of death for young African-American men between 15 and 24 years old (Centers for Disease Control, 1985).

Nonfatal interpersonal violence is less well documented than homicide but also is endemic. Emergency rooms and school data provide the best available sources of rates of interpersonal violence, but these data are underestimates because not all incidents of interpersonal violence are seen in the emergency room or take place on school grounds (Prothrow-Stith, & Spivak, 1992).

The determinants of adolescent violence are many and interactive. Poverty, racial injustice, drug and alcohol use, the glamorous portrayal of violence on television and in the movies, peer pressure, and family influences have all been cited as causes of adolescent violence.

Designing prevention strategies in the face of the many negative socioeconomic and cultural influences experienced by at-risk adolescents is quite difficult. The Violence Prevention Project for Urban Youth in Boston is an example of a program that has been implemented successfully at elementary, high school, and college levels. Through outreach and education, this community-based primary prevention effort is endeavoring to change individual behavior and community attitudes toward violence (Prothrow-Stith, Spivak, & Hausman, 1987). The project includes a curriculum designed to achieve the following ideals:

- Provide statistical information on adolescent violence and homicide
- Present anger as a normal, potentially constructive emotion
- Create awareness in the student of alternatives to fighting by discussing the potential gains and losses of fighting
- Have students analyze situations preceding a fight and practice avoiding fights by using role playing and videotapes
- Create a nonviolent classroom ethos that values violence prevention behavior

Drug and alcohol abuse

Figure 16-1 shows the national percentage of high school seniors using alcohol, tobacco, and other drugs during a 30-day period. Using these figures and a summary of other survey studies, Dryfoos (1990) estimated the percentages of high school seniors using these substances as follows:

- 12% engaged in heavy cigarette smoking (a half pack or more per day)
- 15% engaged in heavy drinking (five or more drinks, three or more times per week)

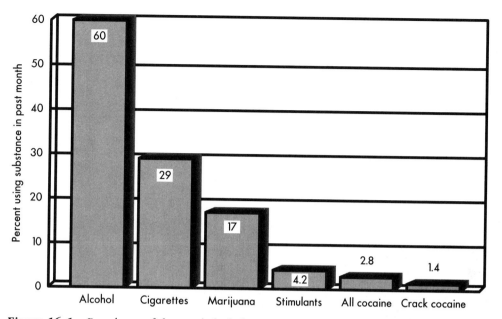

Figure 16-1. Prevalence of drug and alcohol use among high school seniors over a 30-day period.
(Modified from *Press Release of the 1989 National High School Senior Survey,* by L. Johnson, & P. O'Malley, 1990, Ann Arbor, MI: University of Michigan.)

- 5% regularly used marijuana (20 or more times within the last month)
- 3% frequently used cocaine (three or more times within the last month)

These statistics illustrate that substance abuse is relatively common. They also illustrate that drugs garnering a large amount of media attention (such as crack cocaine) are used by a very small percentage of students and that the drugs of choice are instead alcohol, cigarettes, and marijuana.

The literature on the antecedents of adolescent drug use suggests that social, environmental, personality, and behavioral factors are the most important determinants of future drug use (Kelder & Perry, 1992). Because these factors are dynamic and interacting, substance abuse prevention programs should be designed to influence all four sets of factors. Box 16-2 lists psychosocial factors that can be used to develop prevention programs.

Depression and suicide

Depression among adolescents is serious and potentially life threatening. Depression may present directly in the form of overt sadness or indirectly in the form of somatic complaints or school avoidance (Muscari, 1992). The diagnosis and treatment of depression in adolescents is problematic. A small number of teenagers will acknowledge depression and seek help. However, denial is much more common, and adolescents who are chronically depressed may be so used to a depressed mood that they don't recognize it as a disorder. Families will frequently miss signs of depression because labile moods are common in adolescence. In fact, only one third to one half of depressions are recognized by primary care practitioners (Depression Guideline Panel, 1993).

In addition to the common symptoms of depression such as hopelessness and sadness, signs of depression in adolescence may include school

---

Box 16-2. Adolescent substance abuse prevention—psychosocial factors

Environmental factors

Parental influence: Parental involvement and support

Cultural norms: Promotion of a nonuse norm

Opportunities: Appealing substance-free activities

Role models: Peer leaders, influential person's behavior

Social support: From families and peers

Personality factors

Knowledge: Harmful consequences and alternatives

Values: Relative importance of drugs versus abstinence

Self-efficacy: Confidence in being able to resist peer pressure

Locus of control: Perception of being in charge of self

Meanings: Functions that drugs serve

Behavioral factors

Behavioral capability: Skills to refuse, engage in alternative activities

Intentions: Statements about remaining substance free

Behavior repertoire: Communication, decision making

Reinforcements: Tangible rewards for nondrug alternatives

Modified from "Substance Abuse Prevention," by S. Kelder, & C. Perry, 1992, in *Principles and Practice of Student Health* (Vol. 2) (p. 413), by H. Wallace, K. Patrick, G. Parcel, & S. Igoe (Eds.), Oakland, CA: Third Party Publishing.

failure, disruptive or destructive behavior, defiance, truancy, eating disorders, drug and alcohol abuse, and repeated accidents. Antidepressant medications and psychotherapy are effective treatments for depression once symptoms are recognized. The importance of diagnosis and treatment is underlined by the fact that clinical depression is the disorder most commonly linked to suicide.

From 1960 to 1985 the suicide rate among boys 10 to 14 years old and among both young men and women 15 to 19 years old more than doubled (O'Carroll, Saltzman, & Smith, 1992). Concern about this escalating rate of adolescent suicide has prompted some states to mandate suicide prevention programs in high schools. Voluntary programs exist in most other states (Puskar, Lamb, & Norton, 1990). One of the difficulties in developing suicide prevention programs is a lack of good data on the factors that play a role in suicide. Clinical depression and alcoholism are highly associated with suicide, and an increasing body of literature addresses biological and genetic risk factors for suicide (Roy, 1989). Increasingly common suicide clusters among teenagers have stimulated interest in "contagion"—the notion that suicides may be caused by exposure to the suicide or suicidal behavior of others (Centers for Disease Control, 1988; Davidson & Gould, 1989). A study by Fisher et al. (1992) found that suicidal ideation was a significant problem in high schools in which the majority of students were African American and Hispanic and in which the resources for treating depression were limited. It has been documented that adolescent depression accompanied by suicidal thoughts predicts future adjustment problems in high school completion, maintaining employment, substance use, delinquent behavior, being arrested, being convicted of a crime, and being in a car accident (Lewinsohn et al., 1993). An additional link among anger, depression, and suicidal acts finds that suicide may be one of life's most angry actions. People who internalize their anger and aggression have high suicide rates and people who externalize anger have high homicide rates (Jones, Peacock, & Christopher, 1992).

Data available on risk factors associated with adolescent suicide indicate that suicide prevention programs using a multidisciplinary, collaborative approach focusing on teacher, parent, and student awareness will be most effective. An excellent example of this approach is illustrated by the suicide prevention program in Fairfax County, Virginia. Public schools there formed an advisory council that includes teachers, nurses, social workers, and guidance counselors from within the school system and mental health professionals, parents, and police from the community. The program provides teacher training on topics such as suicide awareness, identification of at-risk adolescents, and knowledge of community referral sources. Parent workshops focus on suicide awareness and community resources. Student workshops and regular classroom sessions focus on stressful life issues. Peer support and counseling groups are held for students (Puskar, Lamb, & Norton, 1990).

MODEL PROGRAMS

Burke High School, Charleston, South Carolina

In 1994 the first school-based clinic in South Carolina opened, operated by the Medical University of South Carolina College of Nursing and Department of Pediatrics. The clinic is nurse managed and located on the campus of Burke High School, which serves an inner city adolescent population of 1060 students, of whom 98% are African American. The poverty rate of the families living in the census tracts that feed into the school is 26.8%. A 1993 profile report of the population living within a 10-mile radius of the school indicates that only 33.5% of the population has graduated from high school. Only 6% of families with children between 6 and 17 years old were not in the workforce. The survey found 35% of people were concerned about maintaining personal health and 38.9% were concerned about finding adequate health care. Survey results showed 32% of families were dealing with drug abuse and 23% dealing with teen and child problems (V. Jann Owens, personal communication, 1993). Of the children attending Burke School, 85% do not have a health care provider.

The opening of the clinic was not without controversy, and approval by the school board was granted by a very narrow margin. Opposition to the clinic was expressed by parents, religious

groups, and members of the school board. Religious groups feared that the clinic would provide or prescribe contraceptives. Religious opposition was overcome by reassurance that the clinic would not provide contraceptive advice and that, except for emergencies, no children would be served in the clinic who did not have a signed parent consent form. Philosophical opposition to the clinic was voiced by one school board member who claimed that it was not the mission of the school system to be the primary health care provider for students. In spite of the controversy, 70% of parents signed the consent forms for their children to receive primary care at the Burke High School clinic.

Staffing

The clinic is directed by a full-time nurse practitioner who holds a faculty position at the College of Nursing; the staff consists of another full-time nurse practitioner and a baccalaureate prepared nurse. The Director of Adolescent Medicine, Department of Pediatrics, serves as a medical director and consultant.

Services

The clinic offers primary health care including treatment of physical symptoms, complete medical examinations, referrals to other health care providers when necessary, health education, and nutrition counseling. Students are given the opportunity to discuss concerns such as depression, abuse, problems with peers and family, and other emotional problems with the psychiatric clinical nurse specialist. Student nurses rotate through the clinic and provide services under the supervision of the clinic director. The nursing students also have developed a health curriculum and have taught courses on basic health principles and nutrition to the high school students. They serve as role models for these inner city high school students and encourage the students to stay in school. The freshman class of 1994-1995 will be evaluated over its 4 years at Burke to determine the effect the clinic has on students' education and health. Adolescents who do not complete high school are at increased risk for many health, economic, and social problems including unemployment, welfare dependency, and homelessness (Lear et al., 1991).

Family Services Center, Gainesville, Florida

The Family Services Center differs from the Burke School model in that it offers school-based services to both students and their families in a middle school in an impoverished area of Gainesville, Florida. The philosophy underlying the establishment of the center was that a familiar, accessible site such as a school was needed to help disadvantaged families solve their interrelated educational, social, economic, and health care problems (Uphold & Graham, 1993). The center was developed by the county school board and the Florida Department of Health and Rehabilitative Services. A number of service providers, such as the University of Florida, a local community college, many social service agencies, and city, county, and federal government programs, cooperate in the provision and financing of services at the center.

When a family seeks services at the center, a needs assessment is completed and a contract with the family is developed that addresses such issues as parenting skills, literacy, substance abuse, and health care. A family liaison specialist is assigned to each family; the specialist conducts home visits and works with the family to promote self-esteem and responsible decision making. Job training, job placement services, and literacy classes are available to the adults in the family. After-school programs for the middle school child focus on developing life, coping, and academic skills through individualized tutoring and enrichment programs. A mental health professional provides psychosocial evaluation and counseling. A full-service health clinic is available to students, their families, and the school staff. The clinic is managed by a family nurse practitioner with medical consultation provided by a physician on the faculty at the university.

ROLE OF THE PSYCHIATRIC NURSE IN SCHOOLS

When school-based clinic providers are asked what the largest unmet need is among their clients, they most frequently mention mental health services (Dryfoos, 1994). The demand for mental health counseling has led to the development of school clinics that exist primarily to screen and treat psychosocial problems. As the number of school-based clinics proliferates, excellent opportunities will arise for psychiatric clinical specialists to expand their practice into these settings. However, psychiatric nurses will have to recognize these opportunities and aggressively pursue them. Dryfoos (1994) reviewed a number of school-based mental health programs across the country and found no mention of psychiatric nurses were made in any of these reviews. Instead, these programs were developed, managed, and staffed by psychiatrists, social workers, and psychologists, a finding that is especially troubling when one considers that the majority of school-based health programs are managed by school nurses or nurse practitioners. Puskar, Lamb, and Norton (1990) argue for increased collaboration between psychiatric nurses and school nurses. Psychiatric-mental health nurses can help school nurses initiate programs to improve coping and problem-solving skills and develop programs to educate students, staff, and parents about adolescent stresses, depression, and suicide. The mental health nurse can serve as a consultant to school nurses and teaching staff with concerns about particular students.

Dryfoos (1994) refers to unprotected sex, drug use, violence, and depression as the "new morbidities" that threaten the future of today's children. All these problems are within the psychosocial sphere and underline the need for mental health expertise in school-based health services. The psychiatric-mental health nurse consultant with a theoretical base that includes a biopsychosocial approach to human development is a valuable resource to promote mental health in the school-age population.

SUMMARY

A close interrelationship exists between health and education. To attain the educational goals for the country, schools are assuming more responsibility for the traditional family function of overseeing children's health and development. Providing services within an interinstitutional, interdisciplinary model in schools with large high-risk populations is a promising approach for addressing adolescent health needs. School-based clinics that are fully engaged in their host schools also become the centers to which teachers, principals, coaches, and students refer young people who need assistance. This concept is important because adolescents who do not complete high school are at increased risk for many health, economic, and social problems including unemployment, welfare dependency, and homelessness. Evaluation studies have shown that clinic use effectively reduced absence, suspension; and withdrawal and also increased promotion rates (Dryfoos, 1994). Reducing risk while providing health promotion, education, and skills development to adolescents may be the ideal way to help them address their major developmental task of achieving independence.

REFERENCES

Adams, M. (1992). Screening programs. In H. Wallace, K. Patrick, G. Parcel, & J. Igoe (Eds.), *Principles and practice of student health* (Vol. 2). Oakland, CA: Third Party Publishing.

American Medical Association. (1990a, September 4). *Adolescent health: An AMA white paper*. New York: Discovery Channel.

American Medical Association. (1990b). *Healthy youth 2000: National health promotion and disease prevention objectives for adolescents*. Chicago: Author.

American Nurses Association. (1983). *Standards of school nursing practice*. Kansas City, MO: Author.

Centers for Disease Control. (1985). Homicide among young black males: United States, 1970-1983. *Morbidity and Mortality Weekly Report, 32,* 629-633.

Centers for Disease Control. (1988). Clusters of suicide and suicide attempts. *Morbidity and Mortality Weekly Report, 37,* 213-216.

Centers for Disease Control. (1989). Results from the national adolescent student health survey. *Morbidity and Mortality Weekly Report, 38,* 147-150.

Comer, J. (1988). Educating poor minority children. *Scientific American, 259,* 42-48.

Davidson, L., & Gould, M. (1989). Contagion as a risk factor for youth suicide. *Risk factors for youth suicide.* Report of the Secretary's Task Force on Youth Suicide (Vol. 2) (DHHS Publication No. ADM 89-1624). Washington, DC: U.S. Government Printing Office.

Depression Guideline Panel. (1993). *Depression in primary care: Volume I, Detection and diagnosis. Clinical practice guideline, No. 5* (AHCPR Publication No. 93-0550). Rockville, MD: U.S. Department of Health and Human Services, Public Health Service, Agency for Health Care Policy and Research.

Dryfoos, J. (1990). *Adolescents at risk: Prevalence and prevention.* New York: Oxford Press.

Dryfoos, J. (1994). *Full-service schools.* San Francisco: Jossey-Bass.

Fisher, M., Juszczak, L., Friedman, S. B., Schneider, M., et al. (1992). School-based adolescent health care. Review of a clinical service. *American Journal of Diseases of Children, 146,* 615-621.

Furstenberg, F., Brooks-Gunn, J., & Morgan, S. (1987). *Adolescent mothers in later life.* Cambridge: Cambridge University Press.

Hayes, C. (1987). Risking the future. *Adolescent sexuality, pregnancy and childbearing* (Vol. 1). Washington, DC: National Academy Press.

Igoe, J., & Campos, E. (1991). Report of a national survey of school nurse supervisors. *School Nurse, 6,* 8-20.

Igoe, J. & Speer, S. (1992). The community health nurse in the schools. In M. Stanhope, & J. Lancaster (Eds.), *Community health nursing* (3rd ed.). St. Louis: Mosby.

Jessor, R. (1993). Successful adolescent development among youth in high risk settings. *American Psychologist, 48,* 117-126.

Johnson, L., & O'Malley, P. (1990). *Press release of the 1989 national high school senior survey.* Ann Arbor, MI: University of Michigan.

Jones, M. B., Peacock, M. K., & Christopher, J. (1992). Self-reported anger in black high school adolescents. *Journal of Adolescent Health, 13,* 461-465.

Kelder, S., & Perry, C. (1992). Substance abuse prevention. In H. Wallace, K. Patrick, G. Parcel, & J. Igoe (Eds.), *Principles and practice of student health* (Vol. 2). Oakland, CA: Third Party Publishing.

Kirby, D., Waszak, C., & Ziegler, J. (1991). Six school based clinics, their reproductive health services and impact on sexual behavior. *Family Planning Perspectives, 23,* 6-16.

Kornguth, M. (1990). School absences for illness: Who's absent and why. *Pediatric Nursing, 16,* 95-99.

Lear, J. G., Gleicher, H. B., St. Germaine, A., & Porter, P. J. (1991). Reorganizing health care for adolescents: The experience of the school-based adolescent health care program. *Journal of Adolescent Health, 12,* 450-458.

Lewinsohn, P. M., Hops, H., Roberts, R. E., Seeley, J. R., & Andrews, J. A. (1993). Adolescent psychopathology: I. Prevalence and incidence of depression and other *DSM-III-R* disorders in high school students. *Journal of Abnormal Psychology, 102*(1), 133-144.

McCord, M. T., Klein, J. D., Foy, J. M., & Fothergill, K. (1993). School-based clinic use and school performance. *Journal of Adolescent Health, 14,* 91-98.

Miller, C., Fine, A., & Adams-Taylor, S. (1989). *Monitoring children's health: Key indicators* (2nd ed.). Washington, DC: American Public Health Association.

Muscari, M. (1992). The "acting out" adolescent: Identification and management. *Pediatric Nursing, 18,* 362-366.

National Center for Health Statistics. (1988). Advance report of final natality statistics, 1986. *Monthly vital statistics report* (DHHS Publication No. PHS 88-1120). Washington, DC: Author.

National Center for Health Statistics. (1991). *Advance data characteristics of persons with and without health care coverage, United States, 1989* (No. 116). Washington, DC: Author.

O'Carroll, P., Saltzman, L., & Smith, J. (1992). Suicide. In H. Wallace, K. Patrick, G. Parcel, & J. Igoe (Eds.), *Principles and practice of student health* (Vol. 1). Oakland, CA: Third Party Publishing.

Owens, V.J. (1993). Personal communication. Charleston, SC.

Prothrow-Stith, D., & Spivak, H. (1992). Homicide and violence in youth. In H. Wallace, K. Patrick, G. Parcel, J. Igoe (Eds.), *Principles and practice of student health* (Vol. 1). Oakland, CA: Third Party Publishing.

Prothrow-Stith, D., Spivak, H., & Hausman, A. (1987). The violence prevention project: A public health approach. *Science, Technology and Human Values, 12,* 67-69.

Puskar, K., Lamb, J., & Norton, M. (1990). Adolescent mental health: Collaboration among psychiatric mental health nurses and school nurses. *Journal of School Health, 60,* 69-71.

Report of the secretary's task force on black and minority health. (1985). Washington, DC: Office of Minority Health, DHHS.

Robert Wood Johnson Foundation. (1993). *The answer is at school: Bringing health care to our students.* Washington, DC: The School-Based Adolescent Health Care Program.

Rogers, C., & Bianchi, S. (1992). The socioeconomic status of America's children and youth. In H. Wallace, K. Patrick, G. Parcel, & J. Igoe (Eds.), *Principles and practice of student health* (Vol. 1). Oakland, CA: Third Party Publishing.

Roy, A. (1989). Genetics and suicidal behavior. *Risk factors for youth suicide.* Report of the Secretary's Task Force on Youth Suicide (Vol. 2) (DHHS Publication No. ADM 89-1624). Washington, DC: U.S. Government Printing Office.

Sullivan, A., Brooks-Gunn, J., & Schwarz, D. (1992). Adolescents: Improving life chances. In L. Aiken, & C. Fagin (Eds.), *Charting nursing's future* (pp. 340-362). Philadelphia: J.B. Lippincott.

Uphold, C., & Graham, M. (1993). Schools as centers for collaborative services for families: A vision for change. *Nursing Outlook, 41,* 204-211.

U.S. Bureau of the Census. (1990). U.S. population estimates by age, sex, race, and Hispanic origin: 1989. *Current population reports* (Series P-25, No. 1057). Washington, DC: U.S. Government Printing Office.

Zabin, L. (1992). Teenage pregnancy. In H. Wallace, K. Patrick, G. Parcel, & J. Igoe (Eds.), *Principles and practice of student health* (Vol. 2). Oakland, CA: Third Party Publishing.

Zabin, L., Hirsch, M., & Smith, E. (1986). Evaluation of a pregnancy prevention program for urban teenagers. *Family Planning Perspectives, 3,* 119-126.

Zill, N., & Rogers, C. (1988). Recent trends in the well-being of children in the United States and their implications for public policy. In A. Cherlin (Ed.), *The changing American family and public policy.* Washington, DC: The Urban Institute Press.

Chapter 17

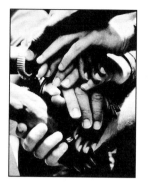

Community Mental Health Centers

Nancy K. Worley

THE CHANGING ROLE OF COMMUNITY MENTAL HEALTH CENTERS

Chapter 1, Political and Economic Perspectives, traces the community mental health center (CMHC) movement from its legislative inception in 1963 to its legislative amendment in 1975. The 1975 amendments to the original legislation were designed to meet the needs of people with chronic mental illness who were not well served by the original legislation. At that time, the community mental health centers were in trouble politically and financially. The Nixon and Ford Administrations declared unequivocal opposition to continuing direct federal support for the CMHC program, arguing that state and local authorities should assume responsibility for the program. Yearly federal appropriations to fund CMHCs were approved over presidential veto from 1972 to 1976. This long battle for survival weakened the centers and was a factor in the loss of many excellent clinicians and administrators. It also was the impetus for several congressional investigations of the CMHC program that documented shortcomings in public mental health care service, organization, and delivery.

Investigators found that CMHCs poorly served chronically mentally ill people discharged and diverted from state and county mental hospitals (Foley & Sharfstein, 1983).

The election of Jimmy Carter breathed new life into the community mental health center movement. As one of his first official acts, President Carter established the President's Commission on Mental Health, which was to undertake a 1-year study of mental health care needs and recommend how these needs might best be met. The commission's report, submitted to President Carter a year later, called for making a priority of meeting the needs of people with chronic mental illness, including the formation of "a national plan for the chronically mentally ill" (PCMH, 1978). President Carter called for a task force to draft the necessary legislation to respond to the recommendations. The result was the Mental Health Systems Act, which Carter signed into law on October 7, 1980. Much of the Act focused on providing a system of care for people with chronic mental illness in the community that would include not only mental health services but also an array of medical, social, rehabilitative, housing, and employment services necessary to sustain a productive life. One month after the enactment of the Mental Health Systems Act, Ronald Reagan was elected. President Reagan and his administration chose not to implement the act and instead recommended to Congress a 25% cut in the CMHC funding level and the conversion of the entire federal mental health service program into a single "block grant" to the states with few restrictions. The effects of this "New Federalism" on community mental health centers were far-reaching and lasting. They included the following:

- The removal of the federal government from the operation of community mental health centers except as a conduit of funds to the states
- The decline of consultation, education, and prevention programs in community mental health centers
- The concentration on people with chronic mental illness as the primary clients of the centers
- The movement of the centers away from a public health model to a medical model of care and treatment

The only section of the Mental Health Systems Act that survived more or less intact under the community mental health center reorganization was the section pertaining to chronically mentally ill adults and severely mentally disturbed children and adolescents. Community mental health centers subsequently became tertiary (rehabilitative) care agencies.

DEFINING CHRONIC MENTAL ILLNESS

The first tasks of the community mental health centers were to identify and count the number of people with chronic mental illness residing in their service areas. This led to considerable debate regarding the definition of chronic mental illness. Without federal government guidelines, states developed their own legal definitions of chronic mental illness; these definitions varied from state to state, making the collection of national epidemiological data extremely difficult. Schinnar et al. (1990) applied the definitions of chronic mental illness from 10 states to a population of public mental health system clients in Philadelphia. They found that prevalence estimates (using the various states' definitions) varied from 38% using Hawaii's definition to 72% using Ohio's definition.

In an effort to overcome this problem the National Institute of Mental Health gathered a small group of clinicians, researchers, and policy officials and charged it with finding a mutually agreeable definition of severe and persistent mental illness. The group sought to operationalize the definition for use across many settings to facilitate service planning and research (Bachrach, 1987). The work group agreed on a definition stressing the three major elements of diagnosis, disability, and duration (Bachrach, 1987):

The severely and persistently mentally ill encompasses persons who suffer severe and persistent mental or emotional disorders [diagnosis] that interfere with their functional capacities in relation to such primary aspects of daily life as self-care, interpersonal relationships and work or schooling [disability] and that often necessitate prolonged or intermittent hospital care [duration].

This definition of severe and persistent mental illness was to be operationalized as indicated in the following sections.

Diagnosis

Psychotic disorders predominate among people with severe and persistent mental illness. The various types of schizophrenia, the major affective disorders, and serious personality disorders are most common. Drug and alcohol abuse disorders among this population have increasingly become secondary complicating factors.

Disability

Most definitions of disability center on the concept of functional incapacity. Four separate functional areas are usually considered in determinations of disability:

1. **Activities of daily living** include adaptive activities such as cleaning, cooking, taking public transportation, paying bills, maintaining a residence, and caring appropriately for grooming and hygiene. People's independence, appropriateness, and effectiveness in performing these activities and their ability to initiate and participate in such activities independent of supervision and direction are taken into account in assessing this functional area.

2. **Social functioning** refers to an individual's capacity to interact appropriately and communicate effectively with other people. Deficits in this area are reflected in a history of altercations, evictions, or firings; fear of strangers; avoidance of interpersonal relationships; and social isolation.

3. **Adaptation or task performance in work or similar situations** refers to an individual's ability to sustain focused attention for a long enough time to complete tasks commonly found in work settings or in similar structured activities that take place in school or home settings.

4. **Deterioration or decompensation in work or similar settings** refers to a person's repeated failure to adapt to the stressful circumstances associated with employment or similar stressors in school or home settings. In such situations the client experiences an exacerbation of signs and symptoms associated with the illness and sometimes withdraws from the stressful environment altogether.

Duration

Some generally accepted criteria for the duration of illness are provided by the Social Security Administration for people diagnosed with schizophrenia (Federal Register, 1985). They include a medically documented history of one or more episodes of acute signs, symptoms, and functional limitations, even though such symptoms or signs might at that time be ameliorated by medication or social support; repeated episodes of deterioration, decompensation, or exacerbation of signs or symptoms; or a documented history of 2 or more years of inability to function outside a highly supportive living situation.

The following case examples illuminate the ways in which the interaction of diagnosis, disability, and duration defines the life courses of people with severe and persistent mental illness.

Case example

Beth had a normal childhood and successful high school career until her senior year. She began to pay less attention to her appearance, withdrew from her friends, dropped out of most of her extracurricular activities, and began to do poorly in school. In response to her family's concern, Beth responded that several of her former friends were trying to harm her by putting poison in her food in the cafeteria and were spreading ugly sexual rumors about her. When her parents questioned her more closely about the validity of these statements, Beth responded, "I know it's all true. I hear voices that tell me all about these things." Beth was subsequently hospitalized and diagnosed as having paranoid schizophrenia. She gradually recovered from the initial episode with the help of medication and supportive psychotherapy. After discharge and some time at home she attempted to return to high school. Her former classmates had all graduated, and she had difficulty acquiring a new group of friends. She worried that the students knew she had been in a mental hospital and were talking about her. This unhappy and stressful situation caused some of her symptoms to return, and she left school and enrolled in a GED program in the community where she could study at her own pace. After obtaining her high school diploma, she found a job as a secretary in a real estate firm. After several months the pressure of the work caused her symptoms to recur, and she was again hospitalized. After discharge she moved into a group home and began to work part-time in a sheltered workshop. For the past 10 years Beth's condition has remained fairly stable. She has had three more brief hospitalizations but has been able to return to the group home and continue her part-time employment between hospitalizations.

Discussion. Schizophrenia typically strikes adolescents and young adults; three fourths of people diagnosed with schizophrenia are between 17 and 30 years old. The early onset of the disease, occurring during high school or college when people are preparing for adult life, is particularly devastating. At a time when most young people are obtaining work skills and enhancing social skills the disruptions caused by schizophrenia often leave the client unable to "catch up" and heighten the disability caused by the disease process. Beth's history of hospitalization over 10 years shows that duration is often a defining characteristic of severe and persistent mental illness.

Case example

Michael is a 44-year-old married attorney with three children. He suffers from severe and recurrent bouts of depression. He was first hospitalized at the age of 25 after a serious suicide attempt, which he attributed to the stress of studying for the bar examination. He was treated with antidepressant medications and made a full recovery. He was again hospitalized at the age of 36 when he was nominated for a partnership in his law firm. Recovery was somewhat slower after this episode, but Michael was eventually able to return to work. About 2 years later he experienced signs of a return of the depression. He was unable to sleep for more than 5 hours a night. His appetite decreased and he lost 25 pounds. He became irritable with his wife and children and had difficulty keeping up with his caseload at the law firm. He was hospitalized after his wife found a loaded gun in the glove compartment of his car.

Discussion. This case example illustrates the symptoms of a severe and persistent affective disorder. Unlike Beth, who has a constant disability, Michael recovers fully from each episode of depression. However, he has experienced major disruptions in his life and is at serious risk of committing suicide.

Case example

David is a 23-year-old high school dropout who became involved with drugs and alcohol while in junior high school. He has been arrested several times for assault and twice for burglary. He has been in a number of drug treatment programs but never completed treatment. He has lived in several group homes but has been discharged because of fighting, drunkenness, or disobeying the rules. He now alternates between living in homeless shelters and in the local jail. He has never been hospitalized.

Discussion. David probably comes closest to the stereotype of the severely and persistently mentally ill person depicted in newspapers and on television. He is a street person, unwashed and unkempt. He aggressively panhandles to buy food, crack cocaine, and alcohol. During his infrequent contacts with the mental health system he has been diagnosed as having a personality disorder (probably schizotypal) complicated by alcohol and cocaine abuse.

TERMINOLOGY

In recent years consumers have objected to the term *chronically mentally ill,* which they feel connotes irreversibility and poor prognosis. In deference to these feelings, agencies such as the National Institute of Mental Health have substituted terms such as *severely and persistently mentally ill* (SPMI) or *severely mentally ill* (SMI). These substitutes seem more acceptable to consumers. The professional literature continues to use all three terms to refer to a functionally impaired population of people who have periodic needs for crisis stabilization and hospitalization and ongoing needs for outpatient care and long-term rehabilitation. This book follows the lead of the professional literature and uses all three terms interchangeably. Regardless of the terminology used, consumers object most to the use of categorical descriptors such as *the chronically mentally ill* or *the seriously mentally ill* and prefer the substitution of "people with" serious, persistent, or chronic mental illness.

EPIDEMIOLOGY

Locating and counting people with severe and persistent mental illness are extremely difficult and expensive tasks in this post-deinstitutionalization era. These tasks are complicated by the dynamic and episodic course of severe mental disorders and by the lack of national consensus on the definition of severe and persistent mental illness. However, there seems to be general agreement that approximately 2 million severely and persistently mentally ill people live in the United States, 70% of whom suffer from schizophrenia. The remaining 30% suffer from severe affective disorders such as bipolar disorder or from severe character disorders. Many are diagnosed with both mental illness and substance abuse. Most studies show that 30% to 50% of people with serious and persistent mental illness are in this category (Raskin & Miller, 1993). A severe shortage of supportive and rehabilitative community programs to meet the needs of people discharged from long-term institutionalization or of younger people with chronic mental illness diverted from mental hospitals has led to public concern about the mental health system's problems. These problems have become apparent as people with severe and persistent mental illness spend less time in the hospital and more time in the community.

A 1984 study by the U.S. Office of Special Education and Rehabilitation Services estimated that approximately 10% of people with severe mental illness are in mental hospitals; 15% in nursing homes; 15% in group homes, supervised residences, or foster care; 40% live with their families; 10% are in jails or shelters or are homeless; and 10% live on their own. This last 10% of people with mental illness are the most visible

and disturbing to the community, to mental health service providers, and to policy makers who struggle to develop effective measures to help them. Homelessness and substance abuse have contributed to the increasing complexity of providing adequate care to people with severe mental illness. The special needs of these two often overlapping groups will be discussed in detail in Chapter 23, Persons with Mental Illness and Substance Abuse, and in Chapter 24, Homeless Persons with Mental Illness.

COORDINATION OF SERVICES

A major system problem became apparent shortly after the beginning of deinstitutionalization. State hospitals had supplied not only mental health treatment but also housing, food, clothing, recreation, medical care, and general safety to patients. Replicating this system of total care in the community, where each service had to be obtained from a different provider, proved an overwhelming task. Many severely and persistently mentally ill people who had recently been discharged from state hospitals had to be readmitted because the stress of attempting to live in the community without the necessary support systems had led to an exacerbation of their symptoms. In the early days of deinstitutionalization as many as 70% of patients discharged from the hospital were readmitted within 1 year. Others, who could not meet the increasingly strict criteria for readmission, were admitted to nursing homes, or, having nowhere to turn, became homeless.

By 1977 the federal government, through the National Institute of Mental Health (NIMH), began to respond to this increasingly serious problem. NIMH helped states and communities to develop comprehensive service systems for recently discharged patients. Planners of comprehensive service systems face three major tasks. They must identify and locate people who need services, make the services available, and ensure that services are coordinated into a coherent individualized service plan.

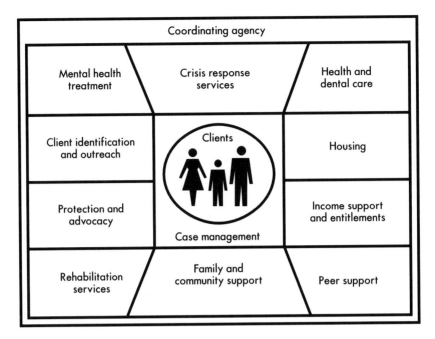

Figure 17–1. Community support system.
(Modified from *Toward a Model Plan for a Comprehensive Community Based Mental Health System,* by the National Institute of Mental Health, Department of Health and Human Services, 1987, Washington, DC: U.S. Government Printing Office.)

COMPONENTS OF A SERVICE SYSTEM FOR PEOPLE WITH CHRONIC MENTAL ILLNESS

Although case management is the "glue" that holds the service system together, case managers generally do not provide clinical services (see Chapter 10, Case Management). Instead, case managers link clients to a network of service providers. Figure 17–1 depicts service components that need to be available in the community to ensure that the needs of people with chronic mental illness are met. Many (if not all) of these services are provided by community mental health centers either directly or through contractual arrangements with other providers. Most of these services are explained in detail in other chapters. The following sections provide a brief overview of these services.

Psychosocial rehabilitation

Psychosocial rehabilitation helps people with psychiatric disabilities master the skills required to live, learn, and work in their communities with minimal support from the mental health system. Similar to physical rehabilitation programs the focus is on restoration of function. The chronically mentally ill person is likely to have deficits in social, self-care, and occupational skills. Rehabilitation interventions focus on teaching needed skills, adapting the skills to the environment in which the client will work and live, and making changes in the environment as necessary. Figure 17–2 illustrates the treatment, rehabilitation, and community supports that should be available to chronically mentally ill people depending on the stage of their illness. See Chapter 12, Psychosocial Rehabilitation, for a detailed discussion of this topic.

Psychoeducation and social skills training

Education of clients and families about mental illness and its management is not a new phenomenon, but the development of a formal curriculum with an underlying theoretical foundation and

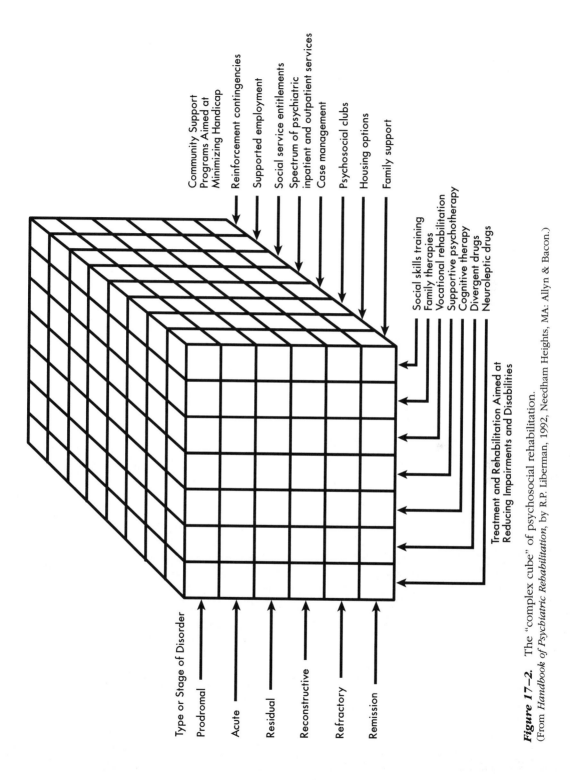

Figure 17–2. The "complex cube" of psychosocial rehabilitation.
(From *Handbook of Psychiatric Rehabilitation*, by R.P. Liberman, 1992, Needham Heights, MA: Allyn & Bacon.)

Table 17–1. Some cognitive deficits experienced by people with schizophrenia and suggestions for remediating them during social skills training*

SCHIZOPHRENIC COGNITIVE DEFICITS	TRAINING PROCEDURES FOR REMEDIATION OF DEFICITS
Showing associative intrusions in speech (this may be explained by a failure to self-edit tentative responses to words). It may be that people with schizophrenia have difficulty ignoring or dismissing inappropriate response options that occur to them, even though they may recognize that they are inappropriate. Thus the person with schizophrenia cognitively perseverates or fixates on the same inappropriate response option until it is actually spoken.	Employ mild censure for inappropriate responding and praise for appropriate responding. Adapt thought stopping or some other intrusive stimulus that can break the person with schizophrenia's perseveration on inappropriate response options. Monitor thought processes by frequent questions and probes and have the person with schizophrenia think aloud.
Having difficulty sustaining focused attention over time.	Keep training tasks and steps brief and focused. Use frequent prompts to regain attentional focus.
Being more susceptible to irrelevant cues, being more likely to misinterpret cues, and being more easily distractible.	Keep the training setting uncluttered and free of distracting stimuli (sound attenuation). Post graphic charts for clear and simple visual cuing of cognitive strategies (for example, post a list of response alternatives to social situations). Post a chart that has social skills training procedures and goals for the person with schizophrenia to look at while listening to the same instructions.
Having cognitive deficits that are made worse by the requirement of speedy responses to presentations of stimuli.	Proceed slowly through the steps of clearly structured training procedures.
Overloading of information that may occur more readily when tasks are complex.	Conduct task analysis and break down tasks into substeps. Reduce novelty by many repetitions before moving on to new material or scenes.
Tending to be influenced by the most immediate stimuli in the environment.	Avoid preceding interferences with learning. Give immediate feedback contingent on performance in training. After overlearning has occurred, gradually introduce delays into feedback and then fade to self-evaluation and feedback.
Developing exacerbation of psychotic symptoms if overstimulated by the environment.	Pace training individually, keeping performance demands low and performance-contingent feedback positive. Examine levels of autonomic responsiveness through psychophysiological recording and potential for information overload by information-processing tests (for example, span-of-apprehension test). Monitor psychopathology by repeated administration of mental status exams and feed back results for clinical decisions on medication dosage and pace of exposure to training. Allow people with schizophrenia to "escape" or take time out from training when necessary.

*Based on work by R.P. Liberman and colleagues at the UCLA Clinical Research Center for Schizophrenia.

rationale has occurred relatively recently. Liberman et al. (1985) pioneered the development of educational programs focused on overcoming cognitive deficits and increasing the skills repertoire of clients with chronic mental illness. Table 17–1 lists the kinds of cognitive deficits common among many people with schizophrenia and the techniques that can be employed to decrease their interference in the learning process.

Anderson, Reiss, and Hogarty (1986) pioneered the development of psychoeducational techniques to help families understand and cope with schizophrenia. They offer 1-day-long "survival skills" psychoeducational workshops for groups of families. Box 17–1 provides an example of the content of a workshop. Chapter 11, Psychoeducation, provides extensive information on psychoeducation.

Family, community, and peer support

Many people with chronic mental illness live with their families. Recent acknowledgment of the important role families play as primary care providers has led to attempts to develop working relationships among clinicians, family members, and clients (Anderson et al., 1986). As evidence mounts that the major mental illnesses have a biological component, theories that faulty family interactions cause mental illness have lost favor. More than any other factor, this questioning of the validity of family pathology as a cause of mental illness has helped create an atmosphere of openness and cooperation between mental health providers and families. In most community settings families are offered information about mental illness and its management rather than therapy.

Consumer self-help groups have proliferated in the past decade. They play an extremely important role in building skills, increasing self-esteem, and providing emotional support for members. Knowledgeable and articulate consumers are increasingly becoming members of mental health care planning bodies and the governing boards of clinical facilities (Hatfield & Lefley, 1993).

Much has been written about the resistance of communities to having people with mental illness living in their midst. Some evidence now indicates

---

Box 17–1. Outline of the psychoeducational workshop day

9:00–9:15	Coffee and informal interaction
9:15–9:30	Formal introductions and explanation of the format
9:30–10:30	Schizophrenia: What is it?
	History and epidemiology
	The personal experience
	The public experience
	Psychobiology
10:30–10:45	Coffee break and informal discussion
10:45–12:00	Treatment of schizophrenia
	Antipsychotic medication
	How it works
	Why it is needed
	Impact on outcome
	Side effects
	Psychosocial treatments
	Effects on course
	Other treatments and management
12:00–1:00	Lunch and informal discussion
1:00–3:00	The family and schizophrenia
	The needs of the client
	The needs of the family
	Family reactions to the illness
	Common problems that clients and families face
	What the family can do to help
	Revise expectations
	Create barriers to overstimulation
	Set limits
	Selectively ignore behaviors
	Keep communication simple
	Support medication regimen
	Normalize the family routine
	Recognize signals for help
	Use professionals
3:30–4:00	Questions regarding problems
	Wrap-up
	Informal interaction

Modified from *Schizophrenia and the Family*, p. 76, by C. Anderson, D. Reiss, and G. Hogarty, 1986, New York: Guildford Press.

that attitudes toward people with mental illness are changing. Television programs and newspaper articles on brain biology and ongoing research into schizophrenia and bipolar disorder have helped debunk some of the myths about mental illness. The active participation of clients and families on mental health boards also has helped demystify mental illness. Psychosocial rehabilitation programs have forged linkages with local businesses and landlords but much remains to be done. Mosher and Burti (1994) advise community mental health centers not to duplicate services the larger community can provide such as vocational, educational, athletic, and recreational programs, to keep the community mental health center firmly embedded within the community. Chapter 3, Family and Consumer Movements, provides extensive information on family and consumer movements.

Partial hospitalization

The most common treatment settings for psychiatric clients have long been either hospitals or outpatient clinics. Partial hospitalization programs were created to fill the need for treatment settings less restrictive than hospitals but more intensive than outpatient clinics. As the name implies, partial hospitalization clients spend part of the day in treatment but spend their nights elsewhere, either with their families or in some other residential facility. See Chapter 18, Partial Hospital Programs, for an extensive discussion of partial hospitalization.

Crisis services

Emergency services were among the original services mandated by the Mental Retardation Facilities and Community Mental Health Centers Construction Act of 1963. In the early years of community mental health centers, emergency service consisted almost entirely of the 24-hour availability of mental health professionals in a hospital emergency room or on call through a special "hot line." As it became apparent that crisis intervention services decreased hospitalization, prevented further decompensation, and provided opportuni-

ties to link clients to appropriate services, crisis services began to expand.

Mobile crisis services

Because hospital-based or agency-based emergency services are facility based, clients who for a variety of reasons cannot or will not avail themselves of these services may have little access to emergency treatment. Mobile crisis services seek to provide outreach mental health assessment and treatment to clients in urgent need. A major goal of mobile crisis teams is to restore clients to a precrisis level of functioning as quickly as possible to allow them to remain in the community if at all possible. The mobile crisis team links clients with needed community services as soon as possible after the initial crisis is resolved. Most mobile crisis teams are interdisciplinary and usually include a psychiatrist, a psychiatric nurse, and a social worker among the team members.

Residential crisis services

A relatively new addition to crisis services available in the community is residential crisis service, which provides a temporary protective and supportive setting in which clients have an opportunity to stabilize. Most of these programs provide physical assessment, psychiatric services, development of a client service plan, crisis-oriented counseling, family and support system consultation, linkage with ongoing community services, social and recreational activities, discharge planning, and follow-up care (Stroul, 1988). Residential crisis services are used when it becomes necessary to temporarily remove people in crisis from their natural environments so that more intensive support, structure, and supervision can be provided during a period of stabilization. Residential crisis services also are used as respite beds when families need relief from the 24-hour-a-day responsibility of caring for a mental ill family member.

Income support and entitlements

Mental health services are funded in a variety of ways: through private health insurance, Medicaid and Medicare, direct allocations from the state, Social Security reimbursement through Supplemental Security Income (SSI) and Social Security and Disability Income (SSDI), housing subsidies, and other categorical programs (Mechanic, 1994). The complexity of reimbursement systems has led many agencies who serve people with mental illness to hire entitlement specialists to ensure that clients receive all the benefits for which they qualify. Mental health professionals need to be familiar with these support mechanisms for their clients.

Private insurance

Most private health insurance policies provide some coverage for both inpatient and outpatient mental health treatment. Coverage is almost always subject to special limits that are more restrictive than for general health care coverage. Inpatient costs are controlled by limits on days of care per admission or per year. Annual and lifetime limits on mental health care are common. Partial hospitalization or residential programs are sometimes covered, often with these benefits counting against the limit on inpatient days (Frank, Goldman, & McGuire, 1992).

Public sector insurance

Many people with severe and persistent mental illness quickly exhaust their private insurance benefits and must depend on the public sector for continuing mental health care. Others who for a variety of reasons have never been eligible for private insurance coverage also depend on publicly funded health insurance. The two major public insurance programs are Medicaid and Medicare. Important distinctions exist between the two programs. Medicaid is a social welfare program in which eligibility depends on certain income and disability criteria. Medicaid is partially state funded and partially federally funded. States have many options regarding eligibility criteria and covered benefits, which results in great variations in treatment options depending on the state in which a client resides. Medicare is a social

insurance program with eligibility based on prior contributions; it primarily finances health care services for people over 65 years old. Two other groups are eligible for Medicare coverage: recipients of Social Security Disability Insurance (SSDI) and people with end-stage kidney disease. Many people with severe mental illness who are younger than 65 years old are eligible for Medicare coverage through the SSDI exception because of their own contributions to Social Security while they were working or as dependents of people eligible for Social Security benefits. Unlike Medicaid, Medicare has a single set of rules governing all participants; the same eligibility and benefit criteria apply in all states (Rubin, 1987).

In addition to providing health care insurance, federal programs provide direct cash payments to people too disabled to work, including people with disabilities from mental illness. Supplemental Security Insurance (SSI) provides income for disabled people who are not eligible for SSDI.

Additional assistance can be provided through the food stamp program, a variety of housing programs, the supplemental food program for women, infants, and children (WIC), and other categorical programs.

The remaining components of a community support system are discussed in detail in other chapters. Client identification and outreach is discussed in Chapter 10, Case Management; protection and advocacy issues are discussed in Chapter 2, Legal and Ethical Issues, and Chapter 3, Family and Consumer Movements. Units 4, Intervention in the Community, and 5, Community Settings, are devoted to mental health treatment and intervention in specific settings.

COMMUNITY MENTAL HEALTH SERVICES FOR CHILDREN AND FAMILIES

During the past 2 decades the recognition that the public service sector is not adequately addressing the mental health needs of children has been increasing. Children and adolescents who receive public services are involved in many bureaucracies—education, social services, juvenile justice, and mental health—all of which have different regulations and many of which do not collaborate well. Problems encountered in the mental health service system for children are analogous in many ways to those encountered in the adult system (difficulties with continuity of care, lack of interagency cooperation, lack of a designated point of responsibility, and overreliance on institutional care). In 1984 NIMH responded to these system problems by initiating the Child and Adolescent Service System Program (CASSP) for young people with serious emotional problems. Modeled on the successful community support systems for adults with serious mental illness, CASSP is developing systems of care involving the five types of agencies designated by law to serve children—child welfare, mental health, public health, education, and juvenile justice.

According to England and Cole (1992), three basic assumptions drive the movement to create multiagency care systems for young people who are seriously emotionally disturbed:

1. The best treatment occurs in the natural setting of the child's family (or surrogate family) and the community.
2. Genuinely intensive care is possible in normal settings such as home and school.
3. Service delivery must be organized to respond consistently to the ever-changing needs of young clients who are growing and developing.

Model programs

The attempt to move away from overreliance on institutional care for children and adolescents with severe emotional disturbances has led to the development of family preservation programs. The goal of these intensive in-home intervention programs is to preserve the family unit while supporting the child through a period of crisis. Clinically trained professionals are available to work with these families 24 hours a day, 7 days a week. Chapter 22, Children and Adolescents, provides a detailed description of a family preservation program.

In those instances in which preservation of the family unit is impossible, alternatives to institutionalization are being developed. Therapeutic foster care that provides an intensive clinical treatment program along with the other services of traditional foster care is becoming more readily available. Group homes in which a small number of children or adolescents live in a home-like setting staffed by professionally trained counselors are growing in popularity.

System coordination

One of the most intractable barriers to developing a coherent care system for children and adolescents is that, unlike in the adult system, five types of agencies have legal responsibilities for children with serious emotional disturbances. The Robert Wood Johnson Foundation recently awarded grants to sites in eight states to develop coherent care systems involving child welfare, mental health, public health, education, juvenile justice, and private sector physical and mental health providers. Each site has an interagency steering committee, a system of long-term care management, in-home services, and an emergency response system; experimentation with innovative financing is common (England & Cole, 1992).

SPECIAL POPULATIONS

Every community includes people with mental illness whose illnesses are complicated by additional social stressors such as homelessness or incarceration, by being members of particularly vulnerable age groups such as children or the elderly, or by having a mental illness complicated by a second medical or psychiatric diagnosis such as HIV infection or substance abuse. In Unit 4, Intervention in the Community, a chapter is devoted to each of these groups that present substantial treatment challenges. A brief introduction to each of these special populations is provided in the following sections.

People who are homeless and mentally ill

A recent national survey on homelessness (Shlay & Rossi, 1994) reports that on average 25% to 30% of homeless people suffer varying degrees of mental illness. The remaining 75% are elderly or have experienced economic difficulties or family violence. The number of children counted among homeless people is rising rapidly. The survey results also note that a large segment of the population is "homeless vulnerable." Chapter 24, Homeless Persons with Mental Illness, discusses this population in detail.

People who are mentally ill and in jail

Torrey et al. (1992) studied the growing trend of incarcerating people with mental illness in local jails and pointed out the relationship between jails and homelessness: "Shelters and jails then comprise an institutional system between which many of the most seriously mentally ill individuals in the United States regularly migrate."

Remarkably little data is available on this phenomenon. Lamb and Grant (1982) are among the few researchers who have studied people with mental illness in jail. Using the Los Angeles jail system as their study site, they found that at the time of arrest, 37% of the men and 42% of the women had been living in homeless shelters, on the streets, or on the beach. Solomon et al. (1992) found similar data in a study of the Philadelphia jail system. They found that 31% of the mentally ill inmates had been homeless at time of arrest. Chapter 26, Persons with Mental Illness in Jail, contains an in-depth discussion of this growing population.

People with mental illness and substance abuse

The phenomenon of concurrent major mental illness and substance abuse disorder is now widely recognized (Drake et al., 1991). At least 50% of the 1.5 to 2 million Americans with severe mental illness abuse illicit drugs or alcohol, compared with 15% of the general population (Ridgely, Osher, & Talbott, 1986). This finding is consistent with a study by Reiger et al. (1990) that found that 47% of people with a lifetime diagnosis of schizophrenia or schizophreniform disorder have met the criteria for some form of substance abuse or dependence. The structural separation of addiction services and mental health services has been a barrier to comprehensive treatment. Recognition of this system problem has led in the past few years to the development of model programs that apply existing psychiatric and substance abuse treatment technology concomitantly. Chapter 23, Persons with Mental Illness and Substance Abuse, discusses working with clients with a dual diagnosis of mental illness and substance abuse.

People with mental illness and HIV infection or AIDS

The impact of HIV infection and AIDS on people with chronic mental illness has received little attention in the psychiatric literature, although psychiatric impairment, substance abuse, and intermittent homelessness put this population at risk for HIV infection. Chapter 25, Persons with Serious Mental Illness and the Issue of HIV Disease, includes a detailed discussion of an educational intervention with this at-risk population.

Children and elderly people with mental illness

Some people with mental illness are particularly vulnerable because of their age. Traditionally, women of childbearing age, infants, and children were considered the most vulnerable members of society (Clemen-Stone, Eigsti, & McGuire, 1995). Information on primary prevention programs for these groups is provided in Chapter 5, Levels of Prevention. Chapter 16, Schools, discusses mental health care in the schools; Chapter 22, Children and Adolescents, contains information on child abuse and neglect, delinquency, and substance abuse.

Almost 31 million people over 65 years old live in the United States (U.S. Bureau of the Census, 1992). Research by the National Institute of Mental

Health estimates that as many as 25% of older people in the community have some degree of mental impairment and could benefit from mental health services. Dementia and depression are significant problems and are discussed in detail in Chapter 27, Elderly Persons with Mental Illness. Of elderly people in the community, 70% describe their health as excellent, very good, or good (American Association of Retired Persons, 1988). Given elderly people's generally positive feelings about their health, primary prevention programs that enhance wellness and help prevent mental disorders are particularly important. Chapter 5, Levels of Prevention, contains information on preventive programs focused on helping elderly people successfully negotiate the developmental tasks and life changes of old age.

THE ROLE OF NURSES IN COMMUNITY MENTAL HEALTH CENTERS

Establishing and maintaining a significant presence in community mental health has not been without problems for psychiatric nurses.

- The early emphasis in community mental health on primary prevention, consultation, and psychotherapy with clients who had problems with activities of daily living rather than major mental illnesses attracted psychologists and social workers rather than more medically oriented professionals such as nurses and psychiatrists.
- A chronic shortage of psychiatric nurses to staff public and private mental hospitals existed, and thus any impetus for psychiatric nurses to move into community mental health was missing.
- The majority of the mental health professionals employed in community mental health centers had graduate degrees in their disciplines. Very few psychiatric nurses were prepared at the graduate level. The Psychiatric and Mental Health Nursing division of the American Nurses Association, which encourages graduate preparation for the specialty, was not established until 1966, 3 years after the passage of the community mental health center legislation.

- Salaries in community mental health centers were not competitive with those earned by psychiatric nurses in hospitals, a further disincentive to leave the hospital setting.

As deinstitutionalization progressed during the 1970s and pressure was exerted on community mental health centers to care for thousands of former patients with chronic mental illness, the centers began to operate under a more medically oriented model. Psychiatric nurses were needed to administer and monitor the psychotropic medications that became common treatment modalities. At the same time the National Institute of Mental Health encouraged advanced preparation for psychiatric nurses by providing training grants. Advanced practice psychiatric nurses with skills in mental and physical health assessment, psychotherapy, case management, medication management, and client education should have fit well on interdisciplinary teams. However, achieving parity in numbers and levels of responsibility with the other core mental health disciplines in community mental health centers continues to be a struggle for psychiatric nurses. Three areas have especially inhibited fuller participation in the centers:

1. Confusion exists on the part of community mental health center administrators regarding the many levels of educational credentialing of nurses (Caverly, 1991). Some community mental health center administrators embrace the "a nurse is a nurse is a nurse" theme. Their interest is in licensure not degrees or credentialing. Nurses must educate administrators about the expanded roles of the advanced practice nurse. One effective way to do this is to place graduate level nursing students in these settings for their clinical practicum.

2. Severe economic inhibitions currently preclude a larger nursing presence in community mental health centers. Although salaries in the centers are generally lower for all disciplines than salaries in institutional settings, this discrepancy is particularly true for nursing salaries.

   Third-party reimbursement is a second economic issue that impacts nursing in community mental health centers. Psychiatrists, psychologists, and social workers have a long history of reimbursement by third-party payers. Nursing is still struggling with this issue. As pointed out by Smith et al. in Chapter 20, Rural Settings, substantial variations occur from state to state; psychiatric nurses must be well aware of the reimbursement regulations in their states and be prepared to lobby for change when necessary.

3. Historical factors have inhibited the movement of nurses into administrative and management positions in community mental health centers. Social workers and psychologists were the early leaders in the community mental health center movement and quickly moved into management positions. This tradition has continued and although nurses have made progress in this area, management positions continue to be dominated by disciplines other than nursing.

In spite of these barriers to full participation by psychiatric nurses in community mental health centers, examples of innovative programs initiated by psychiatric nurses in the centers abound. Borelli and DeLuca (1993) describe a nurse-coordinated day treatment program that stresses client education on physical and mental health and principles of self-care. Chapter 20, Rural Settings, describes an outreach program for the rural elderly people developed and implemented under nursing leadership at a community mental health center in Iowa. COSTAR, a community mobile treatment unit that is part of a community mental health center in Baltimore, is comprised of a multidisciplinary team in which psychiatric nurses play prominent roles (Primm & Houck, 1990).

SUMMARY

A book on mental health nursing in the community written 20 years ago would have been devoted almost entirely to community mental health centers. The fact that this book has one chapter out of 27 devoted to the subject shows the extent to which the range of possibilities for mental health service delivery has expanded in our soci-

ety. Though fiscal and legislative mandates have limited the mission of community mental health centers to the treatment of people with severe and persistent mental illness, the legacy of the centers has been their pioneering of new ways of thinking about treatment and service delivery. CMHCs pioneered the application of public health ideas of "high risk," "at risk," crisis, and transition situations to mental health. The idea that environment has at least as powerful an influence on mental health as intrapsychic processes was developed by the centers. The expansion of service delivery beyond the hospital and outpatient clinic to where people live—in their homes, in schools, and on the streets, and new methods of service delivery such as case management were community mental health center innovations.

As community mental health centers became the most common locus of treatment for people with chronic mental illness, the centers pioneered innovative rehabilitation techniques. Social skills training, psychoeducation, partial hospitalization, and intensive case management became common treatment modalities. When the need for structured living arrangements for some people with severe mental illness became apparent, the centers were at the forefront of experimentation with various types of rehabilitative housing.

Community mental health centers will likely continue to be the "lead" agencies for the care of people with severe mental illness who depend on the public sector for services. Changes in reimbursement mechanisms in the public sector will greatly influence the delivery of services to center clients. Capitated mental health programs for Medicaid beneficiaries are developing in various forms across the country (Dangerfield & Betit, 1993). Under managed care systems, community mental health centers will be able to use treatment modalities that in the past would not have been covered under Medicaid fee-for-service reimbursement. Residential treatment, home care, supported housing, and day treatment programs will proliferate in community mental health centers as alternatives to inpatient treatment are sought.

REFERENCES

American Association of Retired Persons (AARP). (1988). *A profile of older Americans.* Washington, DC: Author.

Anderson, C., Reiss, D., & Hogarty, G. (1986). *Schizophrenia and the family* (Ch. 2). New York: Guilford Press.

Bachrach, L. L. (1987). *Consensus and issues report on a conference to define the chronically mentally ill.* Rockville, MD: National Institute of Mental Health.

Borelli, M., & DeLuca, E. (1993). Physical health promotion in psychiatric day treatment. *Journal of Psychosocial Nursing and Mental Health Services, 31,* 15-18.

Caverly, S. (1991). Coordinating psychosocial nursing care across treatment settings. *Journal of Psychosocial Nursing and Mental Health Services, 29,* 26-29.

Clemen-Stone, S., Eigsti, D., & McGuire, S. (1995). *Comprehensive family and community health nursing,* (4th ed.) (Ch. 14). St. Louis: Mosby.

Dangerfield, D., & Betit, R. (1993). Managed mental health care in the public sector. In W. Goldman, & S. Feldman (Eds.), *Managed mental health care* (New Directions for Mental Health Services, No. 59) (pp. 67-80). San Francisco: Jossey-Bass.

Drake, R., McLauglin, P., Pepper, B., & Minkoff, K. (1991). Dual diagnosis of major mental illness and substance abuse disorder: An overview. In K. Minkoff, & R. E. Drake (Eds.), *Dual diagnosis of major mental illness and substance disorder* (New Directions for Mental Health Services, No. 50) (pp. 3-12). San Francisco: Jossey-Bass.

England, M., & Cole, R. (1992). Building systems of care for youth with serious mental illness. *Hospital and Community Psychiatry, 43,* 630-633.

Federal Register. (1985, August 28). Federal old-age, survivors, and disability insurance: Listing of impairments—Mental disorders: Final Rule 50 (167: 35038-35070).

Foley, H., & Sharfstein, S. (1983). *Madness and government* (Ch. 5). Washington, DC: American Psychiatric Press.

Frank, R., Goldman, H., & McGuire, T. (1992, Summer). A model mental health benefit in private health insurance. *Health Affairs,* 98-117.

Hatfield, A., & Lefley, H. (1993). *Surviving mental illness.* New York: Guilford Press.

Lamb, H., & Grant, R. (1982). The mentally ill in an urban county jail. *Archives of General Psychiatry, 39,* 17-22.

Liberman, R., Massel, H., Mosk, M., & Wong, S. (1985). Social skills training for chronic mental patients. *Hospital and Community Psychiatry, 36,* 396-403.

Mechanic, D. (1994). Establishing mental health priorities. *Milbank Quarterly, 72,* 501-514.

Mosher, L., & Burti, L. (1994). *Community mental health* (Ch. 9). New York: W. W. Norton.

National Institute of Mental Health, Department of Health and Human Services. (1987). *Toward a model plan for a comprehensive community based mental health system.* Washington, DC: U.S. Government Printing Office.

PCMH. (1978). *Report to the President from the President's Commission on Mental Health.* Washington, DC: U.S. Government Printing Office.

Primm, A., & Houck, J. (1990). COSTAR: Flexibility in urban community mental health. In N. Cohen (Ed.), *Psychiatry takes to the streets* (Ch. 6). New York: Guilford Press.

Raskin, V., & Miller, N. (1993). The epidemiology of the comorbidity of psychiatric and addictive disorders: A critical review. *Journal of Addictive Diseases, 3,* 45-67.

Reiger, D., Farmer, M., Rae, D., Locke, B., Keith, S., Judd, L., & Goodwin, F. (1990). Comorbidity of mental disorders with alcohol and other drug abuse. *Journal of the American Medical Association, 264,* 2511-2518.

Ridgely, M., Osher, F., & Talbott, J. (1986). *Chronically mentally ill young adults with substance abuse problems: Treatment and training issues.* Baltimore: Mental Health Policy Studies, University of Maryland School of Medicine.

Rubin, J. (1987). Financing care for the seriously mentally ill. In D. Mechanic (Ed.), *Improving mental health services: What the social sciences can tell us* (New Directions for Mental Health Services, No. 36) pp. 107-116. San Francisco: Jossey-Bass.

Schinnar, A., Rothbard, A., Kantor, R., & Adams, K. (1990). Crossing state lines of mental illness. *Hospital and Community Psychiatry, 41,* 756-760.

Shlay, A., & Rossi, P. (1994). Social science research and contemporary studies of homelessness. *Annual Review of Sociology, 18,* 129-160.

Solomon, P., Draine, J., Marcenco, M., & Myerson, A. (1992). Homelessness in a mentally ill urban jail population. *Hospital and Community Psychiatry, 43,* 169-171.

Stroul, B. (1988). Residential crisis services: A review. *Hospital and Community Psychiatry, 39,* 1095-1099.

Torrey, E., Stieber, J., Ezekiel, J., Wolfe, S., Sharfstein, J., Noble, J., & Flynn, L. (1992). *Criminalizing the seriously mentally ill: The abuse of jails as mental hospitals.* Joint report of the National Alliance for the Mentally Ill and Public Citizens Health Research Group. Washington, DC.

U.S. Bureau of the Census. (1992). *Sixty-five plus in America.* Washington, D.C.: U.S. Government Printing Office.

U.S. Office of Special Education and Rehabilitation Services. (1984). *Digest of data on persons with disabilities.* Washington, DC: U.S. Government Printing Office.

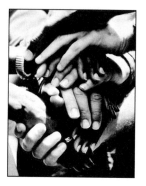

Chapter 18

Partial Hospital Programs

Barbara L. Garrison

The history of partial hospitalization or "day programs" began in Russia in 1933 (Kennedy, 1992). The first psychiatric day hospital in the Western hemisphere was developed in 1946 at the Allen Memorial Institute of Psychiatry in Montreal, Canada. It wasn't until the early 1960s that partial hospitalization became a popular treatment modality for people with serous mental illness in the United States (Goldman & Arvanitakis, 1981). Today partial hospitalization programs have become an important part of the continuum of care for mental health and chemical dependency treatment.

This chapter looks at the history of partial hospitalization programs (PHP) and their evolution since their inception in the United States. The economics of partial hospitalization also will be explored. The staggering costs of health care in this country have resulted in significant changes in the way health care is delivered. By 1996 more than 95% of the people in the United States will have their health care benefits managed through a health maintenance organization (HMO), a preferred provider organization (PPO), or some other form of managed care (Lefkovitz, 1991). Included

in these numbers are those who receive federally funded entitlements such as Medicare and Medicaid. Mental health and chemical dependency programs will be no exception. Nurses must know how to maximize reimbursement for partial hospitalization services; therefore an approach for successfully negotiating with payers also is included.

The role of the nurse in a PHP is examined. For many psychiatric nurses, providing treatment to seriously ill, often high-risk individuals in a PHP instead of an inpatient unit has meant a radical paradigm shift. The diverse needs of clients living in community settings and attending partial hospital programs require that staff be knowledgeable about financial entitlement, housing opportunities, and community support systems in addition to psychiatric treatment. A recent national survey of partial hospital programs indicated that master's-level counselors and social workers and bachelor's-level mental health workers constitute the core full-time service staffs in most programs (Culhane, Hadley, & Kiser, 1994). The ways in which nurses can increase their participation in this important part of the mental health continuum of care will be discussed.

A BRIEF HISTORY OF PARTIAL HOSPITALIZATION

Two different types of partial hospitalization programs have proliferated over the past 2 decades and dominate the field: day hospitals and psychosocial rehabilitation centers (Mosher & Burti, 1994). Because the terms "day hospital," *partial hospital* and *psychosocial rehabilitation programs* often are used interchangeably, considerable confusion remains about the meaning of these terms. Mosher and Burti (1994) define day hospitals and partial hospital programs as medically oriented with a focus on providing specific treatments such as medication and individual, group, and family therapy in the context of a highly organized, structured program format. These programs are similar to inpatient programs, without the room and board provided by hospitals, hence the use of the term *day hospital* or *partial hospital*. Because of their medical orientation, partial hospital programs usually are eligible for third-party reimbursement. They tend to be best suited for a subset of clients who are undergoing a temporary loss of social competence but who have well-established occupations and involved families. Psychosocial rehabilitation programs on the other hand have a rehabilitation orientation, tend to have severely socially and vocationally disabled psychiatric clients, and focus on the acquisition or restoration of social and vocational skills. These programs are discussed in detail in Chapter 12, Psychosocial Rehabilitation. Partial hospital or day hospital programs are the focus of this chapter.

Partial hospital programs and psychosocial rehabilitation centers grew out of different cultures. A brief history of the evolution of these programs will aid in understanding their differences and similarities. In 1963 the United States Congress passed the Mental Retardation Facilities and Community Mental Health Centers Construction Act. This Act mandated and provided funds to establish community mental health centers to serve psychiatric patients (including children, adolescents, adults, older people, and chemically dependent populations). The Act specified five services that had been determined essential for deinstitutionalized people with serious mental illnesses: inpatient treatment, outpatient treatment, emergency services, partial hospitalization, and consultation and education. These early PHPs primarily served individuals with long-term chronic mental illnesses. Community mental health centers attempted to provide a network of programs to provide the necessary support. Sheltered workshops, group homes, and crisis hot lines are examples of other programs that were created to help keep people out of the hospital and living successfully in the community. However, partial hospitalization programs were a major focus of the community mental health centers during the 1970s and promoted community-based care and rehabilitation for individuals discharged from state mental hospitals. The records indicate there were approximately 2000 PHPs in the United States and United Kingdom in 1980 (NIMH, 1984).

Most of the community mental health center PHPs used a rehabilitation model designed to help patients make the transition safely from state mental institutions to living productive lives in the community. The goals of these PHPs were to provide psychosocial skill development and maintenance of functioning within the community. A typical program day focused on activities of daily living (learning to use public transportation, medication education, shopping, cooking, hygiene, social skills, and recreational activities). Community mental health center staff also provided linkages for these former patients by establishing relationships with sheltered workshops, public transportation, and public housing. Community mental health centers provided the ongoing support clients would need to continue to be successful outside the walls of the institution. Providers discovered that treating people in PHPs minimized family disruption, reduced social stigma, and fostered less dependence on the treatment staff. Clients valued the autonomy and social support engendered by the programs.

When federal and state funds began to shrink in the late 1970s, community mental health centers had to turn to other sources of revenue. Programs were developed to attract a higher functioning group of individuals (including homemakers and business professionals) who could afford to pay for mental health or chemical dependency treatment. Services to seriously and persistently mentally ill clients were reduced.

However, as state institutions continued to downsize and bed availability continued to shrink, community mental health centers came under considerable pressure to develop alternatives to inpatient treatment. Through the leadership of NIMH, community support programs (CSPs) for those persons with severe and persistent mental illness were developed in all 50 states. The purpose of CSPs was to develop support networks for individual clients. Psychosocial rehabilitation programs, along with case management and supervised residential programs, have all emerged as principal components of community support systems.

In the 1960s some mental health professionals began to experiment with various PHP models, identifying them as *workshops, educational models, therapeutic community approaches, behavioral models,* and *"eclectic" programs,* to name just a few. These mental health providers discovered the modality worked with various age groups struggling with a wide range of emotional or chemical dependency problems (Dibello et al., 1982):

Most studies focused on patients over 18 years of age, who were not imminently suicidal, violent, or without night supervision of family or significant other. . . . Other patients excluded from study were those who exhibited antisocial behaviors, were addicted to drugs, were severely mentally retarded, or were suffering from organic brain syndrome.

In 1980 a Task Force on Partial Hospitalization wrote the first definition of PH (Casarino, Wilner, & Maxey, 1982):

Partial Hospitalization is an ambulatory treatment program that includes the major diagnostic, medical, psychiatric, psychosocial, and prevocational treatment modalities designed for patients with serious mental disorders who require coordinated intensive, comprehensive, and multidisciplinary treatment not

provided in an outpatient clinic setting. It allows for a more flexible and less restrictive treatment program by offering an alternative to inpatient treatment.

Partial hospitalization was evolving and quickly becoming the preferred treatment modality for many individuals. The successes of people treated in PHPs created a demand for more programs. Programs began to emerge that were designed to work with higher functioning individuals who had become impaired by a significant alteration in their day-to-day functioning. Individuals treated in these new PHPs were typically diagnosed with depression, anxiety, panic attacks, addictions or dependency on drugs or alcohol, and phobias. This increased use of short-term crisis-oriented partial hospital programs generated the need for a method to assess the appropriateness of this type of PHP both for potential referral sources and for the PHP staff faced with admission decisions.

To meet this need, a "Day Therapy Appropriateness Scale" was designed and tested for validity and reliability by Lefkovitz (1982). The scale identified seven critical areas to be considered in helping to determine the appropriateness of an individual for PHP. Individuals who score well on the following dimensions are most likely to have a successful experience in a PHP:

1. Duration of the problem
2. Behavior
3. Suicide or homicide potential
4. Alcohol or drug involvement
5. Motivation
6. Support systems
7. Transportation

Figure 18-1 presents the complete scale and instructions for scoring.

Partial hospitalization was changing from its original definition. This created tension between some treatment professionals who wanted to preserve the original rehabilitation model designed to serve people with serious and persistent mental illness and others who saw an opportunity to evolve an acute, stabilization model to serve a different population. The new models were not

Patient's name _____ Age _____

Person completing scale _____ Date _____

Directions: Rate the patient on each of the seven items listed below. For each item select the point value which most accurately describes the patient. In some instances, a point value between those provided might be most appropriate. Place the appropriate point value in the item score column to the right.

	Point values	Item score

1. Duration of problem
   a. Current episode represents recent crisis. No history of previous difficulties ...   5
   b. Current episode represents recent crisis but patient has experienced similar
      difficulties in the past   3   1. _____
   c. Current episode is reflection of chronic or long-term problem—no recent
      crisis   1

2. Behavior
   a. No overt psychotic or disruptive acting-out behavior present   5
   b. Psychotic behavior present but no disruptive behavior evident   3   2. _____
   c. Disruptive, acting-out behavior present   1

3. Suicide or homicide potential
   a. Little suicidal or homicidal ideation—potential low.   5
   b. Suicidal or homicidal ideation present but no recent attempt and no specific
      plan   3   3. _____
   c. Recent attempt and continued ideation with plan—potential high   1

4. Alcohol or drug involvement
   a. No history of addiction or dependency   5
   b. History of addiction or dependency but not a recent problem.   3   4. _____
   c. Recent problem of addiction or dependency   1

5. Motivation
   a. Patient is highly motivated to be in treatment   5
   b. Patient has adequate motivation to be in treatment   3   5. _____
   c. Patient has little motivation to be in treatment   1

6. Support system
   a. Lives with emotionally supportive family, spouse, or close friend   5
   b. Lives in somewhat supportive environment *or* lives alone and has emotion-
      ally supportive family or friends living nearby   3   6. _____
   c. Does not live with emotionally supportive family or friends and none living
      nearby   1

7. Transportation
   a. Able to drive a car to the Center each day   3
   b. Can arrange to get ride to and from the Center each day or is willing to take
      public transportation   2   7. _____
   c. Transportation to and from the Center is uncertain   1

Item score total   _____

21–33 points—Appropriate candidate for day therapy
17–20 points—Questionable candidate for day therapy
Under 17 points—Poor candidate for day therapy

Figure 18–1. Day therapy appropriateness scale. NOTE: Because of recent developments in the field since original publication, this scale should be used only as a guide for assessment and not as depicted above.
(Modified from "The Assessment of Suitability for Partial Hospitalization. The Day Treatment Appropriateness Scale," by P. Lefkovitz, 1982, *International Journal of Partial Hospitalization, 1,* 45-47.)

meant to replace the original rehabilitation models; rather they were designed to provide greater access to people who needed intense mental health treatment but who didn't need 24-hour care.

The American Association for Partial Hospitalization (AAPH) formally incorporated in 1979. It began as the Federation of Partial Hospitalization Study Groups in the mid 1960s, which over the past 3 decades became a trade association with more than 1000 members. In 1991 AAPH published its first set of standards and guidelines for adult programs. In 1992 the child and adolescent standards and guidelines were published; in 1993 the *Standards and Guidelines for Geriatric Partial Hospitalization* were completed and published. These standards can be obtained by writing to the American Association for Partial Hospitalization, 301 North Fairfax Street, Suite 109, Alexandria, VA 20314, telephone (703) 836-2274.

MARKET FORCES

One of the primary focuses of the 1994 presidential campaign was the high costs of health care in the United States. In 1994 health care expenditures in the United States were estimated to be more than 14% of the gross national product, a significant increase from 9.1% in 1980. Psychiatric and substance abuse services were identified as the major contributors to the increase (Fuller, 1994). Employers, providers, payers, and consumers urged Congress to develop a plan that would ensure accountability and contain costs. The insurance industry effected the current changes by managing the care of beneficiaries and carefully scrutinizing the use of mental health and chemical dependency benefits. By managing the care people receive, the lengths of inpatient and outpatient stays have been reduced. Payers have significantly impacted the number of hospital beds available for inpatient treatment. As the market for behavioral health care has continued to evolve, more emphasis has been placed on the need for short-term, high-quality, efficient, and cost-

effective programs and services to meet the mental health and chemical dependency needs of a diverse American population. The demand for more community-based and in-home services has supported the development of an ambulatory, continuum of care model of treatment that can respond to the wide range of health care needs of all Americans.

In 1993 AAPH published a position paper in response to the need to define the ambulatory continuum of mental health care (Kiser, Lefkovitz, & Kennedy, 1993). The proposed paradigm confirms the need for a continuum of care that can respond to what will be best for the patient, from traditional 24-hour inpatient care to outpatient care to a variety of programs described as intermediate care. The authors proposed some novel concepts: "interventions [should] be defined by function rather than setting" and "services [should] be organized around the individual needs of the patient rather than the practice patterns of the provider." Supporting the use of a continuum of ambulatory care allows the client to be served at the most appropriate and cost-effective level of care (Kiser et al., 1993). Partial hospitalization is one example of a program that fits into a larger scheme known as a *seamless continuum of care*. A continuum of ambulatory mental health care promotes the treatment of all individuals in the least restrictive setting. It also promotes flexibility and movement across a range of diverse programs and services. The promotion and acceptance of levels of care has broadened the creative thinking of providers who are no longer faced with only two choices—inpatient or outpatient treatment. The promotion of a continuum of care has encouraged providers to work together on behalf of clients. PHPs exist in general hospitals, freestanding facilities, managed care offices, physicians' practices, and other nontraditional settings. Providers who have chosen to limit their scope of practice to a couple of modalities (such as outpatient and PH or inpatient and PH) have formed partnerships with the community to address the full range of needs of individuals. For example,

PHP clients who feel unsafe at the end of a treatment day can now be admitted overnight to a 23-hour crisis bed. Often this 23-hour bed provides the structure and safety the individual needs to return to the PHP the next day. Other individuals who would have been hospitalized because of a deteriorating clinical condition can now safely be admitted to a residential treatment program.

THE SHORT-TERM PARTIAL HOSPITALIZATION MODEL

AAPH defines partial hospitalization programs for adults as (Block & Lefkovitz, 1995):

A time-limited, ambulatory, active treatment program that offers therapeutically intensive, coordinated, and structured clinical services within a therapeutic milieu. While specific program variables may differ, all partial hospitalization programs pursue the goal of stabilization with the intention of averting inpatient hospitalization or reducing the length of a hospital stay.

According to AAPH, partial hospitalization is to be used in the treatment of clients as an alternative to 24-hour inpatient care or to prevent inpatient treatment. No longer is it conceived solely as a singular identifiable treatment modality designed to serve a particular set of individuals within a limited number of diagnostic categories in a community mental health center. PHPs provide mental health care and alcohol and drug dependency treatment using an acute, stabilization model.

One of the most recent developments in the field has been the short-term partial hospital program for individuals who need stabilization of their acute crisis but who don't require 24-hour inpatient treatment. Lefkovitz (1988) describes his model of partial hospitalization in a book titled *Differing Approaches to Partial Hospitalization*. He acknowledges the "market forces" that have contributed to the success of these short-term programs. Short-term, crisis stabilization PHPs are cost effective and promote a true partnership with the clients being served. Insurance companies, health maintenance organizations, and preferred provider organizations are increasingly supportive of PHPs as alternatives to costly inpatient care as well as a way to provide transitional care for individuals who were in inpatient programs. People in short-term programs are typically individuals with problems so severe that they interfere with their ability to function day to day. The clients in short-term programs are amenable to treatment and can reasonably be expected to work through this temporary crisis.

Lefkovitz (1988) describes two types of short-term programs—palliative and restorative. The first is similar to the original rehabilitative models of the early community mental health centers. The second model is designed for individuals who don't have a debilitating, chronic mental illness such as schizophrenia. Individuals who are successfully treated in a short-term, restorative PHP usually present with symptoms associated with depression, grief and loss, or financial problems. Some may be struggling with some major life change such as retirement. These stressors significantly interfere with their ability to attend to day-to-day responsibilities such as going to work, caring for children, getting dressed, eating, or bathing. They may become isolated and withdrawn or overly dependent on others. They often feel helpless and hopeless and may allude to thoughts of suicide. No place seems safe, and they appear confused, indifferent, moody, tearful, or unresponsive. Some may have sought help from a counselor or therapist only to find that seeing someone on an individual basis once a week is not helping. Perhaps the therapist has agreed to see the client two or three times a week. When the therapist begins to realize the client needs more help than the therapist can offer on an outpatient basis, a referral to the next intensive level of care, PHP, becomes an important consideration.

A network of supportive family and friends is important for success. Individuals in short-term, restorative PHPs are asked to identify family members, friends, or acquaintances who will provide positive support for the efforts they are making toward change.

Quality short-term, restorative models adhere to the standards and guidelines developed by AAPH. Although these standards and guidelines are not prescriptive, they do provide a framework around which to build a program that provides the intensity needed to overcome the problems that brought the client in for treatment. Typically, a short-term program operates a minimum of 5 days a week, and 6 hours each day. This allows the PHP staff to see the client every day, teaching new skills and evaluating their effective use. It allows staff to continue to monitor the client for potential suicide risk. Proponents of PH also have found that the client's continued interaction with family and friends helps reduce recidivism. As Lefkovitz (1988) points out, PH also offers the client "the maximum opportunity to develop trust and an effective therapeutic alliance with the program."

A model short-term partial hospital program

An example of a short-term, restorative model in a general hospital is used here to help further illustrate the benefit of PH.

Treatment planning

From the first day of admission the client is actively engaged in developing his or her treatment plan, including goals and objectives. Each client's treatment is individualized, and the goals and objectives are recorded on the treatment plan. The treatment plan is the road map for the client's recovery and is reviewed daily by the treatment staff. The treatment plan is a working document, and the client is encouraged to participate in weekly treatment plan review updates. Participation promotes the involvement of clients in their own care and treatment and keeps the staff focused on the goals of treatment.

Staffing

Consistent staffing is important to the success of short-term, restorative PHPs. Predictable, consistent treatment staff provide a safe place for clients to freely express themselves and for clients

to get to know one another. Staff should be qualified through education and experience to lead the various groups; clients benefit greatly from staff who are knowledgeable about group dynamics and group process (Lefkovitz, 1988). Each client is assigned a primary counselor (or case manager) and a primary nurse. The primary counselor is responsible for completing the psychosocial assessment. The nurse is responsible for the medical needs assessment. Medication management becomes the primary responsibility of the PHP client. Clients are encouraged to bring only those doses they will need during the day. The primary nurse records the client's medications in the medical record and keeps the physician informed of any reactions.

Milieu

There is a great deal of discussion about the importance of the client milieu in short-term, restorative PHPs (Lefkovitz, 1988). *Milieu* is defined as "a cohesive, consistent, therapeutic environment, created either within a program or community or through coordination of people, space, materials, equipment and activities" (Kiser et al., 1994). Most short-term, restorative PHPs are milieu driven and Lefkovitz (1988) even goes so far as to say that the milieu is the most important client being treated.

Daily activities

Short-term, restorative PHPs offer clients an integrated daily structured schedule of activities. The primary counselor or case manager and the primary nurse share responsibility for the ongoing care of the client. A tentative discharge date is set, and the client and treatment staff agree on an attendance schedule. The client is given a copy of the attendance schedule and the weekly schedule of activities. Table 18-1 presents an example of a daily schedule.

Common needs and recurrent client issues are identified at the beginning of each treatment day. The day begins with a Goal setting group and community meeting. The PHP staff listen for the

Table 18-1.   St. Vincent Stress Center day therapy program daily schedule

	MONDAY	TUESDAY	WEDNESDAY	THURSDAY	FRIDAY
8:00				Multi-family day group	
9:00	Community meeting and rounds	Community meeting and rounds	Managing your time and your life		Community meeting and rounds
9:30				Transition to group	
10:00	Group therapy	Group therapy	Group therapy	Group therapy	Group therapy
11:00					
12:00	Lunch	Lunch	Lunch	Lunch	Lunch
1:00	Goal setting	Mental health concepts	Self-esteem group	Life-styles	Communication group
2:00	Rational emotive therapy group	Coping skills group	Escape to reality	Assertiveness group	Wrap-up group
3:00	End of day	End of day	End of day	End of day	End of day

Courtesy St. Vincent Hospital and Health Care Center, Indianapolis, Indiana.

common issues and concerns being expressed by the clients. These issues drive the group process throughout a treatment day. Interconnected group therapies provide the context for addressing the core group issue in a variety of ways. For example, if the treatment team decides the overall theme for the day should focus on grief and loss, then the treatment day begins with a didactic or teaching group and staff educate clients about issues associated with grief and loss. Group psychotherapy provides an opportunity for clients and staff to interact, and for input, feedback, and support. Afternoon therapy typically consists of expressive groups, such as art, music, and recreation or activities.

At the end of each treatment day the client group meets with the treatment staff to review the day. Through the group process the treatment staff determine how well the clients have incorporated the teaching and the experiences of the day's activities. This final group also provides an opportunity for the staff to determine some potential themes for the next treatment day. Treatment staff

monitor clients' treatment plans and assess daily the progress toward achieving goals.

Length of stay is determined by the treatment staff with input from the client. Typically, a client is in treatment all day, every day for the first week or two. As the crisis is stabilized and the level of functioning improved, the treatment team considers a reduction in the number of days or hours each day the client will attend. This allows the client to gradually make the transition back to work, home, or school, and when appropriate to continue the work begun by pursuing outpatient treatment.

A minimum attendance of 2 full days a week is required if clients are to continue to achieve the maximum benefit from participation in the program. The number of clients who participate in the program on a part-time schedule should be limited because too many part-time clients can create an ineffective milieu (Lefkovitz, 1988).

Schedule changes are negotiated with each client on the last treatment day each week. An average length of stay for adult clients in a short-term restorative program is between 15 and 20 visits or 3 to 4 weeks. Length of stay for older adults (ages 55 and older) may be 3 to 4 months.

On the day of discharge, clients and treatment staff review the discharge plan and recommendations for continuing care. A detailed discharge plan and a plan for continuing care are essential for optimal success after the client leaves the program. A formal "farewell" group provides the clients who are staying with an opportunity to give the person who is leaving feedback about the accomplishments he or she has made while in the program.

Aftercare

Aftercare or follow-up care is defined as a transitional period after discharge from the PHP, and may be part of an individual's continuing care plan. Aftercare groups are usually led by a member of the PHP staff and generally meet once a week for an hour. The treatment staff encourage clients to talk about any difficulties they are having since their discharge from the PHP. Most aftercare groups are time limited (for example, 4 to 6 weeks).

An indirect value of an aftercare group is the opportunity for current clients to hear about the successes of former clients. One example of a successful aftercare group is a weekly luncheon attended by current and former clients.

For individuals in an intermediate, transitional, or maintenance program designed to serve people with serious and persistent mental illness, an aftercare group is essential. An aftercare group also is important for older adults who benefit from "stepping down" from inpatient to partial hospitalization. As attendance is reduced in the partial hospitalization program from full time to part time, older adults generally benefit from consistent brief contact, which supports and promotes learning. Older adults are usually encouraged to attend at least 1 full day a week for "maintenance" purposes to ensure they are functioning optimally before they are discharged. After they have achieved their goals in attending 1 full day a week, they are encouraged to attend the aftercare group. The aftercare group provides the treatment staff an opportunity to ensure compliance with discharge plans and medication.

A formal aftercare group for higher functioning individuals discharged from an acute stabilization PHP is not as important as it is for other populations. Many of these clients are returning to work, school, or home and have identified resources in their community that will take the place of the aftercare group (such as ongoing weekly therapy with an individual therapist or counselor or participation in a support group).

QUALITY OF CARE AND OUTCOME ISSUES

A high-quality clinical program is essential to the success of a partial hospitalization program. Of equal importance is the financial viability of the program. Experience has shown that "selling" the value of partial hospitalization to insurance companies (HMOs, PPOs, and other third-party payers) for the treatment of a number of psychiatric conditions is becoming easier. Of primary importance to payers is the outcome for the client and the costs associated with the treatment provided. Is the program efficient (does it contain costs) and effective (does it reduce the utilization rate of the mental health or chemical dependency benefit)?

Measuring outcomes is one way of demonstrating a program's efficiency and effectiveness. Rigorous outcome research is still scant in partial hospital programs and most of it has involved the comparison of inpatient care and partial hospitalization for acutely ill, predominately schizophrenic clients (Herz, Herz, & Endicott, 1971; Gudeman et al., 1985; Creed, Black, & Anthony, 1990). Even fewer studies are available for nonschizophrenic clients (Tyrer & Remington, 1979; Dick, Sweeney, & Crombie, 1991). More recently, Piper et al. (1993) evaluated a partial hospital program for clients with affective and personality disorders using randomized assignment to either partial hospitalization or a control group. Seventeen outcome variables covering interpersonal functioning, symptoms, self-esteem, life satisfaction, and defensive functioning were examined. Treated clients showed significantly better outcomes for 7 of the 17 outcome variables including social dysfunction, interpersonal behavior, mood level, life satisfaction, self-esteem, and severity of symptoms.

ROLE OF THE NURSE IN PARTIAL HOSPITAL PROGRAMS

The success of a partial hospitalization program depends on many things. One is the ability of the clinical staff to work together and to see their differences as strengths that contribute to the common good of the whole program. The partial hospital psychiatric team is a multidisciplinary team that generally includes a psychiatrist, psychiatric nurse, social worker, activities therapist, and a vocational counselor. Each member of the team has traditional roles and functions in addition to some overlapping functions. Group psychotherapy is an important component of most partial hospital programs, and psychiatric nurses, social workers, and activity therapists may all function as group psychotherapists or lead activity groups.

Nurses are the sole health and wellness educators yet they collaborate with the recreation therapist to provide information regarding the importance of life-style changes in one's life, creating balance between home and workplace, the importance of rest and relaxation, and how to set healthy habits.

The transition from inpatient treatment to working in partial hospital programs results in more autonomy for the clinical staff. Less direct physician involvement occurs and more treatment decisions are made by the treatment team. As the treatment team develops and becomes more trusting of one another, team members come to depend on one another. The hallmark of a clinically sound treatment team is its ability to give and receive input and feedback from one another and to work together for the good of the clients.

When nurses and other professional staff begin working in the PHP structure, they often experience some anxiety. Without the structure inherent in an inpatient unit they feel more vulnerable and express concerns about the safety of clients and themselves. When a PHP client expresses suicidal thoughts or feelings, staff find they are uneasy supporting a client's departure at the end of a treatment day. Increased education and trust, containment skills, and safety plans help build a therapeutic relationship and confidence between the PHP staff and clients.

Another significant difference between inpatient treatment and partial hospitalization is the changed role of the physician. Most inpatient units require the physician to see clients daily; the PHP may only require the client to be seen weekly. The psychiatric nurse in partial hospital programs must then assume primary responsiblity to assess and identify medical issues that may be contributing to the client's condition. Some clients may have neglected their health care needs. The role of the nurse is essential in helping clients work through their feelings about health care providers. Nurses help clients by promoting self-care and wellness. They engage the client in getting better and in learning life skills by identifying the patterns in their lives.

Psychiatric nurses look at the whole continuum of health care and identify what they think the client needs now and in the future. Similar to a hospital discharge planner or case manager the nurse and the rest of the treatment team help clients identify and access the agencies and facilities in the community that will provide continuing care after they are discharged from the PHP. Examples of community resources include parenting groups, referral to a therapist for ongoing outpatient treatment, a food co-op, or a group home.

The primary modality of treatment in the PHP is group therapy. Some groups are generic to all populations but others need to be tailored to meet the needs of specific client populations. Group therapy is divided between teaching or didactic groups and expressive groups. Examples of teaching groups include assertiveness training, self-esteem, medication education, and nutrition education. Expressive group therapy includes groups such as art, music, recreation, and other activities.

The success of psychiatric nurses in an acute stabilization PHP depends on their ability to work through transference and countertransference issues with PHP clients. Clients with character disorders are challenging to work with in the PHP. These clients typically have issues with boundaries in relationships, tend to push limits, and require a consistent, team-oriented treatment approach. The therapeutic relationship takes on a new meaning as the clinical staff learn to identify and to work through their uncomfortable feelings when borderline clients "act out" their frustrations while attending the PHP. It takes practice and patience to develop the skills necessary to work successfully with a wide variety of disorders. PHPs encourage and support clients' efforts to do for themselves. One nurse commented she often had to stop and ask herself, "Am I doing too much for this client?"

Nurses who work in public health or in community settings are more capable now of identifying individuals who could benefit from admission to a PHP. Home health care and visiting nurses have information about potential signs and symptoms to watch for in individuals assigned to their care. Some of these signs include a noticeable decline in self-care, low self-esteem, expressions of hopelessness or helplessness, and other significant changes in behavior. Some first-time mothers may experience feelings of depression or feel overwhelmed by the demands of their newborn. Mothers with several children at home may be having a difficult time coping. Nurses who provide cholesterol screenings or blood pressure screenings at senior centers have identified recently widowed individuals who are not coping very well. Once active individuals who are faced with cardiac rehabilitation after surgery may be strug-

gling to adjust to a new way of life. Individuals under stress who have not learned how to deal with their stress in healthy ways also may be candidates for PH.

An assessment by the nurse may result in a referral to a mental health professional. Together they may decide the individual could benefit from a brief admission to a PHP. The PHP can provide the necessary structure to promote restoration to the individual's previous level of functioning. The PHP offers clients treatment without stripping them of their dignity. The PHP promotes a partnership with the client and a shared responsibility for getting well again.

SUMMARY

Partial hospitalization has come a long way in 50 years. It has evolved to become an important treatment modality in the full continuum of behavioral health care for every age group (children to older people). Partial hospitalization has proved significant for individuals who struggle with an emotional disorder of a severe and persistent nature as well as for those with an unexpected life crisis. PHPs also have proved effective treatment modalities for individuals with chemical dependency problems. Some PHPs emphasize specialty programming such as cardiac rehabilitation or treatment for eating disorders. Partial hospitalization helps people help themselves by engaging them in a highly structured program of therapeutic activities that promote self-care and education.

Partial hospitalization will become a partner with other forms of ambulatory treatment in the continuum of behavioral health care. The role of the nurse in mental health care will continue to evolve as well. The challenge for nurses will be to remain flexible and open to opportunities to work with a wide range of disciplines. Nurses will be as important to the success of partial hospitalization and other forms of ambulatory health care as other disciplines.

REFERENCES

Block, B., & Lefkovitz, P. (1995). American Association for Partial Hospitalization standards and guidelines for partial hospitalization. Adult programs. *Continuum: Developments in Ambulatory Mental Health Care, 2,* 95-103.

Casarino, J., Wilner, M., & Maxey, J. (1982). American Association for Partial Hospitalization standards and guidelines for partial hospitalization. *International Journal of Partial Hospitalization, 1,* 5-21.

Creed, F., Black, D., & Anthony, P. (1990). Randomized controlled trial of day patient versus inpatient psychiatric treatment. *British Medical Journal, 300,* 1033-1037.

Culhane, D., Hadley, T., & Kiser, L. (1994). A national profile of partial hospitalization programs. *Continuum: Developments in Ambulatory Mental Health Care, 1,* 81-93.

Dibello, G., Weitz, G., Poynter-Berg, D. & Yumark, J. (1982). *Handbook of partial hospitalization* (pp. 20-33). New York: Brunner/Mazel.

Dick, P., Sweeney, L., & Crombie, I. (1991). Controlled comparison of day-patient and out-patient treatment of persistent anxiety and depression. *British Journal of Psychiatry, 158,* 24-27.

Fuller, M. (1994). A new day: Strategies for managing psychiatric and substance abuse benefits. *Health Care Management Review,* 19: 20-24.

Goldman, D., & Arvanitakis, K. (1981). D. Ewen Cameron's day hospital and the day hospital movement. *Canadian Journal of Psychiatry, 26,* 365-368.

Gudeman, J., Dickey, B., Evans, A., & Shore, M. (1985). Four-year assessment of a day hospital-inn program as an alternative to inpatient hospitalization. *American Journal of Psychiatry, 142,* 1330-1333.

Herz, M., Herz, M., & Endicott, J. (1971). Day versus inpatient hospitalization: a controlled study. *American Journal of Psychiatry, 127,* 1371-1382.

Kennedy, L. (1992). Groups in the day hospital. In A. Alonso, & H. Swiller (Eds.), *Group therapy in clinical practice.* Washington, DC: American Psychiatric Press.

Kiser, L., Lefkovitz, P., & Kennedy, L. (1993). *The continuum of ambulatory mental health services: a position paper from the American Association for Partial Hospitalization.* Washington, DC: Author.

Kiser, L., Lefkovitz, P., Kennedy, L., & Knight, M. (1994). The continuum of ambulatory mental health services. *Continuum: Developments in Ambulatory Mental Health Care, 1,* 7-15.

Lefkovitz, P. (1982). The assessment of suitability for partial hospitalization: the day treatment appropriateness scale. *International Journal of Partial Hospitalization, 1,* 45-57.

Lefkovitz, P. (1988). The short-term program. In K. Goldberg (Ed.), *Differing approaches to partial hospitalization* (pp. 31-49). San Francisco: Jossey-Bass.

Lefkovitz, P. (1991). Enhancing third party coverage of partial hospitalization services. In *AAPH seminar series, 1995.* Washington, DC: American Association for Partial Hospitalization.

Mosher, L., & Burti, L. (1994). *Community mental health* (pp. 150-152). New York: Norton and Company.

National Institute of Mental Health. (1984). *The inventory of mental health organizations and general hospital mental health services.* Rockville, MD: Author.

Piper, W., Rosie, J., Azim, H., & Joyce, A. (1993). Randomized trial of psychiatric day treatment for patients with affective and personality disorders. *Hospital and Community Psychiatry, 44,* 757-763.

Tyrer, P., & Remington, M. (1979). Controlled comparison of day hospital and outpatient treatment for neurotic disorders. *Lancet, 1,* 1014-1016.

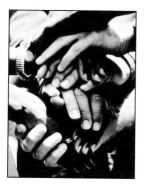

Chapter 19

Residential Treatment

Cynthia A. O'Neil and Philip S. Allard

TARGET GROUPS

Residential program models

Residential programs are a vital component of community-based care for people with serious and prolonged mental illness. The provision of safe, decent, and affordable housing and psychosocial residential treatment have resulted in decreased hospital admissions and improved functioning for this population. Even more important, clients have become viable members of their communities with opportunities for employment, socialization, and self-determination (Hawthorne, Fals-Stewart, & Lohr, 1994).

Since the early years of deinstitutionalization the number of residential programs has dramatically increased and program models have proliferated. In 1977 the number of residential treatment programs was reported as 300 nationwide; in comparison a recent survey identified more than 25,000 residential settings in the United States (Randolph, Ridgway, & Carling, 1991).

Program models have evolved from such restrictive settings as nursing and boarding homes to residential settings offering treatment services in a supervised environment. Residential treatment philosophy also has evolved from providing transitional services that require clients to move through a continuum of packaged programs to providing clients with permanent housing options and individually designed treatment and support plans that offer a more normalized life-style (Shern, Surles, & Waizer, 1989).

Residential program models can be operationally defined as *supported* or *supervised*. Supervised program models provide on-site staffing. They include group homes, board and care homes, halfway houses, respite programs, crisis programs, intermediate care facilities, nursing homes, and shelters. A nationwide survey of residential programs estimated that approximately 64% of clients resided in facilities using the supervised residential program model (Randolph et al., 1991).

Group homes and intermediate care facilities provide varying intensities of staffing and structure to clients. Although on-site staffing patterns may vary, provision is typically made for 24-hour crisis coverage. Services are facility based and provided on site. These homes generally house 4 to 16 clients. Group homes are currently the most prevalent residential models, providing housing for 23% of clients nationwide. Intermediate care facilities, which are the most prevalent models used for the developmentally disabled population, house only 4% of adults with serious mental illness (Randolph et al., 1991). Halfway houses are similar to group homes and intermediate care facilities but limit stays for clients who are expected to move on to more independent living.

Respite and crisis programs provide short-term housing for clients to prevent their rehospitalization and facilitate their referral to more permanent housing. Board and care homes, also referred to as *SROs* (single room occupancy housing), are generally residential hotels or rooming houses that rent out single rooms to clients and may offer other services such as housekeeping and meals. These programs and nursing homes offered alternatives to hospitalization in the early years of deinstitutionalization but were widely criticized for unsafe and unsanitary conditions and for abuse of clients by uncaring landlords. Advantages of SROs for clients include affordability and the opportunity for privacy and independence. SROs that include social service provision by mental health agencies are among the more successful program models (Linhorst, 1991).

The remaining 36% of clients reside in supported residential models including supervised apartments, supportive housing, foster care, and Fairweather Lodges. These programs provide services to clients in community settings such as apartments or homes rather than in group living arrangements.

Supervised apartment programs provide clients with varying levels of staff and peer support. Some programs employ clustered sites in which a number of housing units for clients are located within the same building or adjacent buildings, offering clients opportunities for group activities, peer support, and increased staff accessibility. Clustered sites may include a staff apartment adjacent to client apartments. Other programs offer scattered site apartments located throughout communities, offering clients greater independence.

Supported housing and supportive housing programs involve clients in the selection of housing situations with an emphasis on normalized settings, including single family homes (Figure 19-1). Many programs offer options for home ownership (Shern et al., 1989).

Foster care programs place clients in family homes in the community. Usually these programs screen and train home care providers and provide staff support to clients and caregivers.

The Fairweather Lodge program model was developed by George Fairweather at the Palo Alto Veterans Administration Hospital in 1963. Fairweather Lodges consist of small groups of six to eight clients who share a house and develop a business. Businesses include janitorial services, landscaping, catering, and furniture building. This model has been duplicated in several states. Currently approximately 700 clients live in 110 Fairweather Lodges (Torrey, 1990).

Much debate in the literature has focused on the efficacy of certain models for the entire adult

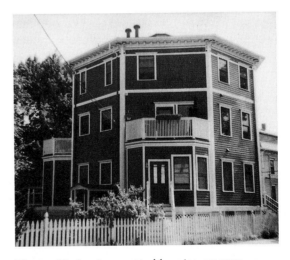

Figure 19-1. A supported housing program owned by New England Fellowship in Rhode Island. (Courtesy New England Fellowship, Lincoln, RI.)

population. In particular, supported housing, with its emphasis on providing services to clients in their own homes or apartments, has been suggested as the preferred program model over staffed settings (Shern et al., 1989). However, recent studies have indicated a need for a variety of models for adults with serious mental illness based on their individual needs for support and structure (Downs & Fox, 1993; Ford et al., 1992).

Adults with serious mental illness

Demographics

A nationwide survey of 59,282 adults with psychiatric disabilities in more than 16,000 residential settings revealed the following demographics (Randolph et al., 1991):

- **Gender:** Men made up 53% of the surveyed population.
- **Age:** Ages ranged from 18 to over 65 years old. Of the clients surveyed, 47% were between 18 and 35 years old, 39% were between 39 and 64 years old, and 14% were 65 years old or older.
- **Race:** Of the survey participants, 78% were white, 15% were African-American, 5% were Hispanic, 1% were Asian or Pacific Islander, and 1% were Native American.
- **Diagnosis:** Schizophrenia was the diagnosis in 65% of the population. Other diagnoses included major affective disorders (16%), personality disorders (8%), and organic disorders (5%). The remaining 6% had other diagnoses or were not given a diagnosis. A six-point scale developed for this survey to measure functioning level indicated that many programs served clients with different levels of disability.

Clients between 18 and 35 years old, the largest category, have been characterized in the literature as the "young adult chronically mentally ill" (Shern et al., 1989). Members of this group are more likely than older clients to have substance abuse problems that exacerbate their mental illness. Clients with a dual diagnosis of mental illness and substance abuse have frequent rehos-

pitalizations, tend to become disaffiliated with their families and support systems, and also may experience homelessness and involvement with the legal system. They require a coordination of substance abuse and psychiatric services that presents a major challenge to residential programming.

Seriously emotionally disturbed children

The population of seriously emotionally disturbed children includes children whose emotional problems affect their ability to function in family, school, and community settings (see Chapter 22). The majority of residential services available for children are provided by inpatient psychiatric facilities. However, as is the case in residential services for adults, the trend toward providing community-based case management services for children and adolescents is growing (Schmitz & Gilchrist, 1991).

INTERVENTIONS
Residential services

Residential services designed to meet the needs of seriously mentally ill people should be delivered in accordance with community support system standards. Services should be comprehensive, ongoing rather than time limited, and individualized to meet the needs and preferences of each client (Baker et al., 1993).

Ideally, all residential programs should offer permanent housing and a comprehensive array of services individualized for each client through a participatory treatment planning process.

The New England Fellowship for Rehabilitation Alternatives (NEFRA) is a nonprofit residential agency that offers a full spectrum of residential services to more than 500 seriously mentally ill adults. All NEFRA residential programs, including supervised and supported models, offer the following services to their clients:

1. **24-hour access to program staff** Whether they are on site, as in staffed program models, or can be reached by an answering service or

pager, staff members are available to clients at all times to provide support or crisis intervention.

2. **Medication monitoring and training in self-medication** Medication plays a significant role in the treatment of mental illness. Clients receive training in administering their own medications and identifying possible side effects to increase their self-sufficiency and ability to live independently.

3. **Symptom identification and control** Clients receive training in symptom identification and control of their illnesses.

4. **Assistance in developing and maintaining personal relationships with family and friends** Programs provide opportunities for socialization through activities, assistance with accessing transportation, and the participatory development of policies to encourage visitors.

5. **Assistance in participation in the community network of activities and support services** In addition to taking part in program-sponsored activities, clients are encouraged to participate in activities and use community services to facilitate their integration into the community. Clients attend community recreational events and use community resources such as public libraries, museums, and community centers.

6. **Integration into other support services** Programs develop both formal and informal linkages with other services and agencies to provide clients a comprehensive choice of resources and ensure continuity of care and treatment. These resources may include psychiatric, emergency, medical, and educational services.

7. **Substance abuse services** To meet the needs of dually diagnosed clients, programs offer support groups with trained facilitators and access to other substance abuse and detoxification services. Clients also are encouraged to participate in community support groups such as Alcoholics Anonymous.

8. **Vocational services** Programs assist clients in obtaining meaningful work in the community to meet their needs for self-esteem. Most people meet this need through work and the development of a career. Clients are assisted in accessing prevocational and vocational activities, volunteer jobs, and competitive employment. Clients who are not interested in working are assisted in identifying meaningful, satisfying, and rewarding ways to spend their time.

9. **Access to entitlements** Programs assist clients in applying for and obtaining all relevant entitlements such as SSI, SSDI, public welfare, food stamps, bus passes, veteran's benefits, and housing subsidies.

10. **Access to health care** All clients have access to primary care physicians. They are encouraged to keep medical and dental appointments and are given training regarding the benefits of appropriate and timely health care.

11. **Housing** Programs assist clients in accessing safe, attractive, and affordable housing. Recognizing the importance of housing as a therapeutic environment for clients, NEFRA programs are committed to providing quality settings that meet standards all people would want for themselves and their families.

Treatment planning

In NEFRA residential programs the assessment and treatment process is an ongoing one. A comprehensive assessment is the basis for initial and subsequent treatment plans and reviews. The assessment includes but is not limited to the following items:

- Cognitive and psychological functioning
- Affect, attitudes, and self-image
- Interpersonal relationships
- Behavioral symptoms, including history and assessment of risk factors
- Description of the course of the illness, expressed as a diagnosis in *DSM-IV* terminology, including any history of substance use or abuse

- Documentation of the need for psychotropic and other medications
- Social and environmental supports, including an evaluation of the client's neighborhood, community, family supports, and key support persons
- Physical health status, including physical, dental, and other evaluations as appropriate and relevant to the client's medical condition
- Vocational and employment history, occupational readiness, skills, and interests
- Educational background, including a history or an evaluation as appropriate of the client's education or schooling and current educational plans if applicable
- Daily living skills, including levels of independence and assistance required to manage health, medication, personal care and grooming, finances, and self-preservation
- Language and communication skills, including the ability to hear, understand, and use the English language; ability to communicate and make needs known in the client's preferred language
- Cultural and ethnic factors, including the client's assessment of applicable racial, ethnic, cultural, and religious backgrounds
- Guardianship status
- Resource availability, including financial entitlements and health insurance

The treatment plan results from a collaborative effort among the client, staff, family members, and other relevant service providers. The typical number of goals is three, and the focus is on concrete, measurable, and observable outcomes.

Staff

Staffing is an important element in residential programming. The literature indicates that in residential programs offering psychosocial rehabilitation services, the relationship between staff and residents is the most beneficial aspect of treatment (Hawthorne et al., 1994). A survey of more than 24,000 residential staff indicates that only a small percentage had professional training. Of the survey participants, 6% were trained in nursing, 5% in social work, and 11.5% in psychology and related disciplines. Of the remaining 77.5%, 28% had paraprofessional training, 24% had no training, and 26% had a bachelor's degree. The programs surveyed offered intensive services such as medication supervision, crisis intervention, and skills training. However, these services were provided by staff who for the most part lacked training in traditional mental health disciplines (Randolph et al., 1991).

With the exception of certain residential models such as Mobile Treatment Teams, funding sources do not mandate or provide sufficient funding for professional staff in residential programs. Low salaries, high expectations, and demanding hours, particularly in staffed models offering daily three-shift coverage, all contribute to high staff turnover. Therefore a major challenge in the delivery of effective residential services is to recruit, train, and retain quality staff.

NEFRA has met this challenge by using a number of effective strategies:

1. **Training** All NEFRA staff receive training in reality therapy, a practical behaviorally based approach that teaches staff to develop involvement (a strong therapeutic relationship between staff and clients) and treatment goals based on individual client needs and preferences. Training is provided by both the Institute for Reality Therapy through its certification process and certified staff on site.
2. **Staff development** NEFRA provides training to prepare current staff for leadership roles within agency management. More than 80% of current management staff began as direct care workers in the agency.
3. **Organizational culture** NEFRA has developed a positive growth-oriented organizational culture with a commitment to quality services by encouraging participation in decision making at all staff levels. Staff also are encouraged to participate in the agency's strategic planning process and receive an annual organizational bonus to celebrate the attainment of agency-wide goals.

4. Utilization review NEFRA has, during the past 10 years, significantly increased its number of professional staff, which now includes social workers, psychiatrists, registered nurses, and occupational therapists. These staff offer supervision and training to residential staff in the assessment and treatment planning process, medication monitoring and maintenance, crisis intervention, and other clinical interventions. Professional staff also conduct utilization reviews of staffing resources, thus providing for more effective allocation of funds.

NEFRA's ability to obtain new contracts through competitive bidding processes and its 4% rehospitalization rate for clients provide strong evidence for its success as a therapeutic residential program agency.

REIMBURSEMENT AND FUNDING OF RESIDENTIAL PROGRAMS

Funding of services for people with serious mental illness is provided through an uncoordinated mix of local, state, and federal efforts, many of whose funding policies favor hospitalization and restrict reimbursement for outpatient and rehabilitation services (Torrey, 1990). Residential services are no exception. Funding is often adequate to staff and operate programs but usually does not include the allowances for inflation and cost of living needed to fund programs for long-term residential care and support. Most often the newest programs are the best funded. Programs that treat clients with comparable needs may vary widely in funding. Frequently this discrepancy is caused by short-term cost-shifting initiatives designed to downsize a particular inpatient psychiatric facility. Although deinstitutionalization is important, programs rarely ask the questions of what the long-range community need is and what will enhance client tenure in the community and rarely plan for the results of those questions. As previously mentioned, funding policies favor reimbursement for hospitalization and inpatient treatments over less expensive but more effective

community treatment. Reimbursement for residential programs is difficult to obtain, even in the face of positive outcomes.

In 1978 the President's Commission on Mental Health concluded that "the level and type of care given to the chronically mentally disabled is frequently based on what services are fundable and not what services are needed or appropriate" (Torrey, 1990). Clearly, new funding mechanisms are needed to keep programs funded at levels that will allow them to continue to provide quality treatment.

States are increasingly using private managed care organizations to manage state Medicaid dollars on a capitated, shared-risk basis. Massachusetts became the first state to establish a comprehensive, privatized, public sector–managed care program (Minkoff, 1994). Future funding seems more likely to come from private managed care organizations such as MHMA (Mental Health Management of America) in Massachusetts. Tying such funding to indicators of quality care and objective outcomes will be an improvement in mental health residential services. Changes in block grant–funding allocation proposed regularly by Congress will further push states toward privatizing payment for residential and community support services.

Clearly, no matter what funding mechanism is used, residential staff and especially nurses will have to provide more specific documentation to justify the cost of each billable unit, therapy session, medication, assessment, treatment plan formulation, and review.

ROLE OF THE NURSE IN RESIDENTIAL PROGRAMS

Nurses play an important role in providing quality residential and rehabilitation services to clients living in residential programs. Because of the lack of medical staff available to work in such programs, the nurse plays a primary role as coordinator of medical services, medication skills training, and medication dispensing and monitoring. Most important, with the notable exception of

Assertive Community Treatment teams, the nurse is usually the only licensed practitioner serving on a residential staff team.

Providers of residential services typically require nurses to have a BSN degree (preferably with 1 year of professional experience working in a mental health facility). They must have a current license with the state or county Board of Registration for Nursing. Nurses must have a working knowledge of the theory and principles of psychiatric nursing and psychopharmacology, including the administering of medication. Nurses also must be familiar with the observation, reporting, and recording of the effects of medication.

Within residential programs, nurses assume responsibility for the nursing care of chronically mentally ill clients. They provide generalized and specialized care, maintain appropriate records, and function as members of an interdisciplinary team. As the influence of managed care in residential programming expands, the ability to carry out treatment plans accurately and effectively and communicate nursing information effectively in both oral and written form will become increasingly important. Nurses provide primary nursing care to clients by assessing health status, recording related health data, administering nursing treatment, evaluating clients' conditions, and adjusting care in conjunction with other treatment providers. Nurses meet clients' nursing care needs by communicating pertinent information to other residential staff to ensure integration, coordination, and continuity of care. Additionally, nurses provide staff training on a range of health issues, including infection control, universal precautions, and OSHA regulations.

Nurses have an important role in providing medication education to clients and staff. Nurses must be able to educate clients by using and demonstrating working knowledge of the classifications of medications and of the dosage and effects of all medications given to clients within a program.

An example of a successful and innovative residential program that employs nurses in key roles is the Louisville Homecare Project (Torrey, 1990). In 1957 this project was funded with an NIMH grant to study whether patients hospitalized for schizophrenia could be treated at home by having public health nurses visit and monitor them regularly. Of the 152 clients studied between 1961 and 1964, 77% of clients taking antipsychotic medications and 34% of clients taking placebo medications were successfully treated at home. Altogether, clients taking antipsychotic medications avoided an estimated 4800 days of hospitalization. Compared with patients treated at the local psychiatric unit, the clients in the project performed better based on measures of mental status, domestic functioning, and social participation (Torrey, 1990). These positive results came at a time when community supports and residential options for people with mental illness were virtually nonexistent compared with the resources currently available for mental health clients. This program, although no longer in operation, points out how effective nurses can be when employed properly in the provision of mental health care services.

FUTURE DIRECTIONS

Current behavioral health care trends that affect mental health services also will have an impact on the future of residential programs. These trends include the new role of clients as consumers of services, a growing preference among states for flexible support services over facility-based programs, and the increased requirements of funding sources for treatment outcome studies (Livingston & Srebnick, 1991). The growing advocacy movement of clients and their families has resulted in client-centered programming. The new program focus seeks to engage clients in a treatment process based on their needs and preferences (Shern et al., 1989). State funding sources have responded to the consumer movement by including clients in state mental health decision-making bodies and supporting client projects and groups with state funds (Livingston & Srebnick, 1991).

A recommendation for states to move toward more flexible services such as supported housing was part of a national policy statement issued by the National Association of State Mental Health Program Directors in 1987 (Livingston & Srebnick, 1991). States responded to this recommendation with initiatives designed to increase the availability of quality affordable housing for clients. Rhode Island established a new housing development agency, Thresholds, which provides grants to vendors and client groups to finance the purchase of supported housing. Several states, including Rhode Island, Delaware, and Washington, provide innovative funding for supported housing through Medicaid.

An example of the dramatic change in focus precipitated by the previously discussed trends is a recent initiative of the Department of Mental Health in Massachusetts. In January 1995, every residential program for adults with serious mental illness was re-bid and private agencies were required to restructure their program models to meet the requirements of a single residential code. This change was designed to facilitate the following goals:

1. Build flexibility into the residential service system
2. Ensure that services were client based and driven
3. Integrate residential services with the department's public managed care approach to service delivery

The new code required that specific services be provided as needed by clients regardless of their residential setting; the program also required flexible staffing that could change or move to meet clients' changing needs. This new program code was a significant transformation in philosophy and treatment model from previous residential codes.

The following values were used as a framework for reorganizing services:

1. All services must be based on the needs and preferences of individual clients.
2. Services should be provided in a way that encourages and empowers clients to take responsibility for themselves.

3. All services must be flexible and responsive to the changing needs and preferences of clients.
4. Service access and provision should be organized and administered to minimize if not eliminate the mandated relocation of clients.
5. To the greatest extent possible, staffing patterns should be flexible and staff services mobile in all residential settings—group homes and individual apartments.
6. All services are based on a psychosocial rehabilitation philosophy that involves creating a supportive environment using situations, tasks, and goals to aid clients in developing employment, housing, and social skills.
7. Residential services are part of the comprehensive community support system (CCSS) and should integrate and coordinate service delivery with other programs in the CCSS to implement the client's service plan.
8. Program effectiveness is measured by the outcomes achieved through the provision of services.

This residential restructuring is too recent to be evaluated in terms of benefit to clients. However, the trend is toward larger, more competitive agencies able and willing to adapt to the change in residential services. Agencies unable to adjust to the changing environment will lose significant contracts or simply will not survive. Residential services will have to adapt to new trends and initiatives to survive in the new behavioral health managed care environment.

SUMMARY

Residential programs are a rapidly growing element in the continuum of care for people with serious mental illness. Residential services and the philosophy that underlies these services have evolved. In the early days of residential services, programs were designed to be transitional based on the premise that most if not all clients would be able to move to increasingly less structured and supervised housing. The new philosophy asserts that client housing should remain stable and treatment and support plans should be individually designed for each client.

Nurses play an increasingly important role in residential programs. They provide primary care to clients and educate staff and clients on a variety of health issues. However, poor funding for residential programs and the lack of a third-party reimbursement mechanism for nurses in many states threaten the availability of nurses for these programs.

REFERENCES

Baker, F., Jodrey, D., Intagliata, J., & Straus, H. (1993). Community support services and functioning of the seriously mentally ill. *Community Mental Health Journal, 29* (4), 321–331.

Downs, M. W., & Fox, J. C. (1993). Social environments of adult homes. *Community Mental Health Journal, 29* (1), 15–23.

Ford, J., Young, D., Perez, B. C., Obermeyer, R. L., & Rohner, D. G. (1992). Needs assessment for persons with severe mental illness: What services are needed for successful community living? *Community Mental Health Journal, 28*: 491–503.

Hawthorne, W. B., Fals-Stewart, W., & Lohr, J. B. (1994). A treatment outcome study of community-based residential care. *Hospital and Community Psychiatry, 45*(2), 152–155.

Linhorst, D. M. (1991). The use of single room occupancy (SRO) housing as a residential alternative for persons with a chronic mental illness. *Community Mental Health Journal, 27*(2), 135–144.

Livingston, J. A., & Srebnick, D. (1991). States' strategies for promoting supported housing for persons with psychiatric disabilities. *Hospital and Community Psychiatry, 42*(11), 1116–1119.

Minkoff, K. (1994). Community mental health in the nineties: Public sector managed care. *Community Mental Health Journal, 30*(4), 317–321.

Randolph, F. L., Ridgway, P., & Carling, P. J. (1991). Residential programs for persons with severe mental illness: A nationwide survey of state-affiliated agencies. *Hospital and Community Psychiatry, 42*(11), 1111–1115.

Schmitz, C. L., & Gilchrist, L. D. (1991). Developing a community-based care system for seriously emotionally disabled children and youth. *Child and Adolescent Social Work, 8*(5), 417–430.

Shern, D. L., Surles, R. C., & Waizer, J. (1989). Designing community treatment systems for the most seriously mentally ill: A state administrative perspective. *Journal of Social Issues, 43*(3), 105–117.

Torrey, E. F. (1990). Economic barriers to widespread implementation of model programs for the seriously mentally ill. *Hospital and Community Psychiatry, 41*(5), 526–531.

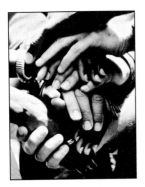

Chapter 20

Rural Settings

Marianne Smith
Kathleen C. Buckwalter
Share DeCroix Bane

The beautiful and tranquil meadows, mountains, and plains of the rural communities of the United States often belie the complexities of rural life. For many residents the romanticized and peaceful vision of country living has been replaced with the realities of economic hardship, inadequate housing and insurance, and unaddressed physical and mental health needs (Norton & McManus, 1989). Almost two decades ago the Panel on Rural Health of the President's Commission on Mental Health (PCMH) described the unique mental health service needs of rural residents (1978):

> Rural communities tend to be characterized by higher than average rates of psychiatric disorders, particularly depression, by severe intergenerational conflicts, by restricted opportunities for developing adequate coping mechanisms for facing stress and for problem solving, by an exodus of individuals who might serve as effective role models for coping, by an acceptance of conditions as being beyond the individual's control, and by an acceptance of fatalistic attitudes and minimal subscription to the idea that change is possible.

Regrettably, only limited progress has been made in meeting the multifaceted physical and mental health needs of people, families, and communities in rural areas since the publication of the PCMH report. In fact the "standard" problems of rural life outlined by the PCMH have been further compounded and exaggerated by the economic hardship and decline that began in the 1980s. The effects of the "farm crisis," which brought the plight of rural America into prominence with "Farm Aid" concerts and events, have extended far beyond the initial traumas experienced during that decade. Although the public, service providers, educational institutions, and policy makers became keenly aware of the need for mental health services in rural communities as a consequence of the farm crisis (Stuve, Beeson, & Hartig, 1989), many barriers to effective physical and mental health service delivery in rural settings still exist.

As with other areas of health and human service in rural communities the practice of community-based psychiatric nursing is heavily influenced by diverse factors characteristic of rural life. Although substantial differences exist among rural communities, a number of challenges are common to sparsely populated regions (Box 20-1). In many rural communities these factors combine to create a social and political climate that views mental illness and emotional problems as either "personal weakness" or criminal behavior, devalues the importance of mental health services, and hence fails to develop service delivery systems to respond to the needs of mentally and emotionally disturbed people.

This chapter describes common challenges psychiatric nurses who practice in rural settings

---

Box 20-1.   Barriers to effective mental health service delivery in rural settings

- **Lack of trained mental health professionals** to provide services, which in turn affects the range and scope of services provided
- **Lack of information** about and insensitivity toward mental health and mental illness by primary health care providers such as general or family practice physicians
- **Values and attitudes** and stigma that deter rural residents from seeking out and using help that may be available
- **Geographic distance** to services, further complicated by a lack of public transportation systems to assist rural residents
- **Economic stress** that results in increasingly scarce material, personal, and human resources to support and sustain rural residents; reduces the likelihood that rural residents will have health insurance; and discourages use of services, particularly for health maintenance or prevention
- **Mental health trends** at the federal, state, and local levels that affect access to services
- **Service delivery barriers,** particularly the lack of innovative service delivery models that respond to the individualized needs of rural communities

---

may encounter. The unique strengths that nursing offers to community mental health care also are discussed, and a brief review is provided of alternative roles, resources, and avenues that may be pursued by community-based psychiatric nurses as they seek to enhance the care, treatment, and support available to the rural communities in which they practice.

Although this chapter focuses on the practice of psychiatric and mental health nursing, reference also will be made to physical health service delivery systems, underscoring the importance of an integrated approach to psychiatric nursing practice in rural communities. The relationship among physical and mental health, the environment, and informal and social systems is important to consider in all populations and settings. However, psychiatric-mental health nurses who practice in rural communities must keep these factors clearly in mind to deal effectively with the challenges faced by rural residents.

COMMON CHALLENGES IN THE RURAL SETTING

Lack of trained mental health professionals

One of the most persistent challenges faced by rural communities is the lack of mental health professionals available to provide basic services to rural communities. Shortages of psychiatrists and psychologists are perhaps more acute than shortages of psychiatric social workers or psychiatric nurses (Meyer, 1990). However, mental health professionals of all disciplines are often dissuaded from selecting rural communities as the focus of their practices.

Many reasons for these shortages exist. Health care providers of all types rarely have the opportunity to explore the advantages and benefits that rural practice affords. In the absence of clinical experiences that promote positive feelings toward sparsely populated areas, many clinicians remain oblivious to the unique attributes and advantages of rural living and practice. Instead, the glamorous large cities, which offer both personal and professional advantages, are preferred because of their resources. Metropolitan areas provide a larger population on which to base a successful and lucrative practice, and Medicare reimbursement rates are higher in urban settings than in rural ones (Meyer, 1990). Movement to managed care and capitated systems will no doubt deepen the disparities between rural and urban practice (WAMI Rural Health Research Center, 1995), thus deterring even more professionals from selecting rural communities.

Because of the scarcity of other mental health professionals, practitioners in rural areas often face competing demands for their time, work long hours, and have fewer opportunities for collegial interaction and educational stimulation (Meyer, 1990). For many the lack of a financial base for services and the need to treat people who have no insurance mean they tend to earn less than their urban counterparts (DeCroix Bane, Rathbone-McCuan, & Galliher, 1994).

Lack of awareness and sensitivity by primary care providers

Another barrier to the provision of effective mental health care in rural settings is the general deficit in knowledge and skills of general health practitioners who may be consulted when mental or emotional problems first occur. In many rural communities, mentally or emotionally disturbed people of all ages—parents concerned for children, adults, and elderly people—turn to their primary care physician when confronted with "stress," "nervous conditions," or the myriad of physical complaints that also are symptomatic of mental disorder.

Primary care (family and general practice) physicians often have the opportunity to identify and treat mental and emotional disorders and make referrals for their patients to be evaluated and treated by mental health professionals. However, in too many cases mental health concerns are not identified as such and treatment is not provided (Meyer, 1990). Busy with providing physical health care and lacking specific knowledge about

mental disorders and their treatment, too many primary care physicians ignore, undertreat, or otherwise "miss" the mental and emotional concerns of their patients (Box 20-2).

Stigma associated with mental illness

Perhaps more disabling and severe than the lack of trained physical and mental health professionals is the effect of the stigma surrounding mental illness. Negative attitudes, beliefs, and myths about mental illness are prevalent in society and may be particularly problematic in rural settings. Thoughts, behaviors, and emotions symptomatic of mental disorder have long been associated with criminal behavior, evil forces, incapacity, and confinement in institutions, prisons, and mental hospitals. Unlike physical illness, mental illness is often perceived as personal weakness rather than as a disorder beyond the person's control. These "myths of madness" are often "well established in the community culture of rural America

---

Box 20-2. Lack of training—
"She's just senile"

Elsie, an 87-year-old nursing home resident, was "confused." Her physician explained to the family that it was senility related to her advanced years. The Elderly Outreach Project's psychiatric nurse urged the family to seek a comprehensive medical workup (which the primary care physician had failed to conduct) to rule out other causes of the confusion. Elsie was found to have a thyroid dysfunction that caused the confusion. Her mental status cleared considerably with medication but was not entirely reversed because the problem had gone untreated for so many years.

Modified from *Mental Health and Illness in Rural Settings: Stigma and Rural Elderly,* by M. Smith, April 12, 1990, Paper presented as testimony for the panel on stigma, National Institute of Mental Health Field Hearing, Marshall, MN.

and are often passed down from one generation to another" (Rathbone-McCuan, 1994) (Box 20-3).

Fear of being labeled as "crazy" or "insane;" of being ostracized by neighbors, family members, or friends; or of being "locked up" in an institution, nursing home, or mental hospital deters many rural residents from receiving needed assistance. For some the word *schizophrenia* still evokes images of "Jekyll and Hyde" and any delusional experience is seen as evidence of permanent insanity (Smith, 1990). Depression is mocked as an everyday occurrence that people should be able to handle, and the words *senile* and *demented* strike fear in the hearts and minds of many rural people, particularly older adults who fear being permanently institutionalized (Buckwalter, Smith,

& Caston, 1994). To the person who values open spaces and independence, institutionalization may loom as a fate worse than death.

Even when mental health services are available and desperately needed, many rural residents may be reluctant to seek assistance because stigma is so powerful and pervasive (Meyer, 1990). The anonymity provided by larger cities is often missing in small rural communities. Even in the urban centers of rural states, educated professionals who accept in-home mental health services from nurses express fear about being seen entering the mental health center and refuse services when asked to do so. The fear of being labeled, ridiculed, avoided, or even abandoned looms large for many rural residents. Lacking clear information about the advantages and benefits of therapy to counter myth and misinformation, many choose to not seek help (Box 20-4).

Rural characteristics and values

Many characteristics influence the demand for and use of mental health services in rural communities. The geography, tax and resource base,

---

Box 20-3. Stigma surrounding mental illness—"I can't walk through those doors"

Henry, a retired school principal, was referred to the Elderly Outreach Project after he experienced a stroke that left him partially paralyzed and extremely depressed. He welcomed the nurse's visits and was receptive to therapy, focusing on his sense of grief and loss. Because he was able to drive, the nurse asked whether he would come to the center (20 miles away) to save the nurse's driving time for people who couldn't drive themselves. He considered the issue but concluded, "I can't. I mean, I can drive, but I can't walk through those doors. I drove to your center and tried to imagine going in. And I couldn't do it. I know it's stupid. I mean, I shouldn't feel this way. But I can't bear the thought of someone seeing me. They'd think I was nuts." He added, "I don't even like to think about you as a mental health person. I never have. You're a nurse, right? You're my visiting nurse!"

Modified from *Mental Health and Illness in Rural Settings: Stigma and Rural Elderly,* by M. Smith, April 12, 1990, Paper presented as testimony for the panel on stigma, National Institute of Mental Health Field Hearing, Marshall, MN.

Box 20-4. Myth and misinformation—"He wasn't a criminal"

A client experienced a reactive depression following his son's suicide. He grieved for the loss of his son but also grieved the perception that his son's death evoked in the minds of his neighbors and friends. He returned to the same sequence over and over again: "He was a good boy. He never hurt anybody. He wasn't a criminal. He didn't use that gun against anybody but himself. But that's not what they think. They think he was bad. They think there was something wrong with him."

Modified from *Mental Health and Illness in Rural Settings: Stigma and Rural Elderly,* by M. Smith, April 12, 1990, Paper presented as testimony for the panel on stigma, National Institute of Mental Health Field Hearing, Marshall, MN.

power structure, and value systems differ from urban to rural regions and affect the mental health service–delivery systems of rural communities (Buckwalter et al., 1994). Geographical landscape, rugged terrain, and distance to travel must be considered. Moreover, sparsely populated communities have limited tax bases, which in turn affect the type and range of services offered (for example, road maintenance outweighing human services). Poor counties frequently have difficulty funding mental health services and may not see them as a priority because of stigma or other demands. Finally, the rural power structure, which is often concentrated in a few people or organizations, often determines which programs are allowed to operate, and conservative ideologies and negative attitudes about mental illness may foster stigma and self-blame.

Of particular concern and interest to psychiatric nurses practicing in the community is the effect of rural values and beliefs. Although further research is needed to clarify and define rural and urban differences, several values and themes seem to dominate in rural settings: subjugation to nature, individualism, an emphasis on primary relationships and family ties, traditionalism, fatalism, a work or "doing" orientation, the "Protestant work ethic," conservative beliefs, and strong religious values (Buckwalter et al., 1994). Individually and collectively these values may come to bear on the practice of mental health nurses (Box 20-5).

Geographical distance

Another extremely common and serious problem faced by rural residents is the often great distances between themselves and the services they may need. Most mental health professionals who practice in rural communities work in urban centers surrounded by sparsely populated counties. As a result, receiving assistance at the mental health center may mean traveling a considerable distance. Even outreach or satellite clinics in remote counties outside the primary care site may be many miles from where clients live.

> ***Box 20-5.*** Values and characteristics— "I don't take charity"
>
> Marie refused to sign a release of information form that allowed the center to bill her insurance for services. This was "charity" and she wanted "none of that." She was quite depressed, appreciated the social worker's assistance, and did not want to terminate services, but she was adamant that she could pay her own way. The center's policy was to charge full fees when people refused to use insurance that was available to them. This meant that Marie would be charged $74 per hour—a fee she could neither understand nor pay.

Modified from *Mental Health and Illness in Rural Settings: Stigma and Rural Elderly,* by M. Smith, April 12, 1990, Paper presented as testimony for the panel on stigma, National Institute of Mental Health Field Hearing, Marshall, MN.

Travel is difficult for a number of reasons. First, few public transportation systems exist on which rural residents can rely to transport them to and from health care services. Lack of private transportation or transportation reliable enough to get them to the city further complicates travel for many rural residents. Long distances to services are often compounded by poor road conditions, adverse weather, and lack of road maintenance and repair in remote areas (Coward & Cutler, 1989). Even when special transportation is available (for example, a bus for seniors or disabled people), many residents resist, complaining they are both physically and emotionally uncomfortable (Buckwalter et al., 1994).

Economic stress

The rural economy, which began to falter with the farm crisis in the 1980s, has shown little improvement in the 1990s. Loss and hardship endured in agricultural communities has contributed to the need for mental health care and simultaneously exacerbated access problems

(Meyer, 1990). Loss of family farms creates a host of difficulties: families must relinquish both their sources of income and their lifelong life-styles. Not only is employment and income lost with the sale of the farm but family homes as well, and an entire heritage dies when a farm is not passed on to the next generation. Small businesses and services that support the agricultural community close because of lack of business. People and families are forced to seek additional employment to help avert losses accrued in farming or find alternative employment to survive dispossession. One farmer who rotates shifts at his full-time job while continuing to farm sadly noted, "I have to keep the job in town to support my 'habit'—farming." Regrettably, the downward spiral of economic distress makes employment opportunities increasingly scarce. Families are forced to relocate to distant communities, leaving friends, relatives, and long-standing support systems behind.

The emotional stress and burden that accompany loss of income, employment, home, and life-style are substantial. Not surprisingly, the incidences of depression, anxiety disorder, child and spouse abuse, and alcohol use reported to rural community mental health centers in the last decade have increased at higher rates in rural communities than in urban ones (Meyer, 1990).

At the same time the financial troubles experienced by rural families, including those in the timber and mining industries and in farming, have led many to cancel their insurance. In turn, access to mental health services—services desperately needed by many people and families—is increasingly limited. Lacking insurance to pay for services and unable to afford the out-of-pocket expense, many rural residents simply go untreated (Zevenbergen & Buckwalter, 1991).

Mental health trends

Initiatives and changes in federal legislation have been influential in the provision of mental health services in rural settings. Between 1965 and 1973 more than 500 community mental health centers (CMHCs) were established; more than 40%

of these were in rural communities (Human & Wasem, 1991). In the following years, amendments to the 1963 Mental Retardation Facilities and Community Mental Health Centers Construction Act provided funding mechanisms to help rural CMHCs explore alternative service structures to better meet the needs of underserved at-risk populations: outreach services were provided where clients congregated (for example, in schools and health, community, and senior centers), peer groups were evaluated as a means to overcome stigma and increase support among adolescents and elderly people, mental health specialists provided low-cost or no-cost education to reduce stigma and increase referrals, and mental health professionals cultivated liaisons with other providers such as ministers and primary care physicians who often encounter people with mental and health problems (Rathbone-McCuan, 1994). "These initiatives were often successful and the 'practical wisdom' of these approaches is now documented in the professional literature" (Rathbone-McCuan, 1994).

Regrettably, progress in rural mental health service provision has been negatively influenced by trends that began in the 1980s (Murray & Keller, 1991). In 1981 the Alcohol, Drug Abuse, and Mental Health block grant statute enacted by Section 901 of the Omnibus Budget Reconciliation Act (OBRA) of 1981 (Pub. L. No. 97-35) mandated transfer of community mental health programs from federal to state and local control, allowing states to reestablish priorities for federal mental health dollars. Categorical community services such as consultation and education, which were the backbone of many innovative service models, were dropped. In addition, OBRA discouraged the National Institute of Mental Health from maintaining a rural mental health focus (Human & Wasem, 1991). In recent years, rural mental health practice has moved farther away from the broad goals of the community mental health center movement of the 1960s, focusing instead on fee-for-service revenues and ability to pay (Murray & Keller, 1991), which perpetuates the "traditional"—and often unsuccessful—outpatient service model.

Service delivery barriers

The economic downturn experienced by rural communities also has been felt in the physical health care system: small community hospitals are in danger of extinction, the shortage of rural health clinics continues, and the disparity between Medicare reimbursement to physicians and health facilities in rural communities compared with urban settings continues to deter professionals from rural practice (Beaulieu, 1992). The wholesale conversion of Medicaid populations to managed care systems has presented a serious threat to the survival of federally certified rural health clinics as some clinics switch from a per-visit fee of $55 to a monthly capitation of $10 (WAMI Rural Health Research Center, 1995). Given the reliance of many rural residents on primary care providers for mental health assistance the loss of health care facilities and services has serious implications.

The situation for mental health services in rural communities is equally bleak. Community mental health centers in rural settings have long struggled with problems of geography and limited population: rural CMHCs are often structured regionally, with one CMHC serving a large geographical area; services are clustered in urban centers, requiring clients to travel long distances; and satellite offices or outreach centers, when available in outlying areas, are often minimally and sporadically staffed (Buckwalter et al., 1994).

Because of professional shortages and funding streams, the range of services provided is often restricted to traditional outpatient services, and priority is given to clients who appear to have the best potential for rehabilitation (especially children). Services for special populations, particularly frail older adults who commonly reside in rural communities, are scarce. Although consultation and education services are a viable means to break down stigma and develop effective working relationships with other human services providers in the community (in schools, jails, and nursing homes), these services are too often viewed as "not income producing" and thus not worthy of attention. In the absence of funding mechanisms to implement and sustain innovative service delivery models, limited outpatient services provided in distant cities are often the norm for rural Americans (Box 20-6).

Regrettably, traditional outpatient service models in which the client asks for assistance with a mental or an emotional problem and is treated in a facility labeled as a mental health or psychiatric clinic are contradictory to the realities of rural life. For reasons outlined in previous sections, many rural residents will not seek help from the mental health center: they are too far away, too expensive, and too threatening; potential benefits of therapy (talking or medication) are not known or well understood; and risks of being ostracized are substantial.

Box 20-6. Service delivery barriers—
"It's our policy"

Mabel, who is legally blind, became severely depressed following the death of her husband. She believed that the food in her refrigerator was poisoned and that her visiting nurse was a "snake detective" who was trying to "put her away." Anorexia combined with her delusions, and her weight reached a dangerously low point of 85 pounds. Her nurse called the mental health center (before the Elderly Outreach Project) and asked for help. The intake technician explained that someone would need to bring Mabel to the center. When Mabel refused, the nurse asked again, "Couldn't someone see Mabel in her home?" Although Mabel lived only a short distance from the center, the answer was "No. If we do it for one, we'll have to do it for everyone and we just don't have time." The visiting nurse was offered two choices: bodily transport Mabel to the emergency room of the local hospital or sign civil commitment papers for her if Mabel was a "danger to herself."

Modified from *Mental Health and Illness in Rural Settings: Stigma and Rural Elderly,* by M. Smith, April 12, 1990, Paper presented as testimony for the panel on stigma, National Institute of Mental Health Field Hearing, Marshall, MN.

IMPLICATIONS FOR PSYCHIATRIC NURSING IN THE RURAL SETTING

Although the list of difficulties and barriers outlined may initially seem discouraging, psychiatric-mental health nurses may use this information to their advantage. Because other disciplines are scarce, nurses may actually have greater opportunities for independent roles, collaboration with physicians and practitioners who would otherwise be inaccessible, and involvement in a wide variety of consultation and liaison work. In fact, psychiatric nurses may have genuine advantages in the rural setting.

By acting as advocates on their own behalf, nurses in many rural states have succeeded in changing their states' nurse practice acts to provide licensure including limited prescriptive authority for advanced practice nurses. As a result, more autonomous practice and group nursing practice are increasingly possible. Psychiatric nurses who are motivated to explore options and alternatives available in community practice, initiate collaborative relationships with others, and lobby on behalf of improved service delivery models for rural residents may find the rural community an exciting and rewarding arena in which to practice. In fact, psychiatric and mental health nurses who practice in rural settings may have some distinct advantages over practitioners of other mental health disciplines.

Physical and mental health skills

Because psychiatric nurses have specialized knowledge about both physical and mental health, opportunities for employment in diverse settings are possible. Unlike the psychologist or psychiatric social worker, whose practice is strictly limited to mental health treatment, psychiatric nurses offer employers both physical and mental health skills. As a result, psychiatric nurses may be affiliated with nursing care centers such as nursing homes and residential facilities, adult day health services, well child or elderly clinics, rural health clinics, and a wide variety of other community-based services that provide both physical and mental health services. In fact, by aligning themselves with physical health providers rather than mental health providers, psychiatric nurses may actually have more opportunities to identify and treat mental and emotional disorders experienced by rural residents.

Acceptance in the community

This alignment with physical health care providers points to another distinct advantage held by psychiatric nurses. Nurses have long been familiar and accepted members of community-based health care. Nurses are commonly encountered in health clinics, doctors' offices, and local hospitals and are the expected "visitor" when home health care services are provided. Even in the most isolated rural communities, visiting nurse and public health nursing services are often available. Unlike other mental health disciplines, nursing care doesn't carry the stigma of "taking welfare," often associated with social workers, or of being "crazy," which is often implied when a psychologist or psychiatrist is involved. Nurses may pass quietly into the lives and homes of rural residents and provide physical and mental health care services without eliciting the fear of stigma associated with other disciplines. Whether in a health center or home visit, seeing the nurse is a much more acceptable option for most rural residents.

Cooperative relationships

The medical education provided in basic nursing education programs also makes nurses natural allies of physicians. Although relationships between doctors and nurses have historically been more power struggle than collegial cooperation, the smaller and more personal environment of rural communities may create opportunities unavailable in other settings. Rural physicians, who are often overwhelmed with medical treatment responsibilities that they understand and accept, may more willingly accept the assistance of a psychiatric nurse who can counsel, support, and educate patients in their practices. Physicians are thus relieved of "wasting time talking" to patients and allowed to do what they do best. At the same time, collaboration with the psychiatric nurse affords them the assurance that patient needs are being met and important concerns such as suicidal ideation are being identified and treated.

Nursing education also may open doors to other cooperative relationships. Because basic nursing education provides skills in working with all age groups and in diverse settings, addressing both health maintenance and illness conditions, psychiatric nurses become the natural liaison to support and assist local schools, human service providers, sheriff's departments (in domestic violence cases), jails, and care facilities. Nurses understand and can provide health promotion and illness care, client education, medication management, and skills other disciplines may learn but that are not central to their educational preparation. Thus psychiatric nurses may be able to open doors that remain closed to others.

Nursing leadership

Psychiatric nurses also may be leaders in the provision of alternative mental health services in rural communities. Because visiting and public health nurses are well understood and accepted in most rural communities, psychiatric nurses also may be the most viable candidates to provide in-home psychiatric assessment and intervention. Given the limitations of traditional outpatient services, the effects of stigma, and problems imposed by long distances to services in rural communities, nurse-led alternative mental health services have provided one of the most promising approaches to care in rural settings.

OPPORTUNITIES FOR PRACTICE IN RURAL SETTINGS

As alluded to in the previous section, a number of unique opportunities may exist for the practice of psychiatric-mental health nursing in rural communities. However, a clear emphasis must be placed on the word *opportunities*. The dearth of existing employment options in most rural communities requires psychiatric nurses to think and work creatively to cultivate relationships, develop and expand existing roles, and explore various options that may exist within the community in which they live or seek to practice.

Restrictions and limitations in state nurse practice acts, state and county funding mechanisms, allocation of federal mental health dollars, and reimbursement mechanisms for both mental health and nursing practice (including Medicaid and Medicare within managed care or capitated systems) are critically important to consider when nurses explore employment and role opportunities. Substantial differences exist from one state to another, even in the interpretation of federal guidelines and policies, producing different options, barriers, and opportunities. Psychiatric nurses must be well aware of various regulatory factors that will influence their practice, as well as sociocultural, economic, and demographic factors that characterize rural communities.

Parallels to urban practice

The type or range of roles played by psychiatric-mental health nurses working in rural communities may easily parallel those of peers working in metropolitan areas. Rural psychiatric nurses may be employed by community mental health centers, partial hospitalization or adult day treatment programs, residential treatment programs, or schools or engaged in private practice. In addition, the type and range of services they provide will no doubt be similar to those offered by mental health nurses in other settings, from education to medication management, supportive therapy to family therapy, and case management to crisis intervention. Rural nurses will certainly encounter the same range of clients who experience diverse social, medical, and mental problems.

In addition to these settings and roles, psychiatric-mental health nurses in rural communities may discover or create new roles, particularly in collaboration with other agencies, services, or human service providers. As Rathbone-McCuan (1994) observed, most program achievements in rural communities have relied on mental health workers incorporating community organization skills into their roles, building mental health systems and services on the existing foundation of the informal helping network, and forging cooperative agreements between mental health providers and other agencies in the service network. By using their existing skills, carefully examining current realities in individual communities, and thinking broadly about resources, limitations, and options, psychiatric-mental health nurses may establish unique and innovative roles that enhance the mental health care provided in rural communities.

Collaborative systems

At present, mental health services in rural areas are often fragmented because of funding and authority patterns. A more effective rural mental health system must maximize limited resources, address unique community needs, provide continuity of care, and use professional, paraprofessional, and lay personnel appropriately (Rathbone-McCuan, 1994). Effective mental health service delivery in rural America requires innovative approaches, coordination, and cooperation among physical health, mental health, and human service providers and workers who have both the vision and persistence to advance alternative strategies to address the unique needs of rural communities.

Psychiatric-mental health nurses may make important contributions to the availability, quality, and accessibility of mental health services in rural communities by advancing the concept of human services integration. Instead of accepting the traditional but limited view of community mental health services as being delivered solely at the mental health clinic, psychiatric nurses in rural communities may lobby for expanded roles that use existing community services and resources as a foundation on which to build. (Box 20-7 lists possible sources of assistance.) From liaisons with primary care providers to educational programs for church members, nurses working in rural communities may better serve their clients by encouraging close collaborative working relationships

among health and human service providers, the informal caregiving network (including community organizations and churches), and the mental health system. By integrating and sharing available resources from each of these domains, nurses may improve the overall delivery of care.

ALTERNATIVES IN RURAL PRACTICE

Although the following description of roles is far from comprehensive, it highlights some options psychiatric nurses who seek to expand their existing roles or establish new opportunities for themselves may explore.

Mental health outreach programs

Outreach programs provide an effective approach for delivery of services, particularly for people residing in rural areas (Buckwalter et al., 1991). Although outreach concepts and strategies may be applied to people of all ages (and certainly are not restricted to use in rural settings), two nurse-led models developed and implemented for older adults are worthy of mention.

Iowa's Mental Health of the Rural Elderly Outreach Project

One effective outreach program, the Mental Health of the Rural Elderly Outreach Project (EOP), was developed and implemented under nursing leadership at a community health center in Iowa. Begun in 1986 with demonstration services research money from NIMH and the Administration on Aging, the EOP was a collaborative effort between a CMHC and an area agency on aging. The outreach project was designed to identify older people in need of mental health care, deliver needed services, and initiate and coordinate referrals to appropriate medical and social service agencies. Because rural elderly people did not present themselves at the mental health center requesting assistance, the outreach model used a wide variety of traditional and nontraditional referral sources: psychosocial screening at local sites, referrals from the county case management

---

Box 20-7.   Possible sources of assistance in rural communities

Health-related services

Physician offices
Multiservice outpatient clinics
Rural health clinics
Well baby clinics
Well elderly clinics
Free clinics
Visiting nurse associations
Home health care programs
Parish nurse programs
Public health services
Nutrition programs
Adult day health programs
Self-help and prevention groups
Community hospitals
Rural assistance programs: Essential access
    community and rural primary care hospitals
    Medical assistance facilities
Community nursing homes

Mental health services

Community mental health centers
Family counseling centers and services
School counselors and psychologists
Case management services
Private practice outpatient services

Pastoral counseling
Counseling by physicians
Peer counseling programs
Self-help, support, and prevention groups
County care facilities (county home)
State psychiatric hospitals
VA psychiatric facilities

Informal social systems

Families, friends, and neighbors
Community and neighborhood groups
Community volunteer programs
Churches and religious organizations
State and county extension services
Community action programs
Area education programs
Area agencies on aging
Social service and welfare programs
Financial assistance programs
Homeless assistance programs
Employment services
Transportation programs
Housing assistance programs
Senior centers
Child care centers and services

---

team and its associated agencies, training of non-traditional referral sources as "gatekeepers" (for example, mail carriers and meter readers) to locate and refer high-risk people, outreach specialists who served as liaisons between the EOP's multidisciplinary team and service agencies in the community, and contact with discharge planning departments of hospitals, clinics, and other mental and physical health care institutions in the community.

Using an approach developed by Raschko (1985), the project trained more than 600 community gatekeepers, people who live and work in rural communities and who can identify and link isolated elderly people with sources of needed assistance. Liaisons were developed with all ser-vice providers for elderly people in the existing case management system (including visiting nurses, home health agencies, and primary care providers), and on-site psychosocial screenings at well elderly clinics were conducted regularly. After referral, clients received a comprehensive in-home assessment from the multidisciplinary EOP team (consisting of geropsychiatric nurses, a social worker, and a psychiatrist), during which medical, psychiatric, and social problems and needs were reviewed. Over a 5-year period more than 800 elderly people were referred to the EOP. This alternative service model also proved cost effective, with per-client per-year costs estimated at approximately $622. (See Buckwalter et al., 1991, for a detailed description of the EOP and its evaluation.) After the grant period the central components of the EOP continued successfully, largely because of cooperative relationships cultivated during the grant period (Smith et al., 1993).

Virginia's Rural Elder Outreach Program

Using the Iowa experience as a guide for action, psychiatric nurses at the University of Virginia joined forces with physicians and community agencies to develop a successful Rural Elder Outreach Program (REOP). The REOP, begun in March of 1991 and supported by grant funds from the Kellogg Foundation, also integrated agencies and professionals from many disciplines in an effort to provide a well-rounded approach to assessment, consultation, case management, and psychosocial support to high-risk clients, their families, and their caregivers (Abraham et al., 1993). A key goal of the REOP was to strengthen the self-reliance of rural communities in caring for their elders and to heighten awareness of aging and mental health issues. Unlike the Iowa EOP model in which professional expertise and resources were more centralized, the REOP featured a multilayered structure of lay, nonprofessional, and professional resources (Buckwalter et al., 1993).

The project served 63 clients in its first year, and the estimated direct cost per client per year was $1015. Most referrals to the REOP were clients with mental health problems too complex for existing resources to manage, problems requiring expertise beyond that provided in community agencies.

Thus psychiatric nurses in both the Iowa and Virginia models helped their communities address unmet needs of rural residents. By using existing community resources, these nurse-led programs identified people in need of assistance, provided an array of mental health and illness services, and helped community members make the best use of existing social and health services. Although the focus of service was on older adults, these concepts and strategies easily translate to other age groups and populations of interest.

Peer counseling programs

Although popularized with older people, the concept of using "peers" to support and assist people with mental health concerns may be applied to all ages. Peer counseling can overcome many barriers to the use of mental health services experienced by people in rural communities, including reluctance to use mental health services because of the stigma associated with mental illness, reimbursement and financial issues, and the feeling of being a failure for needing professional assistance. This relatively new strategy for alleviating the emotional distress of older clients began in the 1970s and uses the life experiences and skills of older adults in a self-help approach. Peer counselors are empathetic and respectful and do not have the negative opinions of many mental health professionals toward working with older people. Moreover, emotionally disturbed older adults (and younger people) are more likely to seek counseling from a peer. This approach removes the stigma from help seeking, promotes rapport, allays fears of negative consequences such as institutionalization, and costs less. An important by-product of the counseling approach is the positive role modeling that peer counselors and helpers provide for older clients.

Psychiatric-mental health nurses in rural communities may find the peer counseling approach a viable strategy for working with clients of all ages. In collaboration with other physical health, mental health, and social service providers, nurse-led peer group or peer counselor programs may provide a means to overcome problems created by myth, finances, or distance. Caring volunteers may be recruited, trained, supervised, and assisted to help people with problems as diverse as coping with adolescence to providing care to a family member with Alzheimer's disease. Whatever the population or special interest at hand, success depends heavily on the careful selection, education, and ongoing supervision of the peer counselors. Nurses, who are both accepted and respected by the community, are often in an excellent position to provide needed leadership to conceptualize and execute programs that effectively recruit, train, and supervise volunteers to provide peer support and counsel.

Self-help and prevention groups

Psychiatric-mental health nurses also may extend their skills to rural community members by advancing "lay" groups designed to assist various at-risk populations who experience mental and emotional distress. Whether based in a community agency or hospital, nurses are often in a key position to take leadership roles in conceptualizing, developing, initiating, and monitoring community agencies designed to provide role models for effective coping, emotional support, methods to reduce unnecessary stress, and strategies to help clients take responsibility for the future course of their lives.

Self-help groups may assist rural residents to progress from perceiving themselves as passive victims of their mental illness (which often coincides with the fatalistic attitudes that pervade rural life) to a more active role in preventing future mental health problems through stress management, medication monitoring, and health care. Prevention groups dealing with bereavement, loss and grief, and managing life change may focus on sustaining mental and physical well-being and promote planning that can facilitate adaptation to various stressors common to a rural environment. From child care to parent care, prevention programs offer rural communities information they need to endure hardship and build on existing resources.

As with other populations and settings, self-help groups may provide emotionally disturbed and mentally ill clients, family members, and caring friends with emotional and social support and group identification. The need for this type of support, which reduces feelings of guilt, stigma, and personal responsibility for problems (countering the myth of being a personal failure), may be particularly evident in rural communities. Given the complex problems imposed by economic trends, geographical isolation, values that resist taking welfare, lack of health insurance, and reduced access to health care services, self-help and prevention groups may offer rural mental health providers a viable alternative and an inroad to clients who may later accept traditional fee-for-service outpatient therapy.

Parish nurse programs

Psychiatric nurses may not initially consider affiliation with a religious organization as a desirable or appropriate pathway to serving emotionally and mentally disturbed rural residents. However, parish nurse programs may offer a viable means to influence mental health care, particularly in rural communities troubled by the barriers outlined in previous sections. A number of churches and groups of churches have hired trained nurses to serve as personal health counselors, health educators, and developers of support groups for older adults and others in their parishes. These nurses also train volunteers and serve as liaisons to the community and its resources. Collectively these methods may glean the benefits of self-help and prevention groups outlined previously.

SUMMARY

A number of barriers exist to providing effective mental health services in rural communities, from stigma to poverty, geographical access to irrelevance of services offered. Psychiatric-mental health nurses bring a number of skills, assets, and abilities to bear in overcoming challenges and problems that pervade sparsely populated areas. Nurses, who are both accepted and understood by rural communities, have unique opportunities to conceptualize, develop, initiate, monitor, supervise, and support programs to improve mental health and illness care. By taking leadership roles in the development of mental health services, psychiatric-mental health nurses may advance principles that are common to successful mental health systems in rural America: incorporating community organization skills into their roles, using multidisciplinary approaches, emphasizing geographical appropriateness, promoting understanding and use of existing lay and community resources, building on the foundation of existing formal and informal resources, coordinating diverse services, and maximizing the benefit of cooperative agreements between mental health providers and other agencies in the service network.

REFERENCES

Abraham, I., Buckwalter, K., Snustad, D., Smullen, D., Thompson-Hiesterman, A., Neese, J., & Smith, M. (1993). Psychogeriatric outreach to rural families: The Iowa and Virginia models. *International Psychogeriatrics, 5,* 203–211.

Beaulieu, B. (1992). Small rural hospitals with long-term care: 1983–1987. *Journal of Rural Health, 8,* 121–142.

Buckwalter, K., Abraham, I., Smith, M., & Smullen, D. (1993). Nursing outreach to the mentally ill rural elderly. *Hospital and Community Psychiatry, 44,* 821–823.

Buckwalter, K., Smith, M., & Caston, C. (1994). Mental and social health of the rural elderly. In R. Coward, N. Bull, G. Kukulka, & J. Gallaher (Eds.), *Health services for rural elders.* New York: Springer Publishing Company.

Buckwalter, K., Smith, M., Zevenbergen, P., & Russell, D. (1991). Mental health of the rural elderly outreach program. *Gerontologist, 31,* 408–412.

Coward, R., & Cutler, S. J. (1989). Informal and formal health care systems for the rural elderly. *Health Services Research, 23,* 785–806.

DeCroix Bane, S., Rathbone-McCuan, E., & Galliher, J. (1994). Mental health services for the elderly in rural America. In J. Krout (Ed.), *Providing community-based services to the rural elderly.* Newbury Park, CA: Sage Publications.

Human, J., & Wasem, C. (1991). Rural mental health in America. *American Psychologist, 46,* 232–239.

Meyer, H. (1990). Rural America: Surmounting the obstacles to mental health care. *Minnesota Medicine, 73,* 24–31.

Murray, J., & Keller, P. (1991). Psychology and rural America: Current status and future direction. *American Psychologist, 41,* 220–231.

Norton, C., & McManus, M. (1989). Background tables on demographic characteristics, health status, and health services utilization. *Health Services Research, 23,* 725–756.

President's Commission on Mental Health. (1978). *Report to the President.* Washington, DC: U.S. Government Printing Office.

Raschko, R. (1985). Systems integration at the program level: Aging and mental health. *Gerontologist, 25,* 460–463.

Rathbone-McCuan, E. (1994). Rural geriatric mental health care: A continuing service dilemma. In C. Bull (Ed.), *Aging in rural America* (pp. 147, 153). Newbury Park, CA: Sage Publications.

Smith, M. (1990, April 12). *Mental health and illness in rural settings: Stigma and rural elderly.* Paper presented as testimony for the panel on stigma, National Institute of Mental Health Field Hearing, Marshall, MN.

Smith, M., Buckwalter, K., Zevenbergen, P., Kudart, P., Springer-Brenneman, D., & Garand, L. (1993). An administrator's dilemma: Keeping innovative mental health and aging programs alive after the grant funds end. *Journal of Mental Health Administration, 20* (3), 212–222.

Stuve, P., Beeson, P., & Hartig, P. (1989). Trends in the rural community mental health work force: A case study. *Hospital and Community Psychiatry, 40,* 932–936.

WAMI Rural Health Research Center. (1995). Rural health clinics facing 1115 waiver issues. *Rural Health News, 2* (1), 10–11.

Zevenbergen, P., & Buckwalter, K. B. (1991, November 23). *The mental health of the rural elderly outreach project: Then and now.* Paper presented at the Gerontological Society of America Annual Conference, San Francisco, CA.

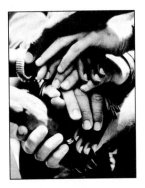

Chapter 21

Independent Practice

Elizabeth A. Huggins

"**I** want to go into private practice" is often the reason given by psychiatric nurses for returning to school to earn a master's degree. The dream of providing therapy to clients within the framework of one's own business is often based on nurses' ideals and ambitions of employing their psychotherapy skills rather than on an understanding of the complexity of developing and maintaining an independent practice.

Independent practice has many advantages. A great deal of autonomy is involved in working outside large bureaucratic health care systems and in managing one's own time. However, with autonomy comes greater responsibility for the business aspects of practice. Thus, in addition to evaluating clinical skills, clinicians must evaluate their business knowledge before embarking on this entrepreneurial venture.

Psychiatric nurses can use their psychotherapy skills within the community in many ways. Some clinical specialists are hired by physicians as part of the physician's practice, and although they are expected to generate income to cover their salary, they retain employee status. Other nurses work within community mental health centers providing therapy both in individual and group work. Some academic appointments also include clinical practice. Nurses in each of these situations practice psychotherapy; many practice with autonomy and independence. However, for the purposes of this chapter, *independent practice* is defined as the practice of psychotherapy by an individual whose source of income is generated through fees for services rendered in direct client contact or consultation. Psychiatric nurses who go into independent practice are responsible for generating revenues large enough to cover income and all the costs of practice. This business aspect of independent practice is often not fully understood or addressed by nurses who dream of becoming "independent practitioners." Successful independent practitioners are those who understand that although their clinical skills are important, they are embarking on a business venture—the business of providing psychotherapy services to people for a fee.

As with any other business the better the preplanning, the better the chance the business will survive. Starting a business without a plan is a sure road to failure. This chapter provides information on the preplanning and decision making necessary before starting a private practice in psychotherapy. It provides business facts and resources available for the individual contemplating private practice. Marketing is discussed as a separate topic. The effects of the changing health care environment on the practice of psychotherapy are considered, and clinical issues for people in private practice are addressed.

PLANNING

A thorough knowledge and understanding of reimbursement, particularly the methods of reimbursement for nurse therapists in the local community, is an important requirement in planning. The nurse also must obtain answers to such questions as "What are the state insurance laws that cover nonphysician providers?" and "What does the state board of nursing require for nurses in independent practice?"

Preliminary planning requires self-assessment from a professional and personal viewpoint. A candid introspective look at one's ability to manage self-employment is essential. Consideration of the adequacy of professional experience and credentials before embarking on independent practice also is indispensable. Certification should be obtained from the American Nurses Association (ANA) in adult or adolescent mental health and psychiatric nursing. This certification establishes that the nurse has had some postgraduate supervision and experience before entering private practice. Lack of certification can restrict access to reimbursement by some third-party payers.

Another consideration is the relative isolation of independent practice. Nurses used to interacting with many people in a busy hospital or clinic often have difficulty practicing without interactive contact with other clinicians for days at a time. With thorough preplanning, however, some of the problems associated with isolation can be overcome. For example, every professional therapist

needs some form of ongoing supervision. Supervision can take many forms, from individual supervision by a colleague to peer supervision with a group of practitioners. Although the primary purpose of supervision is to enhance clinical skills, it also is an excellent way to decrease isolation for the independent practitioner. Continuing education is important to maintain competence and to fulfill requirements for recertification and also is another way to stay in contact with other professionals in the field.

Other issues that require careful consideration are financial and family responsibilities. Nurses who are solely responsible for earning their own income or who may have family financial commitments must consider the financial aspects of independent practice very carefully. In some cases the best plan is to begin part time in private practice and continue working in a salaried position to maintain a stable income. Because the planning and development of a practice are time consuming, family responsibilities and time availability should be considered early in the planning stage. Box 21–1 presents a checklist to assist in determining readiness for independent practice.

Nurses should explore psychotherapy practices in their community and state, especially those that include nurses as part of a group practice and those in which nurses practice independently. Making contact with as many practitioners as possible and asking questions about the cost of practice, methods used to develop referral sources, and the length of time it took for the practice to become self-supporting are important steps in the planning process. Most people are willing to talk about their work and the way they accomplish it. Soliciting recommendations and advice from therapists who are already in practice can be quite helpful.

Developing a business plan

A survey done by *Psychotherapy Finances* (1995) indicated that most full-time clinical practice schedules include 20 to 29 sessions per week, each one lasting an average of 50 minutes for an

---

Box 21–1. Determining readiness for independent practice

Readiness for self-employment   Yes   No

1. Am I willing to accept full responsibility for the success or failure of my practice? ☐ ☐
2. Can I effectively organize my time, plan, and work efficiently without structure? ☐ ☐
3. Do I have complete confidence in my own ability to develop a successful practice? ☐ ☐
4. Am I willing to spend time in practice promotions, public relations, and presentation making to tell my community and other professionals that I have a practice? ☐ ☐
5. Can I make and stick by decisions? ☐ ☐
6. Can I comfortably handle the matter of collecting the fee directly from clients? ☐ ☐
7. Can I afford a potential change in my present tax bracket? ☐ ☐
8. Am I able to persevere in the face of successive setbacks, failures, and adversity? ☐ ☐
9. Am I willing to accept the many administrative duties (such as scheduling, fee collection, insurance billing, bill paying, supply purchasing, insurance coverage, and licensing) and still maintain the highest level of professional performance? ☐ ☐
10. Am I willing to govern my practice in all aspects according to the ethical standards of my profession? ☐ ☐

If after careful and serious consideration of these questions, you find yourself with several "No" answers, you might do well to postpone setting out on your own. Perhaps these questions suggested areas of your life to which you need to give special attention to prepare for your own practice.

If the scales are tipped in the "Yes" direction, you may want to assess your professional personal readiness for private practice.

Professional readiness   Yes   No

1. Do I now possess the professional competence and skills necessary to render mental health services on an independent basis? ☐ ☐
2. Am I duly licensed and qualified to practice in this state and county? ☐ ☐
3. Is there some more experienced or knowledgeable therapist whom I respect who would be willing to supervise or provide feedback to my private work? ☐ ☐
4. In the past has my work with clients indicated that I achieved the following ideals:
    a. Rapid and lasting change resulted from my intervention? ☐ ☐
    b. The incidence of suicide attempts, threats, and emergency psychiatric hospitalizations has been low among my clients? ☐ ☐
    c. The rate of early or premature termination from therapy has been extremely low among my clients? ☐ ☐
5. Can I obtain professional liability insurance to protect me and my family while I am engaged in private practice? ☐ ☐

Box 21-1—cont'd

Personal readiness

	Yes	No
1. An independent practice demands many hours per week in practice promotions and sessions with clients. Will my family accept and support this investment of time and energy outside the home? Is my spouse enthusiastic about the idea?	☐	☐
2. Will my present employer approve of my "moonlighting" in my own practice?	☐	☐
3. Knowing that I am far from an objective observer of myself, are there any personal problems or conflicts in my life that need attention and resolution before I enter private practice?	☐	☐
Would they affect my clients' progress?	☐	☐
4. Will my health permit me to meet the demands of my practice?	☐	☐
5. Do I realistically have the time to devote to a private practice?	☐	☐
6. Do I function well in the midst of frustration, uncertainty, and risk taking?	☐	☐
7. Am I willing to accept infringement on my private or personal time by phone calls from clients on evenings, weekends, and holidays?	☐	☐

Modified from *Private Practice Handbook* (4th ed.), by C. Browning and B. Browning, 1993, Los Alamitos, CA: Duncliff International.

---

individual client and 90 minutes for a group. These hours spent in direct client care are reimbursable. Nonreimbursable hours are spent in marketing, managing paperwork, and making telephone calls to client networks.

Joining an existing group with an established practice makes preplanning much less complicated. Much of this chapter, however, provides information necessary for nurses interested in planning and developing an independent practice. The tasks are much the same as they are for any person opening a small business.

One resource for the small business owner is the Service Corps Of Retired Executives (SCORE), a volunteer, federally funded program that supports small businesses. The Small Business Association also offers courses in developing a small business. Because their services are provided free of charge or at low cost, these two organizations should be the first resources for nurses considering private practice.

Another resource for the small business entrepreneur is the local Internal Revenue Service (IRS) office. A tax identification number and a business tax kit that will aid in starting a tax plan can be obtained there. Unlike personal income tax, busi-

ness taxes must be paid quarterly. Although the IRS can provide some helpful information, tax laws can be exceedingly complicated. Contracting with an accountant for assistance in bookkeeping and tax planning is often well worth the additional expense.

Planning an independent practice should include a written business plan. Formats for creating a business plan can be found in bookstores and libraries. The plan should contain the following elements (Schneider, 1992):

1. A business statement
2. A mission statement
3. A marketing plan
4. A start-up budget
5. A proposed timetable

An important survival tool is a realistic budget that honestly assesses financial resources. In the beginning a private practice may generate very little income; that income also may be sporadic. When possible, nurses who wish to go into private practice should have a 6-month financial reserve to cover living and business expenses. Rent, telephone, water, electricity, taxes, malpractice insurance, janitorial fees, printing, and advertising expenses need to be paid even if the practice does not generate enough income to cover them. Approximately 30% of gross income is needed to maintain a thriving practice, not including overhead funds for such items as health insurance and retirement contributions. The nurse who starts a new business acts as the personnel manager, company bookkeeper, and marketing department. Weaknesses in business knowledge should be identified and plans made to gain that knowledge. Business confidence is as important as clinical confidence (Calmelat, 1993).

Malpractice insurance is a necessity and professional organizations are an excellent source for obtaining it. The American Nurses Association offers a malpractice insurance plan; the cost of the ANA plan should be compared with the cost of other commercial insurance plans. In comparing plans, nurses must ascertain whether the coverage is broad enough and deep enough to provide a safety net in the event of a malpractice suit. Costs vary depending on credentials and scope of practice. Nurses who have prescriptive privileges may find independent practice insurance very expensive.

Selecting a practice site

After completion of a self-assessment, business plan, and budget, the selection of a practice site becomes an important next step. One option, particularly for nurses with a limited budget, is to rent space from other practices. Many practices are willing to rent their offices during times they are not in use, usually in the evening or on weekends. This is a practical way to gradually develop referral sources without the stress of trying to pay full office expenses. An established practice site may charge a flat rate for the use of an office or a percentage of the gross income generated by the nurse (with 40% a common amount). Either arrangement negates the necessity to budget for furnishings, telephone installation, and utilities while building a client base.

For well-financed practitioners and nurses who are ready to move from shared office space, the specific location of a practice also is an important issue that requires some research. Checking the telephone book for the number of people practicing psychotherapy in the area may be helpful. Even in small cities the number of therapists with different professional backgrounds and education who are already in practice may be surprising. Locations close to large medical centers, physicians, and office parks are often ideal because of the ability to network and develop referral sources. The accessibility of public transportation and a good road system also are important considerations in selecting a practice site (Browning & Browning, 1993). Although finances are one consideration, the site with the lowest rental rate is not always the best location for a practice.

MARKETING

Developing an effective marketing plan as part of the business plan is crucial in beginning and maintaining a successful practice. The purpose of a marketing plan is to establish a client base through building reliable referral sources. The two most common sources of referrals are personal contacts with other health care providers and self-referrals from members of the community. Building each referral source requires somewhat different strategies.

Health care providers

One of the most important referral sources is personal contact with other providers. The local mental health center, psychiatric hospitals, physicians in family practice and specialty practices, and pediatricians are all potential referral sources. Building and maintaining these contacts are essential marketing activity. Attending local and national professional meetings is an excellent way to become visible to other providers. Developing a presentation of a topic in an area of expertise is well worth the time invested. For example, a well-presented talk on the signs and symptoms of depression given to a nonpsychiatric group of health care practitioners may result in a number of referrals (Browning & Browning, 1993). Nurses in practice in acute care and home health settings can be good sources for referrals. Volunteering to talk to groups of nurses to provide them with information on the types of appropriate referrals to your practice is an excellent strategy. Acquiring a level of comfort and skill in public speaking is crucial for the independent practitioner. A course in public speaking is a good investment for nurses who have not acquired this skill (Browning & Browning, 1993).

The development of a brochure for direct mailing to target groups of professionals is an excellent marketing strategy. Although brochures can be expensive, methods exist for developing them at a very reasonable cost. An attractive brochure can be created using computer-assisted resources through local computer printing stores. Graphic design college students can be a good source of assistance (Browning & Browning, 1993). Nurses should consider designing two brochures, one for a professional audience and one for a lay audience. A brochure sent to professionals can include professional and academic language, but the one sent to the general population should describe the practice and be understandable to the lay person. For example, a brochure aimed at a professional audience might state "the office has an interdisciplinary team," whereas a brochure aimed at a lay audience might state "practice members include nurses, social workers, and physicians" (Browning & Browning, 1993).

Self-referrals

In addition to establishing a reliable referral base from professional sources, the nurse should become known in the community. One way to do this is by presenting talks and seminars that demonstrate the nurse's clinical expertise to various community groups. Church groups, parent-teacher associations, and neighborhood associations are excellent sources of referrals. Most communities have organizations that consist of families of people who are mentally ill. Consumers of mental health services also have organiza-

tions in most communities. These groups are often looking for speakers and also may be important referral sources. Volunteering to be a consultant for national, state, and local politicians as an expert on mental health in your community can increase visibility in the community while providing a valuable public service.

Devising a method of responding to all referral sources is important. The client data sheet should always include a line for clients to enter their referral source. Personally contacting the referral source to thank them for the referral is professionally responsible and may lead to other referrals.

Advertising can be important to marketing efforts. In the United States, professionals have long resisted advertising. In 1979 the Supreme Court ruled that restraining of honest and truthful advertising by professional organizations was unethical. Professional organizations were to inform all members that advertising is legal and ethical. Some professionals, however, are still reluctant to advertise (Browning & Browning, 1993). One acceptable form of advertising is in the business pages of the telephone book. Business telephone numbers are automatically listed for no extra charge. When potential clients search the business pages of the telephone book looking for help with an individual, marital, or child problem, they're going to be attracted to the advertisement that speaks to them in the most direct way. For example, instead of using "individual psychotherapy," the independent practitioner might consider advertising "counseling for interpersonal relationship problems" or "parent-child conflict." A small newspaper advertisement using language directed at the general public and not other professionals is often a successful marketing tool. Language that best describes the service but is not too academic and reaches out to the person seeking services should be used.

The financial return for time spent on marketing may not be immediately evident. Therefore tracking the effectiveness of various efforts is important to focus on the most productive activities. For example, tracking sources and recording the number of referrals that come through newspaper advertising in a year's time will indicate whether this source generates sufficient referrals to justify the cost.

MANAGING AN INDEPENDENT PRACTICE
Developing a fee schedule

Assessing the fees charged by other psychotherapy practices in the local market is the first step in developing a competitive fee schedule. When building a new practice, the nurse might consider being flexible with fees as a way to develop referral sources. Accepting a limited number of pro bono cases is an excellent way to enhance the image of a new practice. A willingness to do so may assist in the development of referral sources who later may refer paying clients.

Nurses new to private practice should explore the details of Medicare and Medicaid reimbursement and ascertain the rate of reimbursement for nurses. The reimbursement rate for nonphysician providers is often less than that for physicians. Some states will not reimburse nonphysician providers without a physician's signature on the treatment plan. Medicare and Medicaid fees are decided by state or federal regulations. Providers are prohibited from charging clients more than the amount specified by these insurers.

Billing and collection

Nurses contemplating private practice need to consider billing and collection procedures. Some practitioners collect the total fee from clients and expect them to apply for their own insurance reimbursement. Collecting fees at the time of service precludes the time and expense involved in monthly billing and sending reminders to clients with unpaid bills. Although this method of payment simplifies billing and collection procedures for the practitioner, clients often see it as an undue burden. In many cases the practitioner offers the service of applying for reimbursement from the client's insurance, a service that is time consuming and expensive for the practitioner and

involves the risk that the insurance company will deny the claim altogether or reimburse for only a portion of the fee. In dealing with clients who do not have insurance, nurses should be wary of billing for payment for services as opposed to collecting at the time of the session. Some clients will not pay their bills promptly and others will not pay their bills at all unless pressured. Acknowledging this basic business reality is difficult for some in the health care delivery field. Before the practice is financially able to hire a billing clerk or an office manager, the practitioner is going to be responsible for collecting unpaid bills. If the independent practitioner has difficulty asking for payment at the time of the session, payment will be even more difficult to pursue later.

One of the most difficult transitions people in the health care profession must make as they enter independent practice is coping with the importance of collecting fees for their services. The tendency is to provide service to people in need regardless of the payment; although charity should be an element within every practice, it must be balanced with the reality that the practitioner depends on those funds for income and to take care of office expenses.

INDEPENDENT PRACTICE IN A CHANGING HEALTH CARE ENVIRONMENT

Although the majority of the literature on changes in the health care environment and reimbursement has focused on the financial difficulties of hospitals, reimbursement for outpatient services also has been drastically affected. Historically, insurers have not reimbursed for outpatient psychiatric services on the same level as they reimburse for general health care services. As managed care arrangements become more common, restraints on outpatient care have become more severe. The *Psychotherapy Finances* annual report (1995) presents data indicating that income for psychotherapists has dropped gradually over the past few years and that this drop is related to changes in funding. In the past, arrangements between the provider and client were direct. The client paid the provider directly or the provider billed the insurance company for psychiatric services. In either case the client selected the provider. However, in the managed care environment the client must first go through the managed care group to get permission to seek services; those services are often limited and specific. Managed care groups are interested in the most cost-effective treatment that will reduce symptoms in the shortest possible time with very narrowly focused and measurable goals. Most reimburse for a narrow range of diagnoses and often refuse to reimburse for certain diagnostic categories or therapy methods. Practitioners who use a theoretical framework that calls for more in-depth therapy and whose clients subscribe to a managed care system may have difficulty receiving reimbursement for their services.

Individual providers will have difficulty existing without some kind of relationship with managed care groups as an increasing number of companies insure their employees under managed care plans. The independent practitioner who focuses on short-term brief therapy with measurable goals of symptom relief will probably be successful in this new environment.

Documentation

The documentation system initiated by the practitioner should keep the requirements of managed care groups in mind. Most require documented treatment plans in which problems, issues, and outcomes are clearly specified. Outcomes must be measurable and clearly documented, and time limits must be set for achieving those outcomes. The practitioner needs to articulate to the managed care group a cleared precise treatment plan. Vague statements about supportive therapy, such as "I will help this person communicate better," are not going to be acceptable to these providers. A clearly written nursing diagnosis probably best meets the criteria for the managed care group requirement for a treatment plan. Using the North American Nursing Diagnosis Association (NANDA) format is a concise way to develop a treatment plan and meet the requirements of most managed care providers.

For the most part, people in private practice have the leeway to design their own documentation systems. However, incorporating the requirements of managed care companies into any documentation system is always sensible. Maintaining two record-keeping systems, one for fee-for-service clients and another for managed care clients, is neither efficient nor cost effective.

Goodman, Brown, and Deitz (1992) make a case for the use of a Patient Impairment Profile (PIP). They state that a *Diagnostic and Statistical Manual of Mental Disorders* (*DSM-IV*) diagnosis does not give enough specific information to the case manager. For example, not all clients with the diagnosis of major depression have the same therapy issues. A client profile that reflects the behavioral response leads to more effective treatment planning and outcome measurement. In their profile design (Box 21–2), Goodman et al. have made an effort to describe client behaviors that more clearly indicate the direction treatment should take. The PIP method defines therapy issues clearly and succinctly. Although the PIP was designed to meet the demands of payers for justification of inpatient stays, it transfers to the outpatient setting with ease.

Whatever the documentation format, practitioners in the outpatient setting must be responsible for protecting client confidentiality. Records should be locked in a safe place at the end of the day. Office personnel should be trained about information that can and cannot be given out over the telephone. Practitioners should know the laws on confidentiality in the state in which they practice. Practitioners may wish to consult with an attorney for clarification on what can be subpoenaed for court. Client records are not as protected in some states as clinicians might like to believe. The practitioner should seek legal counsel if called to testify in a situation that appears to violate a client's right to confidentiality.

Box 21–2. Patient Impairment Profile

Impairments in the biopsychology sphere

Altered sleep
Compulsions
Concomitant medical condition
Decreased concentration
Deficient frustration tolerance
Delusions
Dissociative states
Dysphoric mood
Dysphoric mood with alexithymia
Eating disorder
Encopresis
Enuresis
Externalization and blame
Fire setting
Gender dysphoria
Grandiosity
Hallucinations
Hyperactivity
Learning disability
Manic thought/behavior

Medical risk factor
Medical treatment noncompliance
Mood lability
Obsessions
Paranoia
Pathological grief
Pathological guilt
Phobia
Promiscuity
Psychomotor agitation
Psychomotor retardation
Psychotic thought and perception
Psychotic thought, perception, and behavior
Rage reactions
Self-mutilation
Somatization
Stealing
Substance abuse
Suicidal thought/behavior

Impairments in the family/significant other sphere

Emotional/physical trauma perpetrator
Emotional/physical trauma victim
Family dysfunction
Family dysfunction with substance abuse
Marital/relationship dysfunction
Marital/relationship dysfunction with physical abuse
Running away

Impairments in the social/interpersonal sphere

Assaultiveness
Egocentricity
Homicidal thought/behavior
Lying
Manipulativeness
Oppositionalism

Paraphilia
Repudiation of adults as helpers
Sexual dysfunction
Social withdrawal
Tantrums
Uncommunicativeness

Sample definitions

Altered sleep   Any disruption of the normative 24-hour sleep-wake cycle, including insomnia, hypersomnia, early morning awakening, and night terrors

Decreased concentration   Any subjectively perceived reduction in ability to direct one's thoughts or efforts or to sustain attention

From *Managing Managed Care: A Mental Health Practitioner's Survival Guide*, pp. 34-37, by M. Goodman, J. Brown, & P. Deitz, 1992, Washington, DC: American Psychiatric Press.

SUMMARY

Independent practice can be a rewarding venture for qualified nurses who understand that their ability to establish and maintain their businesses is as important as their clinical skills. Although it is not for everyone, private practice is one route nurses may take to participate in and contribute to quality care in their communities.

REFERENCES

Browning, C., & Browning, B. (1993). *Private practice handbook* (4th ed.). Los Alamitos, CA: Duncliff International.

Calmelat, A. (1993). Tips for starting your own nurse practitioner practice. *Nurse Practitioner, 18,* 58–68.

Goodman, M., Brown, J., & Deitz, P. (1992). *Managing managed care: A mental health practitioner's survival guide* (pp. 34-37). Washington, DC: American Psychiatric Press.

Practice building: Helpful hints for starting therapy groups. (1995, June). *Psychotherapy Finances, 21* (6), 2-3.

Schneider, B. (1992). Establishing an independent practice. *Professional Insights, 6,* 43–44.

At-Risk Populations

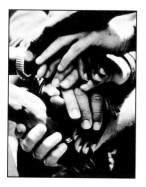

Chapter 22

Children and Adolescents

Phillippe B. Cunningham
Cynthia Cupit Swenson
Scott W. Henggeler

Clinical symptoms resulting from children's exposure to psychosocial hazards have multiple causes and are linked (directly or indirectly) with children's lives and social ecologies (Kazdin, 1995). Unfortunately, recognition of this reality has rarely translated into ecologically valid treatment strategies for children. Existing treatments are often narrowly focused, targeting a limited number of environmental factors linked to maladptive symptoms in children. In response to this narrow focus, a central tenet of this chapter is that treatment strategies systematically addressing the multiple etiological factors associated with children's psychosocial difficulties are needed to make positive changes in at-risk children's developmental progress. Focusing on children with identified problems with delinquency or substance abuse and children who have been abused or neglected, this chapter examines briefly the epidemiology (prevalence and incidence), etiology, and risk factors of these problems. Additionally, this chapter summarizes the current treatment literature on delinquency, substance abuse, and child abuse

and neglect and presents several "model" empirically based treatment programs. The model program sections focus primarily on multisystemic therapy (MST), a family- and community-based treatment approach that explicitly targets the multiple risk factors in the natural environments of children and families. MST has been implemented effectively with each of the three target groups discussed in this chapter: youth with delinquency problems, young people with substance abuse problems, and children and adolescents who have been abused or neglected.*

JUVENILE DELINQUENCY
Epidemiology

Juvenile crime is a major public safety issue facing the United States. Juvenile offenders are responsible for approximately 29% of all crime,

*Preparation of this chapter was supported by the National Institute on Drug Abuse, Grant DA08029, and the National Institute of Mental Health, Grant MH51852-01A1.

and their rate of serious and violent crime has increased dramatically during the past few years (Office of Juvenile Justice and Delinquency Prevention, 1994). For example, the 10-year period between 1982 and 1991 witnessed a 41% increase in juvenile arrests for violent crimes, which included a 93% increase in murder arrests and a 72% increase in aggravated assault arrests (Synder, 1993). Moreover, serious juvenile offenders commit an average of eight violent offenses each year (Elliott, Huizinga, & Morse, 1986).

Epidemiological evidence indicates that delinquent behavior is quite stable over time and is typically committed by boys and that a small number of offenders are responsible for a disproportionately large number of serious and violent juvenile crimes. Wolfgang, Figlio, and Sellin (1972) found, using a Philadelphia birth cohort, that chronic offenders (juveniles with five or more arrests) represented 6% of the cohort and 18% of the delinquents but approximately 80% of the cohort who went on to have extensive adult criminal careers. Additionally, this small subset of offenders was responsible for 62% of all offenses and approximately 64% of all violent offenses. Such findings have been replicated in other longitudinal investigations (Farrington, 1979; Hamparian et al., 1978; Huizinga, Loeber, & Thornberry, 1993; Strasburg, 1978).

Boys and minorities are disproportionately represented in juvenile crime statistics. Boys commit significantly more delinquent acts than girls; this difference is most evident for serious crimes (Henggeler, 1989). Recently, Huizinga et al. (1993), using data derived from a national multisite study of the causes and correlates of delinquency, reported that boys begin committing delinquent acts younger, commit crimes more often, and have longer criminal careers than girls.

Another consistent pattern to emerge from the juvenile delinquency literature is the overrepresentation of minority youth in the juvenile justice system. Although African-American youth represent approximately 15% of the total American youth population, they account for 30% of juveniles arrested for index offenses, 50% of juveniles

arrested for violent offenses, and 42% of juveniles incarcerated (Alwin, 1993; Kristberg et al., 1987). The percentage of African-American youths in correctional custody is almost three times the percentage of African-American youths in the general U.S. population (Alwin, 1993). However, studies of self-reported delinquency have generally failed to find consistent differences between African-American and white youths (Henggeler, 1989). The discrepancy between arrest and self-report data raises questions about whether these findings reflect racial bias in arrest-related decisions or underreporting of offenses by African-Americans (Huizinga & Elliott, 1986).

Although social class influences are central to several sociological models of delinquency, only low associations have been found between social class measured at the individual child level and delinquency (Henggeler, 1991). For example, as part of the National Youth Survey (NYS), a representative national sample of adolescents, Elliott and Huizinga (1983) found few social class differences in self-reported offending. On the other hand, when social class is measured at the neighborhood level, neighborhood crime rates correlate with socioeconomic indicators. Such findings, as indicated in the causal modeling literature, suggest that neighborhood characteristics contribute to youth criminal activity (Henggeler, 1991).

Etiology

The literature on juvenile delinquency has identified a number of factors associated with the development of delinquent behavior. Multidimensional causal models (a research method that examines the relations among several dependent and independent variables) have consistently shown that delinquency has multiple causes and is associated with important characteristics of the individual youth and the systems with which the youth has contact (for example, family, peer group, school, and neighborhood systems). (For comprehensive reviews, see Henggeler, 1991; Kazdin, 1987.) For example, in a longitudinal study as part of the NYS, Elliott, Huizinga, and Ageton (1985) found that delinquency was directly predicted by prior delinquency and association with deviant peers. Furthermore, family and school problems predicted association with deviant peers. Similarly, in a cross-sectional study, Patterson and Dishion (1985) found that delinquency was associated with low parental monitoring, poor academic skills, and association with deviant peers. Concerning violent offenders, Fagan and Wexler (1987) found the strongest predictor of violent behavior was association with deviant peers, which was influenced indirectly by low school integration. Clearly, these studies and others bolster the contention that juvenile delinquency is influenced by mulitiple characteristics of youths and the major social systems with which they interact (Agnew, 1985; Simcha-Fagan & Schwartz, 1986).

Developmental outcomes

Although serious juvenile offenders are responsible for a disproportionately large number of the violent crimes committed in a community and contribute to the public's fear of victimization, they pay a high developmental price for their antisocial behavior (Federal Bureau of Investigation, 1992; Strasburg, 1978). First, serious juvenile offenders compromise their cognitive and emotional development by reducing their access to educational, occupational, and social opportunities (Henggeler, Melton, & Smith, 1992). For example, in a follow-up sample of children referred for conduct disorders, Morris, Escoll, and Wexler (1956) found that 79% suffered from poor social adjustment as adults. Furthermore, "seriously mentally disordered adults commonly develop from the population of youths who engage in antisocial behavior" (Henggeler et al., 1992). Second, antisocial behavior is quite stable over time and generations; a relatively small percentage of families account for a high percentage of the crimes committed in their respective communities (Huesmann et al., 1984; Loeber, 1982; Robins, 1978). Thus serious delinquents are likely to have children who engage in antisocial behavior. Third, serious delinquents are at high risk for a number of related difficulties, including marital conflict, unemployment, alcoholism, and poor interpersonal relationships (Levine et al., 1980; Robins, 1966).

Treatment

Historically, the poor results of treatment outcome studies with delinquents have been rationalized by invoking the intransigent nature of antisocial behavior or its stability over time (Loeber, 1982). However, an alternative explanation for these historically poor results rests with the general failure of existing treatments to consider and address effectively the multiple known determinants of criminal behavior, including family, peer group, school, and neighborhood characteristics. For example, studies have demonstrated that social skills training and behavior modification techniques produce positive behavioral change during the time delinquents are incarcerated but that these effects are short lived once youth return to their natural environments (Henggeler et al., 1995). Given the multiple causes of juvenile delinquency, narrowly focused treatment strategies such as deterrence and fear-based programs (such as shock incarceration programs and boot camps) that remove young offenders from their social ecologies or intervene with only a limited subset of the etiological factors are likely to fail. In contrast, treatment strategies that comprehensively address the known determinants of delinquency in the natural environment of the young person are more likely to succeed, as shown in the following model program.

Model program

Overview of multisystemic therapy

Multisystemic therapy (MST) (Henggeler & Borduin, 1990; Henggeler et al., 1994) is a complex and multifaceted treatment model that has demonstrated short- and long-term reductions in serious delinquency. MST relies on a social-ecological theoretical framework that views behavior as the product of reciprocal transactions between young people and the multiple systems with which they interact (Bronfenbrenner, 1979) (Figure 22-1). Individual, family, peer, and school factors that contribute to delinquent behavior

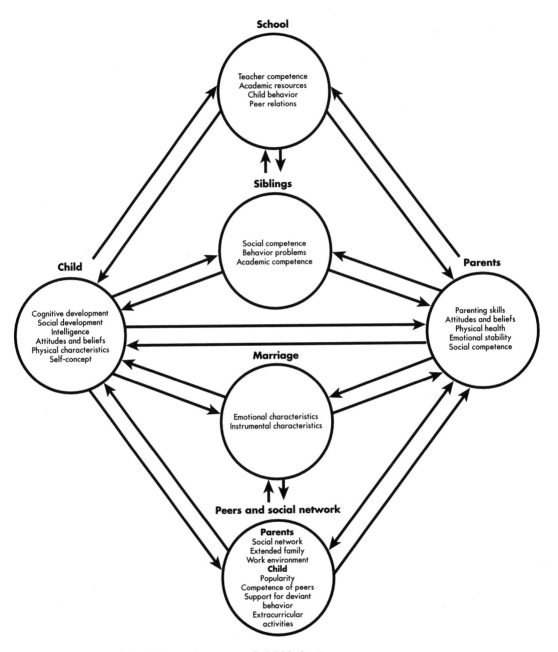

Figure 22-1. The multisystemic context of child behavior.
(From *Family Therapy and Beyond: A Multisystemic Approach to Treating the Behavior Problems of Children and Adolescents,* by S. Henggeler, & C. Borduin, 1990, Pacific Grove, CA: Brooks/Cole.)

become targets for MST interventions (e.g., parental stress and substance abuse, association with deviant peers, inadequate or unsafe housing).

MST does not require a unique set of interventions but rather uses existing pragmatic and goal-oriented treatment strategies that have some empirical support. These strategies include techniques derived from strategic family therapy (Haley, 1976), structural family therapy (Minuchin, 1974), behavior therapy (Blechman, 1985), and cognitive behavior therapy (Kendall & Braswell, 1985). For integration of these treatment techniques across the social ecology of young people, interventions are guided by nine principles that embody the fundamental nature of MST (Box 22-1). In addition, MST treatment programs incorporate a service philosophy (for example, "family preservation") distinct from most traditional mental health approaches. (For a comparison of traditional and MST models of service delivery, see Table 22-1.) Key elements of this philosophy include the following:

1. Therapist and program accountability for engaging families in treatment and for outcome based on tangible evidence of behavioral change
2. Individualization of treatment to meet the strengths and weaknesses of families
3. Empowerment of families with skills and resources to deal effectively and independently with future difficulties
4. Coordination of family interactions with systems such as housing, Social Services, and Department of Juvenile Justice

Controlled evaluations of MST

MST was originally developed to treat delinquency (Henggeler et al., 1986); favorable long-term outcomes in two recent clinical trials of MST with violent, chronic juvenile offenders have taken on national significance (U.S. Department of Justice, 1995). In Simpsonville, South Carolina, 84 serious juvenile offenders (54% of them violent offenders) who were referred by the Department of Youth Services (DYS) because of their immi-

---

> **Box 22-1.** Nine basic principles of multisystemic therapy (MST)
>
> 1. The primary purpose of assessment is to understand the "fit" between the identified problems and their systemic context.
> 2. Therapeutic contact should emphasize the positive and interventions should use systemic strengths as levers for change.
> 3. Interventions should promote responsible behavior and decrease irresponsible behavior.
> 4. Interventions should be present focused and action oriented, targeting specific and well-defined problems.
> 5. Interventions should target sequences of behavior within and among systems.
> 6. Interventions should be developmentally appropriate and fit the developmental needs of the young person.
> 7. Interventions should be designed to require daily or weekly effort by family members.
> 8. Intervention efficacy should be continuously evaluated from different perspectives.
> 9. Interventions should promote treatment generalization and long-term maintenance of therapeutic change.

Modified from *Treatment Manual for Family Preservation Using Multisystemic Therapy*, by S. W. Henggeler, S. K. Schoenwald, S. G. Pickrel, M. J. Brondino, C. M. Borduin, & J. A. Hall, 1994, Charleston, SC: South Carolina Health and Human Services Finance Commission.

---

nent risk for out-of-home placement were randomly assigned to receive MST (*n* = 43) or usual services (*n* = 41) (including court-ordered curfew, mandatory school attendance, and referral to other community agencies) (Henggeler et al., 1992; Henggeler et al., 1993). The judgment of the DYS that these young people were at imminent risk of out-of-home placement was borne out by the finding of 47% of young people receiving usual services being incarcerated after referral and 68% being incarcerated by the 59-week follow-up. Results indicated that MST was significantly more effective than usual services at

Table 22-1. Differences between traditional mental health services and multisystemic therapy (MST)

SERVICE ELEMENT	TRADITIONAL SERVICES	MST
Treatment sites	Clinic (outpatient)	Field (home, school, neighborhood, community)
	Hospital or residential treatment center (inpatient)	
Treatment modality	Individual psychotherapy	Total care
	Group therapy	
	Medication	
Provider	Individual clinician (outpatient)	Generalist team
	Multidisciplinary teams (inpatient)	
Clinical staff/client ratio	1:60-1:100 (outpatient)	1:4-1:6
	Variation in inpatient settings	
Staff availability	Working office hours (outpatient)	Team available 24 hr, 7 days a wk
	Highly variable (inpatient)	
Frequency of contact	Weekly or biweekly (outpatient)	Daily in most cases
	Highly variable (inpatient)	
Family contact	Occasional	Daily in most cases
Treatment outcome	Responsibility of client, family	Responsibility of staff
Case management	Broker of services	Services provider
Expectations of outcome	Gradual change	Immediate, maximal effort by staff and family to attain goals

reducing criminal behavior and out-of-home placement. For example, at the 59-week follow-up, MST youth had significantly fewer arrests (a mean of 0.87 versus 1.52) and fewer weeks incarcerated (a mean of 5.8 versus 16.2) than young offenders receiving usual services. Families receiving MST reported better cohesion after treatment than families receiving usual services. Of interest (particularly for people concerned with juvenile violence) was the finding that families receiving MST reported decreased peer aggression, whereas such aggression remained unchanged for young people receiving usual services. Moreover, a 2.4-year follow-up revealed that almost twice as many MST participants as control subjects were not arrested during that time (Figure 22-2) (Henggeler et al., 1993). Similarly, in

a project conducted in Columbia, Missouri, with 176 serious juvenile offenders, MST substantially reduced violent offending, other criminal behavior, and drug-related offending at a 4-year follow-up, compared with office-based individual therapy (Borduin et al., 1995). These are the first randomized trials with serious juvenile offenders to demonstrate long-term reductions in criminal behavior.

ADOLESCENT SUBSTANCE ABUSE
Epidemiology

Adolescent substance abuse is a major health issue facing the United States (Blau et al., 1988; Matarazzo, 1982; Office of Technology Assessment, 1991; Paulson, Coombs, & Richardson, 1990).

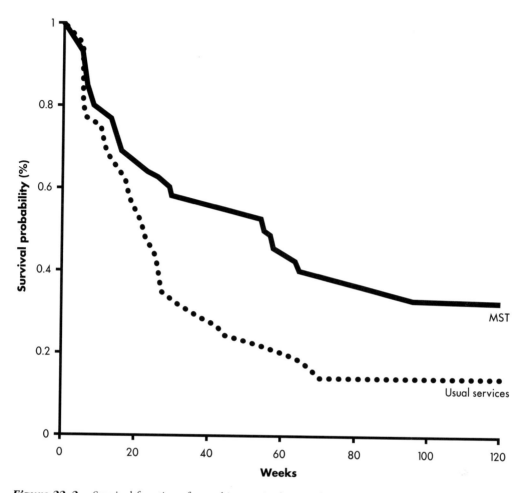

Figure 22-2. Survival functions for multisystemic therapy (MST) youth and usual services youth in a Simpsonville, South Carolina, project. Survival is based on the percentage of participants not rearrested.
(Modified from "Family Preservation Using Multisystemic Therapy: Long-Term Follow-Up to a Clinical Trial with Serious Juvenile Offenders," by S. Henggeler et al., *Journal of Child and Family Studies,* 2(4), 283-293.)

Although the overall rate of substance use among American youth has declined appreciably throughout the 1980s, it remains the highest among similarly aged youth in the industrialized world (Johnston, O'Malley, & Bachman, 1993). Monitoring the Future, a nationwide survey of 8th, 10th, and 12th graders and college students sponsored by the National Institute on Drug Abuse

(NIDA) (1993), revealed that among eighth graders, 69% have tried alcohol; 27% have been drunk; 45% have tried cigarettes; 34%, smokeless tobacco; 17%, inhalants; 11%, marijuana; 11%, stimulants; 4%, tranquilizers; 3%, LSD; 1%, other hallucinogens; 1%, crack; 2%, other cocaine; 1%, heroin; and 1%, steroids. Of particular note in the NIDA survey were the findings that more than

75% of youth have used an illicit drug by their late twenties, more than 30% have used cocaine, and 2.5% of high school seniors and 5% of young adults have used crack cocaine. Additionally, 28% of high school seniors reported they had had 5 or more drinks during the 2 weeks before the survey; the rate was as high as 51% among male college students. Rates of substance use or abuse among high-risk youth (such as the school dropouts that represent 15% to 20% of people between 12 and 17 years old) are even higher. For example, in a sample of young people between 15 and 18 years old drawn from schools and service programs serving adolescents at risk for problem behaviors, the incidence of delinquency and drug use was two to four times the national average (Allen, Leadbeater, & Aber, 1990). These statistics underscore the magnitude of the substance abuse problem facing the United States.

Etiology

The research literature on adolescent substance abuse is quite similar to the delinquency literature in at least two respects: identified correlates and resistance to treatment (Henggeler, 1993). Consistent with the juvenile delinquency literature, cross-sectional and longitudinal studies have concluded that adolescent substance abuse also has multiple determinants and is associated with important characteristics of the individual youth (low self-esteem, low social conformity, and psychiatric symptoms), family relations (ineffective management and discipline, low warmth and high conflict, and parental drug use), peer relations (association with drug-using peers and low association with positive peers), school functioning (low intelligence, achievement, and motivation for achievement), and neighborhood characteristics (disorganization and high crime) (Hawkins, Catalano, & Miller, 1992; Kumpfer, 1989; Office of Technology Assessment, 1991). Buttressing cross-sectional findings, longitudinal multidimensional causal modeling studies have consistently shown that adolescent substance abuse is predicted directly or indirectly by association with drug-using peers, poor family relations, and school difficulties (Brook, Nomura, & Cohen, 1989; Dembo et al., 1994; Dishion, Patterson, & Reid, 1988; Elliott et al., 1985; Oetting & Beauvais, 1987). These studies and others attest to the complex etiology of antisocial behavior in general and substance abuse in particular.

Developmental outcomes

Only scant empirical attention has focused on the long-term consequences of adolescent substance abuse (Farrell & Strang, 1991; Newcomb & Bentler, 1988; Newcomb & Bentler, 1989; Office of Technology Assessment, 1991). The few existing longitudinal studies indicate adolescent substance abuse may result in chronic life-threatening conditions (including liver damage, neurological impairments such as seizures, cardiac arrest, and myocarditis), mental illness (such as depression, decreased concentration, and bizarre and violent behavior), and other drug-related health problems (Cohen, 1979; Czechowicz, 1988; Dupont, 1990; Kandel et al., 1986). For example, alcohol use has been implicated in 40% of adolescent drownings and nearly 35% of fatal pedestrian and bicycle accidents (Howland & Hingson, 1988; Office of Technology Assessment, 1991). In addition, adolescent substance abuse has been associated with negative long-term psychosocial outcomes, including divorce and decreased educational achievement (Kandel et al., 1986; Mensch & Kandel, 1988; Newcomb & Bentler, 1988; Yamaguchi & Kandel, 1985).

The association between drug use and criminal activity is well established. For example, in their longitudinal study, Newcomb and Bentler (1988) reported that the use of hard drugs increased the propensity for aggressive and assaultive behavior. Likewise, Kandel et al. (1986) found the "use of illicit drugs was the strongest predictor of theft among men and women." Emerging evidence suggests that the more a person is involved in crack use and distribution, the more likely a person is to engage in violent crime. For example, in a sample of 611 hard-core adolescent offenders,

Inciardi (1990) found that "those more proximal to the crack distribution market were more involved in violent crime" and were more likely to use drugs regularly.

Treatment

Quasiexperimental and experimental (randomized trial) studies have found minimal support for any particular treatment of adolescent substance abuse (Beschner & Friedman, 1985; Martin & Wilkinson, 1989; Newcomb & Bentler, 1989; Schinke, Botvin, & Orlandi, 1991). Although several quasiexperimental studies have demonstrated positive pre-post changes (changes measured before and after treatment completion) in adolescent substance use, the inherent limitations of study designs preclude determining whether a particular treatment is effective (Friedman, Glickman, & Morrissey, 1986; Henggeler, 1993; Sells & Simpson, 1979). Specifically, pre-post designs cannot demonstrate that a particular treatment is effective without an equivalent or no treatment comparison condition. Single group and quasiexperimental designs fail to rule out alternative explanations for positive treatment effects.

Experimental studies using random assignment to treatment conditions, even though better methodologically, have failed to find strong empirical support for the effectiveness of any treatment for adolescent substance abuse. Several randomized clinical trials have found that adolescent drug use decreased equally across treatments (Amini et al., 1982; Friedman, 1989; Lewis et al., 1990; Szapocznik et al., 1986). For example, Lewis et al. (1990) concluded that family therapy and parent training were equally efficacious treatments for adolescent substance abusers because both treatment conditions produced similar reductions in substance use. However, again, reductions in substance use across conditions can be attributed to extraneous factors unrelated to treatment, including statistical regression, history, and maturation. Thus available treatments for adolescent substance abuse have failed to garner empirical support.

Model program

As noted previously, MST has enjoyed considerable success in treating serious juvenile offenders. One effect of MST across several studies has been a reduction in substance use and abuse among juvenile offenders. Borduin et al. (1995) and Henggeler et al. (1992) found that MST reduced drug use and abuse among serious juvenile offenders. Specifically, Borduin et al. (1995) found that offenders who participated in MST had significantly fewer arrests for drug-related crimes over a 4-year follow-up than their counterparts who participated in individual counseling. Similarly, Henggeler et al. (1992) found that serious offenders who received MST reported significantly less substance use than offenders who received usual services. These findings supported the further development of MST and extension to substance-abusing delinquents.

A 5-year NIDA-funded study is currently comparing the effectiveness of MST with usual community services in treating 118 substance-abusing or substance-dependent juvenile delinquents. Eligible youths were recruited and screened from the Department of Juvenile Justice in Charleston County, South Carolina. Inclusion criteria included the following:

1. A *DSM-III-R* diagnosis of substance abuse or dependence
2. Age between 12 and 17 years
3. Formal or informal probationary status
4. Residence in Charleston County
5. Residence with at least one parent figure

At 6-month follow-up after treatment, results indicated that MST reduced soft and hard drug use, incarceration, and total days in out-of-home placement. Additionally, MST was quite successful in keeping young people and families in treatment. For example, 98% of families in the MST condition received a full course of treatment compared with 78% of families in the usual community services condition (Henggeler et al., in press). This rate is quite favorable compared with the existing substance abuse treatment literature, which is characterized by high rates of treatment dropout (Stark, 1992).

CHILD ABUSE AND NEGLECT

Staggering numbers of children are physically, sexually, and psychologically abused or neglected every day. In 1992, Child Protective Service (CPS) agencies across the United States reported more than 2 million cases of child abuse and neglect (McCurdy & Daro, 1994).

Although physical abuse and neglect require mandated reporting, a broadly accepted operational definition has yet to be developed. Generally, however, child physical abuse involves physical or verbal behavior by an adult toward a child that results in injury to the child. Signs of physical abuse include bruises, welts, cuts, broken bones, skull fractures, burns, poisoning, internal injuries of soft tissue and organs, and injuries to the bone and tissue joints of a child under 18 years old (Caliso & Miller, 1992). Brassard and Gelardo (1987) also categorized threats to kill or injure a child and forcing a child to observe violence toward a loved one as physical abuse. Child neglect involves omissions in child care that result in harm or risk of harm to the child. Examples of neglect include the following (Zuravin, 1991):

1. Failure to provide medical or mental health care
2. Allowing of dirty clothing and poor personal hygiene
3. Failure to provide adequate food or clothing
4. Inadequate supervision
5. Neglect of the home or physical environment

Epidemiology

Several government agencies collect and maintain data on child abuse prevalence and incidence rates. For example, individual state CPS agencies record the number of reports of maltreatment and "indicated and founded" cases involving children. Similarly, the Bureau of Justice Statistics (1992) retains records on reported crime victimization of

children 12 years old and older. In addition to individual agency statistics, national groups such as the American Association for Protecting Children (AAPC) and the National Center on Child Abuse and Neglect (NCCAN) gather and maintain a composite of these data. In general, agency prevalence and incidence rates underestimate the number of children who experience abuse. Factors that contribute to this underestimatation include the following:

1. Discrepancies in the definition of abuse
2. Basing of prevalence reports on the number of families experiencing abuse rather than on the number of children in the family who have been abused
3. Basing of prevalence solely on cases that have been reported to CPS or law enforcement, leaving out many unreported cases

Several national prevalence studies have been conducted to combat the underestimation inherent in agency statistics. Gelles and Straus (1988) interviewed by telephone a national sample of more than 6000 parents of children between 3 and 17 years old. During the interviews, 107 parents per 1000 reported using severe violence (kicking, biting, hitting with fist, beating up) against their children during the previous 1-year period; 19 parents per 1000 reported using very severe violence (the above actions plus using a gun or knife) toward their children during the same period. More recently, Finkelhor and Dziuba-Leatherman (1994) interviewed by telephone 2000 young people between 10 and 16 years old. Within this national sample, 33% of the children reported experiencing a physical assault by someone outside the family and 13% reported a physical assault by a family member. During the interviews, 75% of the young people reported receiving corporal punishment (being slapped, hit, or spanked) from an adult caretaker.

Although child physical abuse rates in the United States are high, child neglect is the most common type of maltreatment, leading to one third of all child fatalities (American Association for Protecting Children, 1988). Neglect accounts for 45% to 55% of reported cases of child maltreatment (AAPC, 1988; McCurdy & Daro, 1994). In 1992, CPS agencies reported more than 1 million cases of child neglect in the United States (McCurdy & Daro, 1994). The combined rates of child physical abuse and neglect highlight the large number of American youth at risk for physical injury and psychosocial difficulties that may interfere with later adult functioning.

Etiology

A substantial body of research indicates a relationship between experiencing family violence and subsequently abusing one's own child (Gelles & Straus, 1987; Pianta, Egeland, & Erickson, 1989). However, research has not supported the simple notion that an abuse experience causes later perpetration of abuse (Kaufman & Zigler, 1987; Widom, 1989). Many parents who were not abused as children become abusive, and many parents who were abused as children do not abuse their children. Based on a review of studies investigating the intergenerational transmission of abuse, Kaufman and Zigler (1987) estimated that one third of people abused or neglected as children abuse or neglect their own children. Many mediating factors (variables that modify the relationship between a predictor and an outcome) influence the likelihood of physical abuse and neglect. As shown in Box 22-2, parent, family, contextual, and child factors have been associated with increased risk for physical abuse and neglect (Finkelhor & Dziuba-Leatherman, 1994; Starr & Wolfe, 1991).

In light of these findings the dominant theoretical models of abuse and neglect emphasize the multidetermined nature of these problems. Within ecological and transactional models, for example, child abuse and neglect is perceived as influenced by factors within the abuser, the family, and the community and the beliefs and values of the culture in which the family, abuser, and child interact (Belsky, 1980; Cicchetti & Rizley, 1981).

Box 22-2. Factors associated with child physical abuse and neglect

Child physical abuse

Parent factors	**Family factors**	**Child factors**	**Contextual factors**
Health problems	Stepparent	Aggression	Poverty
Substance abuse	Spousal abuse or	Aversive behavior	Unemployment
Family violence	domestic violence	Difficult temperament	Geographical region
(in childhood)	Unsatisfactory marital	Age	
Depression	relationships		
	Marital conflict		

Child neglect

Parent factors	**Family factors**	**Child factors**	**Contextual factors**
Substance abuse	Social isolation	Infant temperament	Poverty
	Single-parent families		Unemployment
	Families with large		Inadequate housing
	numbers of children		Dangerous neighborhood

Developmental outcomes

Children who experience physical abuse and neglect may exhibit a variety of emotional and behavioral problems. Table 22-2 summarizes the empirical literature on the short- and long-term effects of physical abuse and neglect. (For a review, see Crouch & Milner, 1993; Kolko, 1993.) These effects can pervade the cognitive and psychosocial functioning of victimized children. How-

ever, not all children who experience physical abuse or neglect show identical behavioral or emotional difficulties. Moreover, if a child exhibits a constellation of symptoms consistent with those noted in Table 22-2, the clinician cannot necessarily assume that the child has been physically abused. Nevertheless, ignoring the possibility of abuse may lead clinicians to erroneous conclusions regarding the etiology of the child's difficulties.

Table 22-2. Developmental outcomes associated with child physical abuse and neglect

AREA AFFECTED	BEHAVIORAL MANIFESTATIONS
Physical abuse	
Aggression	Aggression toward adults and peers persisting into adolescence and adulthood
Social competence	Problems with interpersonal interactions, poor social problem solving
Emotional states	Anxiety/agitation, hypervigilance, depression, posttraumatic stress disorder in some cases
Interpersonal relationships	Insecure attachment, low self-esteem, separation anxiety/problems
Cognitive/neuropsychological functioning	Early developmental delays, neurological soft signs, poor receptive/expressive language, memory impairment, reduced reading ability, perceptual motor deficits, limited ability to use language to solve interpersonal conflicts
Academic performance	Poor school achievement, school discipline problems
Long-term developmental effects	Aggression, violent crime, substance abuse
Child neglect	
Physical development	Failure to thrive (FTT) syndrome in infancy, indicated by growth delay with postural signs (poor muscle tone, persistence of infantile postures); behavioral signs (unresponsiveness, minimal smiling, few vocalizations)
Cognitive functioning	Deficits in language, lower intelligence scores than nonabused children, academic delays
Social and behavioral development	Avoidant and resistant attachment to primary caregiver, passivity, showing of less affection than nonabused children, reduced play interactions with mothers, isolative play (preschool and school aged), withdrawn behavior, increased risk for delinquency and criminal behavior

Modified from "Effects of Child Neglect on Children," by J.L. Crouch, and J.S. Milner, 1993, *Criminal Justice and Behavior,* 20: 49-65; and "Characteristics of Child Victims of Physical Violence," by D.J. Kolko, 1993, *Journal of Interpersonal Violence,* 7: 244-276.

Interventions

Because abused and neglected children often experience difficulty with aggression, social competence, cognitive development, attachment, and academics, multifaceted and integrated interventions addressing these areas appear warranted. Much of the existing research on the treatment of physical abuse and neglect, however, focuses narrowly on either the child or the abusing parent and largely ignores many of the identified etiological and contextual factors contributing to abuse (see Box 22-2).

Child

Existing treatment studies of physical abuse and neglect have focused on improving the social skills of preschool-age abused and neglected children. Two types of direct interventions targeting social skill deficits have been examined: (1) day treatment and (2) a peer social initiation strategy. The effects of day treatment were evaluated in two studies (Culp et al., 1991; Culp, Richardson, & Heide, 1987). First, an assessment was conducted with children who participated in a day treatment program (6 hours daily, 5 days per week, with an average stay of 9 months) that included general classroom work on developing caring peer relationships, play therapy, speech therapy, physical therapy, parent education, individual and family treatment for parents, and a 24-hour crisis phone line. Although this day treatment program provided services for parents and children, the outcome evaluation focused exclusively on the children's social functioning and failed to address contextual variables. Nevertheless, children who completed this program showed increased social, emotional, and cognitive development. In the second study, a subgroup (n = 17) of children who completed the day treatment program was compared with similar peers evaluated but not admitted to the program. Children who completed the program exhibited significantly greater improvements in peer and maternal acceptance than comparison children. Although the second study included a comparison group, neither study randomly assigned

children to treatment conditions, so extraneous factors other than treatment may have accounted for the results.

A peer social initiation strategy was evaluated with physically abused and neglected preschoolers in three studies. Fantuzzo et al. trained abused and neglected children with high levels of adaptive social behavior to initiate play with abused and neglected withdrawn children during eight play sessions over a 3 to 4 week period (Davis & Fantuzzo, 1989; Fantuzzo et al., 1987; Fantuzzo et al., 1988). Withdrawn children were randomly assigned to peer treatment, adult treatment (similar to peer treatment but with an adult), and a control condition. Children who participated in the peer treatment increased their positive social overtures toward peers. Although direct interventions with abused and neglected children hold promise for reducing psychosocial difficulties, additional empirical study of child treatment is needed.

Parent

Because physically abusive parents have difficulty disciplining their children in appropriate, nonviolent ways, interventions have often focused on teaching child management through parent training. The goal of parent training differs for physically abusive and neglectful parents. Training for the former concentrates on reducing rigidity and intrusiveness and increasing knowledge of nonphysical means of discipline. Training for neglectful parents focuses on increasing parent-child interactions and parental responsiveness to children's needs.

Several studies have investigated the efficacy of parent training with abusive parents. These studies indicate parents who complete parent training show increased knowledge of alternatives to physical punishment and understanding of normal child development (Golub et al., 1987). In addition, abusive parents and their children show reduced negative behaviors after parent training (Lorber, Felton, & Reid, 1984). Despite these results, improvements associated with parent training may not generalize to the home setting and may require in vivo work. To help results generalize across settings, Wolfe, Sandler, and Kaufman (1981) taught abusive parents child-management and self-control techniques in the clinic and followed up with work in the home. This combination produced improvements in parenting skills and no reports of further child abuse over a 1-year follow-up period (Wolfe et al., 1981).

Special considerations for work with abusive families

Two issues should be considered by professionals before they initiate treatment with abusive families. First, treating abused children and their families is complex and difficult work. The novice or intermediate therapist should work under the close supervision of an experienced senior clinician to conduct safe and empirically sound treatment. Second, before beginning treatment with abusive families, determining the safety of the child is most important. If the child is living in a household with an untreated offender or has unsupervised visits with an untreated offender, the risk of continuing abuse is high. Also, beginning abuse-specific work when the child is unsafe sets the stage for increased anxiety and behavioral problems in the child. To ensure child safety, the therapist must work closely with the nonoffending parent, CPS, and the family court system to determine the best way to protect the child. After safety issues are resolved, abuse-specific work with the child, parents, and family can begin.

Model programs

Research on factors associated with child physical abuse and neglect underscores the importance of addressing the multiple systems with which these children and their families interact. Programs that provide only child or parent treatment in traditional mental health settings (such as an office, inpatient, or residential treatment center) may yield some improvement in the functioning of each individual but may not generalize to the environments to which these families and children must successfully adapt (for example, family, home, school, and community). Multi-

systemic therapy and Project 12-Ways are model programs that address the multiple systems consistently associated with child physical abuse and neglect (Brunk, Henggeler, & Whelan, 1987; Henggeler & Borduin, 1990; Lutzker, Frame, & Rice, 1982). Short-term evaluations of these programs show promise for physically abusive and neglectful families.

Multisystemic therapy with abusive and neglectful families

MST is consistent with an ecological model of child abuse and neglect; pertinent systems in which the child is involved (including individual, family, school, peer group, and community systems) are targeted for treatment. Brunk et al. (1987) compared the outcome of using home-based MST with that of office-based group parent training (Wolfe et al., 1981) with 43 families who had been investigated for abuse and neglect by CPS and who were randomly assigned to treatment conditions. Results indicated that both MST and parent training were effective in reducing parents' psychiatric symptoms and parental stress and improving family problems. However, families that completed MST showed greater alleviation of their family difficulties than families that completed parent training. Specifically, MST parents demonstrated improvements in effectively controlling their children's behavior. Additionally, neglectful parents in the MST program exhibited increased responsiveness toward their children and in turn these children showed less passive noncompliance. Parents who completed parent training indicated a greater decrease in social problems than MST families, a result that may have been a product of participation in the group format. Thus short-term outcomes tended to favor the more ecologically oriented MST treatment, especially regarding parent-child interactions.

Project 12-Ways

Project 12-Ways is an approach that provides multifaceted, home-based services to abusive and neglectful families. Many risk factors are targeted by Project 12-Ways services, which include parent training, home safety, treatment of parent problems such as substance abuse and stress, financial management, social support, nutrition, education, transportation, and prenatal and postnatal services for young and single parents (Lutzker & Rice, 1984).

Evaluations of the effectiveness of Project 12-Ways have been conducted using quasiexperimental designs. In an initial study, 50 abusive and neglectful families were randomly selected from 150 families served by the project during the previous year and outcomes were compared with those of 47 families who were not served by the project (Lutzker & Rice, 1984). Whether the comparison families received any interventions is unclear. Among Project 12-Ways participants, one family (2%) abused or neglected their child during treatment, compared with five (approximately 11%) of the comparison families. A follow-up assessment, however, indicated that the effects of treatment were reduced over time. Specifically, after termination of treatment, 8% of Project 12-Ways families and 11% of comparison families were involved in continued abuse or neglect of their children (Lutzker & Rice, 1984).

A larger scale evaluation was conducted to assess the recidivism rates of 352 Project 12-Ways families who received services from 1979 through 1984 and 358 comparison families (Lutzker & Rice, 1987). The recidivism rates of Project 12-Ways families were lower than those of comparison families for all years except 1981, when recidivism rates were equal for the two groups. Across the entire time, 21.3% of Project 12-Ways families and 28.5% of comparison families abused or neglected their children after termination of treatment. Lutzker and Rice (1987) suggest that the partial "washing out" of treatment effects over time indicates a need for "booster" services.

SUMMARY

The human toll taken by psychosocial hazards on the lives of children who are abused or neglected, delinquent, or substance abusers is quite alarming. This chapter focused on these children because of their increased risk for poor developmental outcomes. Incidence and prevalence information highlighted the number of children annually exposed to various psychosocial hazards. Etiological factors were consistent across each group. Multiple factors are associated with juvenile delinquency, adolescent substance abuse, and child physical abuse and neglect, including individual, family, peer, and community variables. The treatment literature summarized in each section emphasized that few treatments actually target the various correlates of these problems. Thus that few potent treatment models have been identified is not surprising. One treatment approach that has shown promise with each of these at-risk groups is multisystemic therapy. The results of studies investigating MST suggest its success is linked to its focus on the empirically derived etiological factors of serious clinical problems and its method of delivering ecologically valid services (Henggeler, Schoenwald, & Pickrel, 1995). To improve the developmental progress of at-risk children requires multifaceted and ecologically valid treatment strategies.

REFERENCES

Agnew, R. (1985). Social control theory and delinquency: A longitudinal test. *Criminology, 23,* 47-61.

Allen, J. P., Leadbeater, B. J., & Aber, J. L. (1990). The relationship of adolescents' expectations and values to delinquency, hard drug use, and unprotected sexual intercourse. *Development and Psychopathology, 2,* 85-98.

Alwin, L. F. (1993). *Texas juvenile justice: A system in need of rehabilitation* (SAO Report No. 94-009). Austin, Texas: Office of State Auditor.

American Association for Protecting Children (AAPC). (1988). *Highlights of official child neglect and abuse reporting—1986.* Denver, CO: American Humane Association.

Amini, F., Zilberg, N. J., Burke, E. L., & Salasnek, S. (1982). A controlled study of inpatient vs. outpatient treatment of delinquent drug abusing adolescents: One year results. *Comprehensive Psychiatry, 23,* 436-444.

Belsky, J. (1980). Child maltreatment: An ecological integration. *American Psychologist, 35,* 320-335.

Beschner, G. M., & Friedman, A. S. (1985). Treatment of adolescent drug abusers. *International Journal of the Addictions, 20,* 971-993.

Blau, G. M., Gillespie, J. F., Felner, R. D., & Evans, E. G.(1988). Predisposition to drug use in rural adolescents: Preliminary relationships and methodological considerations. *Journal of Drug Education, 18,* 13-22.

Blechman, E. A. (1985). *Solving child behavior problems at home.* Champaign, IL: Research Press.

Borduin, C. M., Mann, B. J., Cone, L. T., Henggeler, S. W., Fucci, B. R., Blaske, D. M., & Williams, R. A. (1995). Multisystemic treatment of adolescents referred for serious and repeated antisocial behavior. *Journal of Consulting and Clinical Psychology, 63*(4), 569-578.

Brassard, M. R., & Gelardo, M. S. (1987). Psychological maltreatment: The unifying construct in child abuse and neglect. *School Psychological Review, 16,* 127-136.

Bronfenbrenner, U. (1979). *The ecology of human development: Experiments by nature and design.* Cambridge, MA: Harvard University Press.

Brook, J. S., Nomura, C., & Cohen, P. (1989). A network of influences on adolescent drug involvement: Neighborhood, school, peer, and family. *Genetic, Social, and General Psychology Monographs, 115,* 125-145.

Brunk, M., Henggeler, S. W., & Whelan, J. P. (1987). Comparison of multisystemic therapy and parent training in the brief treatment of child abuse and neglect. *Journal of Consulting and Clinical Psychology, 55,* 171-178.

Bureau of Justice Statistics. (1992). *National Crime Survey.* Washington, DC: U.S. Department of Justice.

Caliso, J. A., & Miller, J. S. (1992). Childhood history of abuse and child abuse screening. *Child Abuse and Neglect, 16,* 647-659.

Cicchetti, D., & Rizley, R. (1981). Developmental perspectives on the etiology, intergenerational transmission, and sequelae of child maltreatment. *New Directions for Child Development, 11,* 31-55.

Cohen, S. (1979). Inhalants. In R. I. Dupont, A. Goldstein, & J. O'Donnell (Eds.), *Handbook on drug abuse* (National Institute on Drug Abuse, Alcohol, and Mental Health Administration, U.S. Department of Health, Education, and Welfare, and Office of Drug Policy). Washington, DC: U.S. Government Printing Office.

Crouch, J. L., & Milner, J. S. (1993). Effects of child neglect on children. *Criminal Justice and Behavior, 20,* 49-65.

Culp, R. E., Little, V., Letts, D., & Lawrence, H. (1991). Maltreated children's self-concept: Effects of a comprehensive treatment program. *American Journal of Orthopsychiatry, 61,* 114-121.

Culp, R. E., Richardson, M. T., & Heide, J. S. (1987). Differential developmental progress of maltreated children in day treatment. *Social Work, 42,* 497-499.

Czechowicz, D. (1988). Adolescent alcohol and drug abuse and its consequences: An overview. *American Journal of Drug and Alcohol Abuse, 14,* 189-197.

Davis, S., & Fantuzzo, J. W. (1989). The effects of adult and peer social initiations on social behavior of withdrawn and aggressive maltreated preschool children. *Journal of Family Violence, 4,* 227-248.

Dembo, R., Williams, L., Wothke, W., & Schmeidler, J. (1994). The relationship among family problems, friends' troubled behavior, and high risk youths' alcohol/other drug use and delinquent behavior: A longitudinal study. *International Journal of the Addictions, 29,* 1419-1442.

Dishion, T. J., Patterson, G. R., & Reid, J. R. (1988). Parent and peer factors associated with sampling in early adolescence: Implications for treatment. In E. R. Rahdert, & J. Grabowski (Eds.), *Adolescent drug abuse: Analyses of treatment research* (National Institute on Drug Abuse Research Monograph 77; DHHS Publication No. ADM 88-1523). Washington, DC: U.S. Government Printing Office.

Dupont, R. L. (1990). *Stopping alcohol and other drug use before it starts: The future of prevention* (Office of Substance Abuse Prevention Monograph 1) (DHHS Publication No. ADM 89-1645). Washington, DC: U.S. Department of Health and Human Services.

Elliott, D. S., & Huizinga, D. (1983). Social class and delinquent behavior in a national youth panel. *Criminology, 21,* 149-177.

Elliott, D. S., Huizinga, D., & Ageton, S. S. (1985). *Explaining delinquency and drug use.* Newbury Park, CA: Sage Publications.

Elliott, D. S., Huizinga, D., & Morse, B. (1986). Self-reported violent offending: A descriptive analysis of juvenile violent offenders and their offending careers. *Journal of Interpersonal Violence, 1,* 472-514.

Fagan, J., & Wexler, S. (1987). Family origins of violent delinquents. *Criminology, 25,* 643-669.

Fantuzzo, J. W., Jurecic, L., Stovall, A., Hightower, A. D., Goins, C., & Schachtel, D. (1988). Effects of adult and peer social initiations on the social behavior of withdrawn, maltreated preschool children. *Journal of Consulting and Clinical Psychology, 56,* 34-39.

Fantuzzo, J. W., Stovall, A., Schachtel, D., Goins, C., & Hall, R. (1987). The effects of peer social initiations on the social behavior of withdrawn maltreated preschool children. *Journal of Behavior Therapy and Experimental Psychiatry, 18,* 357-363.

Farrell, M., & Strang, J. (1991). Substance use and misuse in childhood and adolescence. *Journal of Child Psychology and Psychiatry and Allied Disciplines, 32,* 109-128.

Farrington, D. P. (1979). Longitudinal research on crime and delinquency. In N. Morris, & M. Tonry (Eds.), *Crime and justice: An annual review of research* (Vol. 1). Chicago: University of Chicago Press.

Federal Bureau of Investigation. (1992). *Uniform crime reports for the U.S. 1991.* Washington, DC: U.S. Government Printing Office.

Finkelhor, D., & Dziuba-Leatherman, J. (1994). Children as victims of violence: A national survey. *Pediatrics, 94,* 413-420.

Friedman, A. S. (1989). Family therapy vs. parent groups: Effects on adolescent drug abusers. *The American Journal of Family Therapy, 17,* 335-347.

Friedman, A. S., Glickman, N. W., & Morrissey, M. R. (1986). Prediction to successful treatment outcome by client characteristics and retention in treatment in adolescent drug treatment programs: A large-scale cross validation study. *Journal of Drug Education, 16,* 149-165.

Gelles, R. J., & Straus, M. A. (1987). Is violence toward children increasing? *Journal of Interpersonal Violence, 2,* 212-222.

Gelles, R. J., & Straus, M. A. (1988). *Intimate violence.* New York: Simon and Schuster.

Golub, J. S., Espinosa, M., Damon, L., & Card, J. (1987). A videotape parent education program for abusive parents. *Child Abuse and Neglect, 11,* 255-265.

Haley, J. (1976). *Problem solving therapy.* San Francisco: Jossey-Bass.

Hamparian, D. M., Schuster, W. J., Dinitz, S., & Conrad, J. P. (1978). *The violent few.* Lexington, MA: Lexington Press.

Hawkins, J. D., Catalano, R. F., & Miller, J. Y. (1992). Risk and protective factors for alcohol and other drug problems in adolescence and early adulthood: Implications for substance abuse prevention. *Psychological Bulletin, 112,* 64-105.

Henggeler, S. W. (1989). *Delinquency in adolescence.* Newbury Park, CA: Sage Publications.

Henggeler, S. W. (1991). Multidimensional causal models of delinquent behavior and their implications for treatments. In R. Cohen, & A. Siegel (Eds.), *Context and development* (pp. 211-231). Hillsdale, NJ: Lawrence Erlbaum.

Henggeler, S. W. (1993). Multisystemic treatment of serious juvenile offenders: Implications for the treatment of substance abusing youths. In L. S. Onken, J. D. Blaine, & J. J. Boren (Eds.), *Behavioral treatments for drug abuse and dependence* (National Institute on Drug Abuse Research Monograph 137) (NIH Publication No. 93-3684). Rockville, MD: National Institutes of Health.

Henggeler, S. W., & Borduin, C. M. (1990). *Family therapy and beyond: A multisystemic approach to treating the behavior problems of children and adolescents.* Pacific Grove, CA: Brooks/Cole.

Henggeler, S. W., Cunningham, P. B., Pickrel, S. G., & Schoenwald, S. K. (1995). Multisystemic therapy for serious juvenile offenders and their families. In R. R. Ross (Ed.), *Going straight: Effective delinquency prevention and offender rehabilitation* (pp. 109-133). Ottawa: Air Training & Publications.

Henggeler, S. W., Melton, G. B., & Smith, L. A. (1992). Family preservation using multisystemic therapy: An effective alternative to incarcerating serious juvenile offenders. *Journal of Consulting and Clinical Psychology, 60,* 953-961.

Henggeler, S. W., Melton, G. B., Smith, L. A., Schoenwald, S. K., & Hanley, J. H. (1993). Family preservation using multisystemic treatment: Long-term follow-up to a clinical trial with serious juvenile offenders. *Journal of Child and Family Studies, 2,* 283-293.

Henggeler, S. W., Pickrel, S. G., Brondino, M., J., & Crouch, J. L. (1996). Eliminating (almost) treatment dropout: Multisystemic therapy using home-based services with substance abusing/dependent delinquents. *American Journal of Psychiatry, 153*(3), 427-428.

Henggeler, S. W., Rodick, J. D., Borduin, C. M., Hanson, C. L., Watson, S. M., & Urey, J. R. (1986). Multisystemic treatment of juvenile offenders: Effects on adolescent behavior and family interaction. *Developmental Psychology, 22,* 132-141.

Henggeler, S. W., Schoenwald, S. K., & Pickrel, S. G. (1995). Multisystemic therapy: Bridging the gap between university- and community-based treatment. *Journal of Consulting and Clinical Psychology, 63*(5), 709-717.

Henggeler, S. W., Schoenwald, S. K., Pickrel, S. G., Brondino, M. J., Borduin, C. M., & Hall, J. A. (1994). *Treatment manual for family preservation using multisystemic therapy.* Charleston, SC: South Carolina Health and Human Services Finance Commission.

Howland, J., & Hingson, R. (1988). Alcohol as a risk factor for drownings: A review of the literature. *Accident Analysis and Prevention, 20,* 19-71.

Huesmann, L. R., Eron, L. D., Lefkowitz, M. M., & Walder, L. O. (1984). Stability of aggression over time and generations. *Developmental Psychology, 20,* 1120-1134.

Huizinga, D., & Elliott, D. S. (1986). Reassessing the reliability and validity of self-report delinquency measures. *Journal of Quantitative Criminology, 2,* 293-327.

Huizinga, D., Esbensen, F. A., Van Kammen, W. B., & Thornberry, T. P. (1993). Epidemiology. In D. Huizinga, R. Loeber, & T. P. Thornberry (Eds.), *Urban delinquency: Technical report.* Washington, DC: Office of Juvenile Justice and Delinquency Prevention, U.S. Department of Justice.

Huizinga, D., Loeber, R., & Thornberry, T. P. (1993). *Urban delinquency and substance abuse: Technical report.* Washington, DC: Office of Juvenile Justice and Delinquency Prevention, U.S. Department of Justice.

Inciardi, J. A. (1990). The crack-violence connection within a population of hard-core adolescent offenders. In M. De La Rosa, E. Y. Lambert, & B. Gropper (Eds.), *Drugs and violence: Causes, correlates, and consequences* (National Institute on Drug Abuse Research Monograph 103) (pp. 92-111). Rockville, MD: National Institute on Drug Abuse.

Johnston, L D., O'Malley, P. M., & Bachman, J. G. (1993). *National survey results on drug use from the Monitoring the Future study, 1975-1992. Volume 1: Secondary school students* (DHHS Publication No. 93-3597). Rockville, MD: National Institute on Drug Abuse.

Kandel, D. B., Davies, M., Karus, D., & Yamaguchi, K. (1986). The consequences in young adulthood of adolescent drug involvement: An overview. *Archives of General Psychiatry, 43,* 746-754.

Kaufman, J., & Zigler, E. (1987). Do abused children become abusive parents? *American Journal of Orthopsychiatry, 57,* 186-192.

Kazdin, A. E. (1987). Treatment of antisocial behavior in children: Current status and future directions. *Psychological Bulletin, 102*(2), 187-203.

Kazdin, A. E. (1995). Scope of child and adolescent psychotherapy research: Limited sampling of dysfunctions, treatments, and client characteristics. *Journal of Clinical Child Psychology, 24,* 125-140.

Kendall, P. C., & Braswell, L. (1985). *Cognitive-behavioral therapy for impulsive children.* New York: Guilford Press.

Kolko, D. J. (1993). Characteristics of child victims of physical violence. *Journal of Interpersonal Violence, 7,* 244-276.

Kristberg, B., Schwartz, I., Fishman, G., Eisikovits, Z., Guttman, E., & Joe, K. (1987). The incarceration of minority youth. *Crime & Delinquency, 33,* 173-205.

Kumpfer, K. L. (1989). Prevention of alcohol and drug abuse: A critical review of risk factors and prevention strategies. In D. Shaffer, I. Philips, & N. B. Enzer (Eds.), *OSAP prevention monograph 2: Prevention of mental disorders, alcohol and other drug use in children and adolescents.* Rockville, MD: Office of Substance Abuse Prevention, Department of Health and Human Services.

Levine, R. R. J., Watt, N. P., Prentky, R. A., & Fryer, J. H. (1980). Childhood social competence in functionally disordered psychiatric patients and in normals. *Journal of Abnormal Child Psychology, 8,* 132-138.

Lewis, R. A., Piercy, F. P., Sprenkle, D. H., & Trepper, T. S. (1990). Family-based interventions for helping drug-abusing adolescents. *Journal of Adolescent Research, 5,* 82-95.

Loeber, R. (1982). The stability of antisocial and delinquent child behavior: A review. *Child Development, 53,* 1431-1446.

Lorber, R., Felton, D. K., & Reid, J. B. (1984). A social learning approach to the reduction of coercive processes in child abusive families: A molecular analysis. *Advances in Behavior Research and Therapy, 6,* 29-45.

Lutzker, J. R., Frame, R. E., & Rice, J. M. (1982). Project 12-Ways: An ecobehavioral approach to the treatment and prevention of child abuse and neglect. *Education and Treatment of Children, 5,* 141-156.

Lutzker, J. R., & Rice, J. M. (1984). Project 12-Ways: Measuring outcome of a large in-home service for treatment and prevention of child abuse and neglect. *Child Abuse and Neglect, 8,* 519-524.

Lutzker, J. R., & Rice, J. M. (1987). Using recidivism data to evaluate Project 12-Ways: An ecobehavioral approach

to the treatment and prevention of child abuse and neglect. *Journal of Family Violence, 2,* 283-291.

Martin, G. W., & Wilkinson, D. A. (1989). Methodological issues in the evaluation of treatment of drug dependence. *Advances in Behavior Research and Therapy,* 11, 133-150.

Matarazzo, J. D. (1982). Behavioral health's challenge to academic, scientific, and professional psychology. *American Psychologist, 37,* 1-14.

McCurdy, K., & Daro, D. (1994). *Current trends in child abuse reporting and fatalities: The results of the 1993 annual fifty state survey.* Chicago: National Center on the Prevention of Child Abuse.

Mensch, B. S., & Kandel, D. B. (1988). Dropping out of high school and drug involvement. *Sociology of Education, 61,* 95-113.

Minuchin, S. (1974). *Families and family therapy.* Cambridge, MA: Harvard University Press.

Morris, H. H., Escoll, P. S., & Wexler, R. (1956). Aggressive behavior disorders of childhood: A follow-up study. *American Journal of Psychiatry, 112,* 991-997.

National Institute on Drug Abuse. (1993). *National survey results on drug use from the Monitoring the Future study, 1975-1992: Volume I secondary school students* (NIH Publication No. 93-3597). Washington, DC: U.S. Government Printing Office.

Newcomb, M.D., & Bentler, P.M. (1988). *Consequences of adolescent drug use: Impact on the lives of young adults.* Newbury Park, CA: Sage Publications.

Newcomb, M.D., & Bentler, P.M. (1989). Substance use and abuse among children and teenagers. *American Psychologist, 44,* 242-248.

Oetting, E. R., & Beauvais, F. (1987). Peer cluster theory, socialization characteristics, and adolescent drug use: A path analysis. *Journal of Counseling Psychology, 34,* 205-213.

Office of Juvenile Justice and Delinquency Prevention. (1994). *Comprehensive strategy for serious, violent, and chronic offenders: Program summary* (Report No. NCJ 143453). Washington, DC: U.S. Department of Justice, Office of Justice Programs.

Office of Technology Assessment, U.S. Congress. (1991). *Adolescent Health Volume II: Background and the effectiveness of selected prevention and treatment services* (Publication No. OTA-H-466) (pp. 499-578). Washington, DC: U.S. Government Printing Office.

Patterson, G. R., & Dishion, T. J. (1985). Contributions of families and peers to delinquency. *Criminology, 23,* 63-79.

Paulson, M. J., Coombs, R. H., & Richardson, M. A. (1990). School performance, academic aspirations, and drug use among children and adolescents. *Journal of Drug Education, 20,* 289-303.

Pianta, R., Egeland, B., & Erickson, M. F. (1989). The antecedents of maltreatment: Results of the mother-child interaction research project. In D. Cicchetti, & V. Carlson

(Eds.), *Child maltreatment: Theory and research on the causes and consequences of child abuse and neglect* (pp. 203-253). New York: Cambridge University Press.

Robins, L. N. (1966). *Deviant children grown up. A sociological and psychiatric study of sociopathic personality.* Baltimore, MD: Williams & Wilkins.

Robins, L. N. (1978). Sturdy childhood predictors of adult antisocial behavior: Replications from longitudinal studies. *Psychological Medicine, 8,* 611-622.

Schinke, S. P., Botvin, G. J., & Orlandi, M. A. (1991). *Substance abuse in children and adolescents: Evaluation and intervention.* Newbury Park, CA: Sage Publications.

Sells, S. B., & Simpson, D. D. (1979). Evaluation of treatment outcome for youths in the Drug Abuse Reporting Program (DARP): A follow-up study. In G. M. Beschner, & A. S. Friedman (Eds.), *Youth drug abuse: Problems, issues and treatment* (pp. 571-628). Lexington, MA: Lexington Books.

Simcha-Fagan, O., & Schwartz, J. E. (1986). Neighborhood and delinquency: An assessment of contextual effects. *Criminology, 24,* 667-703.

Stark, M. J. (1992). Dropping out of substance abuse treatment: A clinically oriented review. *Clinical Psychology Review, 12,* 93-116.

Starr, R. H., Jr., & Wolfe, D. A. (Eds.). (1991). *The effects of child abuse and neglect.* New York: Guilford Press.

Strasburg, P. A. (1978). *Violent delinquents.* New York: Monarch.

Synder, H. (1993). *Juvenile court statistics: 1990.* Washington, DC: Office of Juvenile Justice and Delinquency Prevention, U.S. Department of Justice.

Szapocznik, J., Kurtines, W. M., Foote, F. H., Perez-Vidal, A., & Hervis, O. (1986). Conjoint versus one-person family therapy: Further evidence for the effectiveness of conducting family therapy through one person with drug-abusing adolescents. *Journal of Consulting and Clinical Psychology, 54,* 395-397.

U. S. Department of Justice, Office of Juvenile Justice and Delinquency Prevention. (1995). *Effective programs for serious, violent, and chronic juvenile offenders: An examination of three model interventions and intensive aftercare initiatives.* National Satellite Teleconference, Richmond, KY.

Widom, C. S. (1989). Does violence beget violence? A critical examination of the literature. *Psychological Bulletin, 106,* 3-28.

Wolfe, D. A., Sandler, J., & Kaufman, K. (1981). A competency-based parent training program for child abusers. *Journal of Consulting and Clinical Psychology, 49,* 633-640.

Wolfgang, M. E., Figlio, R. M., & Sellin, T. (1972). *Delinquency in a birth cohort.* Chicago: University of Chicago Press.

Yamaguchi, K., & Kandel, D. B. (1985). On the resolution of role incompatibility: A life event history analysis of family roles and marijuana use. *American Journal of Sociology, 90,* 1284-1325.

Zuravin, S. J. (1991). Research definitions of child physical abuse and neglect: Current problems. In R. H. Starr, & D. A. Wolfe (Eds.), *The effects of child abuse and neglect: Research issues.* New York: Guilford Press.

Chapter 23

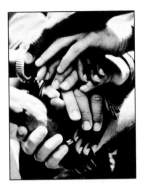

Persons with Mental Illness and Substance Abuse

Sara J. Corse

The treatment of severe mental illness and substance use disorders (SMISD) presents an ongoing challenge for nurses in community mental health. As awareness of the needs of this population has grown, the inadequacies of traditional systems of mental health and drug and alcohol care have become more apparent, leading to efforts to develop effective treatment for people with SMISD. This chapter reviews the history, etiology, and prevalence of SMISD; describes the results of research on innovative treatment models; and discusses the role of the community psychiatric nurse in the assessment, engagement, and ongoing treatment of SMISD. The importance of treating people with SMISD is clear because this combination of chronic, relapsing disorders often results in significant loss of family and social relationships, stable living arrangements, self-esteem and physical well-being, and satisfying life activities. Although such personal losses are associated with both severe mental illness and substance abuse separately, in combination these

disorders interact to create a downward spiral in functioning. However, ways exist to arrest this downward spiral and help people with SMISD undergo recovery and rehabilitation. The role of the community psychiatric nurse is vital in educating, treating, and acting as an advocate for people with SMISD.

EPIDEMIOLOGY
Defining the problem

A variety of terms have been used to describe this population, including *dual diagnosis, MISA (mentally ill substance abuser),* and *MICA (mentally ill chemical abuser).* The term *people with SMISD* is used here to specify the presence of an independent psychiatric disorder and a substance use disorder. SMI stands for *severe mental illness* such as the schizophrenias, schizoaffective disorder, bipolar disorder, and major depressive disorders, which have a chronic course and are often associated with significant compromises in functioning. SD stands for *substance disorders* and includes both substance abuse and dependence. Although the term "dual diagnosis" is often used to describe this group, it lacks specificity in two ways. First, dual diagnosis literally means two diagnoses and has been used to refer to people who have both mental illness and mental retardation. Second, clinically diverse populations have been identified by this one term, including people with SMISD as defined above and people with addictions who experience psychiatric symptoms that are substance induced rather than expressive of an independent psychiatric disorder (Lehman et al., 1994). Psychiatric nurses in community settings may encounter all types of dual diagnosis. However, although the appropriate treatment setting for people whose psychiatric symptoms are substance induced has not yet been determined, people with SMISD are clearly the responsibility of the mental health treatment system (Lehman et al., 1994; White & White, 1989).

Prevalence

Much literature has been written in the mental health field on the prevalence of SMISD, with reports of prevalence ranging from less than 10% to 75% in local studies of psychiatric clients.* These estimates of the prevalence of SMISD are subject to both selection bias (variations based on the client population studied) and ascertainment bias (variations as a consequence of errors, omissions, and inconsistencies in case identification) (Salloum, Moss, & Daley, 1991). For example, Ananth et al. (1989) reported that 75% of 75 clients randomly selected from the acute admissions wards of a large urban state hospital had a drug-related diagnosis according to the research team. In contrast, only 5% of these clients received a diagnosis of substance abuse in the psychiatric emergency room and fewer than 38% were diagnosed in the state hospital.

---

*Alterman et al. (1982), Ananth et al. (1989), Bergman & Harris (1985), Hall et al. (1977), Lehman et al. (1994), Safer (1987), Soyka et al. (1993), and Warner et al. (1994).

Despite their limitations these studies provide evidence that substance use disorders are more prevalent among people with severe mental illness than among the general population (Brown et al., 1989). Although a nationally representative study of the lifetime prevalence of drug dependence among people in the general population between 15 and 54 years of age found a rate of 7.5%, the Epidemiologic Catchment Area survey of 20,000 adults found that 29% of people with mental disorders had a lifetime diagnosis of a substance use disorder, with this number increasing to 64% among clients seeking intensive psychiatric care from emergency rooms or inpatient psychiatric units (Regier et al., 1990; Warner et al., 1995).

ETIOLOGY

Awareness of the increasing prevalence of SMISD grew in the late 1970s (Brown et al., 1989). During the previous 30 years the advancement of pharmacotherapy for severe mental illnesses and the deinstitutionalization movement led to a shift in the goals and locations of mental health treatment. Currently, outpatient care and community-based living are the norm for clients previously considered manageable only within the confines of the large state institutions of the early 1900s (Bassuk & Gerson, 1978; Thompson, Bass, & Witkin, 1982). This change in treatment setting and more important in the residential arrangements of people with severe mental illness increased the accessibility of alcohol and other drugs and the vulnerability to drug and alcohol abuse (McCarrick, Manderscheid, & Bertolucci, 1985). Past generations of people with severe mental illness who were reliant on public funding received care from the "total institution" of the state hospital, which socialized them into the patient role and isolated them from the rest of society, but the "new generation" of people with severe mental illness faced an often painful struggle to survive in the community in the face of poverty and stigma (Minkoff, 1987; Pepper, Kirshner, & Ryglewicz, 1981). Without a strong system of rehabilitative and recovery-oriented services in place in the community mental health system, programs were poorly equipped to address the needs of people with SMISD.

Societal trends in drug and alcohol use also have contributed to the problem of SMISD. "Better living through chemistry" is promoted in contemporary society, with sanctioned use of many kinds of substances to enhance socialization, alleviate distress, control weight, stay up longer, work harder, or relax more quickly. One illustration of this trend is found in a report of the National Comorbidity Survey, which estimated the lifetime and 12-month prevalence of the use of and dependence on drugs (Warner et al., 1995). The overall prevalence of lifetime drug use (use of an illegal drug or nonmedical use of a prescription drug at least once in the lifetime) was 51%. However, when separated by age cohorts, the highest prevalence of lifetime use (70%) was found among survey respondents who were adolescents at the height of the youth drug culture, compared with a lifetime use prevalence of 36% among respondents born before World War II who were past adolescence before the middle 1960s. Data on the lifetime prevalence of drug dependence show similar differences among age cohorts (Warner et al., 1995).

A second indication of increasing drug use in the general population is the increase in the reported involvement of marijuana, cocaine, and heroin in medical incidents reported by emergency rooms and medical examiners from 1976 to 1988 in cities around the country (Gerstein & Harwood, 1990). At the same time that drug and alcohol use is on the rise, so is the use of alcohol-related treatment in the general population (Weisner, Greenfield, & Room, 1995). Thus a variety of factors such as changes in the delivery of mental health care and trends in the availability of illicit drugs have influenced the prevalence of SMISD over the past several decades.

Studies of the reported reasons for and immediate effects of drug or alcohol use by people with SMISD suggest that drugs and alcohol are appealing because of their short-term palliative effects on psychiatric symptoms and their ability to help create superficial social connections (Bergman & Harris, 1985; Dixon et al., 1990). Schizophrenic users of alcohol reported relief of unpleasant but nonpsychotic experiences such as social anxiety, tension, and apathy (Noordsy et al., 1991). In a study of a broader population of psychiatric and substance use disorders, Warner et al. (1994) found that people with SMISD reported social interaction, relief of unpleasant affective states, and boredom as the main reasons for substance use. Khantzian (1985) proposed the "self-medication hypothesis," suggesting that clients choose particular substances to abuse because of the specific psychotropic effects of these drugs on their psychiatric symptoms. For example, opiate use reduces feelings of rage and aggression in angry, violent addicts (Khantzian, 1985). However, subsequent studies have not supported this theory. Most have found that clients used different drugs with different effects and developed different expectations of the consequences of their drug use with no clear patterns related to the reduction of psychiatric symptoms (Castaneda, 1994; Castaneda, Galanter, & Franco, 1989; Schinka, Curtiss, & Mulloy, 1994). Thus many factors influence choice of substance, including drug availability, local patterns of use, and anticipated reduction in symptoms.

Severe mental illnesses such as bipolar disorder and schizophrenia and addictive disorders have been shown to have biological etiologies based on family, adoption, twin, and genetic studies. For example, twin studies of the heritability of schizophrenia suggest a 45% concordance rate among identical twins, meaning that 45% of people with a schizophrenic identical twin also will have schizophrenia. The concordance rate is 10% among fraternal twins whose environment is the same but whose genetic material is no more similar than siblings (Weiner, 1985). More recent research using genetic analysis techniques has implicated the dopamine D2 receptor gene as a genetic risk factor for substance abuse (Comings et al., 1994). Little research has been conducted on the biological etiology of SMISD, but Kendler's (1985) twin study found people with both alcoholism and schizophrenia have an apparent genetic predisposition to both disorders.

INTERVENTION

Recent efforts to improve treatment for people with SMISD, elements of a comprehensive care system, and models of recovery helpful for the assessment, engagement, and treatment of people with SMISD are presented in the following sections.

System barriers to effective treatment

Historically, mental health and substance abuse treatment services have functioned independently under separate legislative, fiscal, and organizational systems. People with SMISD needed to initiate help seeking in each system or risk falling through gaps between the two (Ridgely, Goldman, & Willenbring, 1990). Many people with SMISD are screened out of traditional substance abuse programs or, if admitted, drop out or are discharged prematurely for failure to comply with rules (Galanter, Castenada, & Ferman, 1988; McLellan et al., 1982; Ridgely et al., 1990). People with SMISD get worse rather than better in treatment settings that emphasize confrontation but fail to provide adequate psychiatric evaluation and treatment (LaPorte et al., 1981; McLellan et al., 1983; McLellan et al., 1984). They often have difficulty integrating into community self-help groups such as Alcoholics Anonymous (AA) because of psychiatric symptoms that make them "different" from other group members or conflict over the use of psychotropic medication, although the official position of AA supports the appropriate use of medications for psychiatric or physical disorders (Alcoholics Anonymous, 1984; Wallen & Weiner, 1989).

In traditional mental health settings, substance abuse may often go unrecognized and hence may not be addressed (Ananth et al., 1989; Brown et

al., 1989; Hall et al., 1977). Covert drug abuse was detected in 13.3% of a sample of 195 clients in outpatient treatment in a community mental health center and was associated with greater diagnostic confusion and poorer treatment outcome compared with clients with no or self-reported drug abuse (Hall et al., 1977). Therapists behaved differently with these clients than with diagnostically matched controls, misdiagnosing them 4 times more often, missing appointments with them 7 times more often, and transferring them to other clinicians or agencies 10 times more often (Hall et al., 1977). Substance-abusing clients often fail to engage in treatment and often continue covert substance use during hospitalization (Alterman et al., 1982; McLellan et al., 1981; Solomon & Gordon, 1986-1987). Clients with SMISD who do become involved in psychiatric day treatment programs are four times more likely than clients without substance abuse to be absent or suspended for continued substance abuse or rule infractions (Case, 1991). As of the late 1980s, people with SMISD did not readily fit into existing mental health or substance abuse treatment systems (Ridgely, Goldman, & Talbott, 1986; Ridgely, Osher, & Talbott, 1987; Schwartz & Goldfinger, 1981).

Current treatment approaches

New programs for service delivery and research were initiated in recognition of the need for specialized care for people with SMISD; the most notable of these were a series of NIMH-funded studies begun in the late 1980s and early 1990s. The current literature on effective treatment of people with SMISD emphasizes comprehensiveness, concurrence, and integration of care.* Different approaches to achieving these goals have been designed. Some systems emphasize the use of existing mental health and addiction programs. Treatment for both disorders occurs

---

*Carey (1989), Mercer-McFadden & Drake (in press), Minkoff & Drake (1991), Ridgely et al. (1987), Teague, Schwab, & Drake (1990), and Wallen & Weiner (1989).

sequentially or in parallel, often with case managers working to create and maintain client connections to all necessary treatments. Other systems have created "hybrid" programs that provide simultaneous mental health and substance abuse treatment. These programs operate under one supervisory and administrative umbrella with dually trained staff (Kline et al., 1991; Minkoff, 1991).

The research literature on intervention for people with SMISD has focused on studies of service use and treatment outcome. Findings regarding service use report an association between SMISD and heavy use of costly inpatient and emergency mental health services, nonengagement in community-based treatment, homelessness, and incarceration.[*] On the other hand, outpatient treatment designed to address both the severe mental illness and the substance use disorder has been shown to reduce inpatient hospitalization and length of stay for people with SMISD.[†] Changes in the nature of outpatient treatment have been reported as well, with intensive case management increasing the use of dual diagnosis treatment groups sixfold compared with standard case management (Teague et al., 1990).

Studies of treatment outcome for people with SMISD have focused on changes in substance use, psychiatric symptoms, and psychosocial functioning. With respect to reduction of substance use, findings have been mixed, with some reports indicating treatment fosters abstinence among the majority of program participants (Drake, McHugo, & Noordsy, 1993; Ries & Ellingson, 1989) or leads to reductions in drug and alcohol symptoms (Jerrell & Ridgely, 1995) and other reports showing little or no effect on substance use (Bond et al., 1991; Lehman et al., 1993b). Reductions in psychiatric symptoms as a result of specialized residen-

tial intervention for people with SMISD have been reported in a study comparing treatment for homeless men with SMISD in therapeutic community programs with community residence programs (Rahav et al., 1995); the therapeutic community programs showed greater effectiveness in reducing depressive, psychotic, and functional symptoms. People with SMISD in specialized outpatient treatment (behavioral skills training, case management, and a 12-step recovery model) showed reductions in psychiatric symptoms and improvements in psychosocial functioning in work, independent living skills, and immediate and extended social contacts (Jerrell & Ridgely, 1995). These studies show that specialized interventions designed to address the varied needs of people with SMISD can be effective in engaging people in treatment, reducing substance abuse and psychiatric symptoms, and improving psychosocial functioning.

MODELS OF RECOVERY FROM ADDICTION
Stages of readiness to change

A client's motivation or readiness to change addictive behaviors plays an important role in treatment. A model for understanding readiness to change was developed by Prochaska, DiClemente, and Norcross (1992) through research on a range of addictive behaviors, including overeating, cigarette smoking, and alcohol abuse. Although this model of change has not been studied with respect to people with SMISD, it provides a useful framework for their assessment and treatment because of its emphasis on the role of client motivation in behavioral change and its guidelines on how to motivate clients to change. This model rests on the following suppositions:

1. Change is a process with five identifiable stages.
2. People may cycle through these stages repeatedly on their way to stable behavior change.
3. Some interventions are more effective than others given a person's readiness to change.

---

[*]Bartels et al. (1993), Hadley, Culhane, & McGurrin (1992), Kline et al. (1991), Lamb (1982), Rahav et al. (1995), and Solomon & Gordon (1986-1987).
[†]Bond et al. (1991), Durrell et al. (1993), Hellerstein & Meehan (1987), Jerrell & Ridgely (1995), Kofoed et al. (1986), and Lehman et al. (1993b).

The first stage of change is precontemplation. At this stage, people have no intention of changing their behaviors and often either have no awareness that a problem exists or misidentify the problem. Many people with SMISD who present to the acute care mental health treatment system are precontemplators. The psychiatric nurse who identifies SMISD and presents the diagnosis to the client may be the first person to suggest that the substance use is problematic. People with SMISD in precontemplation may disavow all or part of this assessment. For example, one person might accept a diagnosis of schizophrenia but say personal alcohol use is normal, whereas another person with the same problems may reject the diagnosis of schizophrenia but identify as an alcoholic.

For effectiveness in the precontemplation stage, interventions should emphasize education to raise the client's level of awareness of behaviors and their consequences, communicate that change is possible and worthwhile, and instill hope. Group and individual interventions to persuade people with SMISD to seek treatment for their substance use disorder have been developed in many inpatient and outpatient mental health settings with favorable results (Bond et al., 1991; Galanter et al., 1992; Osher & Kofoed, 1989). Successful interventions for people with SMISD in the precontemplation stage take into account their psychiatric stability and cognitive clarity and present material in various ways such as through psychodrama, videos, and interactive learning sessions.

The second stage of change is contemplation. In this stage the client is aware that a problem exists and seriously considers changing but as yet makes no commitment to take action. People with SMISD in contemplation may vacillate among feeling the pain and loss brought about because of substance use, wanting what a sober life-style might bring to them, and feeling that the effort to change is too great and success too uncertain. Clients may remain at this stage for a very long time before taking any action.

Intervention for contemplators includes education, engagement, and self-evaluation. Miller and Rollnick (1991) suggest using "motivational interviewing" with precontemplators and contemplators to help them move from ambivalence about change to a decision to act. One aspect of this interview method is the avoidance of argumentation and head-to-head confrontation. The psychiatric nurse avoids becoming overidentified with arguments for change in interaction with clients, leaving room for them to formulate their own reasons for change rather than to resist the efforts of the nurse to change them. To use this interviewing style, the nurse must recognize when client resistance has been activated and shift strategies to defuse resistance and promote self-efficacy.

The next stage of change is preparation. People in this stage intend to change soon and have unsuccessfully taken action in the past year (such as reducing but not quitting smoking or limiting alcohol use to weekends only). People in preparation differ from people in contemplation because they have a greater commitment to take action. They have not yet reached the action stage, however, because their attempts to change are inconsistent or incomplete. Commitment-enhancing techniques such as reviewing the pros and cons of changing, setting goals for action (for example, New Year's resolutions), and supporting steps that have been taken toward action are useful for people in preparation.

The central stage of change is action, in which people work to change their behavior. Action entails the most overt behavioral changes, such as abstinence from alcohol or other drugs, and takes considerable time and energy. The action stage has historically received the most attention and has been the focus of treatment programming. It includes cognitive and behavioral change techniques such as restructuring clients' environments or daily activities to reduce contact with drugs or alcohol (for example, heeding the AA advice to the recovering alcoholic or addict to avoid contact with the "people, places and things" that have been associated with the substance use), substituting activities such as relaxation and positive leisure activities for problematic behaviors, and rewarding changes made in problematic behaviors (such as earning a key chain for 30 days of sobriety in AA).

When people with SMISD are in the action phase of change, interventions designed for people without serious mental illness may need to be modified. For example, people with SMISD are often on psychotropic medication and require extensive, ongoing education about the purpose of those medications and the difference between taking such medication as prescribed and either abusing it or using alcohol or illicit drugs. The information may need to be repeated to compensate for cognitive deficits. Furthermore, although clients need information about the risks of mixing alcohol or other drugs with their prescribed medication, the nurse should take great care to determine the way these warnings are being heeded. One client who was told not to drink while taking medication took this to mean medication should be stopped whenever a drink was desired. Being unmedicated and drinking led to a decline in functioning and ultimately a psychotic

break. People with SMISD, even those who are actively abusing substances, fare better than they would if untreated when maintained on their medications with careful treatment of side effects (Siris, 1990).

The next stage of change is maintenance. During this stage, which extends indefinitely, people work to maintain change and prevent relapse. To prepare people with SMISD for maintenance, nurses should provide education during the previous stages of change that includes information about the nature of both addiction and mental illness as relapsing disorders. Because addiction is a disorder in which relapse is common, people may cycle through the various stages many times before achieving stable change. However, gains made during one journey through the stages of change are not completely lost during an episode of relapse. Instead the process of change can be understood as a spiral. The spiral denotes both a circular movement through stages and a linear progression over time (Figure 23-1).

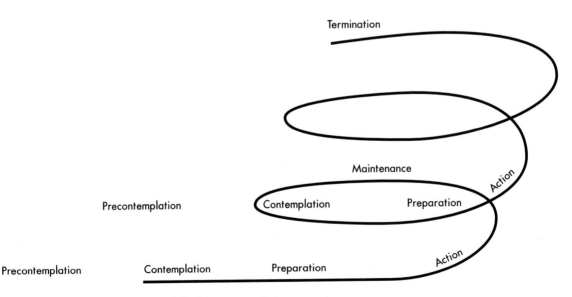

Figure 23-1. A spiral model of the stages of change.
(Modified from "In Search of How People Change: Applications to Addictive Behaviors," by J. O. Prochaska, C. C. DiClemente, & J. C. Norcross, 1992, *American Psychologist, 47*, 1102-1114.)

Developmental models of recovery

Several developmental models of recovery have been proposed by clinical researchers for working with addicted populations, including frequently relapsing alcoholics (Gorski, 1989), alcoholics in inpatient treatment (Wing, 1993), and people with SMISD in mental health settings (Osher & Kofoed, 1989). Many similarities exist among these developmental models and the stages of change model described earlier. A period of denial or fluctuating interest in changing addictive behaviors is followed by some degree of commitment to abstinence, action to achieve abstinence, and relapse prevention. Both Gorski and Wing go on to define further goals for fundamental, progressive, and lasting life changes. Table 23-1 summarizes these three models of recovery to facilitate comparisons among them.

Table 23-1. A comparison of developmental models of recovery

GORSKI RELAPSING ALCOHOLICS	WING ALCOHOLICS IN INPATIENT TREATMENT	OSHER AND KOFOED PEOPLE WITH SMISD
		Stage 1: Engagement **Theme:** Attracting person with SMISD to treatment
Stage 1: Transition **Theme:** Giving up need to control alcohol and other drug use	**Stage 1:** Denial **Theme:** Accepting need for abstinence and deciding to remain abstinent	**Stage 2:** Persuasion **Theme:** Convincing person to accept abstinence-oriented treatment
Stage 2: Stabilization **Theme:** Recuperating from damage caused by addictive use	**Stage 2:** Dependence **Theme:** Finding motivation only in external reasons for abstinence	**Stage 3:** Active treatment **Theme:** Helping people with SMISD develop attitudes and skills necessary for abstinence
Stage 3: Early recovery **Theme:** Making internal changes in way of thinking, feeling, and acting with respect to substance use	**Stage 3:** Behavior change **Theme:** Setting goals for recovery that are internal and growth oriented (self-esteem, trust, coping skills)	**Stage 4:** Relapse prevention **Theme:** Helping clients maintain abstinence over time through ongoing relationship with provider and by working to recognize triggers for relapse
Stage 3: Middle recovery **Theme:** Making external changes, balancing life-style		
Stage 4: Late recovery **Theme:** Delving into childhood and family issues, making life-style changes	**Stage 4:** Life planning **Theme:** Working for life-style goals such as marriage, career, family, and education	
Stage 5: Maintenance **Theme:** Maintaining recovery through effective daily coping, continuing growth		

Modified from *Passages Through Recovery: An Action Plan for Preventing Relapse,* by T. T. Gorski, 1989, San Francisco: Harper & Row; "Treatment of Patients with Psychiatric and Psychoactive Substance Abuse Disorders," by F. C. Osher, and L. L. Kofoed, 1989, *Hospital and Community Psychiatry, 40,* 1025-1030; "Determining Alcohol Treatment Outcomes: A Cost-Effectiveness Perspective," by D. Wing, 1990, *Nursing Economics,* 8: 248-255; and "Applying the 'Model of Recovering Alcoholics' Behavior Stages and Goal Setting' to Nursing Practice," by D. M. Wing, 1993, *Archives of Psychiatric Nursing, 8* (4), 197-202.

Gorski's "Developmental Model of Recovery" (1989) is the most detailed of the three models. In the first stage, transition, the addicted person experiences a period of turbulence. Once seemingly effective means of using alcohol or other drugs while carrying on with life are proving inadequate. Clients experience a growing realization of problems associated with addictive use that help motivate them to consider change. Normal problem solving and strategies for controlling substance use fail. As a sign that this stage is coming to an end, the client accepts the need for abstinence.

The next stage in the Gorski model is stabilization, which begins with a recognition of the need for help in staying abstinent. It also is a time during which the client recovers from the immediate aftereffects of addictive use such as by going through withdrawal and experiencing increased attention span and cognitive clarity. During this stage, destructive preoccupation with substance use is interrupted and the client learns techniques to manage the stresses of everyday life without resorting to substance use. As a signal of the end of this stage, the client feels a greater sense of hope and motivation.

In early recovery, people with addiction become fully cognizant and accepting of the addiction as a disease process and begin to establish a sobriety-centered value system. Much change at this stage is internal and involves changes in the way the client thinks, feels, and acts with respect to drug or alcohol use. Middle recovery entails a focus on making external changes such as repairing relationships damaged by addiction and establishing a balanced life-style and self-regulated recovery program. Late recovery involves deeper intrapsychic work in which people with addiction examine the role of childhood problems and family issues in their recovery. The impact of these childhood problems on adult behavior is examined and substantial life-style changes are effected.

Maintenance, Gorski's final step, involves continued growth and development, effective day-to-day coping, a well-maintained program of recovery, and effective coping through major life transitions. This stage is equivalent to the maintenance stage in Prochaska et al.'s stages of readiness to change (1992). Maintenance is vital because a recovery program is inadequate if it helps someone achieve sobriety but does not contribute to fundamental life change.

Wing's "Model of Recovering Alcoholics' Behavior Stages and Goal Setting" (1993) was developed through her grounded theory research in an inpatient treatment center for alcoholics. She lived in this setting for 28 days and observed a progression to recovery. The first stage, denial, characterizes the addicted person, usually coerced into treatment, who does not admit to a problem with alcohol. Although people in this stage of recovery can successfully complete treatment in an inpatient setting, unless they move through denial to a decision to remain abstinent, relapse to drinking after discharge is highly likely. The second stage is dependence, a condition in which the alcoholic's motivation for abstinence is linked to or dependent on some external object or relationship. In other words the person wishes to remain sober to keep a job or stay married but has not established internal motivation for abstinence. Stage three is behavior change, wherein the desire to make healthy, growth-oriented life changes motivates recovery. During this stage the person with alcoholism works to develop self-esteem, trust, new ways of handling stress, and coping strategies. This stage entails ongoing relapse prevention while new skills are learned. In the final stage, life planning, long-range life goals are pursued in areas such as intimate relationships, parenting, career, and education. A program of relapse prevention is maintained. When the Wing and Gorski models are viewed side by side, the similarities are evident. Early periods of denial, transition, stabilization, and dependence that characterize the person struggling to accept a problem and pursue recovery give way to internal and external changes. The work of recovery in these later stages is to not only maintain abstinent behavior but also foster growth in all arenas of life.

Osher and Kofoed (1989), from their work in a variety of settings, outline four phases of treatment for people with SMISD. Unlike Gorski and Wing their focus is on the treatment environment rather than the addicted mentally ill person, perhaps because the voice of the consumer is only recently being heard in research on people with severe mental illness. The treatment phases are briefly outlined here and described in more detail in later sections in discussions of nursing interventions for people with SMISD.

The first phase of treatment is engagement, or attracting people with SMISD to the treatment program and convincing them that the program has something worthwhile to offer them. In the beginning the enticement to treatment may have little to do with substance abuse, focusing instead on basic necessities such as food, housing, entitlements, or relief from distressing symptoms. No parallel to the engagement stage exists in the Gorski or Wing models because they focus on addicted people already in treatment. Because most people with SMISD do not seek to change their addictive behavior in early stages, the Osher and Kofoed engagement phase describes the way clinical staff might approach people in this stage of readiness.

The next phase of treatment is persuasion, or the process of convincing the person who has become engaged in treatment (but is still in either precontemplation or contemplation) to pursue abstinence and recovery. A variety of interventions are necessary in this phase of treatment, including education about the psychiatric and addictive problems, the link between people's use of substances and adverse consequences they have experienced, and the benefits of recovery. Contact with peers who are already in recovery also is important. Osher and Kofoed advise clinicians to clearly and consistently communicate a goal of abstinence while being aware of the client's readiness to change. Premature commitment to behavioral change can backfire.

Once the client is ready to change addictive behaviors, active treatment begins. This treatment phase is focused on developing recovery tools to remain abstinent in a treatment environment that has a "culture of abstinence" (Osher & Kofoed, 1989). Once abstinence has been achieved, relapse prevention begins; during this ongoing phase of treatment, sobriety is maintained, triggers for relapse are identified and anticipated, and techniques for avoiding relapse are developed. By working effectively with early lapses in a trusting and supportive clinical relationship, nurses may help clients avoid later relapses.

One striking aspect of Table 23-1 is the heavy emphasis on the early phases of recovery for people with SMISD, largely because most work with people with SMISD has focused on clients who are not in treatment for their addiction because of a lack of appropriate treatment programs and the low level of readiness to change of most people with SMISD. For example, in the model program described in a later section, 95% of clinical interventions focus on building motivation to change or helping a person make the transition to a recovery program by making the association between alcohol or drug use and life crises or losses. A useful aspect of developmental models is that they can help nurses form realistic expectations for client progress and time interventions accordingly. This need for realistic staff expectations of client progress is never so pronounced as with people with SMISD. Movement from transition and stabilization to early recovery can be extremely slow, taking many months even among regular program attendees.

STAGES OF NURSING INTERVENTION FOR PEOPLE WITH SMISD
Assessment and diagnosis

Accurate assessment and diagnosis are essential in the treatment of people with SMISD. Diagnostic confusion is often present because symptoms of a severe psychiatric disorder may mimic or mask symptoms of a substance use disorder and vice versa. In addition, patterns of substance use that would be considered mild in the general population may be abusive among people with severe mental illness. Because of the many factors that interfere with them, assessment and diagnosis should be considered multistaged processes that continue through early treatment. Major assessment tools include urine toxicology screening, self-reported data collected through clinical interviews, and information gathered from collateral sources.

Routine toxicology screens, a cornerstone of substance abuse identification, are most effective when conducted at the earliest possible time after drug use and are valid for different lengths of time depending on the substance. Marijuana stays in the system the longest, with derivatives detectable by urine screen for as long as 3 weeks after use. Cocaine derivatives can be detected in urine several days after use, but alcohol use must be screened for less than 48 hours after ingestion. A positive urine screen and observed signs of intoxication are useful in assessment. However, a negative screen should not rule out drug or alcohol use.

Clinical interviewing to obtain a detailed history of substance use patterns and related issues is the next important assessment activity. It should take place when clients are fully able to cooperate, such as after florid psychosis has resolved. Essential data to collect if SMISD is suspected include information about past and current substance use patterns, psychiatric symptoms, treatment history, and information about life history and present activities to assess the premorbid functioning level. Most important, information is needed about the way episodes of substance use and fluctuations in psychiatric symptoms are related to one another. Evaluating the client's premorbid level of functioning can help determine whether functional losses precede or are exacerbated by substance use. Dixon et al. (1993) found that, among state hospital patients, a brief screening for recent regular use of alcohol and drugs (defined as any past period of daily or weekly use plus any use of alcohol or drugs during the past 30 days) was more useful for identifying patients in need of alcohol or drug intervention than *DSM-III-R* diagnosis.

In assessing problematic substance use, the nurse must be sensitive to the impact of low levels of substance use that are usually not a problem in the general population but may cause functional impairment among people with SMISD. In a study of moderate drinking among people with severe mental illness, Drake and Wallach (1993) found that schizophrenic clients have a hard time maintaining a pattern of moderate drinking over time. What begins as moderate drinking leads to an alcohol use disorder in 24.4% of clients. Only 5% of clients initially rated as moderate drinkers were still drinking moderately 7 years after initial evaluation. In contrast, 50% of Americans in the general population drink regularly over time without developing an alcohol use disorder (Hilton, 1987).

Collateral sources may provide useful information about the use patterns of people with SMISD. These can include case managers, residential counselors, other staff, and family or friends. Drake et al. (1990) found that case manager ratings were more sensitive to alcohol use disorders among people in the manager's caseload than research interviews because they were able to incorporate observational data over a period of time, treatment records, information from collateral sources, and interview data.

No single method of assessing or diagnosing SMISD provides complete accuracy or reliability. However, a combination of laboratory tests, self-reported history, observable behavior, and collateral information leads to the most accurate diagnosis. The diagnosis should be reassessed when the client is psychiatrically stable and no longer detoxifying. In a study of the accuracy of self-reporting of drug use by pregnant clients to a certified nurse-midwife (CNM), accuracy improved when clients were treated by the same CNM over time, routine urine toxicologies were performed, the CNMs received special training in the way to assess substance abuse, and on-site substance abuse services were offered (Corse, McHugh, & Gordon, 1995). The CNMs were able to recognize the many subtle ways they had in the past of saying, "Don't tell me about your drug or alcohol use. I don't know how to help you."

Engagement

People with SMISD in the mental health system often do not perceive a problem with their substance use, have not considered changing, do not believe abstinence will lead to desirable outcomes, and even if they do, have not experienced a positive effect from treatment for substance abuse. Thus they may need to be attracted to treatment by something other than the promise of change. Offering concrete help with any aspect of substance use that a client identifies as a problem can foster engagement and active involvement in treatment.

In addition to providing tangible help, clinicians must develop a relationship of trust between clients and themselves. This may take an agonizingly long time and involve many attempts on the part of the psychiatric nurse to engage the client via follow-up phone calls, visits in the emergency room or the inpatient unit when the client decompensates, and home visits. At this stage of treatment the psychiatric nurse emphasizes that change is possible, an idea the client may not yet believe. Although the client is responsible for making the change, the psychiatric nurse must be alert to shifts in the client's readiness to address SMISD and be ready to intervene to help the client take the next step toward recovery. When people are not yet committed to changing their behavior, the most important goal of intervention is to continue communicating. One CNM who works with pregnant addicted women reported an interaction with a client who repeatedly denied cocaine use even after a positive toxicology screen. When the CNM challenged the client's denial, the client essentially closed down and the conversation was finished. At the next appointment the CNM tried a new approach. Without confronting the client's presentation of the situation, the CNM simply asked, "What worries you about knowing there is cocaine in your baby's system?" They then had a meaningful conversation about the client's worries without evoking resistance (Corse et al., 1995).

People with SMISD also must begin to believe in the process of recovery and rehabilitation to engage in the difficult work of treatment. People with severe mental illness are no longer given life sentences to large state institutions. They can be psychiatrically stabilized on appropriate medications, live in community settings, form friendships, marry and have children, and engage in meaningful life activities. However, for people with substance use disorders and perhaps a treatment-resistant mental illness a stable life may have long been elusive. Trust in treatment and hope for a better future do not come easily to staff or clients. When recovery and rehabilitation can be seen in terms of incremental steps rather than giant leaps and expectations are realistic, progress that engenders hope can be seen.

Planning for active treatment

In treatment planning, as with assessment and engagement, the psychiatric nurse must take into account client readiness and capability. As Medzerian (1991) suggests in his work with cocaine addicts, treatment planning should be SMART: Specific, Measurable, Attainable, Relevant, and Time limited:

- Specific: Treatment goals should be clear and specific such as "Attend hour-long recovery group Monday through Friday" and not general such as "Comply with prescribed treatment." This helps keep expectations clear.
- Measurable: When treatment goals are measurable, progress can be tracked. To further this goal, clinicians should always establish a baseline against which to measure progress. As in the previous example, data should be collected to show how many times on average the client attends group therapy per week. Then attendance data should be collected to establish the extent to which the client is successful in meeting the goal of daily attendance compared with the baseline.
- Attainable: Treatment goals for people with SMISD must be within reach and geared to their readiness to change and their recovery phase. When goals are attainable, more feedback about progress can occur. A goal of abstinence is likely to be unattainable by someone who has not identified substance use as a problem.

Attending recovery group or talking to a counselor about consequences of drinking may be more realistic.

- Relevant: Clients must be closely involved in the setting of treatment goals, and the clinician must engage in careful listening and framing so that goals are relevant to the client. For example, for the many people with SMISD who are not yet motivated to seek sobriety, a goal of abstinence is irrelevant. A more relevant goal might be to "obtain stable housing."

- Time Limited: Treatment goals should be attainable within a limited time. A variety of factors may interfere with concentration and attention. If goals require months to achieve, the client may lose motivation without positive feedback about progress.

Active treatment

After assessment, engagement, and treatment planning, active treatment begins. Basic education must be offered regarding substance use and psychiatric disorders, the way they interact, and the aspects of recovery. Clients usually have very limited knowledge about the effects of different substances of abuse on cognitive, motor, and emotional functioning; the effect alcohol or other drugs has on psychiatric symptoms; the meaning of their psychiatric diagnosis; the way medications can help; and the effect of using drugs or alcohol while taking medication. Because of cognitive impairments and denial, clients may need to hear basic information, presented simply, repeatedly. In addition, as with all adult learners, people with SMISD can incorporate new information better if learning is active and many methods for presenting material are used. Skills for remaining sober are developed during this phase. Psychiatric nurses can help clients identify situations and emotions that trigger substance use. Healthier responses to these triggers can be developed by working to fully understand them and creating and practicing alternative responses. As the client tries new behaviors, the nurse can offer support and encouragement, especially if failure is encountered. Interaction with peers in recovery is a critical aspect of active treatment, increasing knowledge and insight, helping to change attitudes, and developing a social network with recovery as the goal. As an illustration of active treatment for people with SMISD, an outpatient program in Philadelphia is described in the following sections.

MODEL PROGRAM: RECOVERY ON 8TH STREET

Over the past 10 years, Philadelphia has developed a citywide care system for people with SMISD, from specialized emergency services to intensive outpatient programs. Services offered by the community mental health centers (CMHCs)—case management, partial hospitalization, counseling, and medication management—provide much of the "glue" that holds treatment together for people with severe mental illness. Recovery on 8th Street is a program designed to address substance abuse in one of Philadelphia's many CMHCs. It uses an integrated approach to provide both mental health and substance abuse services in community treatment.

Recovery on 8th Street is located in an urban CMHC that offers partial hospitalization, social rehabilitation, medication management, supportive counseling, family education, regular and intensive case management, and special programs for homeless people and Southeast Asian clients. Psychiatric emergency, inpatient, and residential programs are affiliated with the CMHC. People with SMISD were not well served by this center in the past.

Components

Recovery on 8th Street was developed when interested staff of the CMHC joined with researchers from the University of Pennsylvania to create and study a model program for treating people with SMISD. The original demonstration grew into an established program of group and individual treatment in which people with SMISD receive special services in addition to standard CMHC treatment.

Specialized case management

The special focus of case management for people with SMISD is on addiction, mental illness, and the interplay of these conditions. The goals of specialized case management include the following:

1. Assessment of the client's psychiatric and substance use disorders to determine which factors may motivate and maintain the client's substance use
2. Engagement of the client as a partner in treatment
3. Encouragement of abstinence
4. Counseling to address underlying issues and external circumstances influencing substance abuse
5. Coordination of and linkage to appropriate services within and outside the CMHC
6. Ongoing monitoring and troubleshooting in all areas of treatment

As with intensive case management, specialized case management emphasizes interaction with clients in their natural surroundings, attention to the practical problems of daily living, support for clients' assertive attempts to satisfy needs within the community, frequent and flexible client contact, and direct assistance with symptom management (Stein & Test, 1980). Caseloads are small (15 to 20 clients), with the specialized case manager well versed in substance use disorders and severe mental illness.

The work of engagement is vital for the case manager. Many people with SMISD are hard to engage in any type of treatment and put up tremendous barriers to care. The case manager may need to assume many roles during engagement such as accompanying the client to other appointments, acting as an advocate for treatment and entitlements, and collaborating with other providers involved in the client's care. As such the functions of the case manager are not limited to the problems of substance abuse and psychiatric dysfunction but may encompass a wide range of activities necessary to achieve full stabilization.

Transition group

A transition group was developed to educate CMHC clients who used drugs or alcohol about their effects and engage people who needed substance abuse treatment in a process of recovery. The 1-hour class is offered daily to any interested client, including clients in the partial hospitalization program and clients in less intensive outpatient care. Daily attendance at Transition Group is encouraged, but nonattendance is not penalized. Since 1992, approximately 500 people have attended transition group. Approximately 35 people attend on any given day, with 60 active cases at a time. The level of functioning of people in this group is quite low; most are diagnosed with schizophrenia or schizoaffective disorder. Substance use disorders include abuse of or dependence on alcohol, cocaine, marijuana, or multiple substances. Most clients also use nicotine and caffeine.

The curriculum of transition group is basic, repetitive, nonconfrontational, and interactive. One goal is to encourage group members to talk about drugs and alcohol in a supportive environment. Educational topics include mental illness and substance use disorders. Clients are given information and encouraged to pursue understanding about their psychiatric diagnoses, their substance use problems, the psychotropic medications they have been prescribed, and the treatments that have been recommended to them. Essential to this learning process is the understanding of the nature of recovery and rehabilitation. Learning activities central to transition group include understanding the effects of different substances on mental, motor, and emotional functioning; making connections between substance use and the undesirable consequences a client may be experiencing; and hearing from people further along in the recovery process about the benefits associated with sobriety and working on recovery. Groups such as this have been developed around the country to draw people who have never even considered recovery along the pathway toward change (Osher & Kofoed, 1989; Sciacca, 1991). Psychiatric nurses are effective group leaders because of their holistic approach and broad knowledge of issues related to SMISD.

Staff involved with the transition group of Recovery on 8th Street must celebrate small successes because large successes are few and far between. For many clients, simply being able to tune into most of the group conversation and add an appropriate comment are major accomplishments. During one session a member inadvertently referred to the group as the "transsexual group" rather than the transition group. In recounting this story the group leader was not focused on the possible meaning of this "Freudian slip" but instead was delighted to note how many group members laughed. The laughter let her know they were paying attention.

Early recovery group

For clients who have made the decision to pursue a program of recovery, early recovery group provides a group therapy experience with greater challenges and depth than the transition group. Early recovery group meets weekly, and regular attendance is expected. In early recovery group, members explore the associations among patterns of substance use, fluctuations of psychiatric symptoms, and immediate and long-term consequences of use. Historical factors also are explored such as childhood physical, emotional, and sexual abuse; traumas; and the more recent experiences of rejection and loss associated with severe mental illness. In addition, group members work in the "here and now," examining their communication patterns, relationships to the group leader, willingness to support one another, and openness to sharing.

Double trouble

Double trouble is a self-help program modeled on Alcoholics Anonymous and designed to support people with SMISD. Double trouble meetings are held twice a week at the CMHC, and all participants in transition group and early recovery group are encouraged to attend. The meetings are a forum for developing support among fellow recovering clients with SMISD. The self-help model empowers its members to be responsible for their own recovery and work on behalf of other recovering addicts. Recovery on 8th Street is located at the same CMHC that provided meeting space for greater Philadelphia's first double trouble meeting and the double trouble intergroup, founded in 1987. The intergroup develops educational materials, responds to requests for information and assistance in starting new groups, and provides a pool of facilitators to speak at or help with double trouble groups. The double trouble meeting at the CMHC operates as a self-help group with staff presence (Caldwell & White, 1991). Members of the group facilitate the meeting, but staff are available to assist if needed.

Leisure time planning

Early in the development of Recovery on 8th Street the need for recreational activities that did not involve alcohol or other drugs was identified. The leisure time planning group focuses on developing interests and skills that are alternatives to substance use and planning activities for clients such as outings to local cultural or sporting events, on-site parties, dances, and community meals.

Ongoing growth and recovery

After people with SMISD have achieved stable abstinence and are engaged in maintenance or relapse prevention, they are ready to pursue other rehabilitative goals in areas such as education, work, relationships, and housing. Clients should be encouraged to use opportunities available to them, knowing that they have somewhere to bring their struggles and frustrations as new challenges trigger old emotions and behaviors.

Over the past 3 years, many clients have benefited from services offered through Recovery on 8th Street. Its effects have been varied. Although some clients dropped out of the program and relapsed, others maintained sobriety. Many experience intervals of sober time and relapses. However, other indicators of the program's success are the numbers of people with SMISD engaging in treatment and the increased attention of clinical staff to assessment and treatment planning for SMISD. Clinical staff refer to Recovery on 8th Street as a "work in progress" to highlight their investment in being open to change and attuned to the needs and interests of clients. Thus new directions and refinements of older methods are always being sought.

SUMMARY

SMISD is a problem that affects approximately 50% of people with serious mental illness in mental health treatment facilities. Promising treatment systems for SMISD are comprehensive, addressing all stages of the recovery process, and integrated, treating both substance use disorders and psychiatric disorders simultaneously and in the same setting. Given that most people with SMISD are not ready to change their patterns of drug or alcohol use, the skilled psychiatric nurse must assess problems over time and work in many different ways to engage clients in a process of recovery and rehabilitation. Work with people with SMISD can be frustrating but need not be so. By focusing on the incremental steps that constitute progress for people with SMISD, both client and psychiatric nurse can remain energized and empowered for the work of recovery.

REFERENCES

Alcoholics Anonymous. (1984). *The AA member: Medication and other drugs.* New York: Alcoholics Anonymous World Services.

Alterman, A. I., Erdlen, D. L., LaPorte, D. J., & Erdlen, F. R. (1982). Effects of illicit drug use in an inpatient psychiatric population. *Addictive Behaviors, 7,* 231-242.

Ananth, J., Vandewater, S., Kamal, M., Brodsky, A., Gamal, R., & Miller, M. (1989). Missed diagnosis of substance abuse in psychiatric patients. *Hospital and Community Psychiatry, 40,* 297-299.

Bartels, S. J., Teague, G. B., Drake, R. E., Clark, R. E., Bush, P. W., & Noordsy, D. L. (1993). Substance abuse in schizophrenia: Service utilization and costs. *Journal of Nervous and Mental Disease, 181,* 227-232.

Bassuk, E. L., & Gerson, S. (1978). Deinstitutionalization and mental health services. *Scientific American, 238,* 46-53.

Bergman, H. C., & Harris, M. (1985). Substance abuse among young adult chronic patients. *Psychosocial Rehabilitation Journal, 9,* 48-54.

Bond, G. R., McDonel, E. C., Miller, L. D., & Pensec, M. (1991). Assertive community treatment and reference groups: An evaluation of their effectiveness for young adults with serious mental illness and substance abuse problems. *Psychosocial Rehabilitation Journal, 15* (2), 31-43.

Brown, V. B., Ridgely, S. M., Pepper, B., Levine, I. S., & Ryglewicz, H. (1989). The dual crisis: Mental illness and substance abuse. *American Psychologist, 44,* 565-569.

Caldwell, S., & White, K. K. (1991). Co-creating a self-help recovery movement. *Psychosocial Rehabilitation Journal, 15,* 91-94.

Carey, K. B. (1989). Emerging treatment guidelines for mentally ill chemical abusers. *Hospital and Community Psychiatry, 40,* 341-342, 349.

Case, N. (1991). The dual-diagnosis patient in a psychiatric day treatment program: A treatment failure. *Journal of Substance Abuse Treatment, 8,* 69-73.

Castaneda, R., Galanter, M., & Franco, H. (1989). Self-medication among addicts with primary psychiatric disorders. *Comprehensive Psychiatry, 30,* 80-83.

Castaneda, R., Lifshutz, H., Galanter, M., & Franco, H. (1994). Empirical assessment of the self-medication hypothesis among dually diagnosed inpatients. *Comprehensive Psychiatry, 35,* 180-184.

Comings, D. E., Muhleman, D., Ahn, C., Gysin, R., & Flanagan, S. D. (1994). The dopamine D2 receptor gene: a genetic risk factor in substance abuse. *Drug and Alcohol Dependence, 34*(3), 175-180.

Corse, S. J., McHugh, M. K., & Gordon, S. M. (1995). Enhancing provider effectiveness in treating pregnant women with addictions. *Journal of Substance Abuse Treatment, 12,* 3-12.

Dixon, L., Dibietz, E., Myers, P., Conley, R., Medoff, D., & Lehman, A. F. (1993). Comparison of *DSM-III-R* diagnoses and a brief interview for substance abuse among state hospital patients. *Hospital and Community Psychiatry, 44,* 748-752.

Dixon, L., Haas, G., Weiden, P., Sweeney, J., & Francis, A. (1990). Acute effects of drug abuse in schizophrenic patients: Clinical observations and patients' self-reports. *Schizophrenia Bulletin, 16,* 69-79.

Drake, R. E., McHugo, G. J., & Noordsy, D. L. (1993). Treatment of alcoholism among schizophrenic outpatients: 4-year outcomes. *American Journal of Psychiatry, 150,* 328-329.

Drake, R. E., Osher, F. C., Noordsy, D. L., Hurlbut, S. C., Teague, G. B., & Beaudett, M. S. (1990). Diagnosis of alcohol use disorders in schizophrenia. *Schizophrenia Bulletin, 16,* 57-67.

Drake, R. E., & Wallach, M. A. (1993). Moderate drinking among people with severe mental illness. *Hospital and Community Psychiatry, 44,* 780-782.

Durell, J., Lechtenberg, B., Corse, S., & Frances, R. J. (1993). Intensive case management of persons with chronic mental illness who abuse substances. *Hospital and Community Psychiatry, 44,* 415-416, 428.

Galanter, M., Castenada, R., & Ferman, J. (1988). Substance abuse among general psychiatric patients: Place of presentation, diagnosis and treatment. *American Journal of Drug and Alcohol Abuse, 142,* 211-235.

Galanter, M., Egelko, S., DeLeon, G., Rohrs, C., & Franco, H. (1992). Crack/cocaine abusers in the general hospital: Assessment and initiation of care. *American Journal of Psychiatry, 149,* 810-815.

Gerstein, D. R., & Harwood, H. J. (1990). *Treating drug problems.* Washington, DC: National Academy Press.

Gorski, T. T. (1989). *Passages through recovery: An action plan for preventing relapse.* San Francisco: Harper & Row.

Hadley, T. R., Culhane, D. P., & McGurrin, M. C. (1992). The identification and tracking of "heavy users" of acute psychiatric inpatient services. *Administration and Policy in Mental Health, 19*(3), 279-290.

Hall, R. C. W., Popkin, M. D., DeVaul, R., & Stickney, S. K. (1977). The effect of unrecognized drug abuse on diagnosis and therapeutic outcome. *American Journal of Drug and Alcohol Abuse, 4,* 455-465.

Hellerstein, D. J., & Meehan, B. (1987). Outpatient group therapy for schizophrenic substance abusers. *American Journal of Psychiatry, 144,* 1337-1339.

Hilton, M. E. (1987). Drinking patterns and drinking problems in 1984: Results from a general population survey. *Alcoholism, Clinical and Experimental Research, 11,* 167-175.

Jerrell, J. M., & Ridgely, M. S. (1995). Evaluating changes in symptoms and functioning of dually diagnosed clients in specialized treatment. *Psychiatric Services, 46*(3), 233-238.

Kendler, K. S. (1985). A twin study of individuals with both schizophrenia and alcoholism. *British Journal of Psychiatry, 58,* 1-14.

Khantzian, E. J. (1985). The self-medication hypothesis of addictive disorders: Focus on heroin and cocaine dependence. *American Journal of Psychiatry, 142,* 1259-1264.

Kline, J., Bebout, R., Harris, M., & Drake, R. E. (1991). A comprehensive treatment program for dually diagnosed homeless people in Washington, D.C. In K. Minkoff, & R. E. Drake (Eds.), *Dual diagnosis of major mental illness and substance disorder* (pp. 95-106). San Francisco: Jossey-Bass.

Kofoed, L., Kania, J., Walsh, T., & Atkinson, R. M. (1986). Outpatient treatment of patients with substance abuse and coexisting psychiatric disorders. *American Journal of Psychiatry, 143,* 867-872.

Lamb, H. R. (1982). Young adult chronic patients: The new drifters. *Hospital and Community Psychiatry, 33,* 465-468.

LaPorte, D. J., McLellan, A. T., O'Brien, C. P., & Marshall, J. R. (1981). Treatment response in psychiatrically impaired drug abusers. *Comprehensive Psychiatry, 22,* 411-419.

Lehman, A. F., Herron, J. D., & Schwartz, R. P. (1993a). Rehabilitation for young adults with severe mental illness and substance use disorders: A clinical trial. *Journal of Nervous and Mental Disease, 181,* 86-90.

Lehman, A. F., Myers, C. P., Corty, E., & Thompson, J. W. (1994). Prevalence and patterns of "dual diagnosis" among psychiatric inpatients. *Comprehensive Psychiatry, 35,* 106-112.

Lehman, A. F., Myers, C. P., Thompson, J. W., & Corty, E. (1993b). Implications of mental and substance use disorders: A comparison of single and dual diagnosis patients. *Journal of Nervous and Mental Disease, 181,* 365-370.

McCarrick, A. K., Manderscheid, R. W., & Bertolucci, D. E. (1985). Correlates of acting-out behaviors among young adult chronic patients. *Hospital and Community Psychiatry, 36,* 848-852.

McLellan, A. T., Childress, A. R., Griffith, J., & Woody, G. E. (1984). The psychiatrically severe drug abuse patient: Methadone maintenance or therapeutic community? *American Journal of Drug and Alcohol Abuse, 10,* 77-95.

McLellan, A. T., Erdlen, F. R., Erdlen, D. L., & O'Brien, C. P. (1981). Psychological severity and response to alcoholism rehabilitation. *Drug and Alcohol Dependence, 8,* 23-35.

McLellan, A. T., Luborsky, L., O'Brien, C. P., Woody, G. E., & Druley, K. A. (1982). Is treatment for substance abuse effective? *Journal of the American Medical Association, 247,* 1423-1428.

McLellan, A. T., Luborsky, L., Woody, G. E., O'Brien, C. P., & Druley, K. A. (1983). Predicting response to alcohol and drug abuse treatments: Role of psychiatric severity. *Archives of General Psychiatry, 40,* 620-625.

Medzerian, G. (1991). *Crack: Treating cocaine addiction.* Blue Ridge Summit, PA: McGraw Hill.

Mercer-McFadden, C., & Drake, R. E. (in press). *A review of 13 NIMH demonstration projects for young adults with severe mental illness and substance abuse problems.* Rockville, MD: Community Support Program, Center for Mental Health Services, U.S. Department of Health and Human Services.

Miller, W. R., & Rollnick, S. (1991). *Motivational interviewing: Preparing people to change addictive behavior.* New York: Guilford Press.

Minkoff, K. (1987). Beyond deinstitutionalization: A new ideology for the postinstitutional era. *Hospital and Community Psychiatry, 38,* 945-950.

Minkoff, K. (1991). Program components of a comprehensive integrated care system for serious mentally ill patients with substance disorders. In K. Minkoff, & R. E. Drake (Eds.), *Dual diagnosis of major mental illness and substance disorder* (pp. 13-28). San Francisco: Jossey-Bass.

Minkoff, K., & Drake, R. E. (1991). *Dual diagnosis of major mental illness and substance disorder.* San Francisco: Jossey-Bass.

Noordsy, D. L., Drake, R. E., Teague, G. B., Osher, F. C., Hurlbut, S. C., Beaudett, M. S., & Paskus, T. S. (1991). Subjective experiences related to alcohol use among schizophrenics. *Journal of Nervous and Mental Disease, 179,* 410-414.

Osher, F. C., & Kofoed, L. L. (1989). Treatment of patients with psychiatric and psychoactive substance abuse disorders. *Hospital and Community Psychiatry, 40,* 1025-1030.

Pepper, B., Kirshner, M. C., & Ryglewicz, H. (1981). The young adult chronic patient: Overview of a population. *Hospital and Community Psychiatry, 32,* 463-469.

Prochaska, J. O., DiClemente, C. C., & Norcross, J. C. (1992). In search of how people change: Applications to addictive behaviors. *American Psychologist, 47,* 1102-1114.

Rahav, M., Rivera, J. J., Nuttborck, L., Ng-Mak, D., Sturz, E. L., Link, B. G., Struening, E. L., Pepper, B., & Gross, B. (1995). Characteristics and treatment of homeless, mentally ill, chemical-abusing men. *Journal of Psychoactive Drugs, 27*(1), 93-103.

Regier, D. A., Farmer, M. E., Rae, D. S., Locke, B. Z., Keith, S. J., Judd, L. L., & Goodwin, F. K. (1990). Comorbidity of mental disorders with alcohol and other drug abuse: Results from the Epidemiologic Catchment Area (ECA) study. *Journal of the American Medical Association, 265,* 2511-2518.

Ridgely, M. S., Goldman, H. H., & Talbott, J. J. (1986). *Chronic mentally ill young adults with substance abuse problems: A review of the literature and creation of a research agenda.* Baltimore: University of Maryland Mental Health Policy Studies Center.

Ridgely, M. S., Goldman, H. H., & Willenbring, M. (1990). Barriers to the care of persons with dual diagnoses: Organizational and financing issues. *Schizophrenia Bulletin, 16,* 123-132.

Ridgely, M. S., Osher, F., & Talbott, J. (1987). *Chronic mentally ill young adults with substance abuse problems: Treatment and training issues.* Baltimore: University of Maryland Mental Health Policy Studies Center.

Ries, R. K., & Ellingson, T. (1989). A pilot assessment at one month of 17 dual diagnosis patients. *Hospital and Community Psychiatry, 41,* 1230-1233.

Safer, D. J. (1987). Substance abuse by young adult chronic patients. *Hospital and Community Psychiatry, 38,* 511-514.

Salloum, I. M., Moss, H. B., & Daley, D. C. (1991). Substance abuse and schizophrenia: impediments to optimal care. *American Journal of Drug and Alcohol Abuse, 17*(3), 321-336.

Schinka, J. A., Curtiss, G., & Mulloy, J. M. (1994). Personality variables and self-medication in substance abuse. *Journal of Personality Assessment, 63,* 413-422.

Schwartz, S. R., & Goldfinger, S. M. (1981). The new chronic patient: Clinical characteristics of an emerging subgroup. *Hospital and Community Psychiatry, 32,* 470-474.

Sciacca, K. (1991). An integrated treatment approach for severely mentally ill individuals with substance disorders. In K. Minkoff, & R. E. Drake (Eds.), *Dual diagnosis of major mental illness and substance disorder* (pp. 69-84). San Francisco: Jossey-Bass.

Siris, S. G. (1990). Pharmacological treatment of substance-abusing schizophrenic patients. *Schizophrenic Bulletin, 16,* 111-122.

Solomon, P., & Gordon, B. (1986-1987). The psychiatric emergency room and follow-up services in the community. *Psychiatric Quarterly, 58,* 119-127.

Soyka, M., Albus, M., Kathmann, N., Finelli, A., Hofstetter, S., Holzbach, R., Immler, B., & Sand, P. (1993). Prevalence of alcohol and drug abuse in schizophrenic inpatients. *European Archives of Psychiatry and Clinical Neuroscience, 242*(6), 362-372.

Stein, L. I., & Test, M. A. (1980). Alternative to mental hospital treatment: I. Conceptual model, treatment program and clinical evaluation. *Archives of General Psychiatry, 37,* 392-397.

Teague, G. B., Schwab, B., & Drake, R. E. (1990). *Evaluating services for young adults with dual diagnoses of severe mental illness and substance use disorder.* Alexandria, VA: National Association of State Mental Health Program Directors.

Thompson, J. W., Bass, R. D., & Witkin, M. J. (1982). Fifty years of psychiatric services: 1940-1990. *Hospital and Community Psychiatry, 33,* 711-717.

Wallen, M. C., & Weiner, H. D. (1989). Impediments to effective treatment of the dually diagnosed patient. *Journal of Psychoactive Drugs, 21,* 161-168.

Warner, L. A., Kessler, R. C., Hughes, M., Anthony, J. C., & Nelson, C. B. (1995). Prevalence and correlates of drug use and dependence in the United States. Results from the National Comorbidity Survey. *Archives of General Psychiatry, 52*(3), 219-229.

Warner, R., Taylor, D., Wright, J., Sloat, A., Springett, G., Arnold, S., & Weinberg, H. (1994). Substance use among the mentally ill: Prevalence, reasons for use and effects on illness. *American Journal of Orthopsychiatry, 64,* 30-39.

Weiner, H. (1985). Schizophrenia: Etiology. In H. I. Kaplan, & B. J. Sadock (Eds.), *Comprehensive textbook of psychiatry* (4th ed.) (pp. 651-680). Baltimore: Williams & Wilkins.

Weisner, C., Greenfield, T., & Room, R. (1995). Trends in treatment of alcohol problems in the U.S. general population, 1979 through 1990. *American Journal of Public Health, 85*(1), 55-60.

White, K. K., & White, D. E. (1989). Dual mental health and substance use problems: A model of four subtypes. *Psychosocial Rehabilitation Journal, 13,* 93-98.

Wing, D. M. (1993). Applying the "Model of Recovering Alcoholics' Behavior Stages and Goal Setting" to nursing practice. *Archives of Psychiatric Nursing, 8*(4), 197-202.

Wing, D.M. (1990). Determining alcoholism treatment outcomes: A cost-effectiveness perspective. *Nursing Economics, 8*: 248-255.

Chapter 24

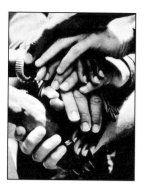

Homeless Persons with Mental Illness

Neil Meisler

The worst sin towards our fellow creatures is not to hate them, but to be indifferent to them. That's the essence of inhumanity.

George Bernard Shaw
The Devil's Disciple,
Act II (1901)

The homeless crisis of the 1980s has become an endemic social problem. Large numbers of Americans have become homeless in the past 10 years. With dramatic changes in federal social policy currently taking place, homeless assistance funding will almost certainly decrease sharply. For example, the 1996 federal budget cut homeless assistance spending by the Department of Housing and Urban Development (HUD) by 27% in 1 year, from $1.12 billion to $823 million.

Spending for social programs to assist low-income families has fallen out of favor. In every budget deficit–reduction scenario, funding for public assistance and low-income housing will be cut. The chief beneficiaries of such funding have been single mothers, their children, and disabled adults. A large number of these people currently dependent on public assistance will likely not obtain employment. Clearly, public and political interest in the problem of homelessness has waned. The United States has adapted to having large numbers of homeless people on its streets and in its shelters. Their numbers are likely to increase.

This chapter explores homelessness as experienced by people with severe mental illness. Homeless mentally ill people are a significant subsample of the homeless population. The relationship of homelessness among people with severe mental illness to economic, social, and treatment factors is explored. Findings from federally sponsored research into homelessness among people with mental illness are reviewed. Finally, key components of a systemic response to be implemented by state mental health authorities are identified.

EPIDEMIOLOGY OF HOMELESS PEOPLE

Since 1980, more than 40 studies have been published estimating the number of homeless people (Jencks, 1994). Most studies have been local, investigating one or more municipalities within a state. Extrapolations have been made from these estimates to derive national estimates varying from 0.2% to 1% of the population (Institute of Medicine, 1988). Several studies also have used more nationally representative samples.

A study by HUD estimated the homeless population in 1984 to be between 250,000 and 350,000 (U.S. Department of Housing and Urban Development, 1984). In 1987 the Urban Institute conducted a systematic study of urban homelessness based on interviews with a random sample of homeless soup kitchen and shelter users in 20 cities representative of all cities with populations greater than 100,000 people (Burt & Cohen, 1989). Extrapolating from the sample, the Institute derived an estimate of approximately 500,000 to 600,000 homeless people in the United States. These and most other studies attempted to count the number of homeless people at one point in time. Such point prevalence studies cannot identify all homeless people.

In a landmark survey of a nationally representative sample of adult members of households with telephones in 1990 (Link et al., 1994), 7.4% of respondents reported having been homeless in their lifetime and 3.1% reported having been homeless within the past 5 years. *Homelessness* was defined as having stayed in a shelter, other temporary housing for the homeless, or nonshelter settings such as parks or abandoned buildings. Of the respondents who had been homeless in their lives, 59% reported having been homeless for more than a month; 13% reported being homeless for more than 1 year. Extrapolated to the 1990 census, the study results indicated that approximately 5.7 million adults had been homeless between 1985 and 1990. These findings are remarkable considering that homeless people and households without telephones were not consulted in the sample.

Taken collectively, the published data suggest a range of 600,000 to 1.2 million homeless adults, 300,000 to 600,000 of whom are long-term homeless (Jenks, 1994). Additionally, 68,000 to 100,000 children are homeless (U.S. General Accounting Office, 1989).

Epidemiology of homeless people with mental illness

Early reports of the number of people with mental illness among the general homeless population estimated that they were the majority of the population (Arce, Tadlock, & Vegare, 1983; Bassuk, Rubin, & Lauriat, 1984; Baxter & Hopper, 1981). However, in a review of 40 local point prevalence surveys of homeless people published since 1981, Shlay and Rossi (1992) derived an estimate of 24% of homeless people having spent some time in a psychiatric hospital and 33% currently experiencing symptoms of mental illness. In their national urban survey of shelter and soup kitchen users, Burt and Cohen (1989) identified 22% of the subjects as having been hospitalized for mental illness.

Deriving a national estimate from local studies that have investigated the prevalence of severe mental illness in homeless populations is hampered by the variance of homelessness across different communities (Tessler & Dennis, 1989). Despite early awareness of the methodological shortcomings of attempts to estimate the number of homeless people with mental illness (Vegare & Arce, 1986), a national study of a representative sample of homeless people has not been performed yet to determine the prevalence of severe mental illness among them.

Taking the 33% estimate derived from the various studies that have attempted to account for mental illness among the homeless population yields a total of 200,000 to 400,000 homeless people with psychiatric histories (Shlay & Rossi, 1992). Because most studies did not distinguish severity of symptoms, a reasonably conservative estimate of homeless people with severe mental illness is 200,000, or approximately 10% of the people with severe mental illness in the U.S. population.

ETIOLOGY OF HOMELESSNESS IN THE GENERAL POPULATION

Three primary factors underlying the overall growth in homelessness since 1970 are population growth, poverty, and lack of access to low-rent housing. Social researchers have identified the dramatic growth in the number of people between 18 and 35 years old since 1970 as the single most significant factor explaining the increase in the homeless population (Baum & Burnes, 1993; Mechanic, 1987). Figure 24-1 illustrates the rise in the birthrate after World War II and its impact on the growth of the adult population. The birthrate increased markedly in 1945 and has remained higher than in preceding decades. Between 1945 and 1964 (the baby boom) the birthrate was 53% higher than between 1925 and 1944. Although the average annual birthrate then declined by 13% between 1964 and 1993, it has remained approximately 40% higher than before the baby boom

(Baum & Burnes, 1993). The number of people in the 25- to 34-year-old cohort increased by 12 million between 1970 and 1980. Not by coincidence, the Urban Institute survey found that the vast majority of homeless people are between 25 and 40 years old (Burt & Cohen 1989). Population growth, combined with an economic recession and an epidemic growth in crack cocaine use during the decade, spurred the growth in the homeless population.

Along with the overall growth in adult population, the number of people and families living below the poverty level has steadily increased. During the economic recession of the early 1980s most state general public assistance programs were eliminated. Also, since the early 1980s the purchasing power of federal and state Aid to Families with Dependent Children (AFDC) program payments and food stamps has declined by more than 20% (Bassuk, 1990; Rosenheck &

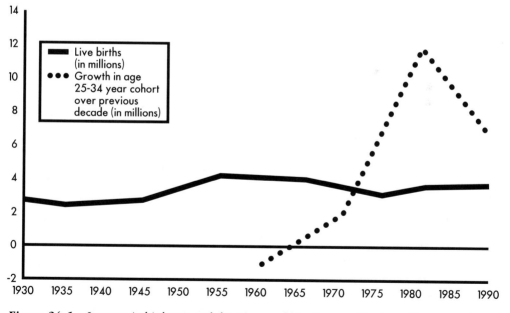

Figure 24-1. Increase in birth rate and the 25-year-old to 34-year-old cohort. The vast majority of adult homeless people fall within this age group.

(Data from *A Nation in Denial: The Truth About Homelessness,* by A. S. Baum, & D. W. Burnes, 1993, Boulder, CO: Westview Press.)

Fontana, 1994). In most states, incomes of families on AFDC are at or below 75% of the poverty level. Approximately 35 million Americans live below the poverty level (Baum & Burnes, 1993); most are children. Although the image of the homeless population has been one of single adults with mental illness, alcoholism, and drug addiction, more than half of the people accounting for the increase in homelessness after 1980 had none of these problems. The most common problem was a lack of sufficient income to pay rent even though many worked.

As the overall number of adults increased after 1970, so did the number of low-income people and families. Moreover, as the real income and purchasing power of low-income people declined during the 1980s, so did the supply of low-rent and government subsidized housing units. By 1985, only 4.7 low-rent units in the United States were available to accommodate every 11.6 low-income families (McChesney, 1990).

Etiology of homelessness among people with mental illness

The growth of homelessness among people with mental illness since the late 1970s has been proportionally greater than the overall increase in the homeless population. Several causes have been postulated to explain this increase, including the following:

1. Demographic and socioeconomic influences
2. Clinical characteristics of the cohort of people with mental illness who become homeless
3. Changing characteristics of the public mental health system

Demographic and socioeconomic influences

The proportion of people with mental illness within the overall homeless population remained constant before and after the sharp increase in homelessness that occurred during the early 1980s (Rossi, 1990). In 1980, approximately 20 million more people were in the 18- to 40-year-old cohort

than in 1970 (Baum & Burnes, 1993). Not coincidentally, studies during the 1980s reported that the vast majority of homeless adults were between 18 and 40 years old (Baum & Burnes, 1993). Applying a conservative 0.928% prevalence estimate to the increase in the 18- to 40-year-old population yields an increase of 186,000 (30%) in the number of adults with severe psychiatric disabilities from 1970 to 1980 (Goldman, Gattozzi, & Taube, 1981).

The increase in the number of adults with mental illness occurred at a time of economic recession and a major reevaluation of the role of the federal government in social welfare. The unemployment rate among people with psychiatric disabilities is 90% (Anthony et al., 1972; Anthony & Jansen, 1984), and most depend on government assistance. Combined effects of high inflation in the late 1970s and federal and state cutbacks in the provision of economic assistance markedly reduced the purchasing power of people on disability income. Furthermore, former U.S. President Reagan campaigned on the pledge to reduce domestic spending by the federal government. His budget message to Congress for fiscal year 1982 proposed an increase in defense spending and drastic reductions in domestic spending to achieve an overall budget decrease of $48.6 billion.

Responding to a U.S. Government Accounting Office (GAO) report of a great increase in the numbers of beneficiaries of Social Security Disability Insurance (SSDI) between 1970 and 1975, Congress passed legislation in 1980 requiring the Social Security Administration to accelerate reviews of recipients' continued eligibility. The Reagan administration set out to save the $2 billion identified by the Office of Management and Budget as being paid to ineligible recipients. Goldman and Gattozzi (1988) found that accelerated review was implemented despite the number of people on SSDI declining without intervention by 1980 to below the 1970 level. Furthermore, although only 10% of all beneficiaries had a psychiatric impairment, 25% of the 130,500 beneficiaries found ineligible for continued benefits in 1981 were mentally disabled (Goldman et al., 1981). In 1982 the disability reviews were extended to Supplemental Security Income beneficiaries and an even larger number of people with psychiatric disabilities were dropped from the rolls. By 1983, when public, legal, and political backlash caused the Social Security Administration to suspend its policy of accelerated review, more than 100,000 people with psychiatric disabilities had lost their benefits. Not coincidentally, this was a period of rapid growth in the homeless population. The Social Security Act, until 1986, prohibited people from qualifying for Social Security and Medicaid benefits without a permanent address. Paradoxically, people who became homeless after losing their Social Security benefits were ineligible to requalify regardless of their disability status.

Another initiative of the Reagan Administration to reduce domestic spending was a sharp reduction in federal revenue sharing and public housing funds. People with mental illness also were disproportionately affected by the 1 million unit reduction in single-room occupancy dwellings that occurred across large American cities throughout the 1970s and 1980s (Kiesler, 1991; Lipton, Sabatini, & Katz, 1983).

Clinical characteristics

A number of studies of homeless people with mental illness provide a profile of their life experiences and clinical characteristics. Reports of these studies provide a description of a population that is seriously ill, severely disabled, and multiply diagnosed and that has entrenched patterns of inability or resistance to engage in available mental health, physical health, and social services. Although the assumption is that such factors contribute to homelessness, no one has proved that they differentiate homeless people from nonhomeless people. To the contrary, empirical evidence points to socioeconomic factors as the major causes of homelessness among people with severe mental illness.

Susser, Lin, and Conover (1991) assessed the

3-month, 3-year, and lifetime prevalence of homelessness for 377 people admitted to a New York state hospital that serves New York City, an urban county, and a suburban county. Overall they found that a substantial number of patients in the sample had been homeless, with a 3-month prevalence of 19%, a 3-year prevalence of 25%, and a lifetime prevalence of 28%. They analyzed the effects of a variety of independent variables on prevalence, including age, gender, race, diagnosis, alcohol or drug use, and county of residence. County of residence was the only variable statistically significantly correlated with homelessness, with New York City residents having the highest prevalence rate. Correlations for drug abuse and age under 40 years old approached significance. Gender, race, alcohol use, and diagnosis had little or no association with prevalence of homelessness. The findings of Susser et al. suggest that although people with severe mental illness are overrepresented in the homeless population, more complex factors than their clinical and personal characteristics place them at risk for homelessness.

In a study of homelessness among Vietnam War veterans, Rosenheck and Fontana (1994) found that vulnerability to homelessness related to a multiplicity of psychiatric and nonpsychiatric factors. No one factor dominated, but factors related to social isolation had the strongest impact on homelessness, although they were considerably more related to homelessness than mental illness.

Sosin and Grossman (1991) reported on a study comparing the characteristics of previously psychiatrically hospitalized homeless people with other disadvantaged previously psychiatrically hospitalized people who were domiciled. The study found that 67% of the currently homeless group and of the domiciled group had been homeless in the past. Sosin and Grossman studied differences between the two groups in a number of independent variables that included age, race, symptoms, hospitalizations, substance use, outpatient mental health service use, and living arrangement after last hospital discharge. The only factors significantly related to homelessness were age, receipt of Supplemental Security Income, receipt of state income assistance, and employment income. Of the homeless group, 21% were currently receiving outpatient services; the figure rose to 36% for the domiciled group. This difference was not significant in the overall analysis.

Herman, Galanter, and Lifshutz (1991) studied 100 consecutive admissions to New York City's Bellevue Hospital of patients with dual diagnoses of mental illness and substance abuse. Through a standardized patient interview, they gathered background information on demographic, educational, employment, economic assistance, residential, psychiatric diagnosis and treatment, and substance use patterns. They found that 46 patients were homeless the day before admission, 34% had been homeless the majority of the time during the 2 months before admission, and 27% had been homeless the majority of the time during the 2 years before admission. Of the total sample, 68% had been homeless for at least 1 month at some point in their lives. The homeless and domiciled groups did not differ significantly in any clinical or epidemiological measure.

Almost 50 studies of homelessness have been reported since 1983. They encompass a wide range of designs and methods, and data can be found to support virtually any argument regarding the representation of people with mental illness among the homeless and the factors more associated with their experience of homelessness than with more heterogenous cohorts of the population. Rossi (1990) attempted to place the contemporary experience of homelessness in historical perspective. He concluded that the incidence of substance abuse, mental illness, and criminal records among people who became homeless in the 1990s is similar to that of homeless people before 1980. The differences he noted included that the homeless population is much larger in number (but not proportion), older, poorer, more diverse in gender and family composition, and more likely to be shelterless than homeless people in past decades.

Mental health system characteristics

The news media, local government officials, and a number of influential mental health academicians have characterized homelessness among people with mental illness as primarily the result of "deinstitutionalization" (Bassuk & Lamb, 1986; Koch, 1988; Lamb, 1990; Lambert, 1987; Torrey, 1989). *Deinstitutionalization* denotes the public policy of the past 30 years to reduce the use of state hospitals in favor of a more abstract construct of care in the community. Critics assert that many mentally ill people in the homeless population would have been housed and cared for in state hospitals in the past (Jencks, 1994).

Ironically, deinstitutionalization began as a federal response to the overcrowded, inhuman conditions common in state hospitals after World War II. Congress passed the Mental Retardation Facilities and Community Mental Health Centers Construction Act of 1963 with the goal of decreasing the state hospital population. Three decades later the number of people with mental illness believed to be homeless roughly corresponds to the reduction in the number of state hospital patients in that period. Whether these circumstances are correlated has been a matter of much debate.

The population of state hospitals has declined from a peak of 550,000 in 1955 to roughly 72,000 currently (Figure 24-2). Half of the reduction occurred between 1960 and 1975, primarily as a result of the shift in the locus of care of elderly and stable long-term patients to nursing homes and residential care facilities financed through Medicaid and Supplemental Security Income (U.S. General Accounting Office, 1977). By 1980, approximately 750,000 people with severe mental illness were residing in nursing homes and residential care facilities (Goldman et al., 1981).

A confluence of diverse influences (including public exposure of deteriorated and overcrowded conditions in state hospital facilities, legal challenges to states' involuntary commitment practices, and the appeal to state officials of transferring state hospital patients to settings largely funded by the federal government) transformed

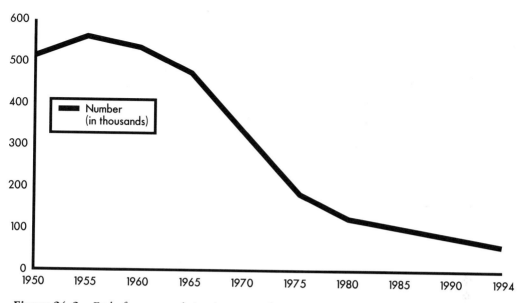

Figure 24-2. End of year population in state and county psychiatric hospitals. (Modified from *Additions and Resident Patients at End of Year, State and County Mental Hospitals, by Age and Diagnosis, by State, United States, 1991,* by Center for Mental Health Services, 1993, Rockville, MD: Author.)

state hospitals. Unlike the first wave of deinstitutionalization the 63% reduction since 1975 occurred independently of availability of financing or alternative care settings (Goldman & Morrissey, 1985). It also occurred during a period of unprecedented growth in the young adult age cohort, a period in which the prevalence of schizophrenia and other severe mental illness was increasing. The continued reduction in the population of state hospitals was influenced by the complex interaction of legal, financial, and ideological factors.

During the 1960s patients' rights litigation became more common, especially concerning standards of institutional care, the right to the least restrictive and most appropriate treatment, and the right to refuse medication. A landmark 1975 Supreme Court decision, *O'Connor v. Donaldson,* ruled that mental illness in the absence of any imminent threat to self or others does not provide sufficient justification for involuntary hospitalization. This ruling and more than 100 other court cases in 39 states by 1975 influenced state legisla-

tures to rewrite their mental health codes. Involuntary commitment was greatly curtailed, and fewer patients admitted for acute psychiatric treatment were held as long-term patients. The people with mental illness affected by these changes were largely younger adults without stable living arrangements, many of whom were unable or unwilling to cooperate with psychiatric treatment outside the structure provided by the state hospital (Goldman & Morrissey, 1985).

As the long-term population of state hospitals declined, hospital buildings (including many that did not meet U.S. standards) were closed or converted to other uses. However, the increase in the number of people with mental illness and a lack of psychiatric treatment programs in the community caused admissions to state hospitals to increase from an annual average of 345,000 during the 1960s to 423,000 during the 1970s, an increase of 23% (Center for Mental Health Services, 1993). Having reduced their bed capacity, state hospitals were overwhelmed with the increased need for acute psychiatric services. They were under constant pressure to maintain a rapid discharge rate to accommodate new admissions. The pressure of an increased volume of hospital admissions, the rapid effect of medication in reducing acute psychiatric symptoms, and stricter standards for involuntary hospitalization interacted to change the professional culture of state hospital staff. These changes fostered a more limited, acute care role for the state hospital. The lack of a permanent residence ceased to be a criterion for continued hospitalization, especially for recently admitted patients. Increasingly, patients were discharged to homeless shelters.

A lag occurred between the changes in the operation of state hospitals and the development of public sector community mental health service systems to address the needs of people with severe mental illness for treatment, rehabilitation, and support. Most state mental health agencies did not anticipate the need to develop local systems of care to substitute for the functions that state hospitals served. Without the assumption of responsibility by a local authority accountable to the state mental health authority, the needs of people with severe mental illness often went unmet even when they were eligible for available health, social, and income assistance.

The only federal legislation enacted with the specific intent of providing federal assistance to promote deinstitutionalization was the Mental Retardation Facilities and Community Mental Health Centers Construction Act of 1963. Former U.S. President Kennedy proclaimed the act a "bold new direction" that would reduce the population confined to state hospitals by half by 1985. Kennedy's vision was fulfilled ahead of schedule but not as intended.

As part of a legislative compromise the focus of the Community Mental Health Centers (CMHC) Act was broadened to include promotion of the mental health of communities. CMHCs tended to be directed and staffed by mental health professionals with little experience or interest in treating severe mental illness. Consequently, during the

formative years of the CMHC program, discharged state hospital patients were underserved by CMHCs. CMHC directors, responding to a survey commissioned by the National Institute of Mental Health in 1972, gave decreasing state hospital use a rank of 9 in the 10 goals of the CMHC program (Baker, Issacs, & Schulberg, 1972).

Another example of erratic implementation of federal mental health policy was restrictions incorporated in the 1965 Social Security amendments creating Medicaid. Out of fear that states would abandon their responsibility for people with mental illness, Congress deliberately restricted the applicability of Medicaid to state hospitals. Moreover, no specific provisions were made to provide financial incentives for CMHCs or other providers of outpatient treatment to establish service networks with state hospitals. However, three general provisions of Medicaid did make it possible to use Medicaid to finance nonhospital treatment for mental illness:

1. Covered services are applicable to all diagnoses.
2. Services can be provided in clinics, hospital outpatient departments, and physician's offices.
3. Rehabilitative services for physical and mental disabilities are covered.

However, states took nearly 20 years to identify and disseminate arrangements to take full advantage of Medicaid payments to fund community treatment for people with severe mental illness (Hadley, Culhane, & McGurrin, 1992; Meisler & Gonzales, in press; National Association of State Mental Health Program Directors, 1993).

Certainly, the growth in homelessness among people with severe mental illness since the 1970s partly resulted from poorly executed federal and state policy to reduce the population of state hospitals. However, attributing the problem entirely to deinstitutionalization is unrealistic. According to Mechanic (1987) the argument that deinstitutionalization was an underlying source of current mental health system problems "has little empirical utility. . . . and the debate is more a source of heat than light."

Although the growth in homelessness coincided with deinstitutionalization, the relationship was not causal. The dramatic increase in the homeless population occurred in the 1980s. During that time, community mental health service expenditures targeted to people with severe mental illness were growing (NASMHPD, 1993). In constant dollars, state mental health agency expenditures for community mental health services increased from $1.5 to $2 billion between 1981 and 1990, while expenditures for state hospital inpatient services decreased from $4 to $3.5 billion. The effect of the increase in community expenditures was amplified by a shift in provision of services from less ill to more severely ill clients (Larsen, 1987). In addition, Medicaid expenditures for community mental health services other than those administered by state mental health agencies increased by approximately $2 billion (NASMHPD, 1993).

Given that the dramatic increase in the number of homeless people with severe mental illness occurred during a period when state and federal expenditures for community support services also were increasing rapidly, the explanation for homelessness cannot rest with characteristics of the mental health system alone. The failure of government to ensure that people with severe mental illness receive humane treatment and assistance with living outside state hospitals has been a contributing factor but not the only factor explaining the growth in homelessness.

FEDERAL GOVERNMENT RESPONSE TO HOMELESSNESS AMONG PEOPLE WITH MENTAL ILLNESS

In 1982 the National Institute of Mental Health (NIMH) was empowered to coordinate federal efforts to address homelessness among people with mental illness. NIMH established an Office of Programs for the Homeless Mentally Ill. However, significant initiatives were not forthcoming until Congress passed the Stewart B. McKinney Homeless Assistance Act in 1987. The McKinney Act funds a homeless mental health services formula grant to state mental health agencies and also funds competitive research and demonstration grants. The McKinney grants have served as vehicles for the Office of Programs for the Homeless Mentally Ill to promote a community support program (CSP) approach among states in organizing homeless assistance and mental health services. Between 1988 and 1990, NIMH also funded 36 research and demonstration projects. The projects produced the following major findings (Center for Mental Health Services, 1994):

1. Outreach to homeless people with mental illness must be linked to housing, mental health, and case management services.
2. Intensive case management must be ongoing.
3. Linking clients to mainstream community mental health services is not a viable approach in most communities.
4. Many homeless people with mental illness have substance use disorders; services for both disorders need to be integrated.
5. Residential stability requires intensive on-site support.
6. Strategies are needed to increase service integration across agencies and organizations that serve homeless people within a given area.

In 1993 the Office of Programs for the Homeless Mentally Ill funded a 9-state, 18-site research demonstration program specifically focused on the effects of adding service integration strategies to intensive case management services. This 5-year, $85 million project is the primary focus of the office through the end of the 20th century.

A MODEL APPROACH TO ADDRESSING HOMELESSNESS AMONG PEOPLE WITH MENTAL ILLNESS

Between 1987 and 1993 the author was director of the Delaware Division of Alcoholism, Drug Abuse, and Mental Health. During this period a systematic approach was implemented by the division to address homelessness and expand the provision of community support services among the population with mental illness. The approach involved the following (Meisler, 1991; Meisler, Detrick & Tremper, 1995):

1. Setting, monitoring, and enforcing policies to ensure that the state mental health service system served those most in need of its care
2. Ensuring that the structure of the public mental health service system facilitated the mission of its component agencies
3. Decentralizing responsibility and resource control for serving "most in need" clients to small, self-contained community support programs

A standard program model was selected for all community support programs based on the Training in Community Living model developed and practiced since 1972 by the Program of Assertive Community Treatment (PACT) in Madison, Wisconsin (Stein & Test, 1980; Test, 1991; Test, Knoedler, & Allness, 1985). In Delaware the programs were called *continuous treatment teams (CTTs)*. Over several years, CTT programs were established throughout the state.

In a continuous treatment team a multidisciplinary team of mental health professionals assumes total responsibility for meeting the needs of a group of as many as 125 clients on a longitudinal basis. The program operates 7 days per week, with staff available on call in the evenings. Programs include a full range of mental health treatment, vocational rehabilitation, supportive housing, and social services. Almost all interventions occur in the client's natural environment rather than in the program offices. In a series of controlled trials at PACT (Stein & Test, 1980; Test et al., 1992) and in several sites replicating the Training in Community Living model (Burns & Santos, 1995), the approach has been repeatedly demonstrated effective in increasing community tenure,

housing stability, and autonomy among people with severe mental illness. The approach also has been demonstrated effective in achieving these results with homeless people with mental illness (Meisler & Gonzales, in press; Morse et al., 1992; Witheridge, 1991). Box 24-1 summarizes the organization, component services, and desired outcomes of the CTT program. The model is the only community support service approach that incorporates all 10 core services of the community support program (Turner & TenHoor, 1978). It also addresses all service issues raised by the findings of homeless services research presented earlier in this chapter.

Figure 24-3 contrasts the organization of case management services within the continuous treatment team program with that of standard case management in which an individual case manager acts as a service broker for a client caseload. The potential for fragmentation of effort and communication failure among multiple providers in the standard case management approach stands in stark contrast to the coherence of the continuous treatment team approach.

CTT programs address a range of domains, including psychiatric symptoms, alcohol and other drug use, education, vocational and social functioning, self-care and independent living capacity, relationships with significant others, psychological states, and health status. Although each client is assigned a primary therapist, the fixed point of responsibility is the team as a whole. Program staff members assume an assertive, "can-do" orientation toward clients' participation in treatment, rehabilitation, and supportive services. A primary emphasis is placed on teaching coping skills (vocational, self-care, and interpersonal) and providing emotional, cognitive, and environmental supports. Emphasis also is placed on collaboration with clients' families, other support networks, and agencies to enhance individual responsibility taking and lessen excessive and destructive dependency. The approach makes minimal use of referrals. The team takes ultimate responsibility for the well-being of its clients.

Box 24-1. Elements of a continuous treatment team

Organization

1. Core services team
   Fixed point of
      accountability
   Direct provision of most
      services
   Multidisciplinary focus
2. Longitudinal care
3. Home and community
   locus of care
4. Around-the-clock
   availability

Services provided

1. Symptom management
   Education about illness
   Medication monitoring
   Supportive counseling
   Individual and group
      psychotherapy
2. Environmental support
   Assistance with meeting
      basic needs
   Education of family
      members
   Support of independent
      living
   Strengthening of social
      network
3. Rehabilitative services
   Social skills training
   Instrumental skills training
   Adult basic education
   Supported employment

Desired outcomes

1. Fewer, less intense
   symptoms
2. Infrequent acute relapse
3. Less subjective distress
4. Greater life satisfaction
5. Positive community
   adjustment
   Employment
   Improved social relations
   Decreased isolation

Modified from "Training in Community Living," by M.A. Test, 1991, in *Handbook of Psychiatric Rehabilitation*, by R.P. Liberman, ed., New York: Pergamon Press.

The CTT program's mission is to help the client establish as normal a daily routine as possible by relieving discomfort from psychiatric symptoms, social isolation, boredom, interpersonal conflict, and material and social impoverishment. This is accomplished by systematic managing of psychotropic medication; teaching, modeling, and reinforcing adaptive behaviors; modifying physical and social environments; and promoting employment.

Test (1991) recommended using the Training in Community Living model as the core CSP organizing concept within an area; Delaware adopted this approach. Although 24-hour supervised living arrangements and group psychosocial rehabilitation also are included in the community support system, such services supplement and are under the control of the continuous treatment team programs.

Application of the model to a population of homeless people with mental illness

In December 1988, Delaware's first CTT program was established in Wilmington, its largest city. Partly funded through a McKinney Homeless Assistance grant to the Division of Alcoholism, Drug Abuse, and Mental Health through the U.S. Department of Labor, this program was charged with serving homeless people with mental illness. Because of the nature of the federal funds, both competitive employment and permanent housing outcomes were the key criteria by which the program was evaluated. At the same time as the program (which was named Connections) was established, the largest emergency shelter in Wilmington (and the only one with no diagnostic or behavioral exclusion criteria) was closed. It had occupied an abandoned fire station in the city's financial district, and media attention to

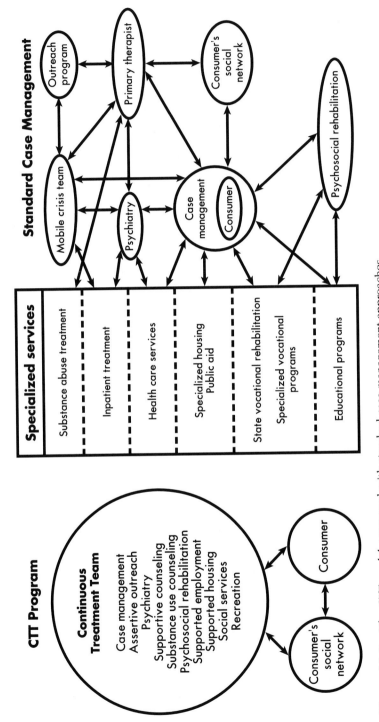

Figure 24-3. The CTT model compared with standard case management approaches. (Modified from "Cost Effectiveness of Assertive Community Treatment," by S.M. Essock, and N.J. Kantos, 1992, October 21–23, Proceedings from the annual meeting of the National Association of State Mental Health Program Directors Research Institute, Baltimore.)

complaints from surrounding businesses about the behavior of the people who congregated around the shelter led the city to accelerate demolition of the building for the development of an office tower that has yet to be built.

In the waning days of the "Firehouse" shelter, Connections staff identified and engaged 32 shelter guests with symptoms and treatment histories of mental illness. By the middle of 1990 the caseload at Connections had grown to 114. A retrospective evaluation of the outcomes of these first 114 people served by Connections has been reported by the author et al. (in press). Of the 114 clients, 59% (67) were dually diagnosed and all of them were using substances at the time of their admission to Connections. All 114 clients were still engaged in treatment at Connections at the end of 1992. The evaluation rated clients on severity of substance use, housing status, employment, psychiatric hospitalization, arrests, and incarcerations.

At the end of 1992, 81% of the clients had attained independent housing; 9% were in transitional housing; 3%, in jail; 4%, hospitalized; and 3%, homeless. At the end of 1992, 43% of the 114 participants were competitively employed. The mean number of psychiatric hospitalizations in 1992 was .3, with 75% having had no psychiatric hospitalizations in 1992. Only 5% had had no psychiatric hospitalizations during the 12 months before enrollment in Connections.

Although this evaluation cannot be applied to all programs that seek to help the homeless because of limitations in its design, the data suggest potential benefits of applying the Training in Community Living approach to the homeless population of adults with severe mental illness. Although only 24% of dually diagnosed clients had been abstinent for a year or longer at the end of 1992, the reduction of homelessness and psychiatric hospital use compared with use before entry to Connections was dramatic. Most remarkable were the vocational outcomes, which compare favorably with outcomes reported for people with mental illness elsewhere, ranging from 8% (Tessler & Goldman, 1982) to 15% (Anthony & Blanch,

1987). They also are consistent with outcomes reported for the Program of Assertive Community Treatment (Knoedler, 1979; Russert & Frey, 1991).

ROLE OF THE NURSE

A small group of nurses has been active in working with homeless people who are mentally ill. They make daily visits to homeless gathering places such as soup kitchens, parks, streets, bridges, and riverbeds. Gulberg (1989) describes a pilot program sponsored by the Veterans Administration. The nursing role in the program consists of a variety of functions, including assertive community outreach. The initial step in working with homeless people involves establishing a therapeutic alliance, an important and sometimes difficult task. Mentally ill people who are homeless are often victimized by other homeless people and have great difficulty trusting others. The nurse must be able to explore fears and listen to painful experiences. Responding to the individual's needs and fears requires sensitivity and timing. Hasty referral to social service agencies will often damage the rapport the nurse is attempting to establish (Berne et al., 1990; Gulberg, 1989; Witt, 1991).

Primm and Houck describe a mobile treatment team that combines case management and psychiatric treatment for people with chronic mental illnesses who reside in hotels and boarding homes and on the street in an inner city catchment area of Baltimore, Maryland. The team is multidisciplinary and includes psychiatrists, psychiatric nurses, social workers, and community workers. Nurses on the team perform triage, physical assessment, medication administration, and staff training in physical illness and medication (Primm & Houck, 1990).

Witt (1991) describes an innovative project that met some of the health care needs of the homeless community in Hartford, Connecticut, and created a unique clinical experience for nursing students. Pairs of students were assigned to each of the eight shelters in Hartford where they provided primary health care and health education; led group discussions; made referrals to appropriate health, mental health, and social service agencies; and assisted the shelter residents in accessing needed services.

Recognizing that nurses can and do provide services to homeless people in a variety of settings, NIMH sponsored a workshop on the "Role of Nurses in Meeting the Health/Mental Health Needs of the Homeless" in 1986. The more than 2 million registered nurses in the United States could play a powerful role in providing care and advocacy for this disenfranchised group.

SUMMARY

Approximately one third of the homeless population has severe mental illness (Task Force on Homelessness and Severe Mental Illness, 1992). One third to one half of these have concurrent substance use disorders (Drake, Osher, & Wallach, 1991). Many people with mental illness within the homeless population are acutely symptomatic because they do not have access to, are too disorganized to seek, or refuse psychiatric treatment or supportive services (Goldfinger, Hopkin, & Surber, 1984; Goldman & Morrissey, 1985; Lipton et al., 1983; Morse & Calsyn, 1986). Their numbers have grown substantially since 1975 and have paralleled a reduction in the population of state hospitals (Jencks, 1994). Research has demonstrated, however, that these factors alone do not explain the growth in homelessness among people with mental illness. On the contrary, empirical evidence suggests that the causes of the increase in homelessness among people with mental illness are the same as for the overall increase in homelessness: population growth, increased poverty, and decreased low-cost housing (Sosin & Grossman, 1991).

Almost 20 years after the emergence of homelessness among adults with psychiatric disabilities as a national health and social crisis, only marginal progress (if any) has been made in reducing its scope. Although a substantial body of literature suggests that noninstitutional service approaches to the problem are viable, dissemination of effective programs has lagged. Consistent, effective public policy to remedy the problem at either the national or local level also has been lacking. Public concern about the problem of homelessness and confidence in government to solve it have waned. An essential rejection is occurring within Congress of a role for the federal government in addressing social problems. Most likely, public spending on housing, income support, and medical care for poor and disabled people will continue to diminish.

REFERENCES

Anthony, W. A., & Blanch, A. (1987). Supported employment for persons who are psychiatrically disabled: A historical and conceptual perspective. *Psychosocial Rehabilitation Journal, 11,* 5-23.

Anthony, W. A., Buell, G. J., Sharratt, S., & Althoff, M. E. (1972). The efficacy of psychiatric rehabilitation. *Psychological Bulletin, 78,* 447-456.

Anthony, W. A., & Jansen, M. A. (1984). Predicting the vocational capacity of the chronically mentally ill. *American Psychologist, 39,* 537-544.

Arce, A. A., Tadlock, M., & Vegare, M. J. (1983). A psychiatric profile of street people admitted to an emergency shelter. *Hospital and Community Psychiatry, 34,* 812-817.

Baker, F., Issacs, C., & Schulberg, H. (1972). *Study of the relationship between community mental health centers and state mental hospitals.* Boston: Socio-Technical Systems Associates.

Bassuk, E. L. (1990). The problem of family homelessness. In E. L. Bassuk, R. W. Carman, and L. F. Weinreb (Eds.), *Community care for homeless families: A program design manual.* Newton Center, MA: The Better Homes Foundation.

Bassuk, E. L., & Lamb, H. R. (1986). Homelessness and the implementation of deinstitutionalization. *New Directions for Mental Health Services, 30,* 7-14.

Bassuk, E. L., Rubin, L., & Lauriat, A. (1984). Is homelessness a mental health problem? *American Journal of Psychiatry, 141,* 1546-1550.

Baum, A. S., & Burnes, D. W. (1993). *A nation in denial: The truth about homelessness.* Boulder, CO: Westview Press.

Baxter, E., & Hopper, K. (1981). *Private lives/public spaces: Homeless adults on the streets of New York City.* New York: Community Service Society.

Berne, A., Dato, C., Mason, D., & Rafferty, M. (1990). A nursing model for addressing the health needs of homeless families. *Image—The Journal of Nursing Scholarship, 22,* 8-13.

Burns, B. J., & Santos, A. B. (1995). Assertive community treatment: An update of randomized trials. *Psychiatric Services, 46,* 669-675.

Burt, M., & Cohen, B. (1989). *America's homeless: Numbers, characteristics, and programs that serve them.* Washington, DC: The Urban Institute Press.

Center for Mental Health Services. (1993). *Additions and resident patients at end of year, state and county mental hospitals, by age and diagnosis, by state, United States, 1991.* Rockville, MD: Author.

Center for Mental Health Services. (1994). *Making a difference: Interim status report of the McKinney demonstration program for homeless adults with serious mental illness.* Rockville, MD: Author.

Drake, R., Osher, F., & Wallach, M. (1991). Homelessness and dual diagnosis. *American Psychologist, 46,* 1149-1158.

Essock, S.M., & Kantos, N.J. (1992, October 21-23). Cost effectiveness of assertive community treatment. Proceedings from the annual meeting of the National Association of State Mental Health Program Directors Research Institute, Baltimore.

Goldfinger, S. M., Hopkin, J. T., & Surber, R. W. (1984). Treatment resisters or system resisters? Toward a better service system for acute care recidivists. *New Directions for Mental Health Services, 21,* 17-27.

Goldman, H. H., & Gattozzi, A. A. (1988). Balance of powers: Social Security and the mentally disabled, 1980-1985. *Milbank Quarterly, 66,* 531-551.

Goldman, H. H., Gattozzi, A. A., & Taube, C. A. (1981). Defining and counting the chronically mentally ill. *Hospital and Community Psychiatry, 32,* 21-25.

Goldman, H. H., & Morrissey, J. P. (1985). The alchemy of mental health policy: Homelessness and the fourth cycle of reform. *American Journal of Public Health, 75,* 727-731.

Gulberg, P. (1989). A psychiatric nurse's role. *Journal of Psychosocial Nursing and Mental Health Services, 27,* 9-13.

Hadley, T. R., Culhane, D. P., & McGurrin, M. C. (1992). Identifying and tracking "heavy users" of acute psychiatric inpatient services. *Administration and Policy in Mental Health, 19,* 279-290.

Herman, M., Galanter, M., & Lifshutz, H. (1991). Combined substance abuse and psychiatric disorders in homeless and domiciled patients. *American Journal of Drug and Alcohol Abuse, 17,* 415-422.

Institute of Medicine. (1988). *Homelessness, health, and human needs.* Washington, DC: National Academy Press.

Jencks, C. (1994). *The homeless.* Cambridge, MA: Harvard University Press.

Kiesler, C. A. (1991). Homelessness and public policy priorities. *American Psychologist, 46,* 1245-1252.

Knoedler, W. H. (1979). How the training in community living program helps patients work. *New Directions for Mental Health Services, 2,* 57-66.

Koch, E. I. (1988, July 11). Lunacies of government: Legal, bureaucratic, ideological. *New York Law Journal, 1.*

Lamb, H. R. (1990). Will we save the homeless mentally ill? *American Journal of Psychiatry, 147,* 649-651.

Lambert, B. (1987, September 1). Psychologists back Koch policy on hospitalizing homeless people. *New York Times,* A1.

Larsen, J. K. (1987). Community mental health services in transition. *Community Mental Health Journal, 23,* 250-259.

Link, B. G., Susser, E., Stueve, A., Phelan, J., Moore, R. E., & Struening, E. (1994). Lifetime and five-year prevalence of homelessness in the United States. *American Journal of Public Health, 84,* 1907-1912.

Lipton, F., Sabatini, A., & Katz, S. (1983). Down and out in the city: The homeless mentally ill. *Hospital and Community Psychiatry, 34,* 817-821.

McChesney, K. Y. (1990). Family homelessness: A systematic problem. *Journal of Social Issues, 46,* 191-206.

Mechanic, D. (1987). Correcting misconceptions in mental health policy: Strategies for improved care of the seriously mentally ill. *Milbank Quarterly, 65,* 203-230.

Meisler, N. (1991). State mental health agency responsibility for outreach. *New Directions for Mental Health Services, 52,* 81-92.

Meisler, N., Blankertz, L., Santos, A.B., & McKay, C. (in press). Impact of assertive community treatment on homeless persons with co-occurring severe psychiatric and substance abuse disorders. *Community Mental Health Journal.*

Meisler, N., Detrick, A., & Tremper, R. (1995). Statewide dissemination of the training in community living program. *Administration and Policy in Mental Health, 23,* 71-76.

Meisler, N., & Gonzales, M. C. (in press). Medicaid financing of community mental health services for adults with serious mental illness. In S. W. Henggeler, & A. B. Santos (Eds.), *Innovative models of mental health treatment for "difficult to treat" clinical populations.* Washington, DC: American Psychiatric Press.

Morse, G., & Calsyn, R. J. (1986). Mentally disturbed homeless people in St. Louis: Needy, willing, but under-served. *International Journal of Mental Health, 14,* 74-94.

Morse, G., Calsyn, R. J., Allen, G., Tempelhoff, B., & Smith, R. (1992). Experimental comparison of the effects of three treatment programs for homeless mentally ill people. *Hospital and Community Psychiatry, 43,* 1005-1010.

National Association of State Mental Health Program Directors. (1993). *Funding sources and expenditures of state mental health agencies, fiscal year 1990.* Alexandria, VA: Author.

Primm, A., & Houck, J. (1990). COSTAR: Flexibility in urban community mental health. In N. Cohen (Ed.), *Psychiatry takes to the streets.* New York: Guilford Press.

Rosenheck, R., & Fontana, A. (1994). A model of homelessness among male veterans of the Vietnam War generation. *American Journal of Psychiatry, 151,* 421-427.

Rossi, P. H. (1990). The old homeless and the new homeless in historical perspective. *American Psychologist, 45,* 954-959.

Russert, M. G., & Frey, J. L. (1991), The PACT vocational model: A step into the future. *Psychosocial Rehabilitation Journal, 14*(4), 11-17.

Shlay, A., & Rossi, P. (1992). Social science research and contemporary studies of homelessness. *Annual Review of Sociology, 18,* 129-160.

Sosin, M. R., & Grossman, S. (1991). The mental health system and the etiology of homelessness: A comparison study. *Journal of Community Psychology, 19,* 337-350.

Stein, L. I., & Test, M. A. (1980). Alternatives to mental hospital treatment, I. Conceptual model, treatment program and clinical evaluation. *Archives of General Psychiatry, 37,* 392-397.

Susser, E. S., Lin, S. P., & Conover, S. A. (1991). Risk factors for homelessness among patients admitted to a state mental hospital. *American Journal of Psychiatry, 148,* 1659-1664.

Task Force on Homelessness and Severe Mental Illness. (1992). *Outcasts on main street: Report of the Federal Task Force on Homelessness and Severe Mental Illness.* Washington, DC: U.S. Department of Health and Human Services.

Tessler, R. C., & Dennis, D. L. (1989). *A synthesis of NIMH-funded research concerning persons who are homeless and mentally ill.* Rockville, MD: National Institute of Mental Health.

Tessler, R., & Goldman, H. H. (1982). *The chronically mentally ill: Assessing community support programs.* Cambridge, MA: Bollinger.

Test, M. A. (1991). Training in community living. In R. P. Liberman (Ed.), *Handbook of psychiatric rehabilitation.* New York: Pergamon Press.

Test, M. A., Knoedler, W. H., & Allness, D. J. (1985). The long-term treatment of young schizophrenics in a community support program. *New Directions for Mental Health Services, 26,* 17-27.

Test, M. A., Knoedler, W., Allness, D., & Burke, S. S. (1992). Training in Community Living (TCL) model: Two decades of research. *Outlook, 2,* 5-8.

Torrey, E. F. (1989, Spring). Thirty years of shame: The scandalous neglect of the mentally ill homeless. *Policy Review.*

Turner, J. C., & TenHoor, W. J. (1978). The NIMH community support program: Pilot approach to needed social reform. *Schizophrenia Bulletin, 4,* 319-349.

U.S. Department of Housing and Urban Development. (1984). *A report to the secretary on the homeless and emergency shelters.* Washington, DC: Author.

U.S. General Accounting Office. (1989). *Children and youths: Report to congressional committees.* Washington, DC: U.S. Government Printing Office.

Vegare, M. J., & Arce, A. A. (1986). Homeless adult individuals and their shelter network. *New Directions for Mental Health Services, 30,* 15-26.

Witheridge, T. F. (1991). The "active ingredients" of assertive outreach. *New Directions for Mental Health Services, 52,* 47-64.

Witt, B. (1991). The homeless shelter. *Nursing and Health Care, 12,* 304-307.

Chapter 25

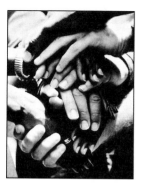

Persons with Serious Mental Illness and the Issue of HIV Disease

James A. Cates and Linda L. Graham

With the pandemic spread of human immunodeficiency virus (HIV) and HIV disease,* a wealth of data has accumulated on the social, psychological, and emotional characteristics of persons who engage in behaviors that increase the risk of infection. However, the emphasis in research is moving from demographic groups at risk for HIV infection (e.g., homosexual men and African-Americans) toward identification of behavioral characteristics that lead the individual within the group to engage in high-risk behaviors. This emphasis works well for behavioral groups with data on infection risk, clearly demarcated boundaries, and defined routes of infection (e.g., men who have sex with men or persons who use injected drugs). For persons with serious mental illness (SMI), however, the lack of clear definitions for group membership, spotty statistical data on prevalence of

infection, and minimal knowledge of characteristics that lead to high-risk behaviors add up to a disturbing lack of evidence to guide intervention efforts. At the same time the ethical mandate to the helping professions remains the same—to provide interventions that will protect clients with SMI.

This chapter discusses existing HIV disease studies and their application to persons with SMI. The data do more to illuminate the lack of information than to provide guidelines for intervention efforts, but the statistics from these data alone suggest the potential epidemic in the population of persons with SMI. From these data the authors extrapolated the need to develop an intervention in a community support program for persons with SMI. The proposed intervention focuses on education, with the target of changing attitudes toward HIV disease. Social-psychological research has long demonstrated the reciprocal relationship between attitudes and behavior; correspondingly,

---

*In this chapter the term *HIV disease* encompasses both HIV-positive status and full-blown AIDS.

the authors hypothesized that changing attitudes would reduce high-risk behaviors. Conceptualizing attitudes within an existing paradigm helped link this research with more mainstream efforts on HIV disease prevention.

EPIDEMIOLOGY

Studies of HIV infection rates among persons with SMI face many obstacles. The most daunting are described in the following sections.

Lack of reliable estimates on the prevalence of HIV disease among persons with SMI

Persons with SMI have been categorized among other "primary" groups based on ethnicity and race (e.g., Hispanic or African-American) or demographic and behavioral characteristics (e.g., homelessness or use of injected drugs). In part, this may be due to the difficulty of defining "serious mental illness." For example, is the individual diagnosed with a schizophrenic disorder whose symptoms are well controlled on medication "seriously" mentally ill? Must the client require inpatient treatment, partial hospitalization, or other extensive support services to qualify? Without clear categorical boundaries the prevalence of risk and disease is equally murky. Researchers are often led to discuss prevalence using such obvious categories as race despite the effort to move to behavioral descriptions.

Seroprevalence rates for HIV disease among persons with SMI hospitalized in psychiatric units, most frequently during periods of acute exacerbation, range from a low of 4.0% in an inpatient unit for long-term patients to a high of 19.4% in a homeless shelter for men (Herman et al., 1994). Most of these data, however, were collected in New York City and therefore the generalizability of the findings is questionable. Nevertheless, they support the finding that persons with SMI are engaging in high-risk behaviors and are being infected with HIV. Statistics collected by the Centers for Disease Control (CDC) have for several years reflected a higher seroprevalence rate for

Hispanics and African-Americans than for whites and, more recently, an increasing seroprevalence rate among women (CDC, 1995). Assuming that these proportions hold true within the population of persons with SMI, a conservative estimate of the HIV infection rate is about 5%, soaring to 20% in certain geographical areas or demographical categories. Persons of color are more likely to engage in high-risk behaviors than whites or (an important distinction) are more likely to engage in high-risk behaviors with infected partners than whites.

Lack of reliable estimates on high-risk behaviors among persons with SMI

Indeed, before the early 1980s the mental health literature on the prevalence and types of sexual behavior among persons with SMI consisted of a handful of articles. In a partial report on a longitudinal study, Test, Burke, and Wallisch (1990) found that within a sample diagnosed with either schizophrenia or schizotypal personality disorder only 7% of women and 2% of men cohabited. During the study, 48% of the women and 70% of the men reported sexual activity. In general, studies reflect a tendency for certain subgroups of persons with SMI characterized by age (with younger individuals being more active), diagnosis, and substance use or abuse to engage in more frequent sexual activity.

Recent research by the authors supports these findings (Cates, Bond, & Graham, 1994). The study compared a sample of 50 persons with SMI in a community support program with 50 persons drawn from the larger community and matched for gender and educational achievement. As part of the criteria, participants were required to be single and not cohabiting at the time of the study; as a result, persons with SMI were significantly older than the comparison sample.

Only 10% of persons with SMI reported themselves sexually abstinent for the past 10 years. Of the remaining 90%, 22% reported engaging in sex with only one partner in that period but 68% reported sexual activity with multiple partners.

Within this two thirds of the sample, only 18% reported consistent condom use. Another 13% reported "often" using condoms. However, the large majority—69%—reported sporadic or no condom use during sexual encounters. Furthermore, only 36% of persons with SMI expressed the intent to reduce the risk of infection.

How do these figures compare with the normative sample? Only 12% of the normative group reported themselves sexually abstinent over the past 10 years. Of the rest of the sample, 20% reported engaging in sex with only one partner in that period and, by coincidence, 68% of this sample reported sexual activity with multiple partners during this time. Of this two thirds of the sample, again, 17% reported consistent condom use. Another 28% reported "often" using condoms. A majority of the participants (55%) reported sporadic or no condom use during sexual encounters. However, 64% of this sample expressed the intent to reduce the risk of infection.

These findings are based on a small, geographically contained sample, and overinterpretation is a significant risk. However, the findings seem to suggest the comparability of sexual behaviors among single persons with SMI and those in the general population in terms of frequency of sexual behavior and approach to risk of HIV disease. What is of greatest concern is the finding that persons with SMI are much less likely than members of the general population to express the intent to reduce their risk.

When these findings are considered in conjunction with data available on homosexual men, persons of color, adolescents, and college students, a recurring pattern emerges. In each group, certain members are sexually abstinent, practice serial monogamy, or consistently use condoms in their sexual encounters. For these people the risk of infection is relatively low. A second subgroup engages in sexual activity with multiple sexual partners; although members of this subgroup use condoms inconsistently, they nevertheless express some concern for the possibility of infection. Members of a third subgroup engage in sexual activity with multiple partners with little or no concern for condom use, exposing themselves to high risk for HIV infection. Studies of persons with SMI replicate these findings but suggest that the high-risk subgroup of persons with SMI is even less intent on changing risky behaviors than its counterpart in the general population.

LEVELS OF PREVENTION
Primary prevention

As noted earlier, the lack of empirical research does not nullify the ethical mandate for health care professionals to provide interventions to persons with SMI. To date, however, models have addressed only primary care interventions (education and prevention). Even so the emphasis remains in the earliest stages; health care professionals themselves provide the education and training. In other populations such as adolescents (Rotheram-Borus, Mahler, & Rosario, 1995) and injection drug users (Siegal et al., 1995), intervention efforts include peer training and enhanced educational interventions so that members of the group can perform educational activities or internalize the dangers or risk behaviors more clearly. The lack of emphasis on secondary interventions (HIV screening and health consciousness) is particularly noticeable among persons with SMI, and tertiary interventions (treating the individual with HIV) are barely addressed.

Secondary prevention

Secondary care of persons with SMI remains an important and largely undiscussed issue. On the one hand is the individual's right and need to know seroconversion status. This knowledge may be socially important (to plan for future sexual behaviors in a responsible manner) or medically important (to provide adequate treatment). On the other hand are the possible detrimental effects of such knowledge. For the person with SMI who has been diagnosed with HIV disease even at the earliest stage of seropositivity, unrealistic fears, misconceptions, and distorted or delusional thinking may contribute to increased difficulties in care and personal anxiety and may fuel existing psychotic processes. This issue is hardly mentioned in the professional literature, and few answers are forthcoming. Areas in need of research include effective means of preparing persons with SMI for knowledge of their HIV status; the impact of this knowledge on social, emotional, and cognitive processes; and the long-term health benefits or detriments that accrue to persons with SMI who learn they have been infected with HIV.

Tertiary prevention

Tertiary care of the person with HIV disease and SMI is even less frequently addressed. Many of the issues concerning tertiary prevention are similar to those noted in secondary care, but issues of death and dying may become more pronounced. At times, extensive medication regimens are required; little research is concerned with the most effective means of assisting persons with SMI with this issue. In the end stage of life the diagnosed mental illness also may combine with dementia secondary to HIV to create significant difficulties in activities of daily living and behavioral management.

INTERVENTIONS
A model intervention for persons with SMI

Granting the need for secondary and tertiary interventions, primary prevention is still a significant concern for persons with SMI. The authors researched and applied an educational intervention in a group home program administered through a community mental health center (CMHC) (Cates & Graham, 1993; Graham & Cates, 1992). The description provided here is twofold. First, it gives a narrative account of the difficulties encountered in developing such a program. Second, it exemplifies the difficulties encountered in facilitating effective interventions for persons with SMI.

The program was assessed for effectiveness in increasing knowledge regarding HIV disease (through preintervention and postintervention

testing) because reduced-risk behaviors are predicated on accurate information on the infection and disease process (particularly transmission routes). To assess the intervention, two attitudinal sets were considered. The first of these is fear of HIV disease, or irrational, negative beliefs regarding HIV, AIDS, and persons infected (Bouton et al., 1987). The second is comfort with discussion, or attitudes toward discussing HIV and AIDS within a group setting, an attitude set that is highly applicable to persons receiving community support services. The primary goals of the study were increased comfort with discussion and diminished fear of HIV disease after educational interventions.

Subjects

Participants in this study were persons with SMI residing in four CMHC group homes in a small Midwestern city. Two group homes housed persons of both genders, and the other two housed either men or women. In all, 35 persons with SMI participated (Box 25-1). The sample was predominantly white. Mean ages were in the middle thirties and the majority had received diagnoses of either schizophrenic disorders or mood disorders. Mean length of time in treatment for serious mental illness was approximately 5 years.

Materials

The materials for the educational intervention included three brief videocassettes, each providing an overview of HIV disease and transmission routes. These videos were selected from the library of the local community-based organization responding to the HIV disease epidemic. The following criteria were used in choosing these videos:

- Brevity (because of short attention span of some residents)
- Clarity of information presented
- Neutrality of tone (non-judgmental or moralizing)
- Easily understood fundamental information on the nature and transmission of HIV disease

Box 25-1. Demographic characteristics of persons with SMI in CMHC group home study

Mean age

35 years old (range: 20 - 65)

Gender

18 Men
17 Women

Race

32 White
 2 African-American
 1 Hispanic

Religion

 7 Catholic
 9 Protestant
 5 No religion
14 Other or not reporting

Average number of years in treatment

5.5 years (range: 1-45)

Diagnosis

 2 Schizophrenia, paranoid
 2 Schizoaffective disorder
22 Schizophrenia, undifferentiated
 1 Major depression
 4 Bipolar disorder
 2 Borderline personality disorder
 1 Personality disorder not otherwise specified
 1 Depressive disorder not otherwise specified

To close the final session, a facilitator demonstrated proper use of a condom on a model penis.

Design and procedure

Before the actual intervention the local community-based organization responding to HIV disease was contacted. The authors facilitated a joint intervention for the group home residents, combining the expertise of this organization and the CMHC staff. The community-based group provided in-service education to the CMHC staff (both direct care staff and administrators) before the intervention. This in-service education updated the information available to staff members on HIV disease, served as a springboard for discussion of the salient issues to be addressed in the intervention, and allowed group discussion of areas of discomfort and uncertainty for staff members in approaching this population. However, the community-based organization had no experience working with persons with SMI. Therefore they deferred to the staff of the CMHC group homes to design and implement an educational intervention based on their assessment of the needs and probable responses of their residents. The intervention eventually designed included three 1-hour group educational sessions at 2-week intervals. The same basic information was offered in each session, but the emphasis was altered to coincide with the primary information to be presented during that session. After a brief formal program focusing on the specific area outlined for that day, the presenter opened the program to questions from the residents (a maximum of 10 in each home). Presenters were a male nurse and a female nurse, each well known to the residents. The male nurse provided training for the male and one mixed gender group home, and the female nurse provided training for the female and one mixed gender group home.

Results

Preintervention and postintervention assessment of knowledge was unchanged; however, residents had a broad and accurate knowledge base before the intervention itself. Likewise, no change occurred in fear of HIV disease despite qualitative observations from the presenters that residents became increasingly comfortable in discussion and in addressing means to reduce their risk. Reports indicated that discussions were more lively and uninhibited in the single-gender group homes; a post hoc analysis comparing preintervention and postintervention attitudes toward discussion potentially supported this finding, although none of the statistical analyses (repeated measures analysis of variance) achieved significance ($p < 0.05$).

Discussion

Persons with SMI differed widely in their responses to the intervention despite the lack of statistical significance. Turning to qualitative analysis of the intervention, acceptance of the information in large part corresponded to the severity of the person's illness and to acute exacerbations at the time of the presentations. Several residents with severe chronic psychoses were unable to tolerate either the videos or discussion periods (and were not included in the formal research). When present, their questions and comments were tangential and unproductive. Interestingly, other residents in the group homes were largely undeterred by these distractions because this type of behavior was pervasive and thus well known in the living environment.

More difficult to manage was the tendency for some residents to incorporate the information provided into their pathology. For example, one female resident maintained the delusion that she had been repeatedly raped under hypnosis. When presented with information regarding HIV disease, she incorporated infection with HIV into her delusional system. Another resident's delusions included persecution by the Roman Catholic Church. He incorporated the information on HIV disease into his delusional system by inferring that the church was now trying to infect him.

Some residents also tended toward somatic complaints; for them, HIV disease became another fear to be addressed. For several older women in the groups, discussion of sex and sexuality triggered memories of past losses and corresponding grief. One male resident with a sexual obsession found the discussions served as "permission" to expound his beliefs.

Although residents seemed relatively comfortable in asking questions, they also recognized that their comments or concerns might be ridiculed. One male resident, after initial hesitation, stammering, and distracting statements, finally admitted he was uncertain whether he should wear a condom throughout the date or only during sexual activity. Some residents diagnosed with schizophrenia experienced difficulty expressing legitimate questions because their tangential, loosely associated style of expression became confusing and difficult to follow.

The use of presenters who were not only knowledgeable about work with persons with SMI but also familiar to these residents was a significant factor in reducing the disruption to the group that these incidents could have caused. Granted, disruption still occurred. Nevertheless, the presenters' skills in acknowledging delusional beliefs without validating them, creating boundaries and structure in discussions without stifling freedom, and recognizing and coping with emotional topics, combined with their rapport with the individual clients, enhanced the education that occurred.

Peripheral concerns stemming from these sessions suggested that some residents may have understood the basic information but lacked the ability to successfully apply it. For example, several persons diagnosed with schizophrenia received injections of fluphenazine (Prolixin). Some were reluctant to allow the injection after the first session on HIV disease in which transmission through injected drugs was discussed. With questioning, staff determined that the clients had understood HIV could be spread through needles but had not grasped the significance of needle sharing to this infection route.

The effort to involve the community-based organization also created unanticipated problems. Its staff and volunteer expertise was in the area of HIV disease, not in the care of persons with SMI. The CMHC staff's expertise was in the area of caring for persons with SMI, not in HIV disease. The joint educational venture required close collaboration and in particular the ability to admit that certain areas were outside of one's competence to work effectively. After the intervention, several persons with SMI chose to be tested for HIV through the local free clinic. Again, the expertise of the clinic staff did not extend to the care of persons with SMI and further collaboration was required.

Theoretical models

Despite the qualitative "success" of the model intervention described, the quantitative analysis indicated no measurable change in attitudes. The authors had directly assessed the attitudes of persons with SMI toward the fear of HIV disease based on previous work specific to HIV disease and had assessed comfort with discussion using items with high face validity. However, was such a focal, direct measure of attitudes the most effective way to measure program success? Was a measure that encompassed a set of attitudes with a conceptual model likely to be more effective? The next study examined attitudes toward HIV disease from this broader perspective.

As noted, attitudes and behavior are theoretically reciprocal. Changes occur through mediating factors both internal and external to the individual (Zimbardo & Leippe, 1991). Thus a change in behavior can precipitate a change in attitude, or, as hypothesized by the majority of risk reduction campaigns, a change in attitude can precipitate a change in behavior.

Health belief model

Of those campaigns that apply an explicit theory, the majority are influenced by variants of the health belief model (HBM) (Rosenstock, 1960, 1974). The primary HBM constructs vary little across time. To motivate a response to a perceived health threat, the individual must identify the following:

- The seriousness of the health risk (described as *severity of threat*)
- The likelihood of its occurrence as a personal threat (described as *probability of occurrence*)
- The efficacy of efforts to respond to the perceived risk (described as *response efficacy*)

After being motivated to respond to a health threat, behavior arises from the internal conflict among motives and potential courses of action. Thus health-related motives and behavior do not logically follow a health risk. Instead, mitigating attitudes disrupt the logical chain of events.

Pragmatic application of the HBM to primary intervention with HIV disease has met with mixed results (Montgomery et al., 1989). In general, a single research sample will support some but not all of the constructs that make up the model (Janz & Becker, 1984). In addition, a frequent criticism is the lack of discussion of self-motivation in responding to a health crisis. A refinement of the HBM incorporates self-efficacy as a component of health beliefs.

Protection-motivation model

Rogers developed the protection-motivation theory (PMT), refining the principles of the HBM (Rogers 1975, 1983) (Figure 25-1). Initial identification of a health risk activates dual cognitive processes. To motivate protective behaviors, the individual must perceive the threat as sufficiently severe to warrant attention (severity of threat). Simultaneously the individual must perceive the threat as sufficiently personal to warrant attention (probability of occurrence). Next, the individual appraises coping responses. Are recommended protective behaviors and techniques (in the case of HIV disease, risk-reduction behaviors) believed to be effective (response efficacy)? Simultaneously, does the individual feel capable of performing risk-reduction behaviors with a positive outcome

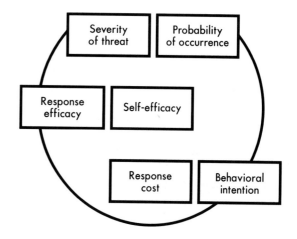

Figure 25-1.   Protection-motivation theory.

(self-efficacy)? Finally, the intent to change behavior is simultaneously considered with response cost or the rewards and reinforcers that will be eliminated if the individual engages in efficacious behavior. Although PMT posits a linear progression through these steps, entry into the decision-making process can occur at any point and lead forward or backward.

Research to date largely supports the validity of PMT as a model to explain attitudes (and thus behaviors) toward HIV disease. In a study using PMT to determine HIV risk with 84 heterosexual men and 147 homosexual men, all of whom had multiple sex partners, PMT accounted for as much as 73% of the variance in high-risk behaviors within the heterosexual sample and 44% of the variance in high-risk behaviors within the heterosexual sample (Van der Velde & Van der Pligt, 1991). In a retrospective study of reduced-risk sexual behaviors among homosexual men, probability of occurrence, response efficacy, self-efficacy, and sexual behavior that occurred before attempts to reduce the risk of infection accounted for 70% of the variance in high-risk behaviors (with severity of threat not reaching significance) (Aspinwall et al., 1991).

Criticism of the HBM focuses on the lack of attention to environmental and cultural factors, and criticism of PMT focuses on the strong emphasis on cognitive responses to fear appeals (Herek & Glunt, 1991; Rippetoe & Rogers, 1987). Nevertheless, research supports the superiority of PMT in predicting preventive health behaviors, largely because of the self-efficacy component (Seydel, Taal, & Wiegman, 1990).

Protection-motivation: application of the theory

Design and procedure

In the previously cited research (Cates et al., 1994) the samples of persons with SMI in a community support program and a normative comparison group were queried regarding their attitudes toward HIV disease, using the constructs of PMT. Knowledge about HIV disease was as-

sessed based on current educational interventions. *Knowledge* was defined as accurate awareness of the known facts regarding HIV disease in three areas: modes of transmission, high-risk behaviors, and medical evidence about the course of the disease. The comprehension subtest of the Wechsler Adult Intelligence Scale (Wechsler, 1981) screened for cognitive impairment to control for potential differences in attitudes created by differences in comprehension of the disease. This information is included in Table 25-1.

Attitude items related to the four areas of PMT and behavioral intention items were rated on a five-point Likert scale (1 = strongly agree, 5 = strongly disagree). Behavioral intention was assessed using a four-item scale constructed for this study. The first item measured intent to remain abstinent; the other three items measured intent to reduce risk if sexual behaviors were pursued. Agreement with the first item did not preclude agreement with the remaining items.

Sexual history was assessed using 20 items that inquired about sexual activity, gender of sexual partners, frequency and consistency of condom use, and the frequency with which participants risked exposure to HIV by sexual transmission

Table 25-1. Comparison of persons with SMI and normative sample on knowledge and attitudes about HIV disease

	SMI (*n* = 50)		NORMATIVE (*n* = 50)	
FACTOR	**M**	**(SD)**	**M**	**(SD)**
Knowledge	31.98	(2.10)	33.66	(1.85)
Attitudes*				
Threat	2.11	(0.40)	2.15	(0.41)
Probability	3.14	(0.59)	3.00	(0.56)
Response	3.45	(0.59)	3.50	(0.60)
Self-efficacy	3.95	(0.58)	3.76	(0.60)

M, Mean; *SD,* standard deviation.
*Potential range of values is 1 to 5; larger values represent greater severity of threat and probability of occurrence and less confidence in response and self-efficacy.

routes. The item on condom use was analyzed separately because it was the only item that indicated a reduction in risk behaviors.

Results

Both samples had a broad knowledge base about HIV disease, with no significant differences between the two. Although persons with SMI exhibited greater cognitive impairment, the correlation between impairment and attitudes or high-risk behaviors was negligible. Based on a multivariate analysis of variance (MANOVA) with Wilks' criterion, the samples were significantly different at the multivariate level (F [1, 95] = 5.08, $p < 0.01$). The samples were significantly different at the univariate level in attitudes toward probability of occurrence (F [1, 98] = 5.98, $p < 0.05$), with persons with SMI perceiving greater risk of infection than the normative sample. Persons with SMI also reported significantly less self-efficacy than the normative sample (F [1, 98] = 11.66, $p < 0.01$). The samples did not significantly differ in attitudes toward severity of threat or response efficacy.

Discussion

Persons with SMI were significantly more concerned by their personal risk (probability of occurrence) and significantly less likely to report a sense of their own ability to respond in an efficacious manner (self-efficacy). This finding (greater fear with less self-efficacy) implies a sense of helplessness and a need for empowerment in the face of HIV disease. This helplessness is particularly alarming given that few differences exist between sexual behavior of people with SMI and the general population. These findings partially replicate previous efforts with both persons in community support programs and inpatient care, suggesting the validity of the findings for persons with SMI.

SUMMARY

Data are scarce on the prevalence of HIV among people with serious mental illness. High-risk sexual behavior among people with serious mental illness seems to mirror that of the general population. However, people with SMI have been found less intent on changing risky behavior than the general population. Therefore primary prevention efforts need to be specifically designed for this population. The studies described in this chapter lead to the following conclusions regarding intervention efforts.

Interventions benefit from the inclusion of a theoretical rationale. Even the most straightforward educational presentations address the twin issues of sexuality and mortality. As such the emotions they engender for both presenter and audience are far more powerful than might be expected on the basis of the material alone. For this reason a logical, cohesive plan for addressing attitudes is essential. An underlying theoretical rationale or premise regarding attitudes ensures greater impartiality in the coverage of material and the dissemination of information.

Interventions with people with SMI need to take into account the probability of heightened fear and greater helplessness. Findings suggest that persons with SMI begin in a "one-down" stance compared with the general public in their attitudes toward HIV disease. Seeing themselves at risk for infection, they lack the concomitant attitudes of self-protection created by beliefs in the efficacy of responses and in the personal potential to act in a manner that reduces risk. Thus educational efforts need to incorporate a message of empowerment. Persons with SMI need practical information on the steps they can take to protect themselves and encouragement that they are able to take these steps.

The cognitive distortions of serious mental illness may apply to information about HIV disease as well. As has been seen, persons with SMI may misinterpret information about HIV disease or incorporate it into an existing set of cognitive distortions. For this reason, information should be not only accessible but also accessible daily from health care personnel who can address their concerns. Rapport with the individual and the audience also is important. Persons with SMI may well have difficulty trusting others; for example, the finding that discussion of HIV issues was more open in single-gender group homes suggests the timidity that may occur when the opposite sex is present. Mental health professionals who are familiar with serious mental illness and with whom the person with SMI is comfortable are essential to effective education.

Interventions with persons with SMI need to recognize and accept their sexuality. The lack of information about sexual behavior for persons with SMI points to the paternalistic attitude maintained toward this population, an attitude that in fairness often seems justified. One of the young men in a study cited earlier identified himself as gay and also was diagnosed with paranoid schizophrenia. He was frequently resistive to his medication regimen, experienced thought insertion and ideas of reference, and at times full-blown delusions. He also was physically a very handsome young man and pleased by the attentions he received from other gay men. During the course of the study the issue of "danger to self" was raised in regard to his multiple sexual partners but without consensus. Eventually his mental disorder came under better control, and he became more efficacious in his behavior, regularly using condoms.

Persons with SMI bring many issues to interventions designed to reduce the risk of HIV disease. In many ways, they are unique. No other population lives with disordered thoughts and a fragmented self, with hope not of recovery but of maintaining. However, as with every population to be addressed, interventions must respect differences and learn to target the most effective style of teaching. At the level of secondary and tertiary intervention, interventions must respect the individual while providing treatment and support.

REFERENCES

Aspinwall, L. G., Kemeny, M. E., Taylor, S. E., Shelley, E., & Schneider, S. G. (1991). Psychosocial predictors of gay men's AIDS risk-reduction behavior. *Health Psychology, 10,* 432-444.

Bouton, R. A., Gallaher, P. E., Garlinghouse, P. A., Leal, T., Rosenstein, L. D., & Young, R. K. (1987). Scales for measuring fear of AIDS and homophobia. *Journal of Personality Assessment, 51,* 606-614.

Cates, J. A., Bond, G. R., & Graham, L. L. (1994). AIDS knowledge, attitudes, and risk behavior among people with serious mental illness. *Psychosocial Rehabilitation Journal, 17,* 19-29.

Cates, J. A., & Graham, L. L. (1993). HIV and serious mental illness: Reducing the risk. *Community Mental Health Journal, 29,* 35-47.

Centers for Disease Control. (1995, Monthly). *HIV/AIDS surveillance report.* Washington, DC: U.S. Government Printing Office.

Graham, L. L., & Cates, J. A. (1992). How to reduce the risk of HIV infection for the seriously mentally ill. *Journal of Psychosocial Nursing and Mental Health Services, 30,* 9-13.

Herek, G. M., & Glunt, E. K. (1991). AIDS-related attitudes in the United States: A preliminary conceptualization. *Journal of Sex Research, 28,* 99-121.

Herman, R., Kaplan, M., Satriano, J., Cournos, F., & McKinnon, K. (1994). HIV prevention with people with serious mental illness: Staff training and institutional attitudes. *Psychosocial Rehabilitation Journal, 17,* 97-103.

Janz, N. K., & Becker, M. H. (1984). The health belief model: A decade later. *Health Education Quarterly, 11,* 1-47.

Montgomery, S. B., Joseph, J. G., Becker, M. H., & Ostrow, D. G. (1989). The health belief model in understanding compliance with prevention recommendations for AIDS: How useful? *AIDS Education and Prevention, 1,* 303-323.

Rippetoe, P. A., & Rogers, R. W. (1987). Effects of components of protection-motivation theory on adaptive and maladaptive coping with a health threat. *Journal of Personality and Social Psychology, 52,* 596-604.

Rogers, R. W. (1975). A protection motivation theory of fear appeals and attitude change. *Journal of Psychology, 91,* 93-114.

Rogers, R. W. (1983). Cognitive and physiological processes in fear appeals and attitude change: A revised theory of protection motivation. In J. T. Cacioppo, & R. E. Petty (Eds.), *Social psychophysiology.* New York: Guilford Press.

Rosenstock, I. M. (1960). What research in motivation suggests for public health. *American Journal of Public Health, 50,* 295-302.

Rosenstock, I. M. (1974). Historical origins of the health belief model. *Health Education Monographs, 2,* 328-335.

Rotheram-Borus, M. J., Mahler, K. A., & Rosario, M. (1995). AIDS prevention with adolescents. *AIDS Education and Prevention, 7,* 320-336.

Seydel, E., Taal, E., & Wiegman, O. (1990). Risk-appraisal, outcome and self-efficacy expectancies: Cognitive factors in preventive behaviour related to cancer. *Psychology and Health, 4,* 99-109.

Siegal, H. A., Falck, R. S., Carlson, R. G., & Wang, J. (1995). Reducing HIV needle risk behaviors among injection-drug users in the Midwest: An evaluation of the efficacy of standard and enhanced interventions. *AIDS Education and Prevention, 7,* 308-317.

Test, M. A., Burke, S. S., & Wallisch, L. S. (1990). Gender differences of young adults with schizophrenic disorders in community care. *Schizophrenia Bulletin, 16,* 331-334.

Van der Velde, F. W., & Van der Pligt, J. (1991).

AIDS-related behavior: Coping, protection motivation, and previous behavior. *Journal of Behavioral Medicine, 14,* 429-451.

Wechsler, D. (1981). *Manual for the Wechsler Adult Intelligence Scale—Revised.* New York: Psychological Corporation.

Zimbardo, P. G., & Leippe, M. R. (1991). *The psychology of attitude change and social influence.* New York: McGraw-Hill.

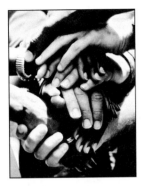

Chapter 26

Persons with Mental Illness in Jail

Joyce K. Laben and Jeff Blum

City and county jails range from very small to large facilities. Generally, jails are "short-term people processing institutions and are not long-term, people changing institutions" (Steadman, 1990), whereas prisons are long-term facilities run by the state or federal government. Jails usually are locally administered confinement units designated to hold individuals awaiting adjudication or those serving sentences of 1 year or less. Nevertheless, with current prison overcrowding, people serving longer sentences are often housed in local jails by contract with the state until space becomes available in a prison. As a result a growing number of convicted felons have been sentenced to local jails (*Bureau of Justice Statistics Bulletin,* 1995). Currently, approximately 3300 jails are operating in the United States, and the majority of detainees are incarcerated in jails. The greatest number are small, holding few inmates, but the larger jails, holding hundreds to thousands, detain half of all men and women in jails. The overall proportion of inmates per 100,000 U.S. residents has increased from 96 in 1983 to 188 in 1994. Between 1983 and 1993 the number of jail inmates increased 106%.

Black non-Hispanics compose 44% of the jail population, followed by whites 39%, Hispanics 15%, and other races 2% (*Bureau of Justice Statistics Bulletin,* 1995). The greatest number of jails are operated by counties, followed by cities, and a small proportion are both a city and county operation (Steadman, McCarty, & Morrissey, 1986). Because of the large volume of people who are processed into jails, they could be considered the most important institutions in the criminal justice system; however, they are among the most neglected aspects of the system (Nielsen, 1979).

HISTORICAL OVERVIEW

In the mid-nineteenth century, Dorothea Dix began her crusade to remove the mentally ill from jails and house them in mental institutions. From 1841 until the late 1880s, many mental hospitals throughout the United States and abroad were built at the instigation of Dix. The mentally ill were removed from penal facilities and almshouses and housed in state hospitals (Deutsch, 1949). The mental health and jail systems did not intersect frequently until almost 30 years later when court clinics in New York and Boston were created to assist the court in determining the most appropriate disposition for specified inmates (Petrich, 1978).

Mental health professionals before the mid 1960s did not give much thought to working with jail systems. Beginning with the deinstitutionalization of mental hospitals in the late 1960s and continuing today, large numbers of people have been discharged from mental hospitals into the community without the necessary programs for treatment, adequate housing, income, vocational training, and family involvement (Report of the Federal Task Force on Homelessness and Severe Mental Illness, 1992). Many of these individuals became homeless and subsequently were charged with petty as well as felonious crimes. Therefore the mentally ill residing in jails reached greater proportions in the 1970s than previously, which continues into the 1990s. In 1983, Cohen lamented, "irresponsible deinstitutionalization" had forced county and local jails into becoming mental hospitals, thereby "returning care of the mentally ill to the deplorable conditions that prevailed more than 300 years ago" (Goldsmith, 1983).

In addition, commitment laws became more stringent as a result of a patients' rights movement (Pogrebin & Poole, 1987; Teplin, 1984). The police found themselves in a quandary when considering an arrest of a mentally ill homeless person, especially if making an arrest was less onerous than waiting in an emergency room, possibly for long periods of time, for commitment of the individual (Teplin, 1984). If the person is taken to the emergency room and does not meet commitment standards, the individual must be released. Police are under pressure to return to their service areas expeditiously. Thus police are then faced with the dilemma of finding an environment safer than the street, which is in all likelihood the jail (Belcher, 1988). "Police have become the most utilized agencies for psychiatric referral in our society" (Pogrebin & Poole, 1987). Teplin stated on the Cable News Network (CNN) program

Mental Health System on the Verge of a Breakdown (1995), "I think for many types of severely mentally ill, the jail has become the dumping ground." One group of authors concerned about the problem asked, "Are jails and prisons the new asylums?" (Shenson, Dubler, & Michaels, 1990).

SCOPE OF THE PROBLEM

Schellenberg et al. (1992) reviewed studies conducted on the arrests of psychiatric clients. Their conclusions were that one half of psychiatric clients had been arrested, 1 in 13 clients every year are arrested after being admitted into mental health treatment, fewer than 20% are arrested for violent crimes, the homeless mentally ill are more likely to be arrested, and a diagnosis of substance abuse increases the probability of being arrested.

Lamb and Grant (1982) studied 102 male inmates referred to a Los Angeles County jail for psychiatric evaluation and found 90% had prior psychiatric hospitalizations and 80% prior arrest records. Of this group, 75% met the criteria for involuntary hospitalization. Using a stratified random sample, Teplin (1990b) studied 728 males, with one-half being charged with felonies and one-half charged with misdemeanors. The prevalence rates were then compared with general population information from the Epidemiologic Catchment Area program. The findings indicated that the prevalence rate of schizophrenia and major affective disorders was two to three times greater than that found in the general population (Teplin, 1990b).

Steadman, McCarty, and Morrissey (1986) reviewed six studies and found that the prevalence rate in local jails for the severely and persistently mentally ill ranged from 1% to 7% and for the nonpsychotic and personality disorders was as high as 20%. Citing one of the studies, they concluded that the prevalence rate was not different from the rate of "psychosis among class-matched community populations." However, considering the mental health care needs for this jail population versus the services available, the findings were sobering.

Lamb and Grant (1983) also studied 101 female inmates in an urban county jail referred for evaluation of psychiatric problems. They found that 85% had a history of psychiatric hospitalization and 94% had a previous criminal record. A majority (58%) of these women had severe and persistent mental illnesses.

Torrey et al. (1992) conducted a study of 1391 jails in the United States, representing 41% of all jails and 62% of the jail inmates. The findings indicated that 7.2% of the inmates were labeled as having a severe mental illness. One startling discovery was that 29% of the jails detain individuals with serious mental illnesses who do not have criminal charges against them. The conclusion was reached that these jails tended to be located in states that were rated as having poor mental health services. If the mentally ill person was charged with a crime, the most likely charges were assault and/or battery, theft, disorderly conduct, or drug and alcohol-related crimes.

Substance abuse

The greatest increase of inmates comes from drug law violators. During 1983, 1 of every 10 inmates was incarcerated in a jail for a drug offense, but in 1989 this number was 1 in 4. This growth accounts for more than 40% of the increase in the jail population (*Bureau of Justice Statistics Bulletin,* 1995).

A study of a randomly selected, stratified sample of 728 male inmates found that one half of the individuals were charged with misdemeanors and the other half with felonies. The findings indicated that substance use disorder rates were 29.1% for current use and 61.8% for a lifetime. Many of the subjects had a dual diagnosis: a substance abuse problem with an accompanying severe and persistent mental illness. Teplin (1994) wrote that the "number of jail detainees who will require treatment in the future—particularly for alcohol and drug abuse—is staggering."

Suicide

Data from 1993 indicate that illness followed by suicide were the leading causes of death in jails (*Bureau of Justice and Statistics Bulletin,* 1995). The rate of suicide is greater than in the general population, with the person communicating in a majority of the cases the intent to commit such action before the act. Usually the psychiatric illness is treatable (DuRand et al., 1995). Suicide was the second leading cause of death in local jails (36%), exceeded by illness (45%), during 1993. The rate of suicide declined from 129 per 100,000 in 1983 to 54 in 1993 (*Bureau of Justice Statistics Bulletin,* 1995).

DuRand et al. (1995) studied 37 suicides in a large urban jail over 25 years; all deaths were by hanging. Those individuals charged with the felonies murder, intent to murder, and manslaughter were 19 times more likely to commit suicide than those accused of other crimes. Many of these decedents had a prior history of attempting suicide. The authors maintain that attention to prevention of suicide is needed (DuRand et al., 1995).

Abuse by other inmates

Torrey et al. (1992) discovered that 40% of the jailed respondents to their questionnaire indicated that mentally ill inmates were abused by other inmates. This abuse included verbal as well as physical assaults and battery and sometimes rape.

ISSUES THAT NEED TO BE CONSIDERED BEFORE INTERVENTION
Mental health professionals

Compounding the problems of large numbers of clients being discharged from state hospitals with little thought to aftercare is most mental health professionals' lack of knowledge about how to negotiate with the legal system if a client is sent to jail. Working therapeutically with an individual suffering from a severe and persistent mental illness is difficult. When a criminal charge is added to the mental illness, some agencies and mental health professionals hesitate to be involved until charges are resolved (Ciccone & Barry, 1976).

The jail is part of the community, and mental health professionals should be aware that as caregivers they have responsibilities to have some knowledge of the criminal justice structure to make an impact on that system when a client is detained with charges. Many mental health centers or case management organizations have individuals specifically trained and designated to work with the local jails to assist the prosecution and the defense about the most appropriate evaluation and disposition of the detainee. Because many complaints are for petty crimes such as theft and shoplifting, judges frequently are willing to drop the charges if the mental health caregiver can provide a plan to assist the individual, especially if the person is homeless (Report of the Federal Task Force, 1992; Roth, 1986).

The jail experience

An individual who enters a local jail usually is faced with overcrowding, poor living conditions, violence among inmates, possible sexual exploitation, and isolation from a support system (Roth, 1986). One sheriff of a local jail remarked as to space availability, "We've been having to put up cots—army cots—and either put them in hallways or set them up in unused drunk tanks" (Margulies, 1995). Petrich (1976) commented that inmates who were violent or acted out in some manner were more likely to be referred for evaluation and services but the more reclusive and quiet inmates suffering from a mental health problem tended to be left unnoticed.

If a jail inmate is psychotic and adequate health care staff including a mental health caregiver are available, the individual is fortunate, but this is the exception rather than the rule. If the person is identified as having a mental health problem, the course of action is often to send the individual for a hospital or an outpatient evaluation, treat briefly, and then return to jail. Sometimes the appropriate

medication is provided, but instructions are not followed or the medication is not continued after discharge and the person returns to the psychotic state (Roth, 1986).

Competency to stand trial and defense of insanity

If the person is charged with a felony or a misdemeanor and has a behavioral problem, the question of competency to stand trial may arise. This issue must be resolved before proceeding with the charges, especially if the crime is a felony. The query concerns the person's current mental condition plus the following questions: Does the defendant understand the charges? Can the defendant appropriately advise counsel? Does the defendant understand the consequence of those charges? An evaluation is conducted by a mental health professional trained to perform these assessments at an inpatient facility, the jail, or an outpatient facility of private mental health practice (Laben & MacLean, 1989). If the person currently is incompetent to stand trial, the mental health provider tries to assist the individual to become competent so that the charges can be moved expeditiously through the court system. To guarantee a fair proceeding, the defendant's counsel and the prosecuting attorney have an obligation to ensure that the person is competent to stand trial. Mental health professionals, including advanced practice nurses in at least one state (Tennessee), can testify to the person's competency to stand trial.

The insanity defense (criminal responsibility) relates to the defendant's mental condition at the time of the commission of the crime. Usually a psychologist or psychiatrist testifies to these issues. The admission of a nurse's testimony depends on each state's requirement about the qualifications needed for a mental health professional to testify about the insanity defense. In some states, guilty but mentally ill is a plea that can be set forth by the defendant. In this situation the person is found guilty but is sent to prison and treated for the mental health condition.

Problems caused by the mentally ill in jail

In Torrey et al.'s (1992) study, the responders were asked about problems the mentally ill caused the jail personnel. One of the issues identified was refusal of medication; 12% said it was a big problem, 48.8% said it was a small problem, and 34.1% said it was not a problem. Health care providers who filled out the survey were more likely to identify medication refusal as an issue.

Outpatient treatment following release from jail

Another factor evaluated by Torrey et al. (1992) was the frequency of mental health treatment after release from jail. Results could not be stated with certainty because many of the respondents did not have knowledge if services were received, but projections from the data indicated that 35.7% did not receive some kind of follow-up. Only 54% of the respondents indicated an estimate of the percentage who received treatment. The majority of the jails commented that more inmates with serious mental illness were being seen now than 10 years ago.

RECOMMENDATIONS FOR INTERVENTIONS

Teplin (1990a) pointed out that interventions with the mentally disordered individual have always been an aspect of police work; however, this role has expanded in recent years. In her evaluation of this situation, Teplin pointed out that disposition of a mentally disordered individual who is causing some kind of "trouble" in the community is greatly influenced by the presence of and successful liaison with local mental health facilities. She recommended that mental health systems and the police work together in cooperative programs, commenting, "police departments must accept their role as street corner psychiatrists" (Teplin, 1990a).

Steadman et al. (1986) have written extensively about jail and early intervention programs. The following are their recommendations. The issue of a mentally ill jail inmate is a community systems issue. Because traditionally mentally ill individuals do not spend long periods of time in jail except in unusual circumstances, developing comprehensive mental health services within the jail itself is not feasible or practical. Other agencies, including community mental health centers, state mental hospitals, psychiatric units of general hospitals, and other community resources, should be used (Steadman et al., 1986).

Steadman et al. (1986) recommend that when the problem of the mentally ill in the criminal justice system presents itself in the community, key providers convene a meeting to work on these issues. Before convening or at initial meetings, providers need to identify problems, including what services are currently available and the costs of these services. Records of the number of services currently provided in the community and what individuals are involved are key information in planning future programs.

Confidential mental health form

When the numbers of the mentally ill in the jail caused a significant problem in Nashville, Tennessee, in 1992, a Mental Health–Criminal Justice Coordinating Committee was convened by a General Sessions Judge. Representatives from the city-county government, including the police department, prosecutor's and public defender's offices, local mental health centers, organizations responsible for case management in the city, state hospital and developmental centers, and the local mental health association, met to problem solve and work on systems problems.

The Confidential Mental Health Information form (Figure 26-1) was developed by a subcommittee of the Mental Health–Criminal Justice Coordinating Committee chaired by a psychiatric-mental health advanced practice nurse. It was implemented in 1993. The form was designed to be used by criminal justice personnel, commencing with the police department at the time of arrest, followed by judges, court commissions, pretrial diversion, and jail intake, to evaluate the defendant. The original idea was that each person in the

NAME			**DATE**		**ATN#**	
DOB / /	**SEX**	**RACE**		**CELL LOCATION**		**S.S.#**
CMHC		**CASEWORKER**			**PHONE**	
PRIOR DIAGNOSIS				**MEDICATION**		

				DATE TIME
POLICE	Inappropriate			
	Behavior (laughter, unresponsive, rambling, disconnected thoughts) . . . . . Yes	No		_____
	Dress, demeanor, hygiene . . . . Yes	No		_____
	Eye contact or attention span . . . . Yes	No		_____
	Evidence of drugs or alcohol . . . . Yes	No		_____
	Witnesses revealed knowledge of mental illness . . . . Yes	No		_____
	Known to police as mentally ill . . . . Yes	No		_____
	Evidence defendant is taking prescribed medication . . . . Yes	No		_____
	Case Management notified at _____ . . . . Yes	No		**OFFICER**

				DATE TIME
COURT	Inappropriate			
	Behavior (laughter, unresponsive, rambling, disconnected thoughts) . . . . . Yes	No		_____
	Dress, demeanor, hygiene . . . . Yes	No		_____
	Eye contact or attention span . . . . Yes	No		_____
	Evidence of drugs or alcohol . . . . Yes	No		_____
	Witnesses revealed knowledge of mental illness . . . . Yes	No		_____
	Known to police as mentally ill . . . . Yes	No		_____
	Evidence defendant is taking prescribed medication . . . . Yes	No		_____
	Case Management notified at _____ . . . . Yes	No		**COMMISSIONER**

				DATE TIME
PRETRIAL	Inmate is threatening to hurt self or others . . . . Yes	No		_____
	Inmate exhibits following behaviors:			_____
	Mute or unresponsive . . . . Yes	No		_____
	Crying . . . . Yes	No		_____
	Inappropriate laughter . . . . Yes	No		_____
	Body tics or jerky movements . . . . Yes	No		_____
	Claims to be hearing voices, is acting grandiose or paranoid . . . . Yes	No		_____
	Rambling, disconnected thoughts or speech patterns . . . . Yes	No		_____
	Drug or alcohol intoxication . . . . Yes	No		_____
	Requesting to see a doctor or psychiatrist . . . . Yes	No		_____
	Case Management notified at _____ . . . . Yes	No		**INTERVIEWER**

				DATE TIME
JAIL INTAKE	Inquiries			
	Presently on medication . . . . Yes	No		_____
	Any allergies to medication . . . . Yes	No		_____
	Do you have seizures . . . . Yes	No		_____
	Any medical or dental problems . . . . Yes	No		_____
	Ever been hospitalized or treated for mental problems . . . . Yes	No		_____
	Ever had TB, hepatitis, or any other communicable disease . . . . Yes	No		_____
	Do you use alcohol or drugs . . . . Yes	No		_____
	Are you pregnant or have you recently given birth . . . . Yes	No		_____
	Observations			_____
	Alert, oriented to time, place, person . . . . Yes	No		_____
	Free of injuries, jaundice, rashes or lice . . . . Yes	No		_____
	Obvious indications of drug abuse . . . . Yes	No		_____
	Obvious deformities or handicaps . . . . Yes	No		_____
	Disposition			_____
	Refer to medical staff . . . . Yes	No		_____
	Place in general population . . . . Yes	No		**INTERVIEWER**

				DATE TIME
PSYCH INTAKE	Known to Psych Services from previous arrests . . . . Yes	No		_____
	History of hospitalization or mental health treatment . . . . Yes	No		_____
	Inmate is threatening violence to others . . . . Yes	No		_____
	Inmate is threatening suicide or self injury . . . . Yes	No		_____
	Mental Health Survey completed . . . . Yes	No		_____
	Inmate considered mentally ill . . . . Yes	No		_____
	Previous diagnosis known to inmate . . . . Yes	No		_____
	Need for medication established and verified . . . . Yes	No		_____
	Drug/alcohol complications . . . . Yes	No		_____
	Inmate referred to Medical Services for assessment . . . . Yes	No		_____
	Assessment completed . . . . Yes	No		_____
	Meets criteria for T.C.A. 33-6-103 . . . . Yes	No		_____
	Medication prescribed . . . . Yes	No		_____
	Caseworker contacted . . . . Yes	No		**INTERVIEWER**

RELEASE	I give permission for the Davidson County Sheriff's Department to release a copy of this interview to the Office of Metropolitan Public Defender of Davidson County	**SIGNATURE** _____
		DATE _____

Figure 26-1. Confidential Mental Health Information form.
(Courtesy Davidson County, Tennessee, Mental Health–Criminal Justice Coordinating Committee, Joyce K. Laben, Chair, Form Subcommittee.)

criminal justice process has a unique perspective that aids in developing an assessment of the defendant.

From the outset, problems were encountered in gaining the cooperation of certain participants in the criminal justice system. Police and Night Court Commissioners, already inundated with paperwork, were loathe to add an additional piece of paper. Pretrial release, a fairly autonomous group in the criminal justice process, failed to use the forms. Despite the lack of cooperation from these departments the form was adopted by the Davidson County Sheriff's Department as its mental health screening form, and currently every person entering the jail is screened using this instrument. What information is not available in the early screening is offset by the consistency of receiving a form on every individual entering the jail system.

Out of an average of 1500 inmates a month who enter the jail in Davidson County, approximately 200 (13%) indicate some type of mental illness on the screening form. Of that number, 50 inmates a year, or an average of 4 a month, are referred to the mental health cooperative (MHC), the case management organization for the city and county. The referral number was much higher in the early days of use of the screening form. The MHC, which was organized around the same time, began to assign large numbers of inmates with mental health problems to case managers. As more people acquired a case manager, referrals decreased and contact with case managers increased.

Each morning a list is faxed to the MHC of those individuals who indicate mental illness on the screening form. A staff person at the MHC reviews this list for consumers under the care of the MHC and alerts the appropriate case manager. The case manager has the responsibility to call the mental health workers at the jail or in the public defender's office to assess the situation and facilitate the consumer's receiving prescribed medications and support. Beyond meeting the immediate needs of the consumer, the mental health providers involved in the criminal justice process work with the case managers to reach an appropriate resolution of the criminal case. Case managed consumers make up about 20% of the people who indicate mental illness on the screening form.

In those few cases when the defendant is actively psychotic and presents a danger to self and others, the crisis team of the MHC is contacted and the individual is assessed for involuntary committal. An average of one person a week is involuntarily committed to the regional mental hospital.

Of the 200 defendants a month identified by the screening form as mentally ill, 5 (2.5%) are referred for an evaluation of competency to stand trial or defense of insanity. This process is used only for serious felony cases, misdemeanors involving persistent violence, and individuals who are seriously psychotic and refuse to cooperate with any treatment in the jail.

The Confidential Mental Health Information form serves as a wide net that alerts jail personnel to the possibility of mental illness. Because the information gathered depends on a defendant's self-reporting to the screener, an unwilling individual who fails to reveal past mental health treatment may pass through the initial screening process unidentified. Many of these individuals are detected elsewhere in the system by case workers or attorneys working with the defendants.

Likewise, a significant percentage of people (75%) who identify some past treatment are not currently in need of any mental health assistance or they are not in the system long enough to warrant or allow any significant intervention. About 25% of those people first identified through the form receive some type of treatment, medication, referral, or evaluation.

Screening

Screening, as mentioned in the Nashville, Tennessee, project, is imperative in the jail setting. In Denver, Colorado, a full-time psychiatric nurse evaluates and screens incoming inmates for signs of mental illness. Based on the recommendation of the nurse, diversions out of the jail can be initiated and half of those received are diverted out. A key staff person in a jail is essential to appropriate diversion (Jemelka, 1990). In addition, use of a screening tool when suicide is expected is very helpful. New York State has developed screening guidelines for suicide prevention (Cox, Landsberg, & Paravati, 1989).

A court program developed in California has demonstrated that 58% of 56 mentally ill defendants charged with misdemeanors who were judicially ordered to receive monitored mental health treatment had a good 1-year outcome, including no subsequent commission of crimes or psychiatric hospitalizations. A psychologist consulted with the court about individuals referred by the defense attorney. A treatment plan was developed for the individual with the approval of the court for diversion follow-up. Lamb, Weinberger, and Reston-Parham (1996) think this was an appropriate function of the criminal justice system and that the judge monitoring the ongoing treatment process thereby reduced the mentally ill offender's "potential to commit other offenses."

The jail

Federal, state, and national guidelines for treatment of the mentally ill in jails should be explored. Jemelka (1990) stated that at least 35 sets of standards concerning the recommended care for the mentally ill in the jails exist. The American Nurses Association (1985) has developed standards for correctional institutions. If any jails are under court order in the state, these guidelines should be examined. Judges must become knowledgeable about mental health services and the problems that are associated with confinement of the mentally ill in jails. The National Commission on Correctional Health Care has developed standards for health services, including mental health services. Minimum staffing requirements are included along with guidelines for mental health care. They specifically state that, "Inmates found to be suffering from serious mental illness or developmental disability are immediately referred for care" (National Commission on Correctional Health Care, 1992). This care can be provided in a mental health facility or a treatment setting within the jail. Because large numbers of people with mental health problems have been detained within the past few years, large jails have developed special units for placement of these individuals. Steadman et al. (1986) do not recommend this strategy except for megajails. One jail in Alexandria, Virginia, has developed a 27-bed critical care mental health unit staffed by "special management deputies" with mental health training. The classification and mental health staff select the occupants for this unit, but the inmate must consent to taking medications. Individual and group therapy and aftercare planning are provided (Fortin, 1993).

One essential standard states written policies and procedures would be in existence relative to assisting inmates who are withdrawing from alcohol or drugs. Observation should be conducted by qualified health professionals. Qualified health professionals include mental health professionals and nurses (National Commission on Correctional Health Care, 1992).

A major point highlighted by the Steadman group (1986) is that jails are correctional facilities and should not be thought of as alternative mental health institutions. Jails are not the appropriate placement for the mentally ill, and caution should be used in developing too wide an array of programs in a jail setting. They recommend, however, that limited quality services be provided within the jail system. The numbers of staff available should relate to the numbers of inmates and the incidence of mental illness. Qualified mental health personnel, which may include nurses, should screen for serious mental illness within 14 calendar days of admission. When appropriate, referral should be immediate (National Commission on Correctional Health Care, 1992).

When providing treatment, courts have asserted that mental health care should be held to the same standard as physical health care. In a

Federal Court of Appeals decision arising out of a prison in Virginia, the court wrote, "We see no underlying distinction between the right to medical care for physical ills and its psychological or psychiatric counterpart. Modern science has rejected the notion that mental or emotional disturbances are the products of afflicted souls, hence beyond the purview of counseling, medication and therapy" (*Bowring v. Godwin,* 1977). Although this decision involved a state prison, a case involving a local jail used the *Bowring* decision as support for its reasoning that mental health care should be kept at the same standard as physical care (*Inmates of the Allegheny County Jail v. Pierce,* 1980). In the United States Supreme Court decision *Estelle v. Gamble* (1976) the court ruled that a Texas prison system was obligated to "provide medical care for those whom it is punishing by incarceration." However, one group of authors states that "Jails which gather the retarded and mentally ill and sequester them without care are clearly beyond the bounds of this requirement," that is, case law involving state facilities may not apply or be complied with in local settings (Shenson et al., 1990).

At the least, early identification, crisis intervention, and case management after discharge should be instituted in each jail. Ideally the early identification would begin when the police officer initially has contact with the detainee. If the police officer does not identify the person as needing assistance at the booking or intake, screening should be accomplished within 72 hours. The public defender's office also can assist in noting individuals to be evaluated. Appointments should not be delayed for evaluation. Many times, however, mental health professionals come to the jails for limited amounts of time during the week. Currently, with the use of more advanced nurse practitioners, especially mental health nurse practitioners with prescriptive privileges, jails could hire on a limited or full-time basis these professionals who could quickly intervene when appropriate. The psychiatrist should be used for consultation or intervention with complex cases.

Collaboration with other providers in the community, especially if the charges are dropped, is imperative so that the person does not get into difficulty upon discharge. Assigning a community case manager when available is an appropriate and usually cost-effective mechanism.

Steadman et al. (1986) emphasized that if the core services are offered and the jail "makes no pretense about its intent or ability to treat the mentally ill, judges may be less inclined to send a disturbed individual to jail for the sole purpose of receiving specialized care." No one "cookbook" approach indicates the best program to implement. Each city or region has to identify the need and explore funding sources and other resources available. Some rural areas have developed regional programs (Steadman et al., 1986).

Dvoskin (1990) suggested the following service components for a jail: some form of mental health evaluation that is built on the screening, referral for competency to stand trial when appropriate, psychotropic medication when necessary and administered safely, substance abuse counseling and referral upon release, short-term supportive therapy if deemed necessary to enable the inmate to endure the jail experience, referral for hospitalization when deemed essential, and case management after release. Other services that he recommended include suicide prevention programs, special housing options for those whose mental status makes them vulnerable to harm either self-inflicted or imposed by others, and consultation and training for the correction staff (Dvoskin, 1990).

Effective postrelease plans for an inmate should begin as soon as possible after the inmate is identified as having a mental health problem. Ideally the inmate should be linked to an aftercare provider while in the jail. A supply of medication should be provided on release along with instructions about the plan of care to be followed in the community. Case management is very desirable when possible (Griffin, 1990).

In a more recent study, Steadman, Barbera, and Dennis (1994) conducted a national survey to determine the numbers of diversion programs for the mentally ill in this country. A mailing was sent to 1263 jails with a census of 50 or more. The final data response was 685 from 1106 eligible jails for a total of a 65% return rate. Telephone interviews with a sample of the respondents also were completed. The following definition was used to determine if a program exists (Steadman et al., 1994):

Programs that screen defined groups of detainees for the presence of mental disorder; use mental health professionals to evaluate all those detainees identified in the screening; and negotiate with prosecutors, defense attorneys, community-based mental health providers, and the courts to produce a mental health disposition outside the jail in lieu of prosecution or as a condition of a reduction in charges.

Added later to the definition was the phrase "that focused all or in part, on the reduction of pretrial jail time" (Steadman et al., 1994). The findings indicated that only 52 jail diversion programs meeting the criteria were currently in existence in this country. The majority of these programs were funded through mental health agencies using county and state funds. Detainees with misdemeanor charges and some who were charged with nonviolent as well as violent crimes were served. Programs that dealt with smaller jails were more willing to serve the violent and nonviolent individual with felony charges. Steadman et al. (1994) stressed that systematic evaluation must take place to determine which programs are successful with which clientele.

In one recently reported study conducted in Portland, Oregon, 47 homeless mentally ill offenders were accepted into a program that provided housing in a single room occupancy hotel. Of the original 47, 38 individuals entered the program, and 14 of these graduated into community housing and were maintaining sobriety. The program resources included active intensive case management, mental health treatment, substance abuse intervention, and supervised housing. Referrals came from county jail or correctional staff in the community and jail. If the individuals resided in the jail, they were seen before release.

The outcomes were evaluated by the number of hospitalizations at the state hospital or incarcerations in the county jail 18 months before instigation of the program and 18 months afterward. The outcomes indicated no statistical difference in before and after use of the state hospital. Researchers noted that many of the clients had not used the state mental hospital in the time before the project. Hospital use, however, increased after the program began at the county jail. If the person was returned to the county jail, the most common offense was violent behavior at the hotel. The authors pointed out that implementing such a project is complicated and that perhaps an intermediate facility should have been developed to assist the clients in managing substance abuse problems. Dangerousness was indicated to be a major issue. The advice of the authors is that "substantial resources" should be allocated before devising a system along with agreement on a treatment philosophy, especially about whether abstinence from alcohol and drugs is to be a criterion or an ideal goal to attain (McFarland & Blair, 1995).

MODEL PROGRAMS

Lucas County (Ohio) Jail Mental Health Project

The Lucas County (Toledo, Ohio) Jail Mental Health Project has several components. If the police detain an individual suspected of having a mental illness and the crime is a misdemeanor, the Rescue Crisis, a community mental health agency, consults and if possible diverts the individual from the criminal justice system (L. A. Ventura, personal communication, October 11, 1995).

If an individual is booked, a medical screening is conducted, including questions related to mental health issues and possible suicidal ideation. Counselors are cross trained as social workers and as deputies; if an immediate intervention is required, it can immediately be implemented. The deputy/social worker can write the application for involuntary commitment if indicated. If this action is not considered necessary, the person can be placed in a special needs unit. A person detained longer than 72 hours has a psychosocial assessment completed with appropriate referrals.

When indicated, mental health services are provided to inmates in the detention center by community mental health centers in partnership with the Lucas County Mental Health Board. The community mental health center team has an office in the Lucas County Corrections Center. Someone is on site at least 6 hours per day during the work week. The mental health provider can refer to the psychiatrist for medication evaluation or follow-up for case management. If case managers are involved, they work closely with the counselors in the jail to coordinate care. The case manager is responsible for reentry plans into the community.

If a person has a substance abuse problem, services are available. A program called *AIM HIGH* provides outreach workers who come into the correctional facility to provide such services as promoting socialization, independent living, and employment readiness skills. All volunteers are former mental health clients.

A study was conducted by the Director of Inmate Services and a clinical psychologist. The hypothesis was if case management and other community mental health services were used, jail recidivism would be reduced. They reviewed the histories of 261 individuals who were diagnosed with a mental disorder. A 3-year follow-up after release from jail was conducted. The factors that proved significant were number of former arrests, age, receptivity to case management in the community, and employment history. In addition, they found that recidivism rates were lower for those who were involved in jail-based case management and subsequently linked to community-based case management (Ventura & Cassel, 1994). These results testify to the importance of intervention as quickly as possible when the person enters a criminal justice system and community follow-up after release.

Henrico County (Virginia) Jail

In Richmond, Virginia, the Henrico County Jail has a collaborative program with mental health professionals, and they work together on mental health and substance abuse issues. A unique substance abuse day treatment program has been established. This treatment initiative is essentially run and managed by inmates. Basic rules and an emphasis on feelings and setting goals guide the program. During weekly group meetings, discussions related to the community, stress management, anger control, and family negotiations take place. Social skills and relapse prevention also are included. In the evening, Alcoholics Anonymous and Narcotics Anonymous gatherings take place. Organization is built around the more senior members, who are considered to have wisdom to share with the community. These senior members participate with staff in interviewing applicants for the program. Both pretrial inmates and those serving sentences can participate in the undertaking (B. Hinkle, personal communication, October 24, 1995). The innovative aspect of this program is primary management by the inmates with staff serving as consultants.

King County, Seattle, Washington

In Seattle, Washington, the King County Mental Health Division, Department of Adult Detention, Division of Alcohol and Substance Abuse Services, Seattle Police Department, and Seattle prosecutor's office have banded together to plan a program for persons with severe and persistent mental illnesses and substance abuse problems who become involved in the criminal justice system. One major goal is to divert those individuals who have mental health problems and are charged with a misdemeanor to alternative programs. Interestingly, in 1994, 59% of the mentally ill who came through the system were transients living on the streets or in cars. One unique aspect of this program is that an assertive effort is exerted to work with individuals who initially reject services. A primary objective is to continue to work with people who initially reject help so that they are ultimately provided mental health services and do not enter the criminal justice system by default because of mental health treatment refusal.

Short stay diversion beds are available, including some for persons with dual diagnoses of mental illness and substance abuse. The Associate Director of Services for the King County Department of Adult Detention writes that "creating diversion programs has resulted in a culture of diversion" (Coleman, 1995). Emphasis is placed on collaboration with all systems involved. A study conducted in 1991 indicated that offenders with mental illness spent three times longer in jail than others in the study population (Coleman, 1995).

New York State suicide prevention program

In the 1970s and 1980s the suicide rate in jail populations was three to nine times higher than the general population (Cox et al., 1989). Because of these statistics and a generally inadequate response to this problem, the New York State Office of Mental Health and the New York State Commission of Correction collaborated with one of the county mental health services, the New York State Division of Criminal Justice Services, and a statewide advisory group to explore these issues. As a result of this strategy to evaluate the problem and develop strategies for interventions, a suicide prevention crisis service model was developed. Included were policy and procedural guidelines for county jails, police lockups, and mental health caregivers. Not only administrative actions but also direct service interventions are provided; therefore staff can screen and intervene appropriately with high-risk mentally ill and suicidal inmates.

Suicide prevention intake screening guidelines that can be used by correctional officers also were developed. An 8-hour training program on suicide and suicide prevention was instituted for jail and lockup officers. In addition, a mental health practitioner's manual was written to provide staff in the jails information related to the problem.

A strong emphasis is placed on interagency communication so that mental health providers, medical staff, the courts, defense attorney, prosecutors, and other correctional agencies are aware of problems of various inmates. Another important aspect of the program is a formal investigation if a suicide does occur to establish corrective action. An independent state commission performs this service (Cox et al., 1989).

Community model for services

The community model for services (Figure 26-2) indicates methods for preventing incarceration of the mentally ill and intervening effectively when an individual is jailed. Formation of a community board to evaluate the problem of the city's or county's mentally ill offender can be effective.

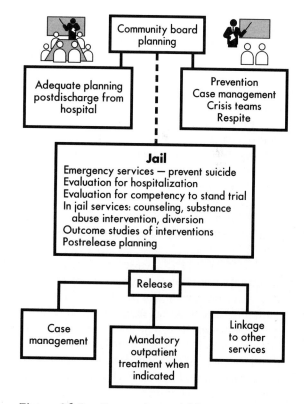

Figure 26-2. Community model for services.

Implementation of prevention and follow-up programs can lead to less time spent in jail. Collaboration of members of the mental health and criminal justice systems as well as the various other social agencies is imperative.

THE ROLE OF THE NURSE

In the process of preparing this chapter and talking with participants in various programs around the country, the authors have noted that psychiatric nurses have not been actively involved in the treatment of the mentally ill in the jail system. Although nurses may be involved in administering medications, possibly screening for mental illness, and providing for the physical care needs of inmates, they did not have active roles in the creative programs that are described here. Reader and Melman (1991) wrote that nurses involved with the mentally ill offender are a "novelty." What can be done to modify this situation?

Schools of nursing

When possible, nursing faculty should be encouraged to provide clinical experiences in the local jails, community mental health centers, outpatient clinics, and homeless shelters. Exposing nursing students to the mentally ill who come in contact with the criminal justice system can demonstrate the rewards that can come from caring for such individuals. Graduate students in psychiatric-mental health nursing should have some contact with such individuals and their problems.

Hospital-based nurses

Mental health nurses working in inpatient facilities can work with members of the health care team to ensure adequate aftercare for individuals being discharged into the community. This would include referral for case management services when indicated. If the individual is to be returned to the jail for resolution of charges, the nurse should ensure that ordered psychotropic medication is continued. Communication with jail personnel is essential.

Community-based nurses

Mental health nurses who work in the community usually are actively involved in case management of their clients. Prevention of criminal charges and subsequent incarceration, especially for minor charges, should be a high-priority goal of the case manager. Encouraging local organizations to provide crisis intervention, respite, and other emergency services is essential to prevent incarceration. Evaluating the financial as well as the housing needs of the client is important. If the clients are actively involved with families, support for those families is imperative, especially if the mentally ill client has a history of difficulty with the criminal justice system.

If the client is incarcerated in a local jail, the nurse should make every effort to contact the nurse in the jail or the personnel who can ensure that the client continues to receive prescribed medication. Communicating to jail personnel or the public defender that a mental health professional in the community is actively following the client can possibly lead to early diversion into the community or appropriate care while in jail. Actively following the client after the jail experience is necessary. Working with the client's family can be most helpful, especially if the family has to obtain a restraining order for assaultive behavior (Solomon & Draine, 1995).

Becoming knowledgeable about the local jail and the kind of treatment provided for the mentally ill should be a high priority for nurses working in the mental health system. Serving on community committees and boards that make recommendations for care of the mentally ill offender in the jail can be most helpful. Nurses who do participate in such activities should be aware of standards of care developed by various organizations, including the American Nurses Association.

Nurses in the jails

"Professional nurses working in corrections are pioneers; they are few in numbers and they rarely publish" (Peternelj-Taylor & Johnson, 1995). The authors of this quotation point out that nurses who work in the correctional systems have been stigmatized and made to feel like a "second class nurse." In addition to this label, nurses working in corrections have been stigmatized by the myth that nurses who worked within a correctional system did so only because they were unsuccessful in gaining employment in other settings (Peternelj-Taylor & Johnson, 1995). In actuality, nurses working in correctional settings, especially jails, must have a sense of self and be able to balance the requirements of security with the values of nursing. Stevens (1993) noted that nurses can have an impact in jails, especially those that do not have a health program or health care staff.

The nurse must not only be able to work with the mentally ill inmate but also deal with the complications of an overlying personality disorder, including possible antisocial traits that the individual exhibits. Being able to assess and treat or refer for treatment the person with dual diagnoses is challenging in the community but can be a daunting experience in the jail (Peternelj-Taylor & Johnson, 1995). Because of the high percentage of substance-abusing inmates, nurses must be very knowledgeable in this area.

Depending on the resources available and the ability to refer to other agencies, nurses working with individuals with mental health problems in jails should be able to provide crisis intervention, initial screening, monitoring of medication, and, with the appropriate education and experience, therapeutic interventions. Inmates have greater anxiety because charges may not be resolved, and fear of violence, especially sexual assault, is present. Overseeing a suicide prevention program, collaborating in team efforts, assisting the correctional officers in interventions to prevent and manage violent behavior, and developing and coordinating substance abuse programs are some of the services that nurses can provide.

Bernier (1986) comments that the ability to resolve disagreements among staff regarding appropriate interventions with inmates is important. Acting as role models to demonstrate to the inmates and staff how to negotiate the resolution of disputes is an important nursing activity. Helping staff members who are victims of assault to prevent such occurrences in the future and assisting them in processing what happened to victimize them in the past is another important duty for the nurse. Learning the legal terminology is imperative when talking with inmates, public defenders, and others in the criminal justice system.

Some problems encountered in working in a jail system can be overcome by networking with other nurses who work in corrections. Having consultation available from mental health consultants in the community can lessen the stress felt by nurses working in such a system. Another strategy is for nurses to negotiate an arrangement to come into a jail or prison and provide a specific service such as group therapy once a week. This strategy enables the nurse to offer expertise in a specific area but not on a full-time basis (Laben, Dodd, & Sneed, 1991; Laben, Sneed, & Seidel, 1995).

Advanced practice psychiatric and mental health nurses with prescriptive authority can be an asset within a jail. Most jails have visitation from a psychiatrist on a limited basis. A nurse who could provide assessment and prescription for psychotropic medications and work collaboratively with a psychiatrist could provide a timely service.

Nursing research

Although research was considered a low priority with nurses working in forensic areas (Niskala, 1986), studies such as those conducted by Morrison (1991) are important to add to the knowledge base of not only nurses but also other professionals. A study was conducted to ascertain the experience of mentally ill inmates in correctional facilities. Although the mentally ill themselves were not interviewed, 13 subjects in a halfway house were interviewed for their perceptions of mentally ill inmates and the way they responded to pressures. As a conclusion to this study,

Morrison (1991) writes, "Health care professionals, particularly mental health professionals, need to be proactive in establishing programs at all levels to provide mental health services to those in need within the prison system."

In his study on jailed mothers, Osborne (1995) emphasized the importance of mental health and maternal-child nurses being employed in prisons as a result of more women being incarcerated. Some of his recommendations could be implemented in a jail setting, especially in jails that house pregnant inmates. Drawing the detainee's attention to the importance of prenatal care could be an important intervention (Osborne, 1995). Both studies described have implications for the practice of nurses in correctional settings.

Diversion or after jail programs

A program has been developed in Milwaukee that attempts to divert the mentally ill from the jail and provides follow-up for those being released from jail. Services include medical and therapeutic services including medication administration and monitoring 5 days a week. Three full-time nurses provide psychological support and when necessary referral to medical services for physical health problems. Other services provided are money management, housing, and daily monitoring of clients in the clinic. For those resistive to treatment, having to comply with legal directives for treatment was felt to be effective (McDonald & Teitelbaum, 1994).

SUMMARY

This chapter discussed the current problems of the mentally ill in jail. The downsizing of mental hospitals and the confinement of some of the mentally ill to jails have led to an outcry. Some model programs have been described and the potential for nurse involvement has been delineated. Opportunities are available for nurses to take an active role in the provision of services for this very needy population.

REFERENCES

American Nurses Association. (1985). *Standards of nursing practice in correctional facilities*. Kansas City, MO: Author.

Belcher, J. R. (1988). Are jails replacing the mental health system for the homeless mentally ill? *Community Mental Health Journal, 24*(3), 185-195.

Bernier, S. L. (1986). Corrections and mental health. *Journal of Psychosocial Nursing and Mental Health Services, 23*(6), 20-25.

Blum, J., Fleming, W., & Laben, J. K. (1993). Confidential Mental Health Information Form. Nashville: Mental Health-Criminal Justice Coordinating Committee.

Bowring v. Godwin, 551 F2d 44, 4th Cir. (1977).

Bureau of Justice Statistics Bulletin. (1995, April). Washington, DC: U.S. Department of Justice Programs.

Ciccone, J. R., & Barry, D. J. (1976). Collaboration between psychiatry and the law: A study of 100 referrals to a court clinic. *Bulletin of the American Academy of Psychiatry and the Law, 4*(3), 275-280.

Coleman, R. (1995). *A choice of diversion or jail for persons with mental illness*. Seattle: King County Department of Adult Detention.

Cox, J. F., Landsberg, G., & Paravati, M. P. (1989). The essential components of a crisis intervention program for jails? The New York local forensic suicide prevention crisis service model. *Psychiatric Quarterly, 60*(2), 103-118.

Deutsch, A. (1949). *The mentally ill in America*. New York: Columbia University Press.

DuRand, C. J., Burtka, M. S., Federman, E. J., Haycox, J. A., & Smith, J. W. (1995). A quarter century of suicide in a major urban jail: Implications for community psychiatry. *American Journal of Psychiatry, 152*(7), 1077-1080.

Dvoskin, J. (1990). Jail-based mental health services. In H. J. Steadman (Ed.), *Jail diversion for the mentally ill: Breaking through the barriers* (pp. 64-90). The National Coalition for the Mentally Ill in the Criminal Justice System.

Estelle v. Gamble, 429 U.S. 97 (1976).

Fortin, C. (1993, October). Jail provides mental health and substance abuse services. *Corrections Today*, pp. 104-105.

Goldsmith, M. F. (1983). From mental hospitals to jail: The pendulum swings. *Medical News, 250*(22), 3017-3018.

Griffin, P. A. (1990). The back door of the jail: Linking mentally ill offenders to community mental health services. In H. J. Steadman (Ed.), *Jail diversion for the mentally ill: Breaking through the barriers* (pp. 91-107). The National Coalition for the Mentally Ill in the Criminal Justice System.

Inmates of the Allegheny County Jail v. Pierce, 487 F.Supp. 638 (1980).

Jemelka, R. (1990). The mentally ill in local jails: Issues in admission and booking. In H. J. Steadman (Ed.), *Jail diversion for the mentally ill: Breaking through the barriers* (pp. 35-59). Seattle: The National Coalition for the Mentally Ill in the Criminal Justice System.

Laben, J. K., Dodd, D., & Sneed, L. (1991). King's Theory of Goal Attainment applied in group therapy for inpatient juvenile sexual offenders, maximum security state offenders, and community parolees, utilizing visual aids. *Issues in Mental Health Nursing, 12*(1), 51-64.

Laben, J. K., & MacLean, C. P. (1989). *Legal issues and guidelines for nurses who care for the mentally ill*. Owing Mills, MD: National Health Publishing.

Laben, J. K., Sneed, L. P., & Seidel, S. L. (1995). Goal attainment in short-term group settings: Clinical implications for practice. In M. A. Frey, & C. L. Sieloff (Eds.), *Advancing King's systems, frameworks, and theory of nursing* (pp. 261-277). Newbury Park, CA: Sage Publications.

Lamb, H. R., & Grant, R. W. (1982). The mentally ill in an urban county jail. *Archives of General Psychiatry, 39*(1), 17-22.

Lamb, H. R., & Grant, R. W. (1983). Mentally ill women in a county jail. *Archives of General Psychiatry, 40*(4), 363-368.

Lamb, H. R., Weinberger, L. E., & Reston-Parham, C. (1996). Court intervention to address the mental health needs of mentally ill offenders. *Psychiatric Services, 47*(3), 275-281.

Margulies, E. (1995, September 20). Jail space hard to come by. *The Tennessean, Wilson*, p. G2.

McDonald, D. C., & Teitelbaum, M. (1994). *Managing mentally ill offenders in the community: Milwaukee's community support program* (pp. 2-11). Washington, DC: U.S. Department of Justice, National Institute of Justice.

McFarland, B. J., & Blair, G. (1995). Delivering comprehensive services to homeless mentally ill offenders. *Psychiatric Services, 46*(2), 179-181.

Morrison, E. F. (1991). Victimization in prison: Implications for the mentally ill inmate and for health professionals. *Archives of Psychiatric Nursing, V*(1), 17-24.

National Commission on Correctional Health Care. (1992). *Standards for health services in jails*. Chicago: Author.

Nielsen, E. D. (1979). Community mental health services in the community jail. *Community Mental Health Journal, 15*(1), 27-32.

Niskala, H. (1986). Competencies and skills required by nurses working in forensic areas. *Western Journal of Nursing Research, 8*, 400-413.

Osborne, O. H. (1995). Jailed mothers: Further explorations in public sector nursing. *Journal of Psychosocial Nursing and Mental Health Services, 33*(8), 23-28.

Peternelj-Taylor, C. A., & Johnson, R. L. (1995). Serving time: Psychiatric mental health nursing in corrections. *Journal of Psychosocial Nursing and Mental Health Services, 33*(8), 12-19.

Petrich, J. (1976). Psychiatric treatment in jail: An experiment in health-care delivery. *Hospital and Community Psychiatry, 27*(6), 413-415.

Petrich, J. (1978). Metropolitan jail psychiatric clinic: A year's experience. *The Journal of Clinical Psychiatry, 3*, 191-195.

Pogrebin, M. R., & Poole, R. R. (1987, Spring). Deinstitutionalization and increased arrest rates among the mentally disordered. *Journal of Psychiatry and the Law, 15*, 117-127.

Reader, D., & Melman, L. (1991). Conceptualizing psychosocial nursing in the jail setting. *Journal of Psychosocial Nursing and Mental Health Services, 29*(8), 40-43.

Report of the Federal Task Force on Homelessness and Severe Mental Illness. (1992). *Outcasts on main street.* Washington, DC: Interagency Council on the Homeless.

Roth, L. (1986). Correctional psychiatry. In *Forensic psychology and psychiatry*. Philadelphia: F. A. Davis.

Schellenberg, E. G., Wasylenki, D., Webster, C. D. & Goering, P. (1992). A review of arrests among psychiatric patients. *International Journal of Law and Psychiatry, 15*(3), 251-264.

Shenson, D., Dubler, R., & Michaels, D. (1990). Jails and prisons: The new asylums? *American Journal of Public Health, 80*(6), 655-656.

Solomon, P., & Draine, J. (1995). Issues in serving the forensic client. *Social Work, 40*(1), 25-33.

Steadman, H. J. (1990). *Jail diversion for the mentally ill: Breaking through the barriers.* Seattle: The National Coalition for the Mentally Ill in the Criminal Justice System.

Steadman, H. J., Barbera, S. S., & Dennis, D. L. (1994). A national survey of jail diversion programs for mentally ill detainees. *Hospital and Community Psychiatry, 45* (11), 1109-1113.

Steadman, H. J., McCarty, D. W., & Morrissey, J. P. (1986). *Developing jail mental health services: Practice and principles.* Rockville, MD: Department of Health and Human Services.

Stevens, R. (1993). When your clients are in jail. *Nursing Forum, 28*(4), 5-8.

Teplin, L. (1984). *Mental health and criminal justice* (vol. 20, Sage Criminal Justice System Annuals). Newbury Park, CA: Sage Publications.

Teplin, L. (1990a). Policing the mentally ill: Styles, strategies and implications. In H. J. Steadman (Ed.), *Jail diversion for the mentally ill: Breaking through the barriers* (pp. 15, 26). Seattle: The National Coalition for the Mentally Ill in the Justice System.

Teplin, L. (1990b). The prevalence of severe mental disorder among male urban jail detainees: Comparison with the Epidemiologic Catchment Area Program. *American Journal of Public Health, 80* (6), 663-669.

Teplin, L. A. (1994). Psychiatric and substance abuse disorders among male urban jail detainees. *American Journal of Public Health, 84* (2), 290-293.

Teplin, L. A. (1995, August 27). Quoted in R. Griffiths (Executive Producer), *Mental health system on the verge of a breakdown.* Atlanta: CNN.

Torrey, E. F., Stieber, J., Ezekiel, J., Wolfe, M., Sharfstein, J., Noble, J. H., & Flynn, L. M. (1992). *Criminalizing the seriously mentally ill: The abuse of jails as mental hospitals.* Arlington, VA: A joint report of the National Alliance for the Mentally Ill and Public Citizens' Health Research Group.

Ventura, L. A., & Cassel, C. A. (1994, November 16-17). *The effects of case management of the 3 year criminal recidivism rate of mentally ill persons released from jail.* Presented at the Ohio Department of Mental Health's Research Result Briefing Conference: Knowledge for a New Era, Columbus, OH.

Chapter 27

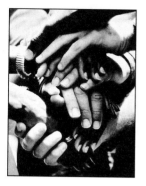

Elderly Persons with Mental Illness

Lore K. Wright

People age 65 and older are generally referred to as *elderly*. Currently, more than 32 million Americans, or 12.6% of the total population, belong to this age group. Although 95% of elderly people continue to live in the community, approximately 23% experience some health problems; 37% have difficulties managing activities of daily living; and 18% to 25% have significant behavioral, social, and mental disorders (Harper, 1991; U.S. Bureau of the Census, 1994).

Physical and emotional problems increase with advancing age, and one problem can precipitate or prolong another. For example, chronic pain often leads to depression, severe depression and social isolation lead to physical neglect and exacerbation of existing health problems, and depression impedes recovery from a variety of medical illnesses (Sadavoy, Lazarus, & Jarvik, 1991; Williamson & Schulz, 1992).

Thus that home health agencies report behavioral, emotional, and mental disorders in 50% to 70% of their clients is not surprising (Harper, 1991). Unfortunately, many home health agencies

and community-based programs do not provide specific mental health interventions; clients' physical problems are their major focus.

This chapter addresses two of the most common mental health problems encountered by community nurses: depression and the wide range of psychiatric disturbances associated with dementia (Wright & Stuart, 1995). Other psychiatric illnesses among community-residing elders are far less common. Active symptoms of schizophrenia and late-onset paranoid states occur in fewer than 0.5% of the population; approximately 4% of elders experience anxiety disorders (including panic, phobia, and obsessional and somatization disorders) (Gurland, 1991).

Although this chapter describes depression and dementia separately, some overlap between the two conditions exists. Elders with depression often have symptoms of memory impairment, and elders with dementia may simultaneously experience depression. In addition, family caregivers of elders with dementia, many of whom are themselves elderly, are at high risk for depression.

DEPRESSION

Epidemiology

The incidence of major depression among community-residing elders older than 65 years is between 2% and 4%. This rate increases to between 10% and 15% if general depressive symptoms, most often associated with bereavement and adjustment disorders, are included (Allen & Blazer, 1991; Blazer, 1986). These rates are considerably lower than those for younger age groups, but the risk of depression increases threefold when elders are physically ill and is three times higher in low socioeconomic status residential areas (American Psychiatric Association, 1994; Hogstel, 1995). In the nursing home population the rate of emotional problems is even higher: 50% to 70% experience depression, anxiety, fearfulness, loneliness, paranoia and other mental disorders (Harper, 1991).

Rates of depression are higher among older women than older men, a pattern similar to that observed in the general population (APA, 1994). Elderly caregiver wives of spouses with Alzheimer's disease, cancer, heart disease, stroke, or other physical illnesses have significantly higher rates of depression than community elders without these responsibilities. Based on standardized depression scales, between 28% and 55% of caregiver wives are clinically depressed (Wright, Clipp, & George, 1993).

Although women have higher rates of depression, men are more likely to commit suicide—6 times more likely than older white women and 24 times more likely than older African-American women (Osgood & Brant, 1991). The suicide rate per 100,000 men between 75 and 79 years old is 42.5, increasing to 50.2 for men older than 85 years (Osgood & Brant, 1991). However, older white men are three times more likely to commit suicide than older African-American men.

Minority elders make up approximately 13% of Americans age 65 years and older, but rates of depression among these community-residing elders are not well researched. Some studies found depressive symptoms more frequent among whites than among African-Americans (Blazer, Hughes, & George, 1987; Husiani et al., 1990; Smallegan, 1989), but others found no significant racial differences (Bojrab et al., 1988; Krause, 1986; Waxman et al., 1985). These discrepancies have been attributed to a complex interplay among sociodemographic, physical, and social risk factors for depression. However, a recent investigation found older African-American women have the highest rates of clinically relevant depressive symptoms, even after controlling for the effects of socioeconomic status (Waid et al., in press).

Etiology

Three major causes of depression need to be considered: (1) past history of depression, (2) social losses associated with aging, and (3) physical health problems, including medication side effects and substance abuse.

Past history of depression

Approximately 50% to 60% of people with a history of one major depression have a second episode. With two previous episodes the probability of having a third increases to 70%; after three episodes the probability of a fourth increases to 90% (APA, 1994). These statistics appear to support the emerging evidence of a hereditary trait for depression (APA, 1994).

Social losses and depression

The later phases of life are associated with losses, especially the following (Hogstel, 1995):

- Loss of economic stability because of retirement
- Loss of social roles because of retirement, death or illness of a spouse, or relocation from one community to another
- Loss of dreams
- Loss of personal freedom associated with becoming a caregiver for an ill spouse or relative
- Loss of strength and agility
- Loss of physical health

Physical health problems and depression

The risk of depression in older people increases threefold with the presence of physical illness, and a wide range of physical disorders are associated with depressive symptoms, especially the following (Hogstel, 1995):

- Congestive heart failure
- Myocardial infarction
- Diabetes mellitus
- Cushing's disease
- Thyroid dysfunction
- Infectious mononucleosis
- Liver dysfunction
- Acquired immunodeficiency syndrome (AIDS)
- Gout
- Rheumatoid arthritis
- Gastrointestinal and metabolic disturbances
- Viral infections
- Various forms of cancer
- Head injury
- Multiple sclerosis
- Multiinfarct dementia
- Alzheimer's and Parkinson's diseases
- Stroke
- Influenza
- Pneumonia
- Tuberculosis

Physical illness can significantly affect an older person's quality of life and thus become a social hindrance. For example, illnesses such as arthritis or osteoporosis can cause chronic pain and reduced mobility, which may in turn lead to social isolation, poor self-esteem, loss of hope, and depression. However, caregivers and health care professionals must recognize that depressed older people may not be aware of underlying physical problems, especially nutritional disorders such as avitaminosis (decreased levels of ascorbic acid, folate, iron, niacin, pyridoxine, thiamine, or zinc), dehydration, pernicious anemia, or protein deficiency.

Side effects from prescribed or over-the-counter (OTC) medications also can contribute to depression. Older adults take an average of 3.54 medications per day (2.23 prescription, 1.31 OTC), twice the amount taken by younger people (Hanlon et al., 1992). Interestingly, Hanlon et al. (1992) also found a racial difference: African-American elders take significantly fewer medications than white elders (3.14 and 3.77 per day, respectively). Use of alcohol was not included in this survey.

The nurse must be aware that elders may use alcohol or drugs to blunt or block feelings associated with depressed moods (Hogstel, 1995). (Medications and drugs that can contribute to and relieve depressive symptoms are discussed in Chapter 13.)

Diagnostic criteria of depression

The *Diagnostic and Statistical Manual of Mental Disorders,* fourth edition *(DSM-IV),* differentiates among major depressive episodes, mood disorders caused by a general medical condition, substance-induced mood disorders, dysthymic disorders, and other disorders that produce depressed moods (APA, 1994).

The diagnosis of major depressive episode applies if at least five symptoms from the following list have been present for 2 weeks and continue to be present daily or almost daily (APA, 1994):

- Depressed moods most of the day
- Markedly diminished interest in activities
- Weight loss or gain amounting to a 5% change in a month
- Insomnia or hypersomnia
- Observable psychomotor agitation or retardation
- Fatigue or loss of energy
- Diminished ability to concentrate or think
- Feelings of worthlessness or excessive or inappropriate guilt
- Recurrent thoughts of death
- Suicidal ideation, plan, or attempt

The first two symptoms, depressed mood and markedly diminished interest, must be present for the diagnosis of major depressive episode to apply.

The diagnosis of mood disorder caused by a general medical condition applies if the persistent mood disturbance and other symptoms typically associated with major depression are caused by a medical condition (APA, 1994). However, not all criteria for major depression must be met.

The diagnosis of substance-induced mood disorder applies if depressed moods or expansive, irritable moods occur immediately after drug intoxication or within 4 weeks of withdrawal from substances and the symptoms are "judged to be in excess of those usually associated with the intoxication or withdrawal syndrome" (APA, 1994).

The diagnosis of dysthymic disorder applies to chronically depressed people whose symptoms persist for at least 2 years. Such people describe themselves as sad or "down in the dumps"; however, they must have at least two other symptoms associated with major depression to be dianosed as having dysthymic disorder. Low interest, self-criticism, and a perception of the self as uninteresting or incapable are prominent features of dysthymic disorder (APA, 1994).

In addition to these diagnoses, an adjustment disorder with depressed moods should be considered if one or several specific precipitating stressors (such as marital or financial problems) can be identified and depressed moods develop within 3 months of the stressors' occurrence (APA, l994).

Depressed moods after the death of a loved one are a normal expression of grief and should not be classified as an adjustment disorder (APA, 1994). If suicidal ideation occurs, evaluation and treatment for a major depressive episode become necessary.

Assessment of depression

Assessment scales

Commonly used standardized depression scales include the Hamilton Depression Rating Scale (Ham-D) (see Appendix F), Geriatric Depression Scale (GDS) (see Appendix H), Zung Self-Rating Depression Scale (SDS), Center for Epidemiologic Studies Depression Scale (CES-D), and Beck Depression Inventory (Weiss, Nagel, & Aronson, 1986). Typically, depression scales assess self-reports or interviewer-assisted responses to questions related to depressive symptoms. (Response options typically range from 0 = not at all to 3 = always.)

The GDS requires only *yes* or *no* responses. However, given the difficulty of assessing depression in elders with dementia, even valid yes/no responses may be difficult to obtain. The Cornell Scale for Depression in Dementia provides a useful alternative (Alexopoulos et al., 1988). Ratings on this scale are based on the clinician's observations.

Clinical assessment of depression

Standardized scales are helpful for obtaining a measure of the severity (or level) of depression, but they do not replace a skilled and sensitive clinical interview. An important point to keep in mind is that the present cohort of elders embraces an ethos of self-reliance and views psychiatric illness as a stigma. Consequently, older adults frequently deny feeling depressed and instead focus on physical symptoms; they also tend to become highly critical of others. The term *masked depression* has been used to describe this phenomenon (Allen & Blazer, 1991).

Clinicians must therefore pay close attention to nonverbal cues of depression such as lack of variation in facial expressions and tone of voice, disheveled clothing, poor hygiene, and untidy, dark rooms with curtains drawn. Additional cues are social isolation, lack of energy, fatigue, and chronic pain.

Some memory impairment, especially delayed recall of events or names, can be observed in depressed older people (Lichtenberg et al., l995). However, this impairment differs from impaired cognition associated with a rarer form of depression referred to as *dementia syndrome of depression* or *pseudodementia* (Allen & Blazer, l991). Characteristics of pseudodementia include rapid onset of memory problems with symptoms of short duration. The client's mood is consistently depressed, and "don't know" answers are typical. The client highlights disabilities, and level of cognitive impairment fluctuates. A client with these symptoms does have dementia but is depressed. In contrast, symptoms of dementia include insidious onset of memory problems, symptoms of long duration, and mood and behavior fluctuation. "Near miss" answers are typical, the client tries to conceal disabilities, and level of cognitive impairment is relatively stable (Allen & Blazer, 1991). A client with these symptoms requires a different assessment (see p. 393).

Clinical assessment of suicidal ideation

Suicidal ideation must always be assessed, but elders may not overtly express such thoughts (Hogstel, 1995). The clinician should be alert to indirect verbal, behavioral, or situational cues (Osgood & Brant, 1991).

A verbal cue may be a statement such as "My family would be better off without me" or a request made to a neighbor or friend to look after a pet "in case something should happen to me." Behavioral cues may take the form of giving away prized possessions, stockpiling pills, performing uncharacteristic behaviors such as waving or kissing goodbye, appearing suddenly calm and resolved after weeks of being upset, or scheduling an appointment with a clinic or physician's office either for no apparent physical problem or very shortly after the last visit. Situational cues include the death of a spouse, loss of a business, chronic pain, and terminal illness (Osgood & Brant, 1991). An elder who is in constant pain or has a fatal illness may consider suicide an honorable choice, and debate is growing over whether society should accept "rational suicide" (Battin, 1991; Moore, 1993; Richman, 1992; Siegel, 1986; Valente, 1993-1994).

Clinicians should ask direct questions about suicidal ideation. A series of graded questions has been suggested by Blazer (1986); if the first question is answered affirmatively, the clinician proceeds with the next question. The first question is "Have you ever thought life is not worth living?" If the answer is "yes," the clinican asks "Have you ever considered harming yourself?" If the answer is "yes," the clinician asks, "Do you have plans for harming yourself?" If the answer is "yes," and the plan is described, the clinician asks, "Have you ever begun to act on that plan?" and "Have you ever made a suicide attempt (even years ago)?"

The suicide plan may be active, for example, taking an overdose or using a gun. However, the plan may possibly be passive, for example, deliberately neglecting a diabetic condition or refusing treatment for cancer. Older people who have a plan and have begun preparations are at high risk for committing suicide. Gurland (1991) expressed the risk of suicide succinctly when he stated that elders tend to be "deadly serious in their suicidal actions; their first attempt is likely to be their last."

Nursing interventions

Nursing interventions begin during the assessment phase, and the nurse establishes rapport while gathering information from a client. A skilled mental health nurse uses problem-focused interventions but above all conveys an attitude of genuine respect, empathy, hopefulness, and caring (Leszcz, 1991). As few as one to three sessions with a nurse can reduce an older person's depressed moods, and if other social support can be arranged, this may be all that is necessary to alleviate distress. A client who is suicidal, however, requires immediate and structured interventions.

Antisuicide contract

At a minimum, clients are asked to make a verbal promise to contact a professional or significant other before acting on feelings to end their lives. A written contract also is advised. Such a contract states, "No matter what happens, I will not kill myself, accidentally or on purpose, at any time" (Neville & Barnes, 1985).

If the client is unwilling to make such a contract, the nurse must stay with the client, call a local crisis unit, or make other emergency arrangements for the client's admission to a hospital.

Clients who are willing to make an antisuicide contract may be left with a responsible, competent adult. Treatment for major depression must be initiated, and additional supervisory help to cover critical periods such as weekends and holidays needs to be arranged.

Interventions for major depression

Clients who meet the criteria for a major depressive episode should receive psychotherapy and antidepressant medications. Clients who are unresponsive to such interventions should be referred for evaluation for electroconvulsive therapy (ECT). This treatment involves a series of mild electrical currents applied to a client's temples or forehead under general anesthesia. ECT has proved effective and safe for older clients (National Institutes of Health, l991).

Psychotherapy modalities include supportive therapy, interpersonal therapy, cognitive-behavioral strategies, and reminiscence or life review (Haight, 1991, 1992; Haight & Dias, 1992; Harper, 1991; Lazarus, Sadavoy, & Langsley, 1991). Elders respond well to individual or group therapies that address current living conditions and past or present family problems. After trust is established, elders willingly share life experiences and engage in role play. They learn from practicing communication strategies, which they may later use in difficult interpersonal relationships. Life review, however, brings unresolved conflicts into focus. A qualified therapist is needed to help clients examine, resolve, and accept past events (Haight, 1992; Hogstel, 1995).

Antidepressant medications such as nortriptyline, desipramine, doxepin, fluoxetine, and trazodone may be prescribed in addition to psychotherapy. These antidepressants can be given in lower doses than those given younger clients and still achieve therapeutic effects. Tertiary-amine tricyclic antidepressants such as imipramine and amitriptyline are less well tolerated by elders and may cause anticholinergic side effects and orthostatic hypotension (U.S. Department of Health and Human Services, l993).

The client and other family members need to know about the appropriate dosage of antidepressants, and they must be able to recognize side effects such as falls, constipation, disorientation, and sudden changes in behavior. The nurse also should alert the family that the risk of suicide may increase when a major depression begins to lift because clients may regain the energy to carry out the self-destructive act.

Interventions for other mood disorders and adjustment reactions

The nurse's assessment provides the focus for interventions. Underlying medical conditions and the removal or careful reduction of licit or illicit drugs may need to take priority. For dysthymic clients, antidepressant medications and cognitive-behavioral therapy can help them challenge and rethink negative views of themselves (Leszcz, 1991). Reminiscence and life review also can be effective (Haight, 1991, 1992; Haight & Dias, 1992).

Clients whose depressed moods are related to specific stressors also benefit from antidepressant medication and supportive or interpersonal therapy or life review. Grieving clients generally do not require medications, but they do need opportunities to express and mourn their loss.

Conclusion

Depression in elders is a complex issue. In 1991, experts from various disciplines attended the National Institutes of Health (NIH) Consensus Development Conference and reached the following conclusions (NIH, 1991):

- Depression in late life occurs in the context of numerous social and physical problems
- Careful clinical assessment is essential
- Depressed elderly people should be treated vigorously with antidepressants (unless contraindicated by medical conditions)
- Psychosocial treatments and ECT can be effective

DEMENTIA

Epidemiology

Dementia is a global term applied to a number of conditions characterized by persistent cognitive impairment. The most common cause of progressive dementia is Alzheimer's disease. Approximately 4 million Americans are diagnosed with this disease; by the middle of the next century, 14 million Americans will be afflicted with Alzheimer's disease unless a cure or preventive method is found (Alzheimer's Association, l993).

The onset of Alzheimer's disease is age related. The latest estimates based on community samples show a prevalence rate of 10% for people between age 65 and 74 years, increasing to 19% for people between 75 and 84 years old; for people age 85 years and older, the rate is 47% (Evans et al., 1989). Prevalence rates among minorities are less well documented, although some studies indicate that based on level of cognitive impairment (not diagnosis), dementing diseases occur earlier and more frequently among African-American and Hispanic populations than in the white population (NIH, l993).

Demographic projections show that by 2030, 66 million Americans (22% of the population) will be 65 years old or older (Harper, 1991). Americans are living longer, and people older than 85 years make up the fastest-growing segment of American society. Given the high prevalence of Alzheimer's disease among people older than 85 years, this disease poses major health and social problems for the decades ahead.

At present, more than 80% of afflicted people are cared for in their homes by family members. Approximately one third to one half of these informal caregivers are spouses; the others are predominantly daughters and daughters-in-law (Wright et al., 1993).

Etiology

Dementia

More than 70 different conditions can cause dementia; however, Alzheimer's disease (also re-ferred to as *senile dementia of the Alzheimer's type, SDAT,* or simply *AD*) accounts for approximately 66% of all cases. Vascular dementias (also referred to as *multiinfarct dementias* or *MID*) account for fewer than 15% of all cases, although the percentage appears higher among African-American elders (NIH, 1993). Another 15% of cases show a mixed diagnosis of SDAT and vascular dementia, and a small percentage of people are afflicted with Alzheimer's disease before they reach 65 years of age, a condition referred to as *early-onset AD* (Alzheimer's Association, l993). Various other illnesses can cause or simulate dementia, including the following (Office of Technology Assessment, 1987; Read, 1991):

- AIDS
- Creutzfeldt-Jakob disease
- Parkinson's disease
- Huntington's disease
- Pick's disease
- Brain tumors
- Psychiatric disorders, especially depression
- Drug reactions
- Nutritional disorders
- Metabolic disorders

Alzheimer's disease

As yet, no cause or cure is known for Alzheimer's disease. The disease is named after a German neurologist, Alois Alzheimer, who in 1907 identified characteristic brain tissue changes of this disease that can be observed at autopsy. Neurofibrillary tangles (or simply *tangles*) and neuritic plaques (or simply "plaques") can be observed microscopically. Tangles are hairlike structures wrapped around one another, and plaques are spherical structures with the protein amyloid in the center. Structural brain changes also are found in older people without dementia, but the density of plaques and tangles distinguishes Alzheimer's disease from changes associated with normal aging (Cohen & Eisdorfer, 1986).

Possible causes of Alzheimer's disease include aluminum toxicity, severe head trauma with loss of consciousness, neurotransmitter deficiencies, and a slow virus (Read, 1991). To date, research evidence supports none of these causes conclusively; however, a growing body of evidence suggests a genetic predisposition. Early-onset AD has been associated with abnormalities on chromosome 21 and chromosome 14. Currently, β-amyloid deposits, the plaques of Alzheimer's disease, are the focus of intense genetic research efforts. In 1993, chromosome 19 and its allele apolipoprotein E (apo E)—and in particular apo E-IV—were implicated in late-onset Alzheimer's disease. Apo E-IV is one of three alleles (E-II, E-III, E-IV) that code for apolipoprotein E; because one allele is inherited from each parent, different combinations occur. Of interest, 50% of clients with familial or sporadic (no family history) Alzheimer's disease had the E-II/E-IV or E-III/E-IV allele combination, but those with the E-IV/E-IV combination had denser and larger plaques; their risk for Alzheimer's disease increased to 90% (Corder et al., 1993; Saunders et al., 1993).

Diagnostic criteria

The *Diagnostic and Statistical Manual of Mental Disorders,* fourth edition *(DSM-IV),* differentiates among senile dementia of the Alzheimer's type, vascular dementia, dementia caused by other general medical conditions, substance-induced persisting dementia, and dementia caused by multiple etiologies (APA, 1994). The characteristic feature of all dementias is *memory impairment,* defined as a deficit in "the ability to learn new information or to recall previously learned information" (APA, 1994). One or more cognitive deficits also are present, including language disturbance (aphasia); impaired ability to carry out motor activities (apraxia); failure to recognize or identify objects (agnosia); and difficulties with planning, organizing, sequencing, and abstracting. The impairments lead to significant decline in social and occupational functioning (APA, 1994).

The diagnosis of senile dementia of the Alzheimer's type applies if, in addition to the above criteria, onset is gradual, cognitive decline is continual, and other causes of dementia have been ruled out (APA, 1994). A distinction of early or late onset is made based on whether illness onset occurred in a client younger or older than 65 years of age. Both early- and late-onset senile dementia of the Alzheimer's type can be specified as occurring with delirium, delusions, or depressed moods or as uncomplicated. For the first time in history, senile dementia of the Alzheimer's type can be coded as a clinical syndrome on axis I of the *DSM-IV* and as a medical illness on axis III.

The diagnosis of vascular dementia (formerly called "multiinfarct dementia") applies if memory impairment, other cognitive deficits, and impaired social functioning are present; however, its distinguishing features are a typically abrupt onset and steplike progression with rapid changes (APA, 1994). However, insidious onset and gradual decline may occur in some individuals. Neurological signs and symptoms (e.g., exaggerated reflexes) can be observed, and infarctions (e.g., focal atrophy) may be seen on brain scans. Delirium, delusions, and depressed moods also can occur with vascular dementia.

The diagnosis of dementia caused by other general medical conditions applies if a specific medical condition (e.g., HIV disease, head trauma, Parkinson's disease, Huntington's disease, Pick's disease, Creutzfeldt-Jakob disease) has been diagnosed and symptoms of memory impairment, other cognitive deficits, and impaired social functioning are thought to be caused by the medical condition (APA, 1994).

The diagnosis of substance-induced persisting dementia applies if, in addition to memory impairment, other cognitive deficits, and impaired social functioning, evidence suggests substance use (either use of medications or drug abuse) and symptoms continue beyond the period of intoxication or withdrawal. Thus, this diagnosis does not apply to substance intoxication delirium. Delirium differs from dementia in that the former is likely to be associated with reduced awareness of the environment, language and perceptual disturbances, and a short (hours to days) period of onset (APA, 1994).

The diagnosis of dementia caused by multiple etiologies applies if evidence from history, physical examination, or laboratory tests supports multiple causes of dementia (for example, senile dementia of the Alzheimer's type and vascular dementia).

Assessment of senile dementia of the Alzheimer's type

Assessment scales

Reisberg's Global Deterioration Scale (1983) provides an excellent description of the progression of senile dementia of the Alzheimer's type (see Appendix I). However, Reisberg (1983) points out that some overlap between phases exists and that not all people progress through the stages and clinical phases uniformly. Commonly used standardized scales for assessing cognitive and functional impairments are the Mini-Mental State Examination (MMSE) and Pfeiffer's Short Portable Mental Status Questionnaire (SPMSQ) (Folstein, Folstein, & McHugh, 1975; Pfeiffer, 1975). Elders with suspected dementia are questioned directly to obtain the information. By contrast, information for the Blessed Dementia Rating Scale (BDRS) is obtained from the elder's caregiver (Blessed, Tomlinson & Roth, 1968). Behavioral problems or level of agitation can be assessed with the Cohen-Mansfield Agitation Inventory (Cohen-Mansfield, 1986). The Hachinski Ischemia Scale helps differentiate between AD and vascular dementia (Hachinski et al., 1975), and the Cornell Depression Scale, described in the previous section, assesses depression in people suffering from dementia (Alexopoulos et al., 1988).

Clinical assessment of senile dementia of the Alzheimer's type

As yet a definitive diagnosis of Alzheimer's disease can be made only at autopsy; therefore tentative diagnosis is made by exclusion of all other possible causes of dementia. Standardized assessment scales help determine the level of impairment or "stage" of AD, but more important

are the behavioral disturbances associated with AD, which occur in 70% of community-residing people with dementia (Evans, 1991; Rabins, Mace, & Lucas, 1982; Wright, 1993). These behaviors include the following:

- Repetitive questions (such as "What day is it?" and "What time is it?" and "Where are we going?")
- Clinging and demanding behavior (wanting the caregiver physically close at all times)
- Aimless wandering (sometimes for hours without resting)
- Hiding and hoarding objects (including placing objects in inappropriate places, e.g., hiding toothbrushes in the freezer)
- Anger, stubbornness, crying, and combativeness in response to seemingly insignificant events (referred to as *catastrophic reactions*)
- Exacerbation of confusion in late afternoon (referred to as *sundown syndrome*)
- Poor hygiene and grooming (including resistance to caregiver's assistance with grooming).

These behavioral problems and guidelines for interventions are summarized in Table 27-1.

Clinical assessment of caregiver stress, depression, and health

In addition to assessing signs and symptoms of dementia, the clinician must assess the family caregiver's reaction to troublesome behaviors. Indeed the subjective interpretation of behaviors displayed by afflicted people is more detrimental to caregivers than frequency of troublesome behaviors (Wright, 1994a). Several standardized scales are available to measure caregiver stress; the most frequently used are the Burden Interview (Zarit & Zarit, 1990) and the Caregiving Hassles Scale (Kinney & Stephens, 1989). Caregivers with high levels of subjective stress could become abusive toward the elder with dementia.

Typically, the early and middle phases of AD are most stressful to caregivers, who not only deal with the behavioral problems of the person with

Table 27-1. Problems associated with dementia and guidelines for intervention

PROBLEM	GUIDELINES FOR INTERVENTION
Repetitive questions	Recognize repetitive questions as a sign of short-term memory problems and the seeking of reassurance, answer the questions, do not say, "I just told you," recognize that large clocks and calendars may help
Clinging, demanding behavior	Recognize such behavior as a need for attachment to someone better able to cope; try to sense expressed worry, fear, or need; respond by saying, "I am here"; introduce a substitute caregiver slowly, without leaving the first few times
Aimless wandering, pacing, wandering off	Distinguish between agitated restlessness and aimless, happy wandering; check for possible underlying physical problems (e.g., urinary tract, ear infections); recognize that walking can relieve stiffness, keep joints mobile, and improve cardiovascular function; provide for safe walks; camouflage doors or install a signal system; monitor weight loss caused by burning off calories; provide extra nourishment (including diet supplements such as *Ensure*)
Hiding and hoarding objects	Recognize hiding and hoarding as expressive of a need for security (even though hiding places are not remembered); learn about hiding places, check them regularly; make extra objects for hoarding available
Catastrophic reactions: crying, anger, increased pacing, combativeness, stubborn response to benign event or request	Recognize such reactions as inability to cope with environmental demands; remain calm; identify triggering events and verify them, simplify home environment; keep the same routines; limit choices, ask questions that require only "yes" or "no" responses; acknowledge underlying feelings, then redirect attention, then ask a simple question, for example, "That TV noise really upset you. Look (pointing), the light is on in the kitchen. Do you want some juice?" remember that elders tend to respond in "like kind" emotionally and that a cheerful, pleasant mood will elicit the same
Sundown syndrome: increased agitation and confusion in the late afternoon	Recognize sundown syndrome as increasing stress and decreased tolerance to environmental demands, turn lights on before darkness, provide snacks and fluids in the afternoon, play soft music, engage elder in low-stimulation activities, use touch
Poor hygiene and grooming, resistance to caregiver's assistance	Recognize poor hygiene as a sign of memory impairment and decreased ability to respond to instructions; have a set routine; let elder use tub rather than shower; experiment with different styling methods—after bath, blow dryers tend to have calming effects on women; guide toothbrush; simplify wardrobe (such as by providing velcro fasteners); lay out clothing in sequence; if elder is too resistive, do not insist, try later; accept that elder may be more cooperative with a respite worker or different relative; maintain a sense of humor

Modified from "Nursing Care and Management of Behavioral Problems in the Elderly, by L. K. Evans, 1991, in *Management and Care of the Elderly,* by M. S. Harper, ed., pp. 191–206, Newbury Park, CA: Sage Publications; "Alzheimer's Disease: Wandering Behaviors," by M. E. McCarthy, E. M. Johnson, & R. W. Hamill, 1995, in *Encyclopedia of Home Care for the Elderly,* by A. Romain-Davis, J. Boondas, & A. Lenihan, eds., pp. 47–51, Westport, CT: Greenwood Press; and *Alzheimer's Disease and Marriage: An Intimate Account,* by L. K. Wright, 1993, Newbury Park, CA: Sage Publications.

dementia but also assume new roles as business and money managers (Wright, 1993). A crucial question included in the caregiver assessment is "Who handles the family finances, and what long-term financial arrangements have you made?" (Wright, 1993).

Caregiver wives have the greatest risk for high stress and negative health consequences. Similar risks exist for daughters and daughters-in-law, who have been described as the *women in the middle* because of their multiple and often competing role demands (Brody, 1991; Wright, 1994a; Wright et al., 1993). For these reasons, questions about the caregiver's formal and informal social support must be asked.

Available research evidence suggests that prolonged stress associated with caregiving is likely to lead to dysphoria and in vulnerable individuals to depression; depression may in turn compromise the immune system, which may lead to poor physical health (Wright et al., 1993). Thus the caregiver's emotional and physical health must be assessed. Emotional health can be assessed with one of the depression scales already described. A brief assessment of the caregiver's physical health can be accomplished by asking, "How do you describe your own health—excellent, good, fair, or poor?" The clinician can then ask questions addressing specific health problems if indicated.

Nursing interventions

Interventions for senile dementia of the Alzheimer's type

To date, tacrine (Cognex) is the only approved medication to treat mild to moderate AD. The drug slows the progression of memory loss, but its beneficial effects diminish as the disease progresses. Side effects include elevated levels of liver enzymes, which must be monitored every 6 weeks initially and every 3 months at maintenance dosages (Laraia, 1995).

Behavioral disturbances (e.g., agitation, assaultiveness) and psychotic symptoms associated with

AD can be treated with neuroleptics (including haloperidol) in low dosages. Neuroleptics relieve but do not entirely eliminate behavioral symptoms, and they increase the risk of falls (Young & Meyers, 1991).

The most important interventions for people with AD increase safety, prevent excess disability, and enhance quality of life. Safety is increased by ordering a VIP (very important person) identification bracelet; discussing when to cease driving and handling of power tools and potentially dangerous kitchen equipment; and providing other safety features such as locks, bolts, an uncluttered environment, and nonslip floors.

Excess disability is prevented by simplifying tasks and focusing on what people with dementia can do rather than what they can no longer do (Wright, 1993). Even if the diagnosis is AD, physical problems such as urinary tract and ear infections, tooth abscesses, hearing or visual problems, malnutrition, and thyroid dysfunction and psychiatric problems such as depression or paranoia can exacerbate memory and behavioral problems and should be treated.

Quality of life in most situations is enhanced if people with AD are cared for at home instead of in a nursing home. The focus should be on simple, pleasurable activities and interactions that convey respect and caring. People with dementia need to be treated as people who still have feelings and are aware of love or rejection (Wright, l994b).

Interventions for caregivers' stress, depression, and ill health

Stress results from caring for the never-ending demands of elders with dementia, demands Mace and Rabins (1991) aptly describe as leading to a "36-hour day." Three interventions can help reduce this stress:

1. Teaching caregivers to use behavioral approaches to prevent agitation in people with dementia or prevent agitation from escalating: A key principle is acknowledgment of the

person with dementia's underlying feelings or needs, followed by diversion and redirection. Approaches to common behavior problems are summarized in Table 27-1.

2. Mobilizing formal and informal support: Names of respite helpers and day care programs should be made available, and caregivers should be taught the way to ask for help from neighbors, friends, and relatives directly and straightforwardly (Robinson, 1988, 1990; Wright, 1993). Caregivers should be encouraged to attend a local support group. Many groups are offered through the Alzheimer's Association, which offers information about groups and other services through its toll-free telephone number, 1-800-272-3900.

3. Advising caregivers to seek financial and legal counsel from professionals specializing in caregiver concerns: Issues such as durable power of attorney for financial aspects and health care power of attorney for future health care decisions need to be addressed.

Depression is a common consequence of prolonged stress. Supportive therapy and antidepressant medications are effective in reducing or stabilizing depression in caregivers. However, many caregivers do not have the time, energy, and money to seek formal therapy. They continue their caregiving responsibilities even if scores on standardized scales indicate significant depression.

The community nurse who visits a person with dementia in the home plays a crucial role in such situations. Caregivers need affirmation of their efforts and recognition that they are doing their best under difficult circumstances. Caregivers should be encouraged to accept help from others and engage in pleasurable activities at least once a week—without feeling guilty. Eventual nursing home placement and feelings of guilt surrounding that issue should be discussed.

The nurse also should be alert to passive suicidal behavior in caregivers; for example, a caregiver wife may deliberately neglect her own serious health condition, rationalizing that after her death her husband's long-term care will be

covered through money he will receive from her life insurance. Intervention in such situations includes bringing into the open issues, thoughts, and feelings; discussing alternatives; providing supportive therapy; and monitoring the situation.

Ill physical health can result from prolonged stress, depression, and exacerbation of prior health problems. The community nurse is in an excellent position to monitor the caregiver's physical health and medication regimen and teach the importance of nutrition, rest, and exercise. The nurse must insist on regular physical examinations and indicated tests. The nurse can encourage health-seeking behavior by asking, "How do you meet your own needs?" If the answer is "I have no time," the nurse can explain, "We have learned from many other people in situations similar to yours that if you do not take care of your own health, you will not be able to take care of _____, and instead of only one ill person, there will be two." Caregivers tend to respond to this logic, particularly if continued support is offered.

Model intervention programs by nurses

Innovative nursing outreach programs for elders with mental illness who live in rural areas have been established in Iowa and Virginia (Buckwalter et al., 1993). In these programs, geropsychiatric nurses are pivotal members of a multidisciplinary team. They successfully intervene with ill elders and family caregivers; the most common problems treated are depression, dementia, and problems in coping with chronic illness (Buckwalter et al., 1993).

Another innovative intervention program designed by nurses is currently being tested in South Carolina (Wright et al., 1995). Using the concept of continuum of care, master's level nurses provide in-home interventions to caregivers of people with dementia after an acute episode of agitation has occurred in which the elder was hospitalized. For 1 year, nurses teach caregivers to use new approaches to difficult behaviors and mobilize community resources. They also provide supportive counseling (Wright et al., 1995).

Conclusion

As yet, no cause or cure is known for Alzheimer's disease. Behavioral and environmental manipulation are the most important interventions for people with AD. Invariably this requires attention to the caregiver's stress, depression, and physical health and mobilization of community resources.

ABUSE AND NEGLECT

Epidemiology

Mistreatment of elders includes physical, psychological, and material abuse and active and passive neglect (Fulmer & O'Malley, 1987; Peirce & Fulmer, 1995). Between 700,000 and 1.2 million elderly people are abused or neglected each year; 64% are women (Fulmer, 1994; Goldstein, 1995). The national prevalence rate of abuse is estimated at 32 per 1000 elders, and neglect is even more common (Fulmer, 1994). However, many cases are never reported, and the true prevalence rate is likely much higher. Elders with dementia and those who have complex care needs are especially at risk for abuse and neglect; the most likely abusers are spouses (Fulmer, 1994; Fulmer & O'Malley, 1987).

Clinicians must distinguish between a caregiver's fear of becoming abusive or violent and actual abusive or violent behavior (Pillemer & Suitor, 1992). In one study, 20% of family caregivers to people with dementia feared becoming violent, but only 6% admitted to actually having engaged in violent behavior (Pillemer & Suitor, 1992).

Etiology

Five causes or explanations for elder abuse have been advanced:

1. Stressed caregiver theory
2. Impairment (dependency) of the elder
3. Exchange theory
4. Transgenerational violence theory
5. Psychopathology of the abuser

The stressed caregiver theory provides the most plausible explanation for abuse of elders with AD and other dementias. An elder's progressive decline leads to increasing demands on the caregiver. Loss of freedom, social isolation, minimal support, and high stress can contribute to abusive behavior toward a dependent elder (Fulmer, 1994; Peirce & Fulmer, 1995).

The impairment (dependency) of the elder theory is similar to the stressed caregiver theory. However, the underlying problem is more likely to be the dependency of the caregiver on the elder rather than the elder's dependency on the caregiver (Wolf, Godkin, & Pillemer, 1984).

Exchange theory asserts that abuse continues if the caregiver gains rewards from the actions and that abuse ceases if it fails to gain rewards. Rewards may be psychological; for example, the caregiver may perceive abuse as "evening up a score" for previously conflicted relationships (Peirce & Fulmer, 1995).

Transgenerational violence theory asserts that violence is learned behavior; adult children who abuse their parents may have been abused earlier in life. However, underlying psychopathology of the abuser should be considered in abusive people with a history of alcohol or drug abuse, severe psychiatric illness, or subnormal intelligence (Goldstein, 1995).

Diagnostic criteria

The *Diagnostic and Statistical Manual of Mental Disorders,* fourth edition *(DSM-IV),* recognizes physical abuse of adult as a clinical problem (APA, 1994). The focus of attention may be either the abuser and the relational unit in which abuse occurs or the victim of abuse (APA, 1994).

Assessment of abuse and neglect

Assessment scales

Particularly helpful to community nurses is the index for assessing the Risk of Elder Abuse in the Home (REAH) (Hamilton, 1989). The REAH combines two assessments: the vulnerability assessment score of the aged person (VASAP) and the stress assessment score of the caregiver (SASC). Scores range from 0 to 41 (Hamilton, 1989). A high

REAH index in the presence of a maladaptive family system suggests high risk for elder abuse (Hamilton, 1989). (The REAH and SASC scales are provided in Appendixes J and K, respectively.)

A comprehensive and well-researched elder assessment instrument (EAI) was developed by Fulmer, Street, and Carr (1984). This instrument includes physical, medical, and social indicators of abuse.

Clinical assessment of abuse and neglect

The community nurse is likely to observe indicators of abuse and neglect. However, signs may not indicate abuse but instead result from an elder's frail physical condition or gait problems, which may cause falls and injuries. However, clinicians should suspect abuse if injuries are unexplainable.

Indicators of physical abuse include unexplained bruises and welts, burns, fractures, and lacerations or abrasions (Fulmer & Edelman, 1991). Unexplained bruises and welts may be observed on the face, lips, mouth, torso, back, buttocks, and thighs. Bruises tend to show various stages of healing, recur at regular intervals, be present on several different surface areas, and reflect the shape of the article used to inflict the bruise (e.g., electric cord, belt buckle) or the hand used to slap the elder (Fulmer & Edelman, 1991).

Unexplained burns may be caused by cigarettes or cigars and are most often seen on soles, palms, back, or buttocks. Burns also can be caused by immersion; such burns appear socklike or glovelike or are in the shape of a doughnut on buttocks or genitalia. Electric burns may reflect the shape of an iron or burner. Rope burns are most often found on arms, legs, neck, or torso (Fulmer & Edelman, 1991).

Unexplained fractures may be present in various stages of healing. Multiple fractures involving the skull, nose, and facial structure may be seen. In addition, unexplained lacerations or abrasions may be observed on the mouth, lips, gums, eyes, and external genitalia (Fulmer & Edelman, 1991).

Sexual abuse should be suspected if the elder has difficulty walking or sitting; has torn, stained, or bloody underclothing; or complains of pain or itching in the genital area. Bruises or bleeding in external genital, vaginal, or anal areas also may indicate sexual abuse (Fulmer & Edelman, 1991).

Physical neglect can be active or passive (Goldstein, 1995). Indicators of physical neglect are poor hygiene, inappropriate dress, consistent hunger, and constant fatigue or listlessness in a dependent elder. Neglectful caregivers do not attend to the physical problems or medical needs of the elder. The elder does not receive appropriate supervision from the caregiver, especially during dangerous activities. The elder may have been abandoned (Fulmer & Edelman, 1991).

Psychological abuse includes name-calling and frightening, humiliating, intimidating, or threatening the elder. Although the nurse may question the elder and caregiver about such occurrences, direct observation of interactions between elder and caregiver provides better assessment data. Indicators of emotional abuse include depression and withdrawal, sucking, biting, rocking, antisocial and destructive behaviors, and sleep disturbances. However, many of these behaviors are associated with the progression of dementia and therefore may not indicate abuse (Fulmer & Edelman, 1991; Goldstein, 1995).

Material abuse refers to exploitation of the elder's financial resources. Caregivers, relatives, financial consultants, or salespersons may steal money and other resources. Indicators are suspicious signatures on paperwork, evidence of threats of withholding services, and any unexplained decrease in savings or standards of living (Peirce & Fulmer, 1995).

Nursing interventions

Reporting suspected abuse or neglect

In most states, mandatory reporting laws require professionals to report abuse and neglect, usually to the department of Adult Protective Services (APS). For the community nurse, ethical considerations may guide the decision to report or not report suspected abuse. For example, the elder may not want the incident to be reported, alternative care may be unavailable, and the caregiver may appear to be trying to overcome abusive tendencies (All, 1994; Fulmer & O'Malley, 1987; Goldstein, 1995; Peirce & Fulmer, 1995).

Abuse and neglect situations requiring immediate intervention

Three situations require immediate intervention to prevent further harm to the elder (Fulmer & O'Malley, 1987):

1. Life-threatening medical problems
2. Unsafe living environment
3. Unlimited access to the elder by someone who has in the past seriously harmed the elder

In life-threatening situations the nurse arranges for emergency room medical evaluations. If the environment is unsafe, the nurse may be able to correct the situation or may have to place the elder with a relative, friend, or shelter. Access to the elder by a previously abusive caregiver may have to be restricted by obtaining an emergency court order, having someone else who can provide protection move in, or moving the elder to a different location (Fulmer & O'Malley, 1987).

Preventing abuse and neglect

Recognizing high-risk situations and providing continued professional contact, support, and education to caregivers is most important. The nurse first acknowledges the caregiver's efforts and stress associated with caregiving and then asks, "Who is taking care of you?" (Fulmer & O'Malley, 1987). After the caregiver's needs have been discussed, the focus shifts to the elder: "One of the ways that we can help you (the caretaker) is to see if there aren't things that can be done for your parent to make it less difficult for you" (Fulmer & O'Malley, 1987). The same nonjudgmental approach, focusing on "care needs," should be used when talking with the elder (Fulmer & O'Malley, 1987).

Elder neglect and abuse is a serious and poorly recognized problem. Mandatory reporting laws vary from state to state; the nurse should be familiar with local policies. The hallmark indicators of abuse are unexplained injuries or behaviors in a dependent elder, high caregiver stress, poor resources, and previous conflicted relationships. The nurse's goal is to prevent abuse and neglect or stop its continuation.

SUMMARY

The care of community-residing elders with mental illness is invariably linked to other family members. Interventions should take the elders' and family members' quality of life into consideration because understanding complex social, psychological, and physical conditions leads to appropriate interventions. Cure may not be possible, but the nurse's assessment skills and knowledge of appropriate interventions can reduce suffering and bring comfort and support to elders with mental illness and their families.

REFERENCES

Alexopoulos, G. S., Abrams, R. C., Young, R. C., & Shamoian, C. A. (1988). Cornell Scale for Depression in Dementia. *Society of Biological Psychiatry, 23,* 271-284.

All, A. C. (1994) A literature review: Assessment and intervention in elder abuse. *Journal of Gerontological Nursing, 20*(7), 25-32.

Allen, A., & Blazer, D. G. (1991). Mood disorders. In J. Sadavoy, L. W. Lazarus, & L. F. Jarvik (Eds.), *Comprehensive review of geriatric psychiatry* (pp. 337-351). Washington, DC: American Psychiatric Press.

Alzheimer's Association. (1993). *Alzheimer's disease: Statistics.* Chicago: Author.

American Psychiatric Association. (1994). *Diagnostic and statistical manual of mental disorders* (4th ed.). Washington, DC: Author.

Battin, M. P. (1991). Rational suicide: How can we respond to a request for help? *Crisis, 12*(2), 73-80.

Blazer, D. (1986). Depression: Paradoxically, a cause for hope. *Generations, 10*(3), 21-23.

Blazer, D., Hughes, D. C., & George, L. K. (1987). The epidemiology of depression in an elderly community population. *Gerontologist, 27*(3), 281-287.

Blessed, G., Tomlinson, B. E., & Roth, M. (1968). The association between quantitative measures of dementia and of senile changes in the cerebral gray matter of elderly subjects. *British Journal of Psychiatry, 114,* 797-811.

Bojrab, S. L., Sipes, G. P., Weinberger, M., Hendrie, H. C., Hayes, J. R., Darnell, J. C., & Martz, B. L. (1988) A model for predicting depression in elderly tenants of public housing. *Hospital and Community Psychiatry, 39,* 304-309.

Brody, E. M. (1991). "Women in the middle" and family help to older people. *Gerontology, 21*(5), 471-480.

Buckwalter, K. C., Abraham, I. L., Smith, M., & Smullen, D. E. (1993). Nursing outreach to rural elderly people who are mentally ill. *Hospital and Community Psychiatry, 44,* 821-823.

Cohen, D., & Eisdorfer, C. (1986). *The loss of self.* New York: Penguin.

Cohen-Mansfield, J. (1986). Agitated behaviors in the elderly. *Journal of the American Geriatrics Society, 34*(1), 722-727.

Corder, E. H., Saunders, A. M., Strittmatter, W. J., Schmechel, D. E., Gaskell, P. C., Small, G. W., Roses, A. D., Haines, J. L., & Pericak-Vance, M. A. (1993). Gene dose of apolipoprotein E type 4 allele and the risk of Alzheimer's disease in late onset families. *Science, 261,* 921-923.

Evans, D. A., Funkenstein, H. H., Albert, M. S., Scherr, P. A., Cook, N. R., Chown, M. J., Herbert, L. E., Hennekens, C. H., & Taylor, J. O. (1989). Prevalence of Alzheimer's disease in a community population of older persons: Higher than previously reported. *Journal of the American Medical Association, 252,* 2551-2556.

Evans, L. K. (1991) Nursing care and management of behavioral problems in the elderly. In M. S. Harper (Ed.), *Management and care of the elderly: Psychosocial perspectives.* Newbury Park, CA: Sage Publications.

Folstein, M. F., Folstein, S. E., & McHugh, P. R. (1975). Mini-Mental State. *Journal of Psychiatric Research, 12,* 189-198.

Fulmer, T. T. (1994). Elder mistreatment. *Annual Review of Nursing Research, 12,* 51-64.

Fulmer, T. T., & Edelman, C. L. (1991). Adult day care. In M. S. Harper (Ed.), *Management and care of the elderly: Psychosocial perspectives.* Newbury Park, CA: Sage Publications.

Fulmer, T. T., & O'Malley, T. A. (1987). *Inadequate care of the elderly.* New York: Springer Publishing.

Fulmer, T., Street, S., & Carr K. (1984). Abuse of the elderly: Screening and detection. *Journal of Emergency Nursing, 10,* 131-140.

Goldstein, M. Z. (1995). Abuse of the elderly: Kings of abuse. In A. Romaine-Davis, J. Boondas, & A. Lenihan (Eds.), *Encyclopedia of home care for the elderly.* Westport CT: Greenwood Press.

Gurland, B. (1991). Epidemiology of psychiatric disorders. In J. Sadavoy, L. W. Lazarus, & L. F. Jarvik (Eds.), *Comprehensive review of geriatric psychiatry* (pp. 25-40). Washington, DC: American Psychiatric Press.

Hachinski, V., Iliff, L., Zilhka, E., DuBoulay, G., McAllister, V., Marshall, J., Russell, R. W. R., & Symon, L.

(1975). Cerebral blood flow in dementia. *Archives of Neurology, 32,* 632-637.

Haight, B. K. (1991). Reminiscing: The state of the art as a basis for practice. *International Journal of Aging and Human Development, 33*(1), 1-32.

Haight, B. K. (1992). Long-term effects of a structured life review process. *Journal of Gerontology, 47*(5), 312-315.

Haight, B. K., & Dias, J. K. (1992). Examining key variables in selected reminiscing modalities. *International Psychogeriatrics, 2,* 279-290.

Hamilton, G. P. (1989). Using a family system approach: Prevent elder abuse. *Journal of Gerontological Nursing, 15*(3), 21-26.

Hanlon, J. T., Fillenbaum, G. G., Burchett, B., Wall, W. E., Jr., Service, C., Blazer, D. G., & George, L. K. (1992). Drug-use patterns among black and nonblack community-dwelling elderly. *Annals of Pharmacotherapy, 26,* 679-685.

Harper, M. S. (1991). An overview: Mental disorders of the elderly. In M. S. Harper (Ed.), *Management and care of the elderly: Psychosocial perspectives* (pp. 3-23). Newbury Park, CA: Sage Publications.

Hogstel, M. O. (1995). *Geropsychiatric nursing* (2nd ed.). St. Louis: Mosby.

Husaini, B. A., Castor, R. S., Linn, J. G., Moore, S. T., Warren, H. A., & Whitten-Stoval, R. (1990). Social support and depression among the African-American and white elderly. *Journal of Community Psychiatry, 18,* 12-18.

Kinney, J. M., & Stephens, M. A. P. (1989). Caregiving Hassles Scale: Assessing the daily hassles of caring for a family member with dementia. *Gerontologist, 29,* 328-332.

Krause, N. (1986). Life stress as a correlate of depression among older adults. *Psychiatry Research, 18,* 227-237.

Laraia, M. (1995). Psychopharmacology. In G. W. Stuart, & S. J. Sundeen (Eds.), *Principles and practice of psychiatric nursing.* St. Louis: Mosby.

Lazarus, L W., Sadavoy, J., & Langsley, P. R. (1991). Individual psychotherapy. In J. Sadavoy, L. W. Lazarus, & L. F. Jarvik (Eds.), *Comprehensive review of geriatric psychiatry.* Washington, DC: American Psychiatric Press.

Leszcz, M. (1991). Group therapy. In J. Sadavoy, L. W. Lazarus, & L. F. Jarvik (Eds.), *Comprehensive review of geriatric psychiatry* (pp. 527-546). Washington, DC: American Psychiatric Press.

Lichtenberg, P. A., Ross, T., Millis, S. R., & Manning, C. A. (1995). The relationship between depression and cognition in older adults: A cross-validation study. *Psychological Sciences, 50B,* 25-32.

Mace, N. L., & Rabins, P. V. (1991). *The 36-hour day.* Baltimore: Johns Hopkins University Press.

McCarthy, M. E., Johnson, E. M., & Hamill, R. W. (1995). Alzheimer's disease: Wandering behaviors. In A. Romain-Davis, J. Boondas, & A. Lenihan (Eds.),

Encyclopedia of home care for the elderly (pp. 47-51). Westport, CT: Greenwood Press.

Moore, S. L. (1993). Rational suicide among older adults: A cause for concern? *Archives of Psychiatric Nursing, 7*(2), 106-110.

National Institutes of Health. (1991, November 4-6). *Diagnosis and treatment of depression in late life. NIH Consensus Development Conference Consensus Statement, 9*(3).

National Institutes of Health. (1993). *Advisory Panel on Alzheimer's Disease: Fourth report of the Advisory Panel on Alzheimer's Disease, 1992.* Washington, DC: U.S. Government Printing Office.

Neville, D., & Barnes, S. (1985). The suicidal phone call. *Journal of Psychosocial Nursing and Mental Health Services, 23*(8), 14-18.

Office of Technology Assessment. (1987). *Losing a million minds: Confronting the tragedy of Alzheimer's disease and other dementias.* Washington, DC: U.S. Government Printing Office.

Osgood, N. J., & Brant, B. A. (1991). Suicide among the elderly in institutional and community settings. In M. S. Harper (Ed.), *Management and care of the elderly: Psychosocial perspectives* (pp. 37-71). Newbury Park, CA: Sage Publications.

Peirce, A., & Fulmer, T. (1995). Abuse of the elderly: Mistreatment, assessment, & intervention. In A. Romaine-Davis, J. Boondas, & A. Lenihan (Eds.), *Encyclopedia of home care for the elderly.* Westport, CT: Greenwood Press.

Pfeiffer, E. (1975). SPMSQ: Short Portable Mental Status Questionnaire. *Journal of the American Geriatrics Society, 23,* 433-441.

Pillemer, K., & Suitor, J. J. (1992). Violence and violent feelings: What causes them among family caregivers? *Journal of Gerontology: Social Sciences, 47*(4), S165-172.

Rabins, P. V., Mace, N. L., Lucas, M. J. (1982). The impact of dementia on the family. *Journal of the American Medical Association, 248,* 333-335.

Read, S. (1991). The dementias. In J. Sadavoy, L. W. Lazarus, & L. F. Jarvik (Eds.). *Comprehensive review of geriatric psychiatry.* Washington, DC: American Psychiatric Press.

Reisberg, B. (1983). Clinical presentation, diagnosis & symptomatology of age-associated cognitive decline and Alzheimer's disease. In *Alzheimer's disease: The standard reference* (pp. 173-187). New York: Free Press.

Richman, J. (1992). A rational aproach to rational suicide. *Suicide and Life-Threatening Behavior, 22*(1), 130-141.

Robinson, K.M. (1990). The relationships between social skills, social support, self-esteem and burden in adult caregivers. *Journal of Advanced Nursing, 15,* 788-795.

Robinson, K. M. (1988). A social skills training program for adult caregivers. *Advances in Nursing Science, 10*(2), 59-72.

Sadavoy, J., Lazarus, L. W., & Jarvik, L. F. (Eds.) (1991). *Comprehensive review of geriatric psychiatry.* Washington, DC: American Psychiatric Press.

Saunders, A. M., Strittmatter, W. J., Schmechel, D., St. George-Hyslop, P. H., Pericak-Vance, M. A., Joo, S. H., Rosi, B. L., Gusella, J. F., Crapper-MacLachlan, D. R., Alberts, M. J., Hulette, C., Crain, B., Goldgaber, D., & Roses, A. D. (1993). Association of apolipoprotein E allele ϵ4 with late-onset familial and sporadic Alzheimer's disease. *Neurology, 43,* 1467-1472.

Siegel, K. (1986). Psychosocial aspects of rational suicide. *American Journal of Psychotherapy, 40*(3), 405-418.

Smallegan, M. (1989). Level of depressive symptoms and life stresses for culturally diverse older adults. *Gerontologist, 29,* 45-50.

U.S. Bureau of the Census. (1994). *Statistical abstract of the United States* (114th ed.). Washington, DC: U.S. Department of Commerce.

U.S. Department of Health and Human Services. (1993). *Depression in primary care.* Washington, DC: Author.

Valente, S. M. (1993-1994). Suicide and elderly people: Assessment and intervention. *Omega, 28*(4), 317-331.

Waid, L. R., Hummer, J. T., Sutherland, S. E., & Keil, J. E. (in press). Prevalence and correlates of depressive symptoms among elderly African-Americans and whites.

Waxman, H. M., McCreary, G., Weinrit, R. M., & Carner, E. A. (1985). A comparison of somatic complaints among depressed and non-depressed older persons. *Gerontologist, 25,* 501-507.

Weiss, I. K., Nagel, C. L., & Aronson, M. K. (1986). Applicability of depression scales to the old, old person. *Journal of the American Geriatrics Society, 34*(3), 215-218.

Williamson, G. M., & Schulz, R. (1992). Pain, activity restriction, and symptoms of depression among community-residing elderly adults. *Journal of Gerontology, 47,* 367-372.

Wolf, R., Godkin, M., & Pillemer, K. (1984). *Elder abuse and neglect: Final report from the three model projects.* Worchester, MA: University of Massachusetts, Center on Aging.

Wright, L. K. (1993). *Alzheimer's disease and marriage.* Newbury Park, CA: Sage Publications.

Wright L. K. (1994a, September). Alzheimer's disease and caregiver stress. *Journal—South Carolina Medical Association,* 424-428.

Wright, L. K. (1994b). Alzheimer's disease afflicted spouses who remain at home: Can human dialectics explain the findings? *Social Science Medicine, 8,* 1037-1046.

Wright, L. K., Clipp, E. C., & George, L. K. (1993). Health consequences of caregiver stress. *Medicine, Exercise, Nutrition, and Health, 2,* 181-195.

Wright, L. K., DeAndrade, S., Chance, L., & Sampson, R. (1995). *Alzheimer's disease: A continuum of care model.* Medical University of South Carolina, Progress Report to the Duke Endowment.

Wright, L. K., & Stuart, G. W. (1995). Psychological and psychiatric disorders and the elderly. In A. Romaine-Davis, J. Boondas, & A. Lenihan (Eds.), *Encyclopedia of home care for the elderly* (pp. 301-306). Westport, CT: Greenwood Press.

Young, R. C., & Meyers, B. S. (1991). Psychopharmacology. In J. Sadavoy, L. W. Lazarus, & L. F. Jarvik (Eds.), *Comprehensive review of geriatric psychiatry.* Washington, DC: American Psychiatric Press.

Zarit, S. H., & Zarit, J. M. (1990). *The memory and behavior problems checklist and the burden interview.* Gerontology Center, College of Health and Human Development, College Station, PA: Pennsylvania State University.

Appendixes

Appendix A

DSM-IV Classification

NOS = Not Otherwise Specified.

An χ appearing in a diagnostic code indicates that a specific code number is required.

An ellipsis (. . .) is used in the names of certain disorders to indicate that the name of a specific mental disorder or general medical condition should be inserted when recording the name (e.g., 293.0 Delirium Due to Hypothyroidism).

If criteria are currently met, one of the following severity specifiers may be noted after the diagnosis:

Mild

Moderate

Severe

If criteria are no longer met, one of the following specifiers may be noted:

In Partial Remission

In Full Remission

Prior History

DISORDERS USUALLY FIRST DIAGNOSED IN INFANCY, CHILDHOOD, OR ADOLESCENCE

Mental retardation

Note: **These are coded on Axis II.**

317	Mild Mental Retardation
318.0	Moderate Mental Retardation
318.1	Severe Mental Retardation
318.2	Profound Mental Retardation
319	Mental Retardation, Severity Unspecified

Learning disorders

315.00	Reading Disorder

From *Diagnostic and Statistical Manual of Mental Disorders,* ed. 4, by the American Psychiatric Association, 1994, Washington, DC: Author.

315.1	Mathematics Disorder
315.2	Disorder of Written Expression
315.9	Learning Disorder NOS

Motor skills disorder

315.4	Developmental Coordination Disorder

Communication disorders

315.31	Expressive Language Disorder
315.31	Mixed Receptive-Expressive Language Disorder
315.39	Phonological Disorder
307.0	Stuttering
307.9	Communication Disorder NOS

Pervasive developmental disorders

299.00	Autistic Disorder
299.80	Rett's Disorder
299.10	Childhood Disintegrative Disorder
299.80	Asperger's Disorder
299.80	Pervasive Developmental Disorder NOS

Attention-deficit and disruptive behavior disorders

314.xx	Attention-Deficit/Hyperactivity Disorder
.01	Combined Type
.00	Predominantly Inattentive Type
.01	Predominantly Hyperactive-Impulsive Type
314.9	Attention-Deficit/Hyperactivity Disorder NOS
312.8	Conduct Disorder
	Specify type: Childhood-Onset Type/ Adolescent-Onset Type
313.81	Oppositional Defiant Disorder
312.9	Disruptive Behavior Disorder NOS

Feeding and eating disorders of infancy or early childhood

307.52   Pica
307.53   Rumination Disorder
307.59   Feeding Disorder of Infancy or Early Childhood

Tic disorders

307.23   Tourette's Disorder
307.22   Chronic Motor or Vocal Tic Disorder
307.21   Transient Tic Disorder
       Specify if: Single Episode/Recurrent
307.20   Tic Disorder NOS

Elimination disorders

___ . ___   Encopresis
787.6   With Constipation and Overflow Incontinence
307.7   Without Constipation and Overflow Incontinence
307.6   Enuresis (Not Due to a General Medical Condition)
       Specify type: Nocturnal Only/Diurnal Only/Nocturnal and Diurnal

Other disorders of infancy, childhood, or adolescence

309.21   Separation Anxiety Disorder
       Specify if: Early Onset
313.23   Selective Mutism
313.89   Reactive Attachment Disorder of Infancy or Early Childhood
       Specify type: Inhibited Type/Disinhibited Type
307.3   Stereotypic Movement Disorder
       Specify if: With Self-Injurious Behavior
313.9   Disorder of Infancy, Childhood, or Adolescence NOS

DELIRIUM, DEMENTIA, AND AMNESTIC AND OTHER COGNITIVE DISORDERS

Delirium

293.0   Delirium Due to . . . *[Indicate the General Medical Condition]*

___.___   Substance Intoxication Delirium *(refer to Substance-Related Disorders for substance-specific codes)*
___.___   Substance Withdrawal Delirium *(refer to Substance-Related Disorders for substance-specific codes)*
___.___   Delirium Due to Multiple Etiologies *(code each of the specific etiologies)*
780.09   Delirium NOS

Dementia

290.xx   Dementia of the Alzheimer's Type, With Early Onset *(also code 331.0 Alzheimer's disease on Axis III)*
   .10   Uncomplicated
   .11   With Delirium
   .12   With Delusions
   .13   With Depressed Mood
       Specify if: With Behavioral Disturbance
290.xx   Dementia of the Alzheimer's Type, With Late Onset *(also code 331.0 Alzheimer's disease on Axis III)*
   .0   Uncomplicated
   .3   With Delirium
   .20   With Delusions
   .21   With Depressed Mood
       Specify if: With Behavioral Disturbance
290.xx   Vascular Dementia
   .40   Uncomplicated
   .41   With Delirium
   .42   With Delusions
   .43   With Depressed Mood
       Specify if: With Behavioral Disturbance
294.9   Dementia Due to HIV Disease *(also code 043.1 HIV infection affecting central nervous system on Axis III)*
294.1   Dementia Due to Head Trauma *(also code 854.00 head injury on Axis III)*
294.1   Dementia Due to Parkinson's Disease *(also code 332.0 Parkinson's disease on Axis III)*
294.1   Dementia Due to Huntington's Disease *(also code 333.4 Huntington's disease on Axis III)*

290.10   Dementia Due to Pick's Disease *(also code 331.1 Pick's disease on Axis III)*

290.10   Dementia Due to Creutzfeldt-Jakob Disease *(also code 046.1 Creutzfeldt-Jakob disease on Axis III)*

294.1   Dementia Due to . . . *[Indicate the General Medical Condition not listed above] (also code the general medical condition on Axis III)*

____.__   Substance-Induced Persisting Dementia *(refer to Substance-Related Disorders for substance-specific codes)*

____.__   Dementia Due to Multiple Etiologies *(code each of the specific etiologies)*

294.8   Dementia NOS

Amnestic disorders

294.0   Amnestic Disorder Due to . . . *[Indicate the General Medical Condition]*
         Specify if: Transient/Chronic

____.__   Substance-Induced Persisting Amnestic Disorder *(refer to Substance-Related Disorders for substance-specific codes)*

294.8   Amnestic Disorder NOS

Other cognitive disorders

294.9   Cognitive Disorder NOS

MENTAL DISORDERS DUE TO A GENERAL MEDICAL CONDITION NOT ELSEWHERE CLASSIFIED

293.89   Catatonic Disorder Due to . . . *[Indicate the General Medical Condition]*

310.1   Personality Change Due to . . . *[Indicate the General Medical Condition]*
         Specify type: Labile Type/Disinhibited Type/Aggressive Type/Apathetic Type/Paranoid Type/Other Type/Combined Type/Unspecified Type

293.9   Mental Disorder NOS Due to . . . *[Indicate the General Medical Condition]*

SUBSTANCE-RELATED DISORDERS

[a] *The following specifiers may be applied to Substance Dependence:*

With Physiological Dependence/Without Physiological Dependence
    Early Full Remission/Early Partial Remission
    Sustained Full Remission/Sustained Partial Remission
    On Agonist Therapy/In a Controlled Environment

The following specifiers apply to Substance-Induced Disorders as noted:

[I]With Onset During Intoxication/[W]With Onset During Withdrawal

Alcohol-related disorders

Alcohol use disorders

303.90   Alcohol Dependence[a]
305.00   Alcohol Abuse

Alcohol-induced disorders

303.00   Alcohol Intoxication
291.8   Alcohol Withdrawal
         Specify if: With Perceptual Disturbances
291.0   Alcohol Intoxication Delirium
291.0   Alcohol Withdrawal Delirium
291.2   Alcohol-Induced Persisting Dementia
291.1   Alcohol-Induced Persisting Amnestic Disorder
291.x   Alcohol-Induced Psychotic Disorder
   .5   With Delusions[I,W]
   .3   With Hallucinations[I,W]
291.8   Alcohol-Induced Mood Disorder[I,W]
291.8   Alcohol-Induced Anxiety Disorder[I,W]
291.8   Alcohol-Induced Sexual Dysfunction[I]
291.8   Alcohol-Induced Sleep Disorder[I,W]
291.9   Alcohol-Related Disorder NOS

Amphetamine (or amphetamine-like)-related disorders

Amphetamine use disorders

304.40   Amphetamine Dependence[a]
305.70   Amphetamine Abuse

Amphetamine-induced disorders

292.89   Amphetamine Intoxication
          Specify if: With Perceptual Disturbances
292.0   Amphetamine Withdrawal
292.81   Amphetamine Intoxication Delirium
292.xx   Amphetamine-Induced Psychotic
          Disorder
    .11   With Delusions[I]
    .12   With Hallucinations[I]
292.84   Amphetamine-Induced Mood Disorder[I,W]
292.89   Amphetamine-Induced Anxiety
          Disorder[I]
292.89   Amphetamine-Induced Sexual
          Dysfunction[I]
292.89   Amphetamine-Induced Sleep Disorder[I,W]
292.9   Amphetamine-Related Disorder NOS

Caffeine-related disorders

Caffeine-induced disorders

305.90   Caffeine Intoxication
292.89   Caffeine-Induced Anxiety Disorder[I]
292.89   Caffeine-Induced Sleep Disorder[I]
292.9   Caffeine-Related Disorder NOS

Cannabis-related disorders

Cannabis use disorders

304.30   Cannabis Dependence[a]
305.20   Cannabis Abuse

Cannabis-induced disorders

292.89   Cannabis Intoxication
          Specify if: With Perceptual Disturbances
292.81   Cannabis Intoxication Delirium
292.xx   Cannabis-Induced Psychotic Disorder
    .11   With Delusions[I]
    .12   With Hallucinations[I]
292.89   Cannabis-Induced Anxiety Disorder[I]
292.9   Cannabis-Related Disorder NOS

Cocaine-related disorders

Cocaine use disorders

304.20   Cocaine Dependence[a]
305.60   Cocaine Abuse

Cocaine-induced disorders

292.89   Cocaine Intoxication
          Specify if: With Perceptual Disturbances
292.0   Cocaine Withdrawal
292.81   Cocaine Intoxication Delirium
292.xx   Cocaine-Induced Psychotic Disorder
    .11   With Delusions[I]
    .12   With Hallucinations[I]
292.84   Cocaine-Induced Mood Disorder[I,W]
292.89   Cocaine-Induced Anxiety Disorder[I,W]
292.89   Cocaine-Induced Sexual Dysfunction[I]
292.89   Cocaine-Induced Sleep Disorder[I,W]
292.9   Cocaine-Related Disorder NOS

Hallucinogen-related disorders

Hallucinogen use disorders

304.50   Hallucinogen Dependence[a]
305.30   Hallucinogen Abuse

Hallucinogen-induced disorders

292.89   Hallucinogen Intoxication
292.89   Hallucinogen Persisting Perception
          Disorder (Flashbacks)
292.81   Hallucinogen Intoxication Delirium
292.xx   Hallucinogen-Induced Psychotic Disorder
    .11   With Delusions[I]
    .12   With Hallucinations[I]
292.84   Hallucinogen-Induced Mood Disorder[I]
292.89   Hallucinogen-Induced Anxiety
          Disorder[I]
292.9   Hallucinogen-Related Disorder NOS

Inhalant-related disorders

Inhalant use disorders

304.60   Inhalant Dependence[a]
305.90   Inhalant Abuse

Inhalant-induced disorders

292.89   Inhalant Intoxication
292.81   Inhalant Intoxication Delirium
292.82   Inhalant-Induced Persisting Dementia
292.xx   Inhalant-Induced Psychotic Disorder
    .11   With Delusions[I]
    .12   With Hallucinations[I]

292.84	Inhalant-Induced Mood Disorder[I]
292.89	Inhalant-Induced Anxiety Disorder[I]
292.9	Inhalant-Related Disorder NOS

Nicotine-related disorders

Nicotine use disorder

305.10	Nicotine Dependence[a]

Nicotine-induced disorder

292.0	Nicotine Withdrawal
292.9	Nicotine-Related Disorder NOS

Opioid-related disorders

Opioid use disorders

304.00	Opioid Dependence[a]
305.50	Opioid Abuse

Opioid-induced disorders

292.89	Opioid Intoxication
	Specify if: With Perceptual Disturbances
292.0	Opioid Withdrawal
292.81	Opioid Intoxication Delirium
292.xx	Opioid-Induced Psychotic Disorder
.11	With Delusions[I]
.12	With Hallucinations[I]
292.84	Opioid-Induced Mood Disorder[I]
292.89	Opioid-Induced Sexual Dysfunction[I]
292.89	Opioid-Induced Sleep Disorder[I,W]
292.9	Opioid-Related Disorder NOS

Phencyclidine (or phencyclidine-like)-related disorders

Phencyclidine use disorders

304.90	Phencyclidine Dependence[a]
305.90	Phencyclidine Abuse

Phencyclidine-induced disorders

292.89	Phencyclidine Intoxication
	Specify if: With Perceptual Disturbances
292.81	Phencyclidine Intoxication Delirium
292.xx	Phencyclidine-Induced Psychotic Disorder
.11	With Delusions[I]
.12	With Hallucinations[I]

292.84	Phencyclidine-Induced Mood Disorder[I]
292.89	Phencyclidine-Induced Anxiety Disorder[I]
292.9	Phencyclidine-Related Disorder NOS

Sedative-, hypnotic-, or anxiolytic-related disorders

Sedative, hypnotic, or anxiolytic use disorders

304.10	Sedative, Hypnotic, or Anxiolytic Dependence[a]
305.40	Sedative, Hypnotic, or Anxiolytic Abuse

Sedative-, hypnotic-, or anxiolytic-induced disorders

292.89	Sedative, Hypnotic, or Anxiolytic Intoxication
292.0	Sedative, Hypnotic, or Anxiolytic Withdrawal
	Specify if: With Perceptual Disturbances
292.81	Sedative, Hypnotic, or Anxiolytic Intoxication Delirium
292.81	Sedative, Hypnotic, or Anxiolytic Withdrawal Delirium
292.82	Sedative-, Hypnotic-, or Anxiolytic-Induced Persisting Dementia
292.83	Sedative-, Hypnotic-, or Anxiolytic-Induced Persisting Amnestic Disorder
292.xx	Sedative-, Hypnotic-, or Anxiolytic-Induced Psychotic Disorder
.11	With Delusions[I,W]
.12	With Hallucinations[I,W]
292.84	Sedative-, Hypnotic-, or Anxiolytic-Induced Mood Disorder[I,W]
292.89	Sedative-, Hypnotic-, or Anxiolytic-Induced Anxiety Disorder[W]
292.89	Sedative-, Hypnotic-, or Anxiolytic-Induced Sexual Dysfunction[I]
292.89	Sedative-, Hypnotic-, or Anxiolytic-Induced Sleep Disorder
292.9	Sedative-, Hypnotic-, or Anxiolytic-Related Disorder NOS

Polysubstance-related disorder

304.80	Polysubstance Dependence[a]

Other (or unknown) substance-related disorders

Other (or unknown) substance use disorders

304.90 Other (or Unknown) Substance
Dependence[a]

305.90 Other (or Unknown) Substance Abuse

Other (or unknown) substance-induced disorders

292.89 Other (or Unknown) Substance
Intoxication
Specify if: With Perceptual Disturbances

292.0 Other (or Unknown) Substance Withdrawal

292.81 Other (or Unknown) Substance-Induced
Delirium

292.82 Other (or Unknown) Substance-Induced
Persisting Dementia

292.83 Other (or Unknown) Substance-Induced
Persisting Amnestic Disorder

292.xx Other (or Unknown) Substance-Induced
Psychotic Disorder

   .11 With Delusions[I,W]

   .12 With Hallucinations[I,W]

292.84 Other (or Unknown) Substance-Induced
Mood Disorder[I,W]

292.89 Other (or Unknown) Substance-Induced
Anxiety Disorder[I,W]

292.89 Other (or Unknown) Substance-Induced
Sexual Dysfunction[I]

292.89 Other (or Unknown) Substance-Induced
Sleep Disorder[I,W]

292.9 Other (or Unknown) Substance-Related
Disorder NOS

SCHIZOPHRENIA AND OTHER PSYCHOTIC DISORDERS

295.xx Schizophrenia

The following Classification of Longitudinal Course applies to all subtypes of Schizophrenia:

Episodic With Interepisode Residual Symptoms (*specify if:* With Prominent Negative Symptoms)/ Episodic With No Interepisode Residual Symptoms

Continuous (*specify if:* With Prominent Negative Symptoms)

Single Episode In Partial Remission (*specify if:* With Prominent Negative Symptoms)/Single Episode In Full Remission

Other or Unspecified Pattern

   .30 Paranoid Type

   .10 Disorganized Type

   .20 Catatonic Type

   .90 Undifferentiated Type

   .60 Residual Type

295.40 Schizophreniform Disorder
Specify if: Without Good Prognostic
Features/With Good Prognostic Features

295.70 Schizoaffective Disorder
Specify type: Bipolar Type/Depressive Type

297.1 Delusional Disorder
Specify type: Erotomanic Type/Grandiose
Type/Jealous Type/Persecutory Type/Somatic
Type/Mixed Type/Unspecified Type

298.8 Brief Psychotic Disorder
Specify if: With Marked Stressor(s)/Without
Marked Stressor(s)/With Postpartum Onset

297.3 Shared Psychotic Disorder

293.xx Psychotic Disorder Due to . . . *[Indicate
the General Medical Condition]*

   .81 With Delusions

   .82 With Hallucinations

___.__ Substance-Induced Psychotic Disorder
(*refer to Substance-Related Disorders
for substance-specific codes*)
Specify if: With Onset During Intoxication/
With Onset During Withdrawal

298.9 Psychotic Disorder NOS

MOOD DISORDERS

Code current state of Major Depressive Disorder or Bipolar I Disorder in fifth digit:

1 = Mild

2 = Moderate

3 = Severe Without Psychotic Features

4 = Severe With Psychotic Features
Specify: Mood-Congruent Psychotic
Features/Mood-Incongruent Psychotic
Features

5 = In Partial Remission

6 = In Full Remission

0 = Unspecified

The following specifiers apply (for current or most recent episode) to Mood Disorders as noted:

[a]Severity/Psychotic/Remission Specifiers/[b]Chronic/[c]With Catatonic Features/[d]With Melancholic Features/[e]With Atypical Features/[f]With Postpartum Onset

The following specifiers apply to Mood Disorders as noted:

[g]With or Without Full Interepisode Recovery/[h]With Seasonal Pattern/[i]With Rapid Cycling

Depressive disorders

296.xx	Major Depressive Disorder,
.2x	Single Episode[a,b,c,d,e,f]
.3x	Recurrent[a,b,c,d,e,f,g,h]
300.4	Dysthymic Disorder

     Specify if: Early Onset/Late Onset

     Specify: With Atypical Features

311	Depressive Disorder NOS

Bipolar disorders

296.xx	Bipolar I Disorder,
.0x	Single Manic Episode[a,c,f]

     Specify if: Mixed

.4	Most Recent Episode Hypomanic[g,h,i]
.4x	Most Recent Episode Manic[a,c,f,g,h,i]
.6x	Most Recent Episode Mixed[a,c,f,g,h,i]
.5x	Most Recent Episode Depressed[a,b,c,d,e,f,g,h,i]
.7	Most Recent Episode Unspecified[g,h,i]
296.89	Bipolar II Disorder[a,b,c,d,e,f,g,h,i]

     Specify (current or most recent episode): Hypomanic/Depressed

301.13	Cyclothymic Disorder
296.80	Bipolar Disorder NOS
293.83	Mood Disorder Due to . . . *[Indicate the General Medical Condition]*

     Specify type: With Depressive Features/With Major Depressive-Like Episode/With Manic Features/With Mixed Features

___.__	Substance-Induced Mood Disorder *(refer to Substance-Related Disorders for substance-specific codes)*

     Specify type: With Depressive Features/With Manic Features/With Mixed Features

     Specify if: With Onset During Intoxication/With Onset During Withdrawal

296.90	Mood Disorder NOS

ANXIETY DISORDERS

300.01	Panic Disorder Without Agoraphobia
300.21	Panic Disorder With Agoraphobia
300.22	Agoraphobia Without History of Panic Disorder
300.29	Specific Phobia

     Specify type: Animal Type/Natural Environment Type/Blood-Injection-Injury Type/Situational Type/Other Type

300.23	Social Phobia

     Specify if: Generalized

300.3	Obsessive-Compulsive Disorder

     Specify if: With Poor Insight

309.81	Posttraumatic Stress Disorder

     Specify if: Acute/Chronic

     Specify if: With Delayed Onset

308.3	Acute Stress Disorder
300.02	Generalized Anxiety Disorder
293.89	Anxiety Disorder Due to . . . *[Indicate the General Medical Condition]*

     Specify if: With Generalized Anxiety/With Panic Attacks/With Obsessive-Compulsive Symptoms

___.__	Substance-Induced Anxiety Disorder *(refer to Substance-Related Disorders for substance-specific codes)*

     Specify if: With Generalized Anxiety/With Panic Attacks/With Obsessive-Compulsive Symptoms/With Phobic Symptoms

     Specify if: With Onset During Intoxication/With Onset During Withdrawal

300.00	Anxiety Disorder NOS

SOMATOFORM DISORDERS

300.81	Somatization Disorder
300.81	Undifferentiated Somatoform Disorder
300.11	Conversion Disorder

Specify type: With Motor Symptom or Deficit/ With Sensory Symptom or Deficit/With Seizures or Convulsions/With Mixed Presentation

307.xx	Pain Disorder
.80	Associated With Psychological Factors
.89	Associated With Both Psychological Factors and a General Medical Condition

Specify if: Acute/Chronic

300.7	Hypochondriasis

Specify if: With Poor Insight

300.7	Body Dysmorphic Disorder
300.81	Somatoform Disorder NOS

FACTITIOUS DISORDERS

300.xx	Factitious Disorder
.16	With Predominantly Psychological Signs and Symptoms
.19	With Predominantly Physical Signs and Symptoms
.19	With Combined Psychological and Physical Signs and Symptoms
300.19	Factitious Disorder NOS

DISSOCIATIVE DISORDERS

300.12	Dissociative Amnesia
300.13	Dissociative Fugue
300.14	Dissociative Identity Disorder
300.6	Depersonalization Disorder
300.15	Dissociative Disorder NOS

SEXUAL AND GENDER IDENTITY DISORDERS

Sexual dysfunctions

The following specifiers apply to all primary Sexual Dysfunctions:

Lifelong Type/Acquired Type
Generalized Type/Situational Type
Due to Psychological Factors/Due to Combined Factors

Sexual desire disorders

302.71	Hypoactive Sexual Desire Disorder
302.79	Sexual Aversion Disorder

Sexual arousal disorders

302.72	Female Sexual Arousal Disorder
302.72	Male Erectile Disorder

Orgasmic disorders

302.73	Female Orgasmic Disorder
302.74	Male Orgasmic Disorder
302.75	Premature Ejaculation

Sexual pain disorders

302.76	Dyspareunia (Not Due to a General Medical Condition)
306.51	Vaginismus (Not Due to a General Medical Condition)

Sexual dysfunction due to a general medical condition

625.8	Female Hypoactive Sexual Desire Disorder Due to . . . *[Indicate the General Medical Condition]*
608.89	Male Hypoactive Sexual Desire Disorder Due to . . . *[Indicate the General Medical Condition]*
607.84	Male Erectile Disorder Due to . . . *[Indicate the General Medical Condition]*
625.0	Female Dyspareunia Due to . . . *[Indicate the General Medical Condition]*
608.89	Male Dyspareunia Due to . . . *[Indicate the General Medical Condition]*
625.8	Other Female Sexual Dysfunction Due to . . . *[Indicate the General Medical Condition]*
608.89	Other Male Sexual Dysfunction Due to . . . *[Indicate the General Medical Condition]*
___.__	Substance-Induced Sexual Dysfunction *(refer to Substance-Related Disorders for substance-specific codes)*

Specify if: With Impaired Desire/With Impaired Arousal/With Impaired Orgasm/ With Sexual Pain
Specify if: With Onset During Intoxication

302.70	Sexual Dysfunction NOS

Paraphilias

302.4	Exhibitionism
302.81	Fetishism
302.89	Frotteurism
302.2	Pedophilia

Specify if: Sexually Attracted to Males/ Sexually Attracted to Females/Sexually Attracted to Both
Specify if: Limited to Incest
Specify type: Exclusive Type/Nonexclusive Type

302.83	Sexual Masochism
302.84	Sexual Sadism
302.3	Transvestic Fetishism

Specify if: With Gender Dysphoria

302.82	Voyeurism
302.9	Paraphilia NOS

Gender identity disorders

302.xx	Gender Identity Disorder
.6	in Children
.85	in Adolescents or Adults

Specify if: Sexually Attracted to Males/ Sexually Attracted to Females/Sexually Attracted to Both/Sexually Attracted to Neither

302.6	Gender Identity Disorder NOS
302.9	Sexual Disorder NOS

EATING DISORDERS

307.1	Anorexia Nervosa

Specify if: Restricting Type; Binge-Eating/ Purging Type

307.51	Bulimia Nervosa

Specify type: Purging Type/Nonpurging Type

307.50	Eating Disorder NOS

SLEEP DISORDERS

Primary sleep disorders

Dyssomnias

307.42	Primary Insomnia
307.44	Primary Hypersomnia

Specify if: Recurrent

347	Narcolepsy
780.59	Breathing-Related Sleep Disorder
307.45	Circadian Rhythm Sleep Disorder

Specify type: Delayed Sleep Phase Type/Jet Lag Type/Shift Work Type/Unspecified Type

307.47	Dyssomnia NOS

Parasomnias

307.47	Nightmare Disorder
307.46	Sleep Terror Disorder
307.46	Sleepwalking Disorder
307.47	Parasomnia NOS

Sleep disorders related to another mental disorder

307.42	Insomnia Related to . . . *[Indicate the Axis I or Axis II Disorder]*
307.44	Hypersomnia Related to . . . *[Indicate the Axis I or Axis II Disorder]*

Other sleep disorders

780.xx	Sleep Disorder Due to . . . *[Indicate the General Medical Condition]*
.52	Insomnia Type
.54	Hypersomnia Type
.59	Parasomnia Type
.59	Mixed Type
___.__	Substance-Induced Sleep Disorder *(refer to Substance-Related Disorders for substance-specific codes)*

Specify type: Insomnia Type/Hypersomnia Type/Parasomnia Type/Mixed Type
Specify if: With Onset During Intoxication/ With Onset During Withdrawal

IMPULSE-CONTROL DISORDERS NOT ELSEWHERE CLASSIFIED

312.34	Intermittent Explosive Disorder
312.32	Kleptomania
312.33	Pyromania
312.31	Pathological Gambling
312.39	Trichotillomania
312.30	Impulse-Control Disorder NOS

ADJUSTMENT DISORDERS

309.xx Adjustment Disorder
  .0   With Depressed Mood
  .24   With Anxiety
  .28   With Mixed Anxiety and Depressed Mood
  .3   With Disturbance of Conduct
  .9   With Mixed Disturbance of Emotions and Conduct
  .9   Unspecified
          Specify if: Acute/Chronic

PERSONALITY DISORDERS

Note: *These are coded on Axis II.*

301.0   Paranoid Personality Disorder
301.20 Schizoid Personality Disorder
301.22 Schizotypal Personality Disorder
301.7   Antisocial Personality Disorder
301.83 Borderline Personality Disorder
301.50 Histrionic Personality Disorder
301.81 Narcissistic Personality Disorder
301.82 Avoidant Personality Disorder
301.6   Dependent Personality Disorder
301.4   Obsessive-Compulsive Personality Disorder
301.9   Personality Disorder NOS

OTHER CONDITIONS THAT MAY BE A FOCUS OF CLINICAL ATTENTION
Psychological factors affecting medical condition

316 . . . *[Specified Psychological Factor]* Affecting . . . *[Indicate the General Medical Condition] Choose name based on nature of factors:* Mental Disorder Affecting Medical Condition
Psychological Symptoms Affecting Medical Condition
Personality Traits or Coping Style Affecting Medical Condition
Maladaptive Health Behaviors Affecting Medical Condition
Stress-Related Physiological Response Affecting Medical Condition
Other or Unspecified Psychological Factors Affecting Medical Condition

Medication-induced movement disorders

332.1   Neuroleptic-Induced Parkinsonism
333.92 Neuroleptic Malignant Syndrome
333.7   Neuroleptic-Induced Acute Dystonia
333.99 Neuroleptic-Induced Acute Akathisia
333.82 Neuroleptic-Induced Tardive Dyskinesia
333.1   Medication-Induced Postural Tremor
333.90 Medication-Induced Movement Disorder NOS

Other medication–induced disorder

995.2   Adverse Effects of Medication NOS

Relational problems

V61.9   Relational Problem Related to a Mental Disorder or General Medical Condition
V61.20 Parent-Child Relational Problem
V61.1   Partner Relational Problem
V61.8   Sibling Relational Problem
V62.81 Relational Problem NOS

Problems related to abuse or neglect

V61.21 Physical Abuse of Child
        (code 995.5 if focus of attention is on victim)
V61.21 Sexual Abuse of Child
        (code 995.5 if focus of attention is on victim)
V61.21 Neglect of Child
        (code 995.5 if focus of attention is on victim)
V61.1   Physical Abuse of Adult
        (code 995.81 if focus of attention is on victim)
V61.1   Sexual Abuse of Adult
        (code 995.81 if focus of attention is on victim)

Additional conditions that may be a focus of clinical attention

V15.81	Noncompliance With Treatment
V65.2	Malingering
V71.01	Adult Antisocial Behavior
V71.02	Child or Adolescent Antisocial Behavior
V62.89	Borderline Intellectual Functioning
	Note: *This is coded on Axis II.*
780.9	Age-Related Cognitive Decline
V62.82	Bereavement
V62.3	Academic Problem
V62.2	Occupational Problem
313.82	Identity Problem
V62.89	Religious or Spiritual Problem
V62.4	Acculturation Problem
V62.89	Phase of Life Problem

ADDITIONAL CODES

300.9	Unspecified Mental Disorder (nonpsychotic)
V71.09	No Diagnosis or Condition on Axis I
799.9	Diagnosis or Condition Deferred on Axis I
V71.09	No Diagnosis on Axis II
799.9	Diagnosis Deferred on Axis II

MULTIAXIAL SYSTEM

Axis I	Clinical Disorders Other Conditions That May Be a Focus of Clinical Attention
Axis II	Personality Disorders Mental Retardation
Axis III	General Medical Conditions
Axis IV	Psychosocial and Environmental Problems
Axis V	Global Assessment of Functioning

Appendix B

Psychiatric History and Mental Status Exam

I. History

A. Identification: Name, age, marital status, gender, occupation, language if other than English, race, nationality, religion, previous admissions to a hospital for same or a different condition, address, telephone number.

B. Chief complaint

C. Appearance and behavior during interview

D. History of present illness

E. Previous illnesses:
1. Emotional or mental disturbances
2. Psychophysiological disorders
3. Medical conditions
4. Neurological disorders

F. Past personal history:
1. Early childhood (through age 10 years)
2. Later childhood (from prepuberty through adolescence), including psychosexual history.
3. Adulthood, including occupational, sexual, and social history.

G. Family history

H. Marital history

I. Current social situation

II. Mental Status

A. General description:
1. Appearance
2. Behavior and psychomotor activity
3. Attitude toward examiner

B. Speech

C. State of consciousness

D. Affective or emotional state

E. Anxiety level

F. Stream of thought

G. Content of thought

H. Orientation

I. Memory

J. Information and intelligence

K. Concentration

L. Abstract thinking

M. Judgment

N. Insight

    O. Dreams, fantasies, and value systems
    P. Other tests as indicated
    Q. Reliability

III. Further Diagnostic Studies
    A. Physical examination
    B. Additional diagnostic interviews
    C. Interviews with family members, friends, neighbors
    D. Psychological tests
    E. Specialized tests

IV. Summary of Positive Findings (Strengths and Weaknesses)

V. Diagnosis According to *DSM-IV*

VI. Prognosis

VII. Recommendations

Appendix C

Global Assessment of Functioning (GAF) Scale

Consider psychological, social, and occupational functioning on a hypothetical continuum of mental health–illness. Do not include impairment in functioning due to physical (or environmental) limitations.

Code (**Note:** Use intermediate codes when appropriate, e.g., 45, 68, 72.)

100 | **Superior functioning in a wide range of activities, life's problems never seem to get out of hand,**
| **is sought out by others because of his or her many positive qualities. No symptoms.**
91 |

90 | **Absent or minimal symptoms** (e.g., mild anxiety before an exam), **good functioning in all areas,**
| **interested and involved in a wide range of activities, socially effective, generally satisfied with life,**
81 | **no more than everyday problems or concerns** (e.g., an occasional argument with family members).

80 | **If symptoms are present, they are transient and expectable reactions to psychosocial stressors**
| (e.g., difficulty concentrating after family argument); **no more than slight impairment in social,**
71 | **occupational, or school functioning** (e.g., temporarily falling behind in schoolwork).

70 | **Some mild symptoms** (e.g., depressed mood and mild insomnia) **OR some difficulty in social,**
| **occupational, or school functioning** (e.g., occasional truancy, or theft within the household), **but**
61 | **generally functioning pretty well, has some meaningful interpersonal relationships.**

60 | **Moderate symptoms** (e.g., flat affect and circumstantial speech, occasional panic attacks) **OR moderate**
| **difficulty in social, occupational, or school functioning** (e.g., few friends, conflicts with peers or
51 | co-workers).

50 | **Serious symptoms** (e.g., suicidal ideation, severe obsessional rituals, frequent shoplifting) **OR any**
| **serious impairment in social, occupational, or school functioning** (e.g., no friends, unable to keep
41 | a job).

40 | **Some impairment in reality testing or communication** (e.g., speech is at times illogical, obscure, or
| irrelevant) **OR major impairment in several areas, such as work or school, family relations,**
| **judgment, thinking, or mood** (e.g., depressed man avoids friends, neglects family, and is unable to
31 | work; child frequently beats up younger children, is defiant at home, and is failing at school).

30 | **Behavior is considerably influenced by delusions or hallucinations OR serious impairment in**
| **communication or judgment** (e.g., sometimes incoherent, acts grossly inappropriately, suicidal
| preoccupation) **OR inability to function in almost all areas** (e.g., stays in bed all day; no job, home,
21 | or friends).

20 | **Some danger of hurting self or others** (e.g., suicide attempts without clear expectation of death;
| frequently violent; manic excitement) **OR occasionally fails to maintain minimal personal hygiene**
11 | (e.g., smears feces) **OR gross impairment in communication** (e.g., largely incoherent or mute).

10 | **Persistent danger of severely hurting self or others** (e.g., recurrent violence) **OR persistent inability**
| **to maintain minimal personal hygiene OR serious suicidal act with clear expectation of**
1 | **death.**
0 | Inadequate information.

From *Diagnostic and Statistical Manual of Mental Disorders,* ed. 4, by the American Psychiatric Association, 1994, Washington, DC: Author.
The rating of overall psychological functioning on a scale of 0-100 was operationalized by Luborsky in the Health-Sickness Rating Scale (Luborsky L: "Clinicians' Judgments of Mental Health." *Archives of General Psychiatry* 7:407-417, 1962). Spitzer and colleagues developed a revision of the Health-Sickness Rating Scale called the Global Assessment Scale (GAS) (Endicott J, Spitzer RL, Fleiss JL, Cohen J: "The Global Assessment Scale: A Procedure for Measuring Overall Severity of Psychiatric Disturbance." *Archives of General Psychiatry* 33:766-771, 1976). A modified version of the GAS was included in *DSM-III-R* as the Global Assessment of Functioning (GAF) Scale.

Appendix D

Specific Level of Functioning Scale

INSTRUCTIONS:

Circle the number that best describes this person's *typical* level of functioning on each item listed below. Be as accurate as you can. If you are not sure about a certain rating, ask someone who may know or consult the case record. Mark only one number for each item. Be sure to mark all items.

Self-Maintenance

A. PHYSICAL FUNCTIONING	NO PROBLEM	PROBLEM, BUT NO EFFECT ON GENERAL FUNCTIONING	SLIGHT EFFECT ON GENERAL FUNCTIONING	RESTRICTS GENERAL FUNCTIONING SUBSTANTIALLY	PREVENTS GENERAL FUNCTIONING
1. Vision	5	4	3	2	1
2. Hearing	5	4	3	2	1
3. Speech impairment	5	4	3	2	1
4. Walking, use of legs	5	4	3	2	1
5. Use of hands and arms	5	4	3	2	1

B. PERSONAL CARE SKILLS	TOTALLY SELF-SUFFICIENT	NEEDS VERBAL ADVICE OR GUIDANCE	NEEDS SOME PHYSICAL HELP OR ASSISTANCE	NEEDS SUBSTANTIAL HELP	TOTALLY DEPENDENT
6. Toileting (uses toilet properly; keeps self and area clean)	5	4	3	2	1
7. Eating (uses utensils properly; eating habits)	5	4	3	2	1
8. Personal hygiene (body and teeth; general cleanliness)	5	4	3	2	1
9. Dressing self (selects appropriate garments; dresses self)	5	4	3	2	1
10. Grooming (hair, make-up, general appearance)	5	4	3	2	1
11. Care of own possessions	5	4	3	2	1
12. Care of own living space	5	4	3	2	1

Social Functioning

C. INTERPERSONAL RELATIONSHIPS	HIGHLY TYPICAL OF THIS PERSON	GENERALLY TYPICAL OF THIS PERSON	SOMEWHAT TYPICAL OF THIS PERSON	GENERALLY UNTYPICAL OF THIS PERSON	HIGHLY UNTYPICAL OF THIS PERSON
13. Accepts contact with others (does not withdraw or turn away)	5	4	3	2	1
14. Initiates contact with others	5	4	3	2	1
15. Communicates effectively (speech and gestures are understandable and to the point)	5	4	3	2	1
16. Engages in activities without prompting	5	4	3	2	1
17. Participates in groups	5	4	3	2	1
18. Forms and maintains friendships	5	4	3	2	1
19. Asks for help when needed	5	4	3	2	1

D. SOCIAL ACCEPTABILITY	NEVER	RARELY	SOMETIMES	FREQUENTLY	ALWAYS
20. Verbally abuses others	5	4	3	2	1
21. Physically abuses others	5	4	3	2	1
22. Destroys property	5	4	3	2	1
23. Physically abuses self	5	4	3	2	1
24. Is fearful, crying, clinging	5	4	3	2	1
25. Takes property from others without permission	5	4	3	2	1
26. Performs repetitive behaviors (pacing, rocking, making noises)	5	4	3	2	1

Community Living Skills

E. ACTIVITIES	TOTALLY SELF-SUFFICIENT	NEEDS VERBAL ADVICE OR GUIDANCE	NEEDS SOME PHYSICAL HELP OR ASSISTANCE	NEEDS SUBSTANTIAL HELP	TOTALLY DEPENDENT
27. Household responsibilities (house cleaning, cooking, washing clothes)	5	4	3	2	1
28. Shopping (selection of items, choice of stores, payment at register)	5	4	3	2	1
29. Handling personal finances (budgeting, paying bills)	5	4	3	2	1
30. Use of telephone (getting number, dialing, speaking, listening)	5	4	3	2	1
31. Traveling from residence without getting lost	5	4	3	2	1
32. Use of public transportation (selecting route, using timetable, paying fares, making transfers)	5	4	3	2	1
33. Use of leisure time (reading, visiting friends, listening to music)	5	4	3	2	1
34. Recognizing and avoiding common dangers (traffic safety, fire safety)	5	4	3	2	1
35. Self-medication (understanding purpose, taking as prescribed, recognizing side effects)	5	4	3	2	1
36. Use of medical and other community services (knowing whom to contact, how, and when to use)	5	4	3	2	1
37. Basic reading, writing, and arithmetic (enough for daily needs)	5	4	3	2	1

Community Living Skills—**cont'd**

F. WORK SKILLS	HIGHLY TYPICAL OF THIS PERSON	GENERALLY TYPICAL OF THIS PERSON	SOMEWHAT TYPICAL OF THIS PERSON	GENERALLY UNTYPICAL OF THIS PERSON	HIGHLY UNTYPICAL OF THIS PERSON
38. Has employable skills	5	4	3	2	1
39. Works with minimal supervision	5	4	3	2	1
40. Is able to sustain work effort (not easily distracted, can work under stress)	5	4	3	2	1
41. Appears at appointments on time	5	4	3	2	1
42. Follows verbal instructions accurately	5	4	3	2	1
43. Completes assigned tasks	5	4	3	2	1

Other Information

44. From your knowledge of this person, are there other skills or problem areas not covered on this form that are important to this person's ability to function independently? If so, please specify.

45. How well do you know the skills and behavior of the person you just rated? (Circle one)

Very Well		Fairly Well		Not Very Well at All
5	4	3	2	1

46. Have you discussed this assessment with the client? (Circle one)   Yes   No

If yes, does the client generally agree with the assessment? (Circle one)   Yes   No

From "SLOF: A Behavioral Rating Scale for Assessing the Mentally Ill," by L. Schneider, & E. Struening, 1983, *Social Work Research and Abstracts.*

Brief Psychiatric Rating Scale

	NOT PRESENT	MILD	MODERATE	SEVERE	NOT RATABLE
1. Somatic concern: Degree of concern over present bodily health. Rate the degree to which physical health is perceived as a problem by the patient, whether complaints have a realistic basis or not.	1	Occasional 2 3	Exaggerated 4 5	Preoccupied 6 7	0
2. Anxiety-anxiety statements: Worry, fear, or overconcern for present or future. Rate solely on the basis of verbal report of patient's own subjective experiences. Do not infer anxiety from neurotic defense mechanisms.	1	Worried 2 3	Fearful 4 5	Panicked 6 7	0
3. Emotional withdrawal: Deficiency in relating to others; seclusiveness. Rate only the degree to which the patient gives the impression of failing to be in emotional contact with other people.	1	Doesn't initiate 2 3	Withdraws from 4 5	Repels contact 6 7	0
4. Conceptual disorganization/ disorganization in speech: Degree to which the thought processes are confused, disconnected, or disorganized. Rate on the basis of integration of the verbal products of the patient; do not rate on the basis of the patient's subjective impression of his own level of functioning.	1	Vague 2 3	Unclear 4 5	Incoherent Talk 6 7	0

5. Guilt feeling/guilt statements: Overconcern or remorse for past behavior. Rate on the basis of the patient's subjective experiences of guilt as evidenced by verbal report with appropriate affect; do not infer guilt feelings from depression, anxiety, or neurotic defenses.	**Overconcern**	**Preoccupied**	**Delusions of guilt**	
1	2 3	4 5	6 7	0

6. Tension/tension behavior: Physical and motor manifestations of tension, "nervousness," and heightened activation level. Tension should be rated solely on the basis of physical signs and motor behavior and not on the basis of subjective experiences of tension reported by the patient.	**Seems tense**	**Restless**	**Agitated**	
1	2 3	4 5	6 7	0

7. Mannerisms and posturing: Unusual and unnatural motor behavior which causes certain mental patients to stand out in a crowd of normal people. Rate only abnormality of movements; do not rate simple heightened motor activity.	**Occasional**	**Frequent**	**Pervasive**	
1	2 3	4 5	6 7	0

8. Grandiosity/grandiose statements: Exaggerated self-opinion, conviction of unusual ability or powers. Rate only on the basis of patient's statements about himself or self in relation to others, not on the basis of his demeanor.	**Expansive**	**Special abilities**	**Delusional state**	
1	2 3	4 5	6 7	0

9. Depressive mood: Despondency in mood, sadness. Rate only degree of despondency; do not rate on the basis of inferences concerning depression based upon general retardation and somatic complaints.	**Sad**	**Despondent**	**Despairing**	
1	2 3	4 5	6 7	0

10. Hostility—statements of behavior:		Annoyed		Hostile		Raging		
Animosity, contempt, threats, belligerence, disdain for other people. Rate solely on the basis of reported feelings and of actions of the patient toward others; do not infer hostility from neurotic defenses, anxiety, or somatic complaints.	1	2 3		4 5		6 7		0

11. Suspiciousness:		Seems guarded		Says doesn't trust		Paranoid delusions		
Belief (delusional or otherwise) that others have now, or have had in the past, malicious or discriminatory intent toward the patient. On the basis of verbal report and behavior, rate only those suspicions currently held, whether they concern past or present circumstances.	1	2 3		4 5		6 7		0

12. Hallucinatory behavior/ hallucination statements:		Occasional and with insight		Often and no insight		Pervasive		
Perceptions without normal external stimulus correspondence. Rate only those experiences which are reported to have occurred during the rating period and which are described as distinctly different from the thought and imagery process of normal people.	1	2 3		4 5		6 7		0

13. Motor retardation/behavior:		Slowed		Retarded		Catatonic		
Reduction in energy level, evidenced in slowed movements and speech, reduced body tone, decreased number of movements. Rate on the basis of observed behavior of the patient only; do not rate on the basis of patient's subjective impression of own energy level.	1	2 3		4 5		6 7		0

	Resents	Resists	Refuses	
14. Uncooperativeness: Evidences of resistance, unfriendliness, resentment, and lack of readiness to cooperate with ward procedures and with others. 1	2 3	4 5	6 7	0

	Odd	Bizarre	Impossible	
15. Unusual thought content: Unusual, odd, strange, or bizarre thought content. Rate here the degree of unusualness, not the degree of disorganization of thought processes. 1	2 3	4 5	6 7	0

	Lowered feeling	Flat	Mechanical	
16. Blunted affect: Reduced emotional tone, apparent lack of normal feeling or involvement. 1	2 3	4 5	6 7	0

	Increased emotion	Intense	Off the wall	
17. Excitement: Heightened emotional tone, increased reactivity, agitation, impulsivity. 1	2 3	4 5	6 7	0

	Muddled	Confused	Disoriented	
18. Disorienation: Confusion or lack of proper association for person, place, or time. 1	2 3	4 5	6 7	0

	Mild loss	Moderate loss	Severe loss	
19. Loss of functioning*: Rate general level of functioning 1	2 3	4 5	6 7	0

From "The Brief Psychiatric Rating Scale," by J. E. Overall and D. R. Gorham, 1962 (Modified 1966), *Psychological Reports, 10,* 799-812.

*Item 19 is a global scale that is not added in with the other items. Items 1 to 18 are added together to give the total score.

Hamilton Depression Rating Scale

For each item, select the one "answer" that best characterizes the patient and check the corresponding numbered box.

1. Depressed mood (sadness, hopeless, helpless, worthless)

0	1	2	3	4

  0 = Absent
  1 = These feeling states indicated only on questioning
  2 = These feeling states spontaneously reported verbally
  3 = Communicates feeling states nonverbally—i.e., through facial expression, posture, voice, and tendency to weep
  4 = Patient reports VIRTUALLY ONLY these feeling states in his spontaneous verbal and nonverbal communication

2. Feelings of guilt

0	1	2	3	4

  0 = Absent
  1 = Self-reproach, feels he has let people down
  2 = Ideas of guilt or rumination over past errors or sinful deeds
  3 = Present illness is a punishment. Delusions of guilt
  4 = Hears accusatory or denunciatory voices and/or experiences threatening visual hallucinations

3. Suicide

0	1	2	3	4

  0 = Absent
  1 = Feels life is not worth living
  2 = Wishes he were dead or any thoughts of possible death to self
  3 = Suicide ideas or gesture
  4 = Attempts at suicide (any serious attempt rates 4)

4. Insomnia early

0	1	2

  0 = No difficulty falling asleep
  1 = Complains of occasional difficulty falling asleep—i.e., more than $\frac{1}{2}$ hour
  2 = Complains of nightly difficulty falling asleep

5. Insomnia middle

0	1	2

  0 = No difficulty
  1 = Patient complains of being restless and disturbed during the night
  2 = Waking during the night—any getting out of bed rates 2 (except for purposes of voiding)

6. Insomnia late

0	1	2

  0 = No difficulty
  1 = Waking in early hours of the morning but goes back to sleep
  2 = Unable to fall asleep again if he gets out of bed

7. Work and activities

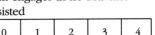

| 0 | 1 | 2 | 3 | 4 |

- 0 = No difficulty
- 1 = Thoughts and feelings of incapacity, fatigue or weakness related to activities, work or hobbies
- 2 = Loss of interest in activity—hobbies or work—either directly reported by patient, or indirect in listlessness, indecision, and vacillation (feels he has to push self to work or activities)
- 3 = Decrease in actual time spent in activities or decrease in productivity. In hospital, rate 3 if patient does not spend at least three hours a day in activities (hospital job or hobbies) exclusive of ward chores
- 4 = Stopped working because of present illness. In hospital rate 4 if patient engages in no activities except ward chores, or if patient fails to perform ward chores unassisted

8. Retardation (slowness of thought and speech; impaired ability to concentrate; decreased motor activity)

| 0 | 1 | 2 | 3 | 4 |

- 0 = Normal speech and thought
- 1 = Slight retardation at interview
- 2 = Obvious retardation at interview
- 3 = Interview difficult
- 4 = Complete stupor

9. Agitation

| 0 | 1 | 2 |

- 0 = None
- 1 = "Playing with" hands, hair, etc.
- 2 = Hand-wringing, nail-biting, hair-pulling, biting of lips

10. Anxiety—psychic

| 0 | 1 | 2 | 3 | 4 |

Physiological concomitants of anxiety, such as:
Gastrointestinal—dry mouth, wind, indigestion, diarrhea, cramps, belching
Cardiovascular—palpitations, headaches
Respiratory—hyperventilation, sighing
Urinary frequency
Sweating

- 0 = Absent
- 1 = Mild
- 2 = Moderate
- 3 = Severe
- 4 = Incapacitating

11. Somatic symptoms—gastrointestinal

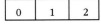

| 0 | 1 | 2 |

- 0 = None
- 1 = Loss of appetite, but eating without staff encouragement. Heavy feelings in abdomen
- 2 = Difficulty eating without staff urging. Requests or requires laxatives or medication for bowels or medication for GI symptoms

12. Somatic symptoms—general

| 0 | 1 | 2 |

- 0 = None
- 1 = Heaviness in limbs, back of head. Backaches, headaches, muscle aches. Loss of energy and fatigability
- 2 = Any clear-cut symptom rates 2

13. Genital symptoms

| 0 | 1 | 2 |

Symptoms such as: loss of libido, menstrual disturbances

- 0 = Absent
- 1 = Mild
- 2 = Severe

From "Development of a Rating Scale for Primary Depressive Illness," by M. Hamilton, 1967, *British Journal of Social Clinical Psychology, 6,* 278-296.

14. Hypochondriasis

| 0 | 1 | 2 | 3 | 4 |

0 = Not present
1 = Self-absorption (bodily)
2 = Preoccupation with health
3 = Frequent complaints, request for help, etc.
4 = Hypochondriacal delusions

15. Loss of weight—rate either A or B

| 0 | 1 | 2 | 3 |

A. When rating by history:
0 = No weight loss
1 = Probable weight loss associated with present illness
2 = Definite (according to patient) weight loss
3 = Not assessed

B. On weekly ratings by ward psychiatrist, actual weight changes:

| 0 | 1 | 2 | 3 |

0 = Less than 1 lb. weight loss in week
1 = Greater than 1 lb. weight loss in week
2 = Greater than 2 lb. weight loss in week
3 = Not assessed

16. Insight

| 0 | 1 | 2 |

0 = Acknowledges being depressed and ill
1 = Acknowledges illness but attributes cause to bad food, climate, overwork, virus, need for rest, etc.
2 = Denies being ill at all

17. Diurnal variation

**A. Note whether symptoms are worse in morning or evening.
If NO diurnal variation, mark "None."**

| 0 | 1 | 2 |

0 = No variation
1 = Worse in A.M.
2 = Worse in P.M.

**B. When present, mark the severity of the variation. Mark "None" if
NO variation.**

| 0 | 1 | 2 |

0 = None
1 = Mild
2 = Severe

**18. Depersonalization and derealization
Such as: feelings of unreality, nihilistic ideas**

| 0 | 1 | 2 | 3 | 4 |

0 = Absent
1 = Mild
2 = Moderate
3 = Severe
4 = Incapacitating

19. Paranoid symptoms

| 0 | 1 | 2 | 3 |

0 = None
1 = Suspicious
2 = Ideas of reference
3 = Delusions of reference and persecution

20. Obsessional and compulsive symptoms

| 0 | 1 | 2 |

0 = Absent
1 = Mild
2 = Severe

This scale is used for rating the severity of depression. A score of less than 11 suggests that no depression is present.

Appendix G

Michigan Alcoholism Screening Test

POINTS			YES	NO
	0.	Do you enjoy a drink now and then?	———	———
(2)	1.	Do you feel you are a normal drinker? (By normal we mean you drink less than or as much as most other people.)*	———	———
(2)	2.	Have you ever awakened the morning after doing some drinking the night before and found that you could not remember a part of the evening?	———	———
(1)	3.	Does your wife, husband, a parent or other near relative ever worry or complain about your drinking?	———	———
(2)	4.	Can you stop drinking without a struggle after one or two drinks?*	———	———
(1)	5.	Do you ever feel guilty about your drinking?	———	———
(2)	6.	Do friends or relatives think you are a normal drinker?*	———	———
(2)	7.	Are you able to stop drinking when you want to?*	———	———
(5)	8.	Have you ever attended a meeting of Alcoholics Anonymous (AA)?	———	———
(1)	9.	Have you gotten into physical fights when drinking?	———	———
(2)	10.	Has your drinking ever created problems between you and your wife, husband, a parent, or other relative?	———	———
(2)	11.	Has your wife, husband (or other family member) ever gone to anyone for help about your drinking?	———	———
(2)	12.	Have you ever lost friends because of your drinking?	———	———
(2)	13.	Have you ever gotten into trouble at work or school because of drinking?	———	———
(2)	14.	Have you ever lost a job because of drinking?	———	———
(2)	15.	Have you ever neglected your obligations, your family, or your work for two or more days in a row because you were drinking?	———	———
(1)	16.	Do you drink before noon fairly often?	———	———
(2)	17.	Have you ever been told you have liver trouble? Cirrhosis?	———	———
(2)	18.	After heavy drinking have you ever had delirium tremens (DTs) or severe shaking, or heard voices or seen things that really weren't there?†	———	———

From "The Michigan Alcoholism Screening Test (MAST): The Quest for a New Diagnostic Instrument," by M. L. Selzer, 1971, *American Journal of Psychiatry, 3,* 176-181.

NOTE: *Scoring System:* In general, five points or more would place the subject in an "alcoholic" category. Four points would be suggestive of alcoholism. Three points or less would indicate the subject was not alcoholic.

Programs using the above scoring system find it very sensitive at the five-point level and it tends to find more people alcoholic than anticipated. However, it is a screening test and should be sensitive at its lower levels.

*Alcoholic response is negative.

†5 points for delirium tremens.

POINTS			YES	NO
(5)	19.	Have you ever gone to anyone for help about your drinking?	_____	_____
(5)	20.	Have you ever been in a hospital because of drinking?	_____	_____
(2)	21.	Have you ever been a patient in a psychiatric hospital or on a psychiatric ward of a general hospital where drinking was part of the problem that resulted in hospitalization?	_____	_____
(2)	22.	Have you ever been seen at a psychiatric or mental health clinic or gone to any doctor, social worker, or clergyman for help with any emotional problem, where drinking was part of the problem?	_____	_____
(2)	23.	Have you ever been arrested for drunk driving, driving while intoxicated, or driving under the influence of alcoholic beverages?‡	_____	_____
(2)	24.	Have you ever been arrested, or taken into custody, even for a few hours, because of other drunk behavior?‡ (If YES, how many times_____)	_____	_____

‡2 points for *each* arrest.

Appendix H

Geriatric Depression Scale

Choose the best answer for how you felt over the past week

1.	Are you basically satisfied with your life?	yes / no
2.	Have you dropped many of your activities and interests?	yes / no
3.	Do you feel that your life is empty?	yes / no
4.	Do you often get bored?	yes / no
5.	Are you hopeful about the future?	yes / no
6.	Are you bothered by thoughts you can't get out of your head?	yes / no
7.	Are you in good spirits most of the time?	yes / no
8.	Are you afraid that something bad is going to happen to you?	yes / no
9.	Do you feel happy most of the time?	yes / no
10.	Do you often feel helpless?	yes / no
11.	Do you often get restless and fidgety?	yes / no
12.	Do you prefer to stay at home, rather than going out and doing new things?	yes / no
13.	Do you frequently worry about the future?	yes / no
14.	Do you feel you have more problems with memory than most?	yes / no
15.	Do you think it is wonderful to be alive now?	yes / no
16.	Do you often feel downhearted and blue?	yes / no
17.	Do you feel pretty worthless the way you are now?	yes / no
18.	Do you worry a lot about the past?	yes / no
19.	Do you find life very exciting?	yes / no
20.	Is it hard for you to get started on new projects?	yes / no
21.	Do you feel full of energy?	yes / no
22.	Do you feel that your situation is hopeless?	yes / no
23.	Do you think that most people are better off than you are?	yes / no
24.	Do you frequently get upset over little things?	yes / no
25.	Do you frequently feel like crying?	yes / no
26.	Do you have trouble concentrating?	yes / no
27.	Do you enjoy getting up in the morning?	yes / no
28.	Do you prefer to avoid social gatherings?	yes / no
29.	Is it easy for you to make decisions?	yes / no
30.	Is your mind as clear as it used to be?	yes / no

NOTE: For scoring, reverse answers 1, 5, 7, 9, 15, 19, 21, 27, 29, 30. Each yes = 1 score

Score between 0 and 10 = not depressed
Score of 11 = possible depression
Score of 15 = mild depression
Score of ≥20 = severe depression

From "Development and Validation of a Geriatric Depression Screening Scale: A Preliminary Report," by J. A. Yesavage and T. L. Brink, 1983, *Journal of Psychiatric Research, 17*(1), 37-49.

Global Deterioration Scale

GDS STAGE	CLINICAL PHASE	CLINICAL CHARACTERISTIC
1 No cognitive decline	Normal	No subjective complaints of memory deficit. No memory deficit evident on clinical interview.
2 Very mild cognitive decline	Forgetfulness	Subjective complaints of memory deficit, most frequently in following areas: a) forgetting where one has placed familiar objects; b) forgetting names one formerly knew well. No objective evidence of memory deficit on clinical interview. No objective deficits in employment or social situations. Appropriate concern with respect to symptomatology.
3 Mild cognitive decline	Early confusional	Earliest clear-cut deficits. Manifestations in more than one of the following areas: a) patient may have gotten lost when traveling to an unfamiliar location; b) co-workers become aware of patient's relatively poor performance; c) word and name finding deficits become evident to intimates; d) patient may read a passage or a book and retain relatively little material; e) patient may demonstrate decreased facility in remembering names upon introduction to new people; f) patient may have lost or misplaced an object of value; g) concentration deficit may be evident on clinical testing. Objective evidence of memory deficit obtained only with an intensive interview conducted by a trained geriatric psychiatrist. Decreased performance in demanding employment and social settings. Denial begins to become manifest in patient. Mild to moderate anxiety accompanies symptoms.
4 Moderate cognitive decline	Late confusional	Clear-cut deficit on careful clinical interview. Deficits manifest in following areas: a) decreased knowledge of current and recent events; b) may exhibit some deficit in memory of personal history; c) concentration deficit elicited on serial subtractions; d) decreased ability to travel, handle finances, etc. Frequently no deficit in following areas: a) orientation to time and person; b) recognition of familiar persons and faces; c) ability to travel to familiar areas. Inability to perform complex tasks. Denial is dominant defense mechanism. Flattening of affect and withdrawal from challenging situations occur.

5 Moderately severe decline	Early dementia	Patients can no longer survive without some assistance. Patients are unable during interview to recall a major relevant aspect of their current lives: e.g., the names of close members of their family (such as grandchildren), the name of the high school or college from which they graduated.
		Frequently some disorientation to time (date, day of week, season, etc.) or to place. An educated person may have difficulty counting back from 40 by 4s or from 20 by 2s.
		Persons at this stage retain knowledge of many major facts regarding themselves and others. They invariably know their own names and generally know their spouse's and children's names. They require no assistance with toileting or eating, but may have some difficulty choosing the proper clothing to wear.
6 Severe cognitive decline	Middle dementia	May occasionally forget the name of the spouse upon whom they are entirely dependent for survival. Will be largely unaware of all recent events and experiences in their lives. Retain some knowledge of their past lives, but this is very sketchy. Generally unaware of their surroundings, the year, the season, etc. May have difficulty counting from 10, both backward and sometimes forward. Will require some assistance with activities of daily living, e.g., may become incontinent, will require travel assistance, but occasionally will display ability to travel to familiar locations. Diurnal rhythm frequently disturbed. Almost always recall their own name. Frequently continue to be able to distinguish familiar from unfamiliar persons in their environment.
		Personality and emotional changes occur. These are quite variable and include: a) delusional behavior, e.g., patients may accuse their spouse of being an impostor, may talk to imaginary figures in the environment, or to their own reflection in the mirror; b) obsessive symptoms, e.g., person may continually repeat simple cleaning activities; c) anxiety symptoms, agitation, and even previously nonexistent violent behavior may occur; d) cognitive abulia, i.e., loss of willpower because an individual cannot carry a thought long enough to determine a purposeful course of action.
7 Very severe cognitive decline	Late dementia	All verbal abilities are lost. Frequently there is no speech at all—only grunting. Incontinent of urine; requires assistance toileting and feeding. Lose basic psychomotor skills, e.g., ability to walk. The brain appears to no longer be able to tell the body what to do.
		Generalized and cortical neurologic signs and symptoms are frequently present.

From "Clinical Presentation, Diagnosis, and Symptomatology of Age-Associated Cognitive Decline and Alzheimer's Disease," by B. Reisberg, 1983, in *Alzheimer's Disease: The Standard Reference*, pp. 173-187, New York: Free Press.

Appendix J

REAH: An Index for Assessing the Risk of Elder Abuse in the Home

The REAH is the sum of two components, the vulnerability assessment score of the aged person (VASAP) and the stress assessment score of the caregiver (SASC). Calculate VASAP and SASC, then add them to find the REAH.

REAH (sum of VASAP and SASC, range 0 to 41)	
	____

VASAP—vulnerability assessment score of the aged person				
A. Personal data section (aged person)				
	2 points	1 point	0 points	Score
Age Sex Health	85 or older Frail	75-84 Female Average	74 or younger Male Robust	____ ____ ____
subtotal, A. Personal data (sum of above, range 0 to 5)				____

B. Dependency needs section (aged person)	
1 point for a "yes," 0 points for a "no" or "don't know"	Score
Intellectual or severe mental impairment?	____
Lives in home with caregiver?	____
Needs help bathing?	____
Needs help dressing?	____
Needs help toileting? (or is incontinent or has catheter)	____
Needs help eating?	____
Depends on caregiver for all social interaction?	____
Allows caregiver to assume parental role?	____
Demanding and authoritative to caregiver?	____
Is financially dependent upon caregiver?	____
subtotal, B. Dependency needs (sum of above, range 0 to 10)	____
VASAP (sum of subtotals A and B, range 0 to 15)	____

NOTE: The REAH index should be calculated on a regular basis (e.g., monthly). "With a high REAH index in the presence of an undifferentiated and maladaptive family system, the risk of elder abuse is compounded."

From "Using a Family Systems Approach: Prevent Elder Abuse," by G. P. Hamilton, 1989, *Journal of Gerontological Nursing, 15*(3), 21-26.

Appendix K

SASC: Stress Assessment Score of the Caregiver

A. Personal data section (caregiver)				
	2 points	1 point	0 points	Score
Age	70 and over	45-69	under 45	————
Phys. health	poor	good	excellent	————
Ment. health	poor	good	excellent	————
Finances	under $7000	$7-$14000	$14000 & more	————
Dependents (not elder)	2 or more	1	none	————
subtotal, A. Personal data (sum of above, range 0 to 10)				————

B. Stress factors section (caregiver)	
1 point for a "yes," 0 points for a "no" or "don't know"	Score
Alcoholism or substance abuse?	————
Mental retardation?	————
History or observation of family violence?	————
Change in lifestyle to assume care of aged person?	————
Receives financial help from the elder?	————
Limited time for own personal activities?	————
Personal stresses (i.e. marital problems, empty nest)?	————
Mostly or always at home (unable to leave aged person)?	————
Absence of support system (family, friends, community)?	————
Shows frustrations, resentment in care of aged person?	————
Treats elder as a child?	————
Has limited knowledge of the aging process?	————
Believes any care at home is better than nursing home?	————
Minimizes or denies dependency of aged person?	————
Shows dependency toward the elder?	————
Authoritative manner with the elder?	————
subtotal, B. Stress factors (sum of above, range 0 to 16)	————
SASC (sum of subtotals A and B, range 0 to 26)	————
NOTE: Add SASC score to REAH index.	

From "Using a Family Systems Approach: Prevent Elder Abuse," by G. P. Hamilton, 1989, *Journal of Gerontological Nursing,* *15*(3), 21-26.

Index*

*Page numbers in italics indicate illustrations; *t* indicates
tables.